Medical Terminology
for
Health Professions
Fifth Edition

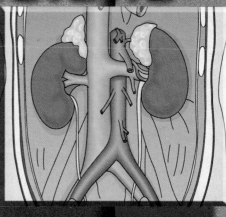

Cells

Ann Ehrlich
Carol L. Schroeder

THOMSON

DELMAR LEARNING ™

Australia Canada Mexico Singapore Spain United Kingdom United States

THOMSON
★
TM
DELMAR LEARNING

Medical Terminology for Health Professions, Fifth Edition
by Ann Ehrlich and Carol L. Schroeder

Vice President,
Health Care Business Unit:
William Brottmiller

Editorial Director:
Cathy L. Esperti

Acquisitions Editor:
Marah Bellegarde

Developmental Editor:
Debra Flis

Marketing Director:
Jennifer McAvey

Editorial Assistant:
Jennifer McGovern

Marketing Coordinator:
Kimberly Duffy

Technology Project Manager:
Victoria Moore

Art/Design Specialist:
Bob Plante

Production Coordinator:
John Mickelbank

Project Editor:
Daniel Branagh

Library of Congress Cataloging-in-Publication Data

Ehrlich, Ann, B.
   Medical terminology for health professions / Ann Ehrlich, Carol L. Schroeder.-- 5th ed.
      p. ; cm.
   Includes index.
   ISBN-13: 978-1-4018-6026-4
   ISBN-10: 1-4018-6026-5
   1. Medicine--Terminology--Programmed instruction. I. Schroeder, Carol L. II. Title.
   [DNLM: 1. Terminology--Programmed Instruction. W 18.2 E33m 2005]
   R123.E47 2005
   610'.1'4--dc22

                    2004051619

Notice to the Reader

Publisher does not warrant or guarantee any of the products described herein or perform any independent analysis in connection with any of the product information contained herein. Publisher does not assume, and expressly disclaims, any obligation to obtain and include information other than that provided to it by the manufacturer.

The reader is expressly warned to consider and adopt all safety precautions that might be indicated by the activities described herein and to avoid all potential hazards. By following the instructions contained herein, the reader willingly assumes all risks in connection with such instructions.

The publisher makes no representations or warranties of any kind, including but not limited to, the warranties of fitness for particular purpose or merchantability, nor are any such representations implied with respect to the material set forth herein, and the publisher takes no responsibility with respect to such material. The publisher shall not be liable for any special, consequential, or exemplary damages resulting, in whole or part, from the readers' use of, or reliance upon, this material.

Contents

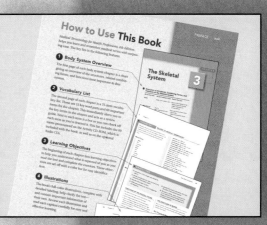

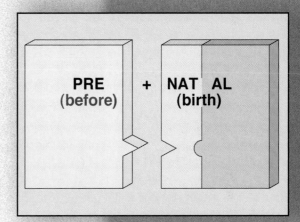

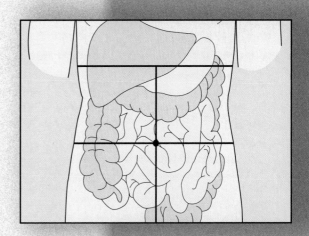

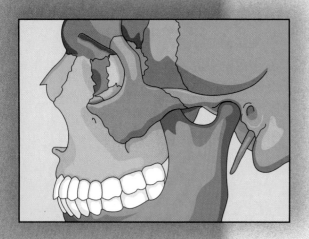

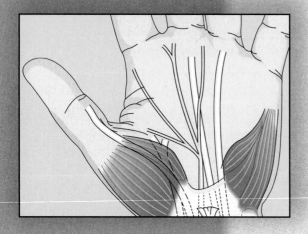

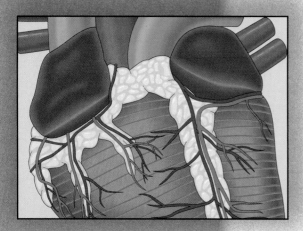

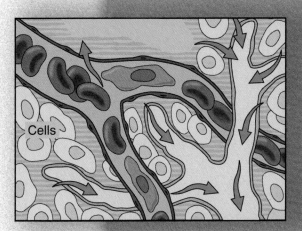

Chapter 6: The Lymphatic and Immune Systems   **159**

Chapter 7: The Respiratory System   **187**

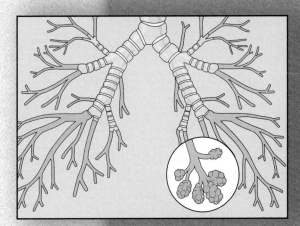

Chapter 8: The Digestive System   **217**

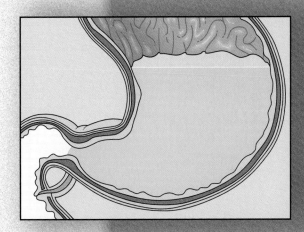

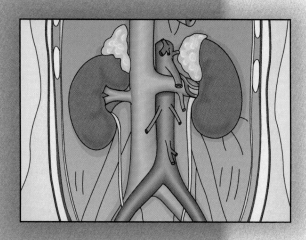

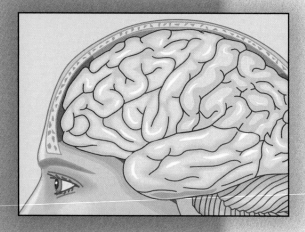

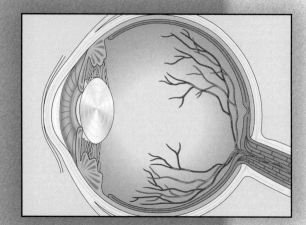

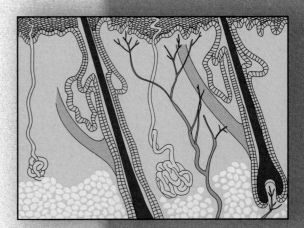

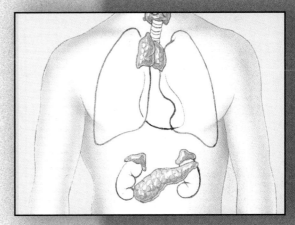

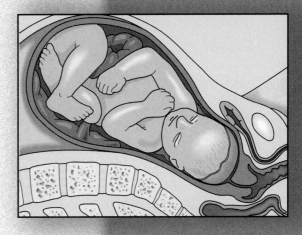

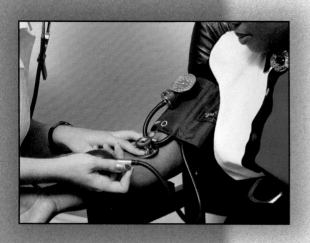

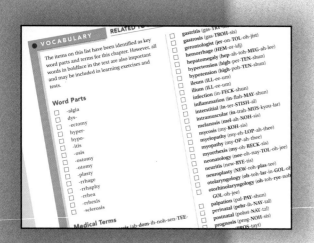

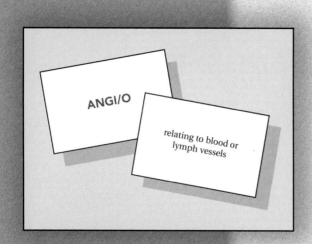

Preface

TO THE LEARNER

Welcome to the world of medical terminology! Learning this special language is an important step in preparing for your career as a health care professional. Here's good news: Learning medical terms is much easier than learning a foreign language because you are already familiar with quite a few of the words, such as *appendicitis* and *tonsillectomy*. Understanding new words becomes easier with the discovery that many of these terms are made up of interchangeable word parts that are used in different combinations. Once you understand this, you'll be well on your way to translating even the most difficult medical terms, including words you have never seen before. You'll be amazed to see how quickly your vocabulary will grow!

This book and the accompanying teaching materials are designed to make the process as simple as possible. Review the introductory sections—including "How to Use This Book," "How to Use *Medical Terminology for Health Professions*, Fifth Edition StudyWARE™," and the rest of this section—so you can find your way around easily. Once you get comfortable with the materials, you'll discover you are learning faster than you ever imagined possible.

CHAPTER ORGANIZATION

The text is organized into 15 chapters, a comprehensive review section, three appendices, and removable flash cards.

Introductory Chapters and Word Part Review

Chapters 1 and 2 provide the foundation that enables you to master the rest of the book. Chapter 1 introduces key word parts—the building blocks of most medical terms. Chapter 2 introduces more word parts and provides an overview of basic terms used throughout the health field.

After reading these chapters, complete the **Word Part Review** that follows Chapter 2. These exercises and the test will help you determine whether you've mastered the concept of these all-important building blocks. If you are having trouble here, it is important to put more effort into learning these basics.

Body System Chapters

Chapters 3 through 14 are organized by body system. Because each body system stands alone, you can study these chapters in any sequence. Each chapter begins with an overview of the structures and functions of that system so you can relate these to the specialists, pathology, and diagnostic and treatment procedures that follow.

Chapter 15 introduces basic diagnostic procedures, imaging procedures and positioning, and pharmacology. This chapter can be studied at any point in the course.

Comprehensive Medical Terminology Review

This section, which is located after Chapter 15, is designed to help you prepare for your final examination. It includes study tips, practice exercises, and a simulated final test.

Appendices

Appendix A: Prefixes, Combining Forms, and Suffixes is a convenient alphabetical reference for medical word parts. When you don't recognize a word part, you can look it up here.

Appendix B: Abbreviations and Their Meanings is an extensive list of commonly used abbreviations and their meanings. Abbreviations are important in medicine and using them *accurately* is essential!

Appendix C: Glossary of Pathology and Procedures is a reference you can use to quickly find any of the pathology, diagnostic, and treatment procedure terms introduced in the text. Also included here are the "Challenge Word Building" exercise terms and their definitions.

LEARNING SUPPLEMENTS

Flash Cards

Improve your knowledge and test your mastery by using the flash cards in the last section of the book. Review the suggestions for games and activities for using these, then carefully remove the pages from the book and separate the cards.

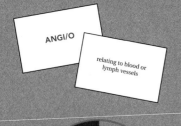
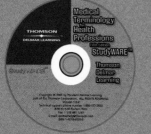

Medical Terminology for Health Professions, Fifth Edition StudyWARE™

The StudyWARE™ CD-ROM offers an exciting way to gain additional practice in working with medical terms. The quizzes and activities help you remember even the most difficult terms. See "How to Use *Medical Terminology for Health Professions*, Fifth Edition StudyWARE™" on page xxi for details.

TO THE INSTRUCTOR

From the very first edition, *Medical Terminology for Health Professions* has attempted to break new ground in this complex discipline by making mastery quick and easy. Now, the fifth edition brings your learners fully updated information and more pedagogical tools than ever before.

CHANGES TO THE FIFTH EDITION

This edition continues the emphasis on the **up-to-date language** of current medicine and includes more than 100 new terms such as SARS and magnetic resonance angiography (MRA). Obsolete terms, or those no longer in common usage, have been deleted.

Although changes have been made, you can convert to this new edition quickly and easily by using the Correlation Guide found on the Electronic Classroom Manager CD-ROM.

Vocabulary List

Each chapter begins with a **vocabulary list**. This includes **15 word parts** and **60 important terms**. All terms on the list are pronounced on the StudyWARE™ CD-ROM as well as the optional Audio CDs.

Primary and Secondary Terms

Throughout the chapters **primary terms** appear in bold face and, when appropriate, are followed by a pronunciation guide. Primary terms are used in the exercises and tests. *Secondary terms*, which appear in italics, are included where needed to clarify the meaning of a primary term. Secondary terms are not used in exercises or tests.

Abbreviations

In response to requests from instructors like you, we have increased the coverage of abbreviations and changed the way in which we introduce them. At the end of the content portion of each chapter, we've included a table that summarizes the abbreviations related to the chapter. The table can be searched by either topic or abbreviation. This is an excellent teaching opportunity to introduce these abbreviations and to help users learn to use them correctly.

Changes in Learning Exercises

All of the Learning Exercises have been reworked to require short written answers. Writing terms, rather than circling a multiple choice option, reinforces learning and provides practice in writing and spelling these terms. To facilitate correcting these exercises, the answer keys are included on the Electronic Classroom Manager CD-ROM. To facilitate correcting exercises in class, the answers are also included as optional slides in the PowerPoint® presentation.

Word Surgery is a new exercise format to help learners master the skill of breaking complex terms down into word parts. All of the reviewers were very enthusiastic about Word Surgery!

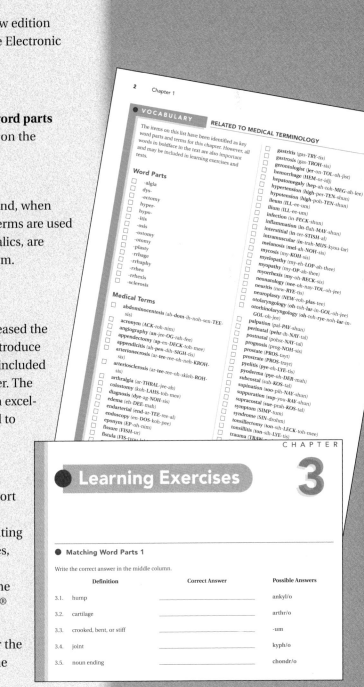

Index

The index has been improved to include all primary and secondary terms plus the terms from Appendix C.

SPECIAL RESOURCES TO ACCOMPANY THE BOOK

Audio CDs

The Audio CDs include the 60 terms from the vocabulary list for each chapter. Each term is pronounced, followed by a pause to allow the learner to pronounce the term. After the pause the term is pronounced again and defined. These Audio CDs are a valuable, flexible learning aid for use whenever and wherever the learner needs to study.

Two Audio CDs, ISBN 1-4018-6027-3

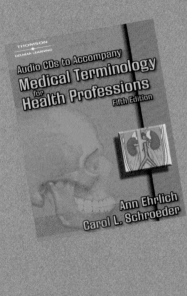

The Electronic Classroom Manager

The Electronic Classroom Manager is a robust computerized tool for your instructional needs! A must-have for all instructors, this comprehensive and convenient CD-ROM contains:

- **Textbook Teaching Resources** is an overview of the teaching resource featured in the text.

- **Conversion Guide** helps you make the change from the fourth to the fifth edition of *Medical Terminology for Health Professions*.

- **Textbook Learning Exercises Answer Keys** are arranged for ease of printing, with one chapter per page. As an additional feature, these answer keys are also available as PowerPoint slides for use when correcting exercises in class.

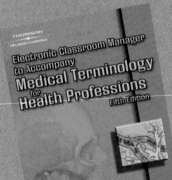

- **Exam View® Computerized Testbank** contains 100 questions per chapter, plus a mid-term test that covers Chapters 1 through 8 and a final test covering the entire text. You can use these questions to create your own review materials or tests.

- **PowerPoint Presentations**, including animations, are designed to aid you in planning your class presentations. If a learner misses a class, a printout of the slides for a lecture makes a helpful review page.

- **The Instructor's Manual** includes a wide variety of valuable resources to help you plan the course and implement activities by chapter. The availability of this manual in an electronic format increases its value as a teaching resource. This manual includes:

  - **Course Planning Tips**, including a sample 16-week syllabus and a sample course outline

  - **Tips for New Teachers** that include practical ideas to help new teachers and their students have a successful experience.

  - The **Teaching Tools by Chapter** feature includes two 25-question chapter quizzes with answer keys, classroom activities, a crossword puzzle and answer, and a case study.

  - **Review activities for mid-term and final tests**

Electronic Classroom Manager, ISBN 1-4018-6028-1

Complete Online Course

Designed as a standalone course, this eliminates the need for a separate book. Everything is online! Content is presented in four major sections: Study, Practice, Tests, and Reports. The Study section includes the content from the text, along with graphics, animations, and audio links. The Practice section includes exercises and games to reinforce learning. The Test section includes tests with a variety of question types for each chapter. A mid-term and a final exam are also available. The Report section features learner reports and instructor reports.

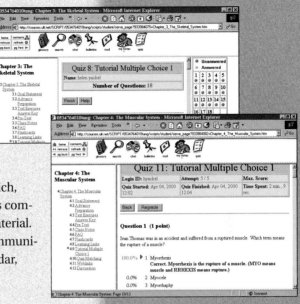

Individual Course, ISBN: 0-7668-2738-0

Educational Course, ISBN: 0-7668-2737-2

WebTUTOR™ Advantage

Designed to complement the book, WebTUTOR™ is a content-rich, Web-based teaching and learning aid that reinforces and clarifies complex concepts. Animations enhance learning and retention of material. The WebCT™ and Blackboard™ platforms also provide rich communication tools to instructors and learners, including a course calendar, chat, email, and threaded discussions.

WebTUTOR™ Advantage on WebCT™, ISBN 1-4018-6031-1

Text Bundled with WebTUTOR™ Advantage on WebCT™, ISBN 1-4018-7645-5

Text Bundled with WebTUTOR™ Advantage on WebCT™ and Audio CDs, ISBN 1-4018-7648-X

WebTUTOR™ Advantage on Blackboard™, ISBN 1-4018-6032-X

Text Bundled with WebTUTOR™ Advantage on Blackboard™, ISBN 1-4018-7647-1

Text Bundled with WebTUTOR™ Advantage on Blackboard™ and Audio CDs, ISBN 1-4018-7642-0

WebTUTOR™ Toolbox

With WebTUTOR™ Toolbox, you get the same rich communication tools and functionality of this Web-based teaching and learning aid. Chapter components include Goal Statements, Advance Preparation, and FAQs.

WebTUTOR™ Toolbox on WebCT™, ISBN 1-4018-6029-X

Text Bundled with WebTUTOR™ Toolbox on WebCT™, ISBN 1-4018-8777-5

Text Bundled with WebTUTOR™ Toolbox on WebCT™ and Audio CDs, ISBN 1-4018-8778-3

WebTUTOR™ Toolbox on Blackboard™, ISBN 1-4018-6030-3

Text Bundled with WebTUTOR™ Toolbox on Blackboard™, ISBN 1-4018-8779-1

Text Bundled with WebTUTOR™ Toolbox on Blackboard™ and Audio CDs, ISBN 1-4018-8780-5

Thomson Delmar Learning's Medical Terminology Audio Library

This extensive audio library of medical terminology includes four Audio CDs with over 3700 terms pronounced, and a software CD-ROM. The CD-ROM presents terms organized by body system, medical specialty, and general medical term categories. The user can search for a specific term by typing in the term or key words, or click on a category to view an alphabetical list of all terms within the category. The user can hear the correct pronunciation of one term or listen to each term on the list pronounced automatically. Definitions can be viewed after hearing the pronunciation of terms.

Institutional Version, ISBN: 1-4018-3223-7

Individual Version, ISBN: 1-4018-3222-9

Delmar's Medical Terminology Image Library CD-ROM, 2nd Edition

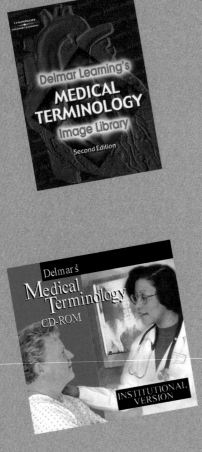

This CD-ROM includes over 600 graphic files. These files can be incorporated into a PowerPoint, Microsoft® Word, or WordPerfect presentation, used directly off the CD-ROM in a classroom presentation, or used to make color transparencies. The Image Library is organized around body systems and medical specialties. The library includes various anatomy, physiology, and pathology graphics of different levels of complexity. You can search and select the graphics that best apply to your teaching situation. This is an ideal resource to enhance your teaching presentation of medical terminology or anatomy and physiology.

ISBN: 1-4018-1009-8

Delmar's Medical Terminology CD-ROM Institutional Version

This is an exciting interactive reference, practice, and assessment tool designed to complement any medical terminology program. Features include the extensive use of multimedia—animations, video, graphics, and activities—to present terms and word-building features. Difficult functions, processes, and procedures are included so that learners can more effectively learn from a textbook.

ISBN: 0-7668-0979-X

Delmar's Medical Terminology Video Series

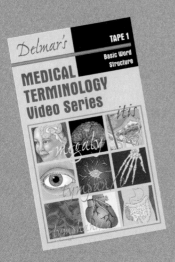

This series of 14 medical terminology videotapes is designed for allied health and nursing students who are enrolled in medical terminology courses. The videos may be used in class to supplement a lecture or in a resource lab by students who want additional reinforcement. The series can also be used in distance learning programs as a telecourse. The videos simulate a typical medical terminology class, and are organized by body system. The on-camera instructor leads students through the various concepts, interspersing lectures with graphics, video clips, and illustrations to emphasize points. This comprehensive series is invaluable to students trying to master the complex world of medical terminology.

Complete Set of Videos, ISBN 0-7668-0976-5 (Videos can also be purchased individually.)

Delmar's Medical Terminology Flash!: Computerized Flashcards

Learn and review over 1,500 medical terms using this unique electronic flashcard program. Flash! is a computerized flashcard-type question-and-answer association program designed to help users learn correct spellings, definitions, and pronunciations. The use of graphics and audio clips make it a fun and easy way for users to learn and test their knowledge of medical terminology.

ISBN: 0-7668-4320-3

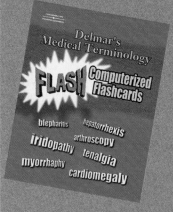

VALUE PACKAGES

You can order the following innovative Thomson Delmar Learning products separately—or package them with *Medical Terminology for Health Professions*, Fifth Edition, in a convenient and affordable package:

Text and Audio CDs Value Package

With these two Audio CDs, users learn the definitions of some of the most difficult medical terms and how to pronounce those terms. The Audio CDs include 60 difficult terms from each chapter that are listed on the vocabulary list.

Text and Audio CDs, ISBN 1-4018-7643-9

Text and Delmar's Medical Terminology CD-ROM Individual Version Value Package

This is an exciting, interactive reference, practice, and assessment tool designed to complement any medical terminology program. Features include the extensive use of multimedia—animations, video, graphics, and activities—to present terms and word-building features. Difficult functions, processes, and procedures are included so that learners can more effectively learn from a textbook.

Text and CD-ROM Individual Version, ISBN 1-4018-7644-7

Acknowledgments

Special thanks to Don Jacobsen for his help in "pronouncing" the terms in this text, and to Dr. Elizabeth McMahon, Katrina Schroeder, and Dr. Linda Cunning for their contributions. Thanks also to the editorial and production staff of Delmar Thomson Learning for their very professional assistance in making this revision possible.

We are particularly grateful to the reviewers who continue to be a valuable resource in guiding this book as it evolves. Their insights, comments, suggestions, and attention to detail were very important in creating this text.

Ann Ehrlich
Carol L. Schroeder

Reviewers

Gloria Ahern, RHIA
Professor Emeritus, Health Information Technology
Central Oregon Community College
Bend, Oregon

Mary Brown, RN, MSN
Instructor
Arapahoe Community College
Englewood, Colorado

Linda R. Delunas, PhD, RN
Associate Professor and Associate Dean
School of Nursing and Health Professions
Indiana University Northwest
Gary, Indiana

Beverlee Jackson, RHIT
Director, Health Information Technology
Central Oregon Community College
Bend, Oregon

Melody Hale, RHIT
Health Information Technology Program
Central Oregon Community College
Bend, Oregon

Maxine Walker Mangum, BS, MS
Office Systems Technology Instructor
Piedmont Community College
Roxboro, North Carolina

Josy M. Petr, MS, RN
Lecturer and Educational Testing Director
Indiana University School of Nursing
Indianapolis, Indiana

Ingrid Sidoror, RN, MSN
Gerontological Clinical Nurse Specialist
Adjunct Faculty
Harcum College
Ardmore, Pennsylvania

Stacey Wilson, MT, PBT (ASCP), CMA
Medical Assisting Program Coordinator
Cabarrus College of Health Sciences
Concord, North Carolina

How to Use **This Book**

Medical Terminology for Health Professions, Fifth Edition, helps you learn and remember medical terms with surprising ease. The key lies in the following features.

1 ## Body System Overview

The first page of each body system chapter is a chart giving an overview of the structures, related combining forms, and functions most important to that system.

2 ## Vocabulary List

The second page of each chapter is a 75-item vocabulary list. These are 15 key word parts and 60 important terms for the chapter. This immediately alerts you to the key terms in the chapter and acts as a review guide. Next to each term is a box so you can check off each term as you've learned it. This list includes the 60 terms pronounced on the *Medical Terminology for Health Professions*, Fifth Edition StudyWARE™ CD-ROM, which is included with the book, as well as on the optional Audio CDs.

3 ## Learning Objectives

The beginning of each chapter lists learning objectives to help you understand what is expected of you as you read the text and complete the exercises. These objectives are set off with a color bar for easy identification.

4 ## Illustrations

The book's full-color illustrations, complete with detailed labeling, help clarify the text—and contain important information of their own. Review each illustration and read each caption carefully for easy and effective learning.

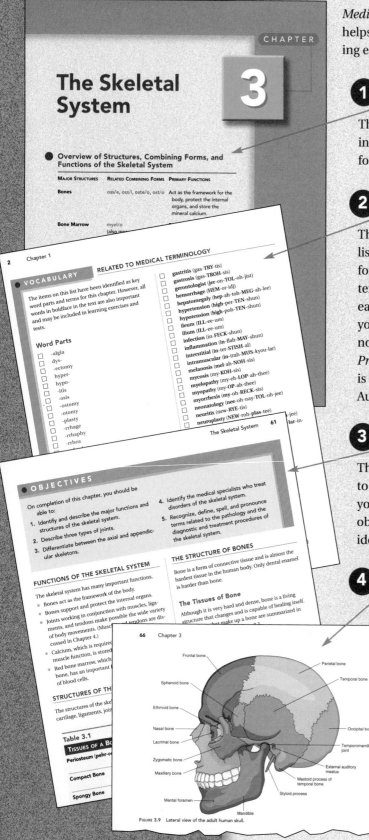

FIGURE 3.9 Lateral view of the adult human skull.

5 Sounds-Like Pronunciation System

The "sounds-like" pronunciation system makes pronunciation easy by respelling the word with syllables you can understand—and say—at a glance. Simply pronounce the term just as it appears in parentheses, accenting the syllables as follows:

- **Primary** (strongest) **accent**: capital letters and bold type
- **Secondary accent**: lowercase letters and bold type

6 Word Parts

Because word parts are so important to learning medical terminology, whenever a term made up of word parts is introduced, the definition is followed (in parentheses) by the word parts highlighted in magenta and defined.

7 Abbreviation Summary

The abbreviations related to each chapter are summarized in a table at the end of the chapter content. Use this table as a review guide and to compare and contrast confusing abbreviations.

Table 3.2

ABBREVIATIONS RELATED TO THE SKELETAL SYSTEM	
acetaminophen = APAP	**APAP** = acetaminophen
bone density testing = BDT	**BDT** = bone density testing
bone marrow biopsy = BMB	**BMB** = bone marrow biopsy
bone marrow transplant = BMT	**BMT** = bone marrow transplant
closed reduction = CR	**CR** = closed reduction
craniostenosis = CSO	**CSO** = craniostenosis
dual x-ray absorptiometry = DXA	**DXA** = dual x-ray absorptiometry
fracture = Fx	**Fx** = fracture
hallux valgus = HV	**HV** = hallux valgus
juvenile rheumatoid arthritis = JRA	**JRA** = juvenile rheumatoid arthritis
magnetic resonance imaging = MRI	**MRI** = magnetic resonance imaging

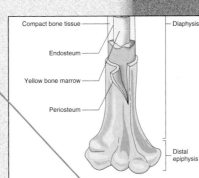

FIGURE 3.1 Anatomic features of a typical long bone.

- **Hemopoietic** (**hee**-moh poy-**ET**-ick), also known as **hematopoietic** (**hee**-mah-toh-poi-**ET**-ick), means pertaining to the formation of blood cells (**hem/o** and **hemat/o** both mean blood and **-poietic** means pertaining to formation).
- **Yellow bone marrow**, which is found in the medullary cavity, is composed chiefly of fat cells and functions as a fat storage area.

Cartilage

- **Cartilage** (**KAR**-tih-lidj) is the smooth, rubbery, blue-white connective tissue that acts as a shock absorber between bones. Cartilage, which is more elastic than

farthest away from the midline.

- A **foramen** (foh-**RAY**-men) is an opening in a b through which blood vessels, nerves, and ligam pass (plural, **foramina**). For example, the spina cord runs through the vertebral foramen show Figure 3.13.
- A **process** is a normal projection on the surface bone that serves as an attachment for muscles tendons. For example, the mastoid process is th bony projection located on each temporal bon behind the ear (Figure 3.9).

JOINTS

Joints, also known as **articulations**, are connection between bones. As used here, *articulation* means join or come together in a manner that allows mo between the parts. *Articulation* also means speaki clearly.

Types of Joints

Different types of joints make a wide range of mo possible. These types of joints include sutures, ca laginous joints, and synovial joints.

Sutures

- A **suture** is an immovable joint. Here bones joi along a jagged line to form a joint that does no move. *Suture* also means to stitch. Figure 3.2 sh the coronal and sagittal sutures across the top

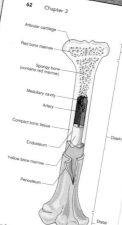

Learning Exercises

Matching Word Parts 1

Write the correct answer in the middle column.

Definition	Correct Answer	Possible Answers
3.1. hump		ankyl/o
3.2. cartilage		arthr/o
3.3. crooked, bent, or stiff		-um
3.4. joint		kyph/o
3.5. noun ending		chondr/o

Matching Word Parts 2

Write the correct answer in the middle column.

Definiti...

The Skeletal System   93

THE HUMAN TOUCH: CRITICAL THINKING EXERCISE

The following story and questions are designed to stimulate critical thinking through class discussion or as a brief essay response. There are no right or wrong answers to these questions.

Dr. Johnstone didn't like what he saw. The x-rays of Gladys Guynn's hip showed a fracture of the femoral neck and severe osteoporosis of the hip. Mrs. Guynn had been admitted to the orthopedic ward of Hamilton Hospital after a fall that morning at Sunny Meadows, an assisted-living facility. The accident had occurred when Sheri Smith, a new aide, lost her grip while helping Mrs. Guynn in the shower.

A frail but alert and cheerful woman of 85, Gladys Guynn has osteoarthritis and osteoporosis that have forced her to rely on a walker. She has been living at Sunny Meadows since her husband's death four years ago. Dr. Johnstone knew that she didn't have any relatives in the area, and he did not think that she had signed a health care power of attorney designating someone to help with medical decisions like this.

A total hip replacement (THP) would be the logical treatment for a younger patient because it could restore some of her lost mobility. However, for a frail patient like Mrs. Guynn, internal fixation of the fracture might be the treatment of choice. This would repair the break but not improve her mobility.

Dr. Johnstone needed to make a decision soon, but Mrs. Guynn was still groggy from the pain medication. With one more look at the x-ray, Dr. Johnstone sighed and walked toward Mrs. Guynn's room.

Suggested Discussion Topics:

1. Gladys Guynn has no children or other relatives in the area and is unable to speak for herself. Who should decide which surgery should be performed?

2. Do you think Sheri Smith or Sunny Meadows should be held responsible for Mrs. Guynn's accident? If so, who should be held responsible?

3. A total hip replacement is more expensive than the internal fixation procedure and has a longer, more strenuous recovery period. Given the patient's condition and the limited dollars available for health care, which procedure should be performed?

4. Would you have answered Question 3 differently if Mrs. Guynn were your mother?

---

8 Learning Exercises

Each chapter includes 100 Learning Exercises in a variety of formats that require a one- or two-word written answer. Writing terms, rather than circling a multiple choice option, reinforces learning and provides practice in writing and spelling these terms.

9 The Human Touch: Critical Thinking Exercise

A "real-life" mini story and related critical thinking questions at the end of each chapter that involve patients and pathology help you apply what you are learning to the real world. There are no right or wrong answers, just questions to get you started thinking about and using the new terms you have learned.

How to Use *Medical Terminology for Health Professions, Fifth Edition* StudyWARE™

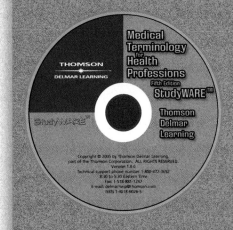

● Minimum System Requirements

- Operating System: Microsoft Windows 95, 98 SE, 2000, or XP
- Processor: Pentium PC 500 MHz or higher (750 MHz recommended)
- RAM: 64 MB of RAM (128 MB recommended)
- Screen Resolution: 800 × 600 pixels
- Color Depth: 16-bit color (thousands of colors)
- Macromedia Flash Player V7.x. (The Macromedia Flash Player is free, and can be downloaded at http://www.macromedia.com.)

● Installation Instructions

1. Insert disc into CD-ROM player. The *Medical Terminology for Health Professions*, Fifth Edition, StudyWARE™ installation program should start up automatically. If it does not, go to step 2.
2. From My Computer, double-click the icon for the CD drive.
3. Double-click the *setup.exe* file to start the program.

● Technical Support

Telephone: 1-800-477-3692, 8:30 a.m. to 5:30 p.m. Eastern Time

Fax: 1-518-881-1247

E-mail: delmarhelp@thomson.com

StudyWARE™ is a trademark used herein under license.

Refer to the license agreement in the back of the book following the index.

● Getting Started

The StudyWARE™ software will help you learn medical terms in *Medical Terminology for Health Professions*, Fifth Edition. As you study each chapter in the text, be sure to explore the activities in the corresponding chapter in the software. Use StudyWARE™ as your own private tutor to help you learn the material in the text.

Getting started is easy. Install the software by inserting the CD and following the on-screen instructions. Enter your first and last name so the software can store your quiz results. Then choose a chapter from the menu and take a quiz or explore one of the activities.

Menus

You can access any of the menus from wherever you are within the program. The menus include Quizzes, Scores, Activities, and Audio Library.

Quizzes. Quizzes include Multiple Choice, True/False, Fill-in, and Word Building questions. You can take the quizzes in both Practice Mode and Quiz Mode. Use Practice Mode to improve your mastery of the material. You have multiple tries to get the answers correct. Instant feedback tells you whether you're right or wrong—and helps you learn quickly by explaining why an answer was correct or incorrect. Use Quiz Mode when you are ready to test yourself and keep a record of your scores. In Quiz Mode, you have one try to get the answers right, but you can take each Quiz as many times as you want.

Scores. You can view your last scores for each quiz and print out your results to hand in to your instructor.

Reports for Jane Jones

Date Taken	Quiz Name	Score	
5/28/2004 (11:41 a.m.)	Chapter 1: Introduction to Medical Terminology	90	View Details
5/28/2004 (11:44 a.m.)	Chapter 2: The Human Body in Health and Disease	90	View Details
5/28/2004 (11:45 a.m.)	Chapter 3: Skeletal System	80	View Details

Activities. Activities include Image Labeling, Spelling Bee, Crossword Puzzles, and a Jeopardy!-style Championship Game. Have fun while increasing your knowledge!

Audio Library. The StudyWARE™ Audio Library is a reference that includes audio pronunciations and definitions for over 950 medical terms! Use the audio library to practice pronunciation and review definitions. Browse terms by chapter and then listen to pronunciations of the terms you select or listen to an entire list of terms.

Introduction to Medical Terminology

● Overview of Introduction to Medical Terminology

Word Parts Are the Key! Introduction to word parts and how they create complex medical terms.

Word Roots The word parts that usually, but not always, indicate the part of the body involved.

Combining Forms Word roots plus a vowel (usually the letter o) added to the end. This form is used when connecting word roots or when the word root is joined to a suffix that begins with a consonant.

Suffixes The word parts that usually, but not always, indicate the procedure, condition, disorder, or disease.

Prefixes The word parts that usually, but not always, indicate location, time, number, or status.

Determining Meanings on the Basis of Word Parts Use knowledge of word parts to decipher medical terms.

Medical Dictionary Use Guidelines to make the use of a medical dictionary easier.

Pronunciation Learn the easy-to-use "sounds-like" pronunciation system.

Spelling Is Always Important Discover how one wrong letter can change the entire meaning of a term!

Using Abbreviations Caution is important when using abbreviations.

Singular and Plural Endings Unusual singular and plural endings used in medical terms.

Basic Medical Terms Terms used to describe disease conditions.

Look-Alike Sound-Alike Terms and Word Parts Clarification of confusing terms that look or sound alike.

● VOCABULARY   RELATED TO MEDICAL TERMINOLOGY

The items on this list have been identified as key word parts and terms for this chapter. However, all words in boldface in the text are also important and may be included in learning exercises and tests.

Word Parts

- [ ] -algia
- [ ] dys-
- [ ] -ectomy
- [ ] hyper-
- [ ] hypo-
- [ ] -itis
- [ ] -osis
- [ ] -ostomy
- [ ] -otomy
- [ ] -plasty
- [ ] -rrhage
- [ ] -rrhaphy
- [ ] -rrhea
- [ ] -rrhexis
- [ ] -sclerosis

Medical Terms

- [ ] **abdominocentesis** (ab-**dom**-ih-noh-sen-**TEE**-sis)
- [ ] **acronym** (**ACK**-roh-nim)
- [ ] **angiography** (**an**-jee-**OG**-rah-fee)
- [ ] **appendectomy** (**ap**-en-**DECK**-toh-mee)
- [ ] **appendicitis** (ah-**pen**-dih-**SIGH**-tis)
- [ ] **arterionecrosis** (ar-**tee**-ree-oh-neh-**KROH**-sis)
- [ ] **arteriosclerosis** (ar-**tee**-ree-oh-skleh-**ROH**-sis)
- [ ] **arthralgia** (ar-**THRAL**-jee-ah)
- [ ] **colostomy** (koh-**LAHS**-toh-mee)
- [ ] **diagnosis** (dye-ag-**NOH**-sis)
- [ ] **edema** (eh-**DEE**-mah)
- [ ] **endarterial** (end-ar-**TEE**-ree-al)
- [ ] **endoscopy** (en-**DOS**-koh-pee)
- [ ] **eponym** (**EP**-oh-nim)
- [ ] **fissure** (**FISH**-ur)
- [ ] **fistula** (**FIS**-tyou-lah)
- [ ] **gastralgia** (gas-**TRAL**-jee-ah)

- [ ] **gastritis** (gas-**TRY**-tis)
- [ ] **gastrosis** (gas-**TROH**-sis)
- [ ] **gerontologist** (**jer**-on-**TOL**-oh-jist)
- [ ] **hemorrhage** (**HEM**-or-idj)
- [ ] **hepatomegaly** (**hep**-ah-toh-**MEG**-ah-lee)
- [ ] **hypertension** (**high**-per-**TEN**-shun)
- [ ] **hypotension** (**high**-poh-**TEN**-shun)
- [ ] **ileum** (**ILL**-ee-um)
- [ ] **ilium** (**ILL**-ee-um)
- [ ] **infection** (in-**FECK**-shun)
- [ ] **inflammation** (**in**-flah-**MAY**-shun)
- [ ] **interstitial** (**in**-ter-**STISH**-al)
- [ ] **intramuscular** (**in**-trah-**MUS**-kyou-lar)
- [ ] **melanosis** (**mel**-ah-**NOH**-sis)
- [ ] **mycosis** (my-**KOH**-sis)
- [ ] **myelopathy** (my-eh-**LOP**-ah-thee)
- [ ] **myopathy** (my-**OP**-ah-thee)
- [ ] **myorrhexis** (**my**-oh-**RECK**-sis)
- [ ] **neonatology** (**nee**-oh-nay-**TOL**-oh-jee)
- [ ] **neuritis** (new-**RYE**-tis)
- [ ] **neuroplasty** (**NEW**-roh-**plas**-tee)
- [ ] **otolaryngology** (**oh**-toh-**lar**-in-**GOL**-oh-jee)
- [ ] **otorhinolaryngology** (**oh**-toh-**rye**-noh-**lar**-in-**GOL**-oh-jee)
- [ ] **palpation** (pal-**PAY**-shun)
- [ ] **perinatal** (**pehr**-ih-**NAY**-tal)
- [ ] **postnatal** (pohst-**NAY**-tal)
- [ ] **prognosis** (prog-**NOH**-sis)
- [ ] **prostate** (**PROS**-tayt)
- [ ] **prostrate** (**PROS**-trayt)
- [ ] **pyelitis** (**pye**-eh-**LYE**-tis)
- [ ] **pyoderma** (**pye**-oh-**DER**-mah)
- [ ] **subcostal** (sub-**KOS**-tal)
- [ ] **supination** (**soo**-pih-**NAY**-shun)
- [ ] **suppuration** (**sup**-you-**RAY**-shun)
- [ ] **supracostal** (**sue**-prah-**KOS**-tal)
- [ ] **symptom** (**SIMP**-tum)
- [ ] **syndrome** (**SIN**-drohm)
- [ ] **tonsillectomy** (**ton**-sih-**LECK**-toh-mee)
- [ ] **tonsillitis** (**ton**-sih-**LYE**-tis)
- [ ] **trauma** (**TRAW**-mah)
- [ ] **triage** (tree-**AHZH**)
- [ ] **viral** (**VYE**-ral)
- [ ] **virile** (**VIR**-ill)

● OBJECTIVES

On completion of this chapter, you should be able to:

1. Identify the roles of the four types of word parts in forming medical terms.

2. Analyze unfamiliar medical terms using your knowledge of word parts.

3. Describe the steps in locating a term in a medical dictionary.

4. Define the commonly used prefixes, word roots, combining forms, and suffixes introduced in this chapter.

5. Pronounce medical terms correctly using the "sounds-like" system.

6. Recognize the importance of always spelling medical terms correctly.

7. State why caution is important when using abbreviations.

8. Recognize, define, spell, and pronounce the medical terms in this chapter.

WORD PARTS ARE THE KEY!

Learning medical terminology is much easier once you understand how word parts work together to form medical terms. This book includes many aids to help you continue reinforcing your word building skills.

- The types of word parts and the rules for their use are explained in this chapter. Learn these rules and follow them!

- Key terms made up of word parts include in their definitions an explanation of the word parts and their meanings. These word parts appear in magenta.

- The Learning Exercises for each chapter include a "Challenge Word Building" section to help develop your skills in working with word parts.

- After Chapter 2 there is a Word Part Review section. This section provides additional word part practice and enables you to evaluate your progress toward mastering the meanings of these word parts.

The Four Types of Word Parts

Four types of word parts may be used to create medical terms. Guidelines for their use are shown in Table 1.1.

- **Word roots** contain the basic meaning of the term. They usually, *but not always*, indicate the involved body part.

- **Combining forms** are word roots with a vowel at the end so that a suffix beginning with a consonant can be added.

- **Suffixes** usually, *but not always*, indicate the procedure, condition, disorder, or disease. A suffix always comes at the end of a word.

- **Prefixes** usually, *but not always*, indicate location, time, number, or status. A prefix always comes at the beginning of a word.

WORD ROOTS

Word roots act as the foundation of most medical terms. They usually, *but not always*, describe the part of the body that is involved (Figure 1.1). They may also indicate color. Some of the word roots that indicate color are shown, in their combining forms, in Table 1.2.

Table 1.1
WORD PART GUIDELINES

1. A word root cannot stand alone. A suffix must be added to complete the term.

2. The rules for the use of creating a combining form by adding a vowel apply when a suffix beginning with a consonant is added to a word root. These rules are explained in Table 1.3.

3. When a prefix is necessary, it is always placed at the beginning of the word.

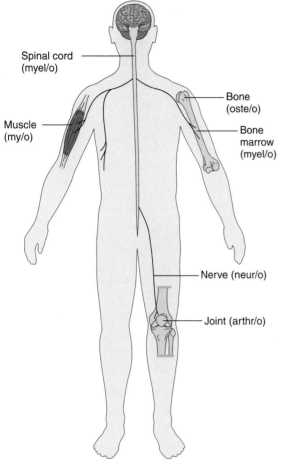

Spinal cord
(myel/o)

Muscle
(my/o)

Bone
(oste/o)

Bone
marrow
(myel/o)

Nerve (neur/o)

Joint (arthr/o)

FIGURE 1.1   A word root (combining form) usually indicates the involved body part.

Combining Vowels

A combining vowel may be needed between the word root and suffix to make the medical term easier to pronounce. The rules for using combining vowels are explained in Table 1.3.

● The letter **o** is the most commonly used combining vowel.

● When a word root is shown with a back slash and a combining vowel, such as **cardi/o**, this format is referred to as a **combining form** (**cardi/o** means heart).

SUFFIXES

A suffix is added to the end of a word root or its combining form to complete the term. Suffixes usually, *but not always*, indicate the procedure, condition, disorder, or disease (Figure 1.2).

● For example, **tonsill/o** means tonsils. A suffix is added to complete the term and to tell what is happening to the tonsils.

● **Tonsillitis** (**ton**-sih-**LYE**-tis) is an inflammation of the tonsils (**tonsill** means tonsils and **-itis** means inflammation).

● A **tonsillectomy** (**ton**-sih-**LECK**-toh-mee) is the surgical removal of the tonsils (**tonsill** means tonsils and **-ectomy** means surgical removal).

Table 1.2

WORD/ROOTS/COMBINING FORMS INDICATING COLOR	
cyan/o means blue	**Cyanosis** (**sigh**-ah-**NOH**-sis) is a blue discoloration of the skin caused by a lack of adequate oxygen (cyan means blue and -osis means condition).
erythr/o means red	**Erythrocytes** (eh-**RITH**-roh-sights) are mature red blood cells (erythr/o means red and cytes means cells).
leuk/o means white	**Leukocytes** (**LOO**-koh-sights) are white blood cells (leuk/o means white and -cytes means cells).
melan/o means black	**Melanosis** (**mel**-ah-**NOH**-sis) is any condition of unusual deposits of black pigment in different parts of the body (melan means black and -osis means condition).
poli/o means gray	**Poliomyelitis** (**poh**-lee-oh-**my**-eh-**LYE**-tis) is a viral infection of the gray matter of the spinal cord that may result in paralysis (poli/o means gray, myel means spinal cord, and -itis means inflammation).

Table 1.3

RULES FOR USING COMBINING VOWELS

1. A combining vowel *is used* when the suffix begins with a consonant.

For example, when neur/o (nerve) is joined with the suffix -plasty (surgical repair), the combining vowel o *is used* because -plasty begins with a consonant.

Neuroplasty (**NEW**-roh-**plas**-tee) is the surgical repair of a nerve (neur/o means nerve and -plasty means surgical repair).

2. A combining vowel *is not used* when the suffix begins with a vowel (*a, e, i, o, u*).

For example, when neur/o (nerve) is joined with the suffix -itis (inflammation), no combining vowel is used because -itis begins with a vowel.

Neuritis (new-**RYE**-tis) is inflammation of a nerve or nerves (neur means nerve and -itis means inflammation).

3. A combining vowel *is always used* when two or more root words are joined.

As an example, when gastr/o (stomach) is joined with enter/o (small intestine), the combining vowel *is used* with gastr/o; however, when the suffix -itis (inflammation) is added, the combining vowel *is not used* with enter/o because -itis begins with a vowel.

Gastroenteritis (**gas**-troh-en-ter-**EYE**-tis) is an inflammation of the stomach and small intestine (gastr/o means stomach, enter means small intestine, and -itis means inflammation).

Suffixes Meaning "Pertaining To"

Some suffixes complete the term by changing the word root into an **adjective** (a word that describes a noun). Many of these suffixes are defined as "pertaining to." The "Pertaining to" table, at the beginning of Appendix A, makes such suffixes easy to find.

- For example, **cardiac** (**KAR**-dee-ack) is an adjective that means pertaining to the heart (cardi means heart and -ac means pertaining to).

Suffixes as Noun Endings

Some suffixes complete the term by changing the word root into a **noun** (a word that is the name of a person, place, or thing). Other suffixes in this group are defined as *noun endings*. These suffixes also are listed in a table at the beginning of Appendix A.

- For example, the **cranium** (**KRAY**-nee-um) is the portion of the skull that encloses the brain (crani means skull and -um is a noun ending).

Suffixes Meaning "Abnormal Condition"

Some suffixes have a general meaning of "abnormal condition or disease." These suffixes are also listed in a table at the beginning of Appendix A.

- For example, -osis means an abnormal condition or disease. **Gastrosis** (gas-**TROH**-sis) means any disease of the stomach (gastr means stomach and -osis means abnormal condition).

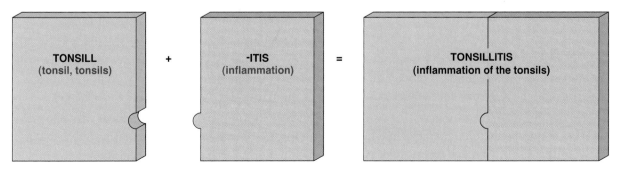

FIGURE 1.2   A word root, without a combining vowel, plus a suffix creates a new term.

Suffixes Related to Pathology

Pathology (pah-**THOL**-oh-jee) means the study of disease, and the suffixes related to pathology describe specific disease conditions (**path** means disease and **-ology** means study of).

- **-algia** means pain and suffering. **Gastralgia** (gas-**TRAL**-jee-ah) means pain in the stomach (**gastr** means stomach and **-algia** means pain).

- **-dynia** also means pain. **Gastrodynia** (gas-troh-**DIN**-ee-ah) also means pain in the stomach (**gastr/o** means stomach and **-dynia** means pain).

- **-itis** means inflammation. **Gastritis** (gas-**TRY**-tis) is an inflammation of the stomach (**gastr** means stomach and **-itis** means inflammation).

- **-malacia** means abnormal softening. **Arteriomalacia** (ar-**tee**-ree-oh-mah-**LAY**-shee-ah) is the abnormal softening of the walls of an artery or arteries (**arteri/o** means artery and **-malacia** means abnormal softening). Notice that **-malacia** is the opposite of **-sclerosis**.

- **-megaly** means enlargement. **Hepatomegaly** (hep-ah-toh-**MEG**-ah-lee) is the abnormal enlargement of the liver (**hepat/o** means liver and **-megaly** means enlargement).

- **-necrosis** means tissue death. **Arterionecrosis** (ar-**tee**-ree-oh-neh-**KROH**-sis) is the tissue death of an artery or arteries (**arteri/o** means artery and **-necrosis** means tissue death).

- **-sclerosis** means abnormal hardening. **Arteriosclerosis** (ar-**tee**-ree-oh-skleh-**ROH**-sis) is the abnormal hardening of the walls of an artery or arteries (**arteri/o** means artery and **-sclerosis** means abnormal hardening). Notice that **-sclerosis** is the opposite of **-malacia**.

- **-stenosis** means abnormal narrowing. **Arteriostenosis** (ar-**tee**-ree-oh-steh-**NOH**-sis) is the abnormal narrowing of an artery or arteries (**arteri/o** means artery and **-stenosis** means abnormal narrowing.)

Suffixes Related to Procedures

Suffixes related to procedures identify a procedure that is performed on the body part identified by the word root.

- **-centesis** is a surgical puncture to remove fluid for diagnostic purposes or to remove excess fluid.

Abdominocentesis (ab-**dom**-ih-noh-sen-**TEE**-sis) is the surgical puncture of the abdominal cavity to remove fluid (**abdomin/o** means abdomen and **-centesis** means a surgical puncture to removal fluid).

- **-graphy** means the process of producing a picture or record. **Angiography** (**an**-jee-**OG**-rah-fee) is a radiographic (x-ray) study of the blood vessels after the injection of a contrast medium (**angi/o** means blood vessel and **-graphy** means the process of recording).

- **-gram** means a picture or record. An **angiogram** (**AN**-jee-oh-**gram**) is the film produced by angiography (**angi/o** means blood vessel and **-gram** means a picture or record).

- **-plasty** means surgical repair. **Myoplasty** (**MY**-oh-**plas**-tee) is the surgical repair of a muscle (**myo** means muscle and **-plasty** means surgical repair).

- **-scopy** means visual examination. **Endoscopy** (en-**DOS**-koh-pee) is the visual examination of the interior of a body cavity or organ by means of an endoscope (**endo-** means within and **-scopy** means visual examination).

The "Double *R*" Suffixes

Suffixes beginning with two *R*s, which are often referred to as the "**double RRs**," are particularly confusing. They are grouped together here to help you understand the word parts and to remember the differences.

- **-rrhage** and **-rrhagia** mean bleeding, bursting forth, or abnormal or excessive flow. A **hemorrhage** (**HEM**-or-idj) is the loss of a large amount of blood in a short time (**hem/o** means blood and **-rrhage** means bursting forth of blood).

- **-rrhaphy** means surgical suturing to close a wound and includes the use of sutures, staples, and surgical glue. **Myorrhaphy** (my-**OR**-ah-fee) is the surgical suturing of a muscle wound (**my/o** means muscle and **-rrhaphy** means surgical suturing).

- **-rrhea** means flow or discharge and refers to the flow of most body fluids. **Diarrhea** (**dye**-ah-**REE**-ah) is the flow of frequent loose or watery stools (**dia-** means through and **-rrhea** means flow or discharge).

- **-rrhexis** means rupture. **Myorrhexis** (**my**-oh-**RECK**-sis) is the rupture of a muscle (**my/o** means muscle and **-rrhexis** means rupture).

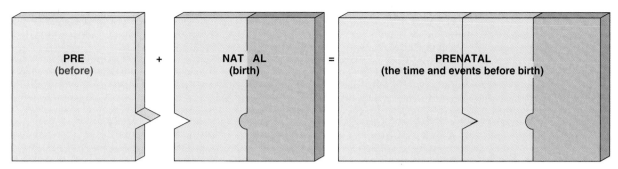

FIGURE **1.3** A prefix added to a word root and suffix changes the meaning of the term.

PREFIXES

A prefix is added to the beginning of a word to influence the meaning of that term (Figure 1.3). Prefixes usually, *but not always*, indicate location, time, or number. The term **natal** (**NAY**-tal) means pertaining to birth (**nat** means birth, and **-al** means pertaining to). The following examples show how a prefix changes the meaning of this term.

- **Prenatal** (pre-**NAY**-tal) means the time and events before birth (**pre-** means before, **nat** means birth, and **-al** means pertaining to) (Figure 1.4).

- **Perinatal** (**pehr**-ih-**NAY**-tal) refers to the time and events surrounding birth (**peri-** means surrounding, **nat** means birth, and **-al** means pertaining to). This is the time just before, during, and just after birth (Figure 1.5).

- **Postnatal** (pohst-**NAY**-tal) refers to the time and events after birth (**post-** means after, **nat** means birth, and **-al** means pertaining to) (Figure 1.6).

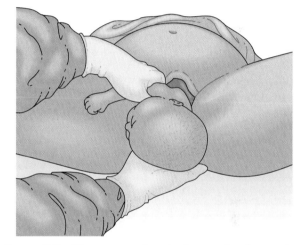

FIGURE **1.5** The term *perinatal* refers to the time and events around birth. As shown here, in a normal delivery, the baby's head emerges first.

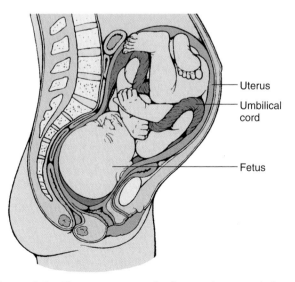

Uterus

Umbilical cord

Fetus

FIGURE **1.4** The term *prenatal* refers to the events that occur before birth. Shown here is a diagram of a developing child in the uterus before birth.

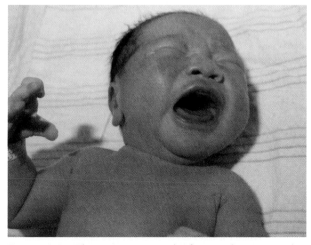

FIGURE **1.6** The term *postnatal* refers to the time and events after birth. As shown here, a healthy newborn has a lusty cry.

Table 1.4

CONTRASTING AND CONFUSING PREFIXES	
ab- means away from.	ad- means toward or in the direction of.
Abnormal means not normal or away from normal.	**Addiction** means drawn toward or a strong dependence on a drug or substance.
dys- means bad, difficult, painful.	eu- means good, normal, well, or easy.
Dysfunctional means an organ or body part that is not working properly.	**Euthyroid** (you-**THIGH**-roid) means a normally functioning thyroid gland.
hyper- means excessive or increased.	hypo- means deficient or decreased.
Hypertension (**high**-per-**TEN**-shun) is higher than normal blood pressure.	**Hypotension** (**high**-poh-**TEN**-shun) is lower than normal blood pressure.
inter- means between or among.	intra- means within or inside.
Interstitial (**in**-ter-**STISH**-al) means between, but not within, the parts of a tissue.	**Intramuscular** (**in**-trah-**MUS**-kyou-lar) means within the muscle.
sub- means under, less, or below.	super-, supra- mean above or excessive.
Subcostal (sub-**KOS**-tal) means below a rib or ribs.	**Supracostal** (**sue**-prah-**KOS**-tal) means above or outside the ribs.

Contrasting and Confusing Prefixes

Some prefixes are confusing because they are similar in spelling but opposite in meaning. The more common prefixes of this type are summarized in Table 1.4.

DETERMINING MEANINGS ON THE BASIS OF WORDS PARTS

Knowing the meaning of the word parts often makes it possible to figure out the definition of an unfamiliar medical term.

Taking Terms Apart

To determine a word's meaning by looking at the component pieces, you must first separate it into word parts.

- Always start at the end of the word, with the suffix, and work toward the beginning.
- As you separate the word parts, identify the meaning of each. Identifying the meaning of each part should give you a definition of the term.
- Because some word parts have more than one meaning, it also is necessary to determine the context in which the term is being used. As used here,

context means to determine which body system this term is referring to.

- If you have any doubt, use your medical dictionary to double-check your definition.

An Example

Look at the term **otorhinolaryngology** as shown in Figure 1.7. It is made up of three combining forms plus a suffix. Here are the word parts as the term is taken apart, beginning at the end.

- The suffix -**ology** means the study of.
- The word root **laryng** means larynx and throat. The combining vowel *is not used* here because the word root is joining a suffix that begins with a vowel.
- The combining form **rhin/o** means nose. The combining vowel *is used* here because **rhin/o** is joining another word root.
- The combining form **ot/o** means ear. The combining vowel *is used* here because **ot/o** is joining another word root.
- Together they form **otorhinolaryngology** (**oh**-toh-**rye**-noh-**lar**-in-**GOL**-oh-jee), which is the study of the ears, nose, and throat (**ot/o** means ear, **rhin/o**

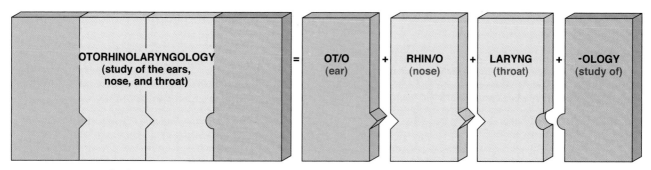

| OTORHINOLARYNGOLOGY (study of the ears, nose, and throat) | = | OT/O (ear) | + | RHIN/O (nose) | + | LARYNG (throat) | + | -OLOGY (study of) |

FIGURE 1.7   A medical term may be taken apart to determine its meaning.

means nose, **laryng** means throat, and **-ology** means study of).

- Because this is such a long name, this specialty is frequently referred to as **ENT** (ears, nose, and throat) or it is shortened to **otolaryngology** (oh-toh-**lar**-in-**GOL**-oh-jee), which is the study of the ears and larynx or throat (**ot/o** means ears, **larynx** means larynx, and **-ology** means study of).

Guessing at Meanings

When you are able to guess at the meaning of a term on the basis of word parts that make it up, you must always double check for accuracy, because some terms have more than one meaning. For example, look at the term **lithotomy** (lih-**THOT**-oh-mee):

- On the basis of word parts, a **lithotomy** is a surgical incision for the removal of a stone (**lith** means stone and **-otomy** means a surgical incision). This meaning is discussed further in Chapter 9.

- However, **lithotomy** is also the name of an examination position in which the patient is lying on the back with the feet and legs raised and supported in stirrups. This term is discussed further in Chapter 15.

- This possible confusion is only one of the many reasons why a medical dictionary is an important medical terminology tool.

MEDICAL DICTIONARY USE

Learning to use a medical dictionary is an important part of mastering the correct use of medical terms. The following tips for dictionary use apply whether you are working with a traditional book-form dictionary or an electronic dictionary on your computer.

If You Know How to Spell the Word

When starting to work with an unfamiliar dictionary, spend a few minutes reviewing its use guide, table of contents, and appendices. The time you spend reviewing now will be saved later when you are looking up unfamiliar terms.

- On the basis of the first letter of the word, start in the appropriate section of the dictionary. Look at the top of the page for clues. The top left word is the first term on the page. The top right word is the last term on the page.

- Next, look alphabetically for words that start with the first and second letters of the word you are researching. Continue looking through each letter until you find the term you are looking for.

- When you think you have found it, check the spelling very carefully letter by letter working from left to right. Terms with similar spellings have very different meanings.

- When you find the term, carefully check *all* of the definitions.

If You Do Not Know How to Spell the Word

- Listen carefully to the term and write it down. If you cannot find the word on the basis of your spelling, start looking for alternative spellings based on the beginning sound as shown in Table 1.5. *Note:* All of these examples are in this text. However, you could practice looking them up in the dictionary!

Look Under Categories

Most dictionaries use categories such as *Diseases* and *Syndromes* to group disorders with these terms in their titles. For example:

- *Venereal disease* would be found under *Disease, venereal*. These sexually transmitted diseases are discussed further in Chapter 14.

- *Fetal alcohol syndrome* would be found under *Syndrome, fetal alcohol*. This condition is discussed further in Chapter 2.

Table 1.5

GUIDELINES TO LOOKING UP THE SPELLING OF UNFAMILIAR TERMS

If it sounds like	It may begin with	Example
F	F	flatus (**FLAY**-tus)
	PH	phlegm (**FLEM**)
J	G	gingivitis (jin-jih-**VYE**-tis)
	J	jaundice (**JAWN**-dis)
K	C	crepitus (**KREP**-ih-tus)
	CH	cholera (**KOL**-er-ah)
	K	kyphosis (kye-**FOH**-sis)
	QU	quadriplegia (**kwad**-rih-**PLEE**-jee-ah)
S	C	cytology (sigh-**TOL**-oh-jee)
	PS	psychologist (sigh-**KOL**-oh-jist)
	S	serology (seh-**ROL**-oh-jee)
Z	X	xeroderma (zee-roh-**DER**-mah)
	Z	zygote (**ZYE**-goht)

- When you come across such a term and cannot find it listed by the first word, the next step is to look under the appropriate category.

Multiple Word Terms

When you are looking for a term that includes more than one word, begin your search with the last term. If you do not find it here, move forward to the next word.

- For example, *congestive heart failure* is sometimes listed under *heart failure, congestive*.

SEARCHING FOR DEFINITIONS ON THE INTERNET

Search engines can help you find medical terms. Type the complete term into the "search box" and add the word "definition." Be cautious and take care to determine that the site you've found is a reputable source for medical information.

PRONUNCIATION

A medical term is easier to understand and remember when you know how to pronounce it properly. To help you pronounce terms, we have identified each new term in the text in **bold.** The term is followed (in parentheses) by a commonly accepted pronunciation and then the definition.

- In this "sounds-like" pronunciation system, the word is respelled using normal English letters to create sounds that are familiar. To pronounce a new word, just say it as it is spelled in the parentheses.
- The part of the word that receives the primary (most) emphasis when you say it is shown in capital letters and bold. For example, **edema** (eh-**DEE**-mah) means excess fluid in body tissues, causing swelling.
- A part of the word that receives secondary emphasis when you say it, is shown in lowercase letters and bold. For example, **appendicitis** (ah-**pen**-dih-**SIGH**-tis) means an inflammation of the appendix (**appendic** means appendix and -**itis** means inflammation).

A Word of Caution

Frequently, there is more than one correct way to pronounce a medical term!

- The pronunciation of many medical terms is based on their Greek, Latin, or other foreign origin. However, there is a trend toward pronouncing terms as they would sound in English.
- The result is more than one "correct" pronunciation for a term. In the text, sometimes an alternative pronunciation is included to reflect these changes.
- Both are correct, and the difference is a matter of preference. However, your instructor will tell you which pronunciation to use in your course.

SPELLING IS ALWAYS IMPORTANT

Accuracy in spelling medical terms is extremely important!

- Changing just one or two letters can completely change the meaning of a word—and this difference literally could be a matter of life or death for the patient.
- The section "Look-Alike Sound-Alike Terms and Word Parts" later in this chapter will help you become aware of some terms and word parts that are frequently confused.

USING ABBREVIATIONS

Abbreviations are frequently used as a shorthand way to record long and complex medical terms; Appendix B contains an alphabetized list of many of the more commonly used medical abbreviations.

- Abbreviations can also lead to confusion and errors! Therefore, it is important that you be very careful when using or translating an abbreviation.
- For example, the abbreviation **BE** means both "below elbow" and "barium enema." Just imagine what a difference a mix-up here would make for the patient!

- Most clinical agencies have policies for accepted abbreviations. It is important to follow this list for the facility where you are working.
- If there is any question in your mind about which abbreviation to use, always follow this rule: *When in doubt, spell it out.*

SINGULAR AND PLURAL ENDINGS

Many medical terms have Greek or Latin origins. As a result of these different origins, there are unusual rules for changing a singular word into a plural form. In addition, English endings have been adopted for some commonly used terms.

- Table 1.6 provides guidelines to help you better understand how these plurals are formed.
- Also, throughout the text, when a term with an unusual singular or plural form is introduced, both forms are included. For example, a **phalanx** (**FAY**-lanks) is one bone of the fingers or toes (plural, **phalanges**) (Figure 1.8).

Table 1.6

GUIDELINES TO UNUSUAL PLURAL FORMS

Guideline	Singular	Plural
1. If the term ends in **a**, the plural is usually formed by adding an **e**.	bursa vertebra	bursae vertebrae
2. If the term ends in **ex** or **ix**, the plural is usually formed by changing the **ex** or **ix** to **ices**.	appendix index	appendices indices
3. If the term ends in **is**, the plural is usually formed by changing the **is** to **es**.	diagnosis metastasis	diagnoses metastases
4. If the term ends in **itis**, the plural is usually formed by changing the **is** to **ides**.	arthritis meningitis	arthritides meningitides
5. If the term ends in **nx**, the plural is usually formed by changing the **x** to **ges**.	phalanx meninx	phalanges meninges
6. If the term ends in **on**, the plural is usually formed by changing the **on** to **a**.	criterion ganglion	criteria ganglia
7. If the term ends in **um**, the plural usually is formed by changing the **um** to **a**.	diverticulum ovum	diverticula ova
8. If the term ends in **us**, the plural is usually formed by changing the **us** to **i**.	alveolus malleolus	alveoli malleoli

*If you are in doubt as to how a plural is formed, **look it up** under the singular in a medical dictionary!*

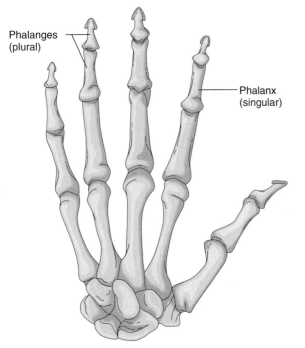

Phalanges
(plural)

Phalanx
(singular)

FIGURE 1.8   A phalanx is one finger or toe bone. Two or more of these bones are called phalanges.

BASIC MEDICAL TERMS

Some of the basic medical terms used to describe diseases and disease conditions are shown in Table 1.7.

LOOK-ALIKE SOUND-ALIKE TERMS AND WORD PARTS

One confusing part of learning medical terminology is dealing with words and word parts that look and sound much alike. This section highlights some frequently used terms and word parts that you may find confusing. Pay particular attention to these terms and word parts as you encounter them in the text.

arteri/o, ather/o, and arthr/o

* **arteri/o** means artery. **Endarterial** (**end**-ar-**TEE**-ree-al) means pertaining to the interior or lining of an artery (**end-** means within, **arteri** means artery, and **-al** means pertaining to).

Table 1.7

BASIC MEDICAL TERMS

A **sign** is objective evidence of disease, such as a fever. *Objective* means that the sign can be evaluated or measured by the patient or others.	A **symptom** (**SIMP**-tum) is subjective evidence of a disease, such as pain or a headache. *Subjective* means that it can be evaluated or measured only by the patient.	A **syndrome** (**SIN**-drohm) is a set of the signs and symptoms that occur together as part of a specific disease process.
A **diagnosis** (**dye**-ag-**NOH**-sis) is the identification of the disease (plural **diagnoses**). To **diagnose** is the process of reaching a diagnosis.	A **differential diagnosis** attempts to determine which one of several diseases may be producing the symptoms. Also known as to **rule out** (R/O).	A **prognosis** (prog-**NOH**-sis) is a forecast or prediction of the probable course and outcome of a disorder (plural, **prognoses**).
An **acute** disease or symptom has a rapid onset, a severe course, and a relatively short duration.	A **chronic** disease or symptom is of long duration. Although such diseases may be controlled, they are rarely cured.	A **remission** is the temporary, partial, or complete disappearance of the symptoms of a disease without having achieved a cure.
Some diseases are named for the **condition described**. For example, **chronic fatigue syndrome** is a persistent overwhelming fatigue that does not resolve with bed rest.	An **eponym** (**EP**-oh-nim) is a disease, structure, operation, or procedure named for the person who discovered or described it first. For example, **Alzheimer's disease** is named for Alois Alzheimer, a German neurologist who lived from 1864 to 1915. (See Chapter 10.)	An **acronym** (**ACK**-roh-nim) is a word formed from the initial letter or letters of the major parts of a compound term. For example, the acronym **laser** stands for **l**ight **a**mplification by **s**timulated **e**mission of **r**adiation. (See Chapter 12.)

- **ather/o** means plaque or fatty substance. An **atheroma** (**ath**-er-**OH**-mah) is a fatty deposit within the wall of an artery (**ather** means fatty substance and **-oma** means tumor).

- **arthr/o** means joint. **Arthralgia** (ar-**THRAL**-jee-ah) means pain in a joint or joints (**arthr** means joint and **-algia** means pain).

-ectomy, -ostomy, and -otomy

- **-ectomy** means surgical removal. An **appendectomy** (ap-en-**DECK**-toh-mee) is the surgical removal of the appendix (**append** means appendix and **-ectomy** means surgical removal).

- **-ostomy** means to surgically create an artificial opening. A **colostomy** (koh-**LAHS**-toh-mee) is the surgical creation of an opening between the colon and the body surface (**col** means colon and **-ostomy** means an artificial opening).

- **-otomy** means cutting into or a surgical incision. A **colotomy** (koh-**LOT**-oh-mee) is a surgical incision into the colon (**col** means colon and **-otomy** means a surgical incision).

Fissure and Fistula

- A **fissure** (**FISH**-ur) is a groove or crack-like sore of the skin. This term also describes normal folds in the contours of the brain.

- A **fistula** (**FIS**-tyou-lah) is an abnormal passage usually between two internal organs, or leading from an organ to the surface of the body.

Ileum and Ilium

- The **ileum** (**ILL**-ee-um) is part of the small intestine. (Remember, il**e**um is spelled with an *e* as in int**e**stine.)

- The **ilium** (**ILL**-ee-um) is part of the hip bone. (Remember, il**i**um is spelled with an *i* as in h**i**p.)

Infection and Inflammation

- An **infection** (in-**FECK**-shun) is the invasion of the body by a pathogenic (disease producing) organism. The infection may remain localized or may be systemic (affecting the entire body).

- **Inflammation** (**in**-flah-**MAY**-shun) is a localized response to an injury or destruction of tissues. The cardinal signs (indications) of inflammation are (1) *redness* (erythema), (2) *heat* (hyperthermia),

(3) *swelling* (edema), and (4) *pain*. These are caused by extra blood flowing into the area as part of the healing process.

- The suffix **-itis** means inflammation. However, it also is often used to indicate infection.

Laceration and Lesion

- A **laceration** (**lass**-er-**AY**-shun) is a torn, ragged wound.

- A **lesion** (**LEE**-zhun) is a pathologic change of the tissues due to disease or injury.

Mucous and Mucus

- **Mucous** (**MYOU**-kus) is an adjective that describes the specialized mucous membranes that line the body cavities.

- **Mucus** (**MYOU**-kus) is a noun and is the name of the fluid secreted by the mucous membranes.

myc/o, myel/o, and my/o

- **myc/o** means fungus. **Mycosis** (my-**KOH**-sis) means any disease caused by a fungus (**myc** means fungus and **-osis** means abnormal condition).

- **myel/o** means bone marrow *or* spinal cord. **Myelopathy** (my-eh-**LOP**-ah-thee) is any pathologic change or disease in the spinal cord (**myel/o** means spinal cord, or bone marrow, and **-pathy** means disease).

- **my/o** means muscle. **Myopathy** (my-**OP**-ah-thee) is any pathologic change or disease of muscle tissue (**my/o** means muscle and **-pathy** means disease).

-ologist and -ology

- **-ologist** means specialist. A **gerontologist** (**jer**-on-**TOL**-oh-jist) is a specialist in diagnosing and treating diseases, disorders, and problems associated with aging (**geront** means old age and **-ologist** means specialist).

- **-ology** means the study of. **Neonatology** (**nee**-oh-nay-**TOL**-oh-jee) is the study of disorders of the newborn (**neo-** means new, **nat** means birth, and **-ology** means study of).

Palpation and Palpitation

- **Palpation** (pal-**PAY**-shun) is an examination technique in which the examiner's hands are used to feel the texture, size, consistency, and location of certain body parts

- **Palpitation** (**pal**-pih-**TAY**-shun) is a pounding or racing heart.

Prostate and Prostrate

- **Prostate** (**PROS**-tayt) refers to a male gland that lies under the urinary bladder and surrounds the urethra.
- **Prostrate** (**PROS**-trayt) means to collapse and be lying flat or to be overcome with exhaustion.

pyel/o, py/o, and pyr/o

- **pyel/o** means renal pelvis (which is part of the kidney). **Pyelitis** (**pye**-eh-**LYE**-tis) is an inflammation of the renal pelvis (**pyel** means renal pelvis and **-itis** means inflammation).
- **py/o** means pus. **Pyoderma** (**pye**-oh-**DER**-mah) is any acute, inflammatory, pus-forming bacterial skin infection such as impetigo (**py/o** means pus and **-derma** means skin).
- **pyr/o** means fever or fire. **Pyrosis** (pye-**ROH**-sis), also known as **heartburn,** is discomfort due to the regurgitation of stomach acid upward into the esophagus (**pyr** means fever or fire and **-osis** means abnormal condition).

Supination and Suppuration

- **Supination** (**soo**-pih-**NAY**-shun) is the act of rotating the arm so that the palm of the hand is forward or upward.

- **Suppuration** (**sup**-you-**RAY**-shun) is the formation or discharge of pus.

Triage and Trauma

- **Triage** (tree-**AHZH**) is the medical screening of patients to determine their relative priority of need and the proper place of treatment. For example, emergency personnel arriving on an accident scene must identify which of the injured require care first and determine where they can be treated most effectively.
- **Trauma** (**TRAW**-mah) means wound or injury. These are the types of injuries that might occur in an accident, shooting, natural disaster, or fire.

Viral and Virile

- **Viral** (**VYE**-ral) means pertaining to a virus (**vir** means virus or poison and **-al** means pertaining to).
- **Virile** (**VIR**-ill) means possessing masculine traits.

ABBREVIATIONS RELATED TO THE INTRODUCTION TO MEDICAL TERMINOLOGY

Table 1.8 presents an overview of the abbreviations related to the terms introduced in this chapter. *Note:* To avoid errors or confusion, always be cautious when using abbreviations.

Table 1.8

ABBREVIATIONS RELATED TO THE INTRODUCTION TO MEDICAL TERMINOLOGY

Alzheimer's disease = AD	**AD** = Alzheimer's disease
appendectomy or **appendicitis** = AP	**AP** = appendectomy or appendicitis
barium enema, below elbow = BE	**BE** = barium enema, below elbow
chronic fatigue syndrome = CFS	**CFS** = chronic fatigue syndrome
cyanosis = C	**C** = cyanosis
diagnosis = DG, Dg, Diag, diag, DX, Dx	**DG, Dg, Diag, diag, DX, Dx** = diagnosis
differential diagnosis = D/D, DD, DDx, diaf. diag	**D/D, DD, DDx, diaf. diag** = differential diagnosis
endoscopy = EN	**EN** = endoscopy
gastroenteritis = GE	**GE** = gastroenteritis
hemorrhage = He	**He** = hemorrhage
inflammation = Inflam, Inflamm	**Inflam, Inflamm** = inflammation
intramuscular = IM	**IM** = intramuscular
pathology = PA, Pa, path	**Pa, PA, Path** = pathology
postnatal = PN	**PN** = postnatal
prognosis = prog, progn, Prx, Px	**prog, progn, Prx, Px** = prognosis
tonsillectomy = TE	**TE** = tonsillectomy
venereal disease = VD	**VD** = venereal disease

Learning Exercises

● Matching Word Parts 1

Write the correct answer in the middle column.

	Definition	Correct Answer	Possible Answers
1.1.	bad, difficult, painful	_____	-algia
1.2.	excessive, increased	_____	dys-
1.3.	liver	_____	-ectomy
1.4.	pain, suffering	_____	hepat/o
1.5.	surgical removal	_____	hyper-

● Matching Word Parts 2

Write the correct answer in the middle column.

	Definition	Correct Answer	Possible Answers
1.6.	abnormal condition	_____	hypo-
1.7.	abnormal softening	_____	-itis
1.8.	deficient, decreased	_____	-malacia
1.9.	inflammation	_____	-necrosis
1.10.	tissue death	_____	-osis

● Matching Word Parts 3

Write the correct answer in the middle column.

Definition	Correct Answer	Possible Answers
1.11. bleeding, bursting forth	_____	-ostomy
1.12. surgical creation of an opening	_____	-otomy
1.13. surgical incision	_____	-plasty
1.14. surgical repair	_____	-rrhage
1.15. surgical suturing	_____	-rrhaphy

● Matching Word Parts 4

Write the correct answer in the middle column.

Definition	Correct Answer	Possible Answers
1.16. visual examination	_____	-rrhea
1.17. rupture	_____	-rrhexis
1.18. abnormal narrowing	_____	-sclerosis
1.19. abnormal hardening	_____	-scopy
1.20. flow or discharge	_____	-stenosis

● Definitions

Select the correct answer and write it on the line provided.

1.21.   The word part meaning plaque or fatty substance is _____ .

   -algia   **angi/o**   **ather/o**   **arthr/o**

1.22.   The prefix meaning surrounding is _____ .

   inter-   **intra-**   **peri-**   **pre-**

1.23.   A _____ is always placed at the end of the term.

   combining form   prefix   suffix   word root

1.24. The combining form meaning white is _____ .

cyan/o erythr/o leuk/o poli/o

1.25. The suffix meaning abnormal softening is _____ .

-malacia -necrosis -sclerosis -stenosis

1.26. Pain, which can be observed only by the patient, is a _____ .

prognosis remission sign symptom

1.27. The prefix meaning deficient or decreased is _____ .

hyper- hypo- peri- supra-

1.28. A _____ is a prediction of the probable course and outcome of a disease.

diagnose diagnosis prognosis syndrome

1.29. The suffix meaning to rupture is _____ .

-rrhage -rrhaphy -rrhea -rrhexis

1.30. The plural of the term appendix is _____ .

appendexes appendices appendixxes appendizes

● Matching Terms and Definitions

Write the correct answer in the middle column.

Definition	Correct Answer	Possible Answers
1.31. examination procedure	_____	laceration
1.32. male gland	_____	lesion
1.33. pathologic tissue change	_____	palpitation
1.34. pounding heart	_____	palpation
1.35. torn, ragged wound	_____	prostate

● Which Word?

Select the correct answer and write it on the line provided.

1.36. The body cavities are lined with specialized _____ membranes.

mucous mucus

1.37. The formation of pus is called _____ .

   supination   suppuration

1.38. The term meaning wound or injury is _____ .

   trauma   triage

1.39. The term _____ means pertaining to a virus.

   viral   virile

1.40. The term describing part of the small intestine is _____ .

   ileum   ilium

● Spelling Counts

Find the misspelled word in each sentence. Then write that word, spelled correctly, on the line provided.

1.41. A disease named for the person who discovered it is known as an enaponym.

   _____

1.42. A localized response to injury or tissue destruction is called inflimmation. _____

1.43. A fisure of the skin is a groove or crack-like sore. _____

1.44. The medical term meaning the surgical repair of a nerve is neuriplasty. _____

1.45. The medical term meaning inflammation of the tonsils is tonsilitis. _____

● Matching Terms

Write the correct answer in the middle column.

Definition	Correct Answer	Possible Answers
1.46. abnormal stomach condition	_____	cardiac
1.47. pertaining to the heart	_____	gastralgia
1.48. rupture of a muscle	_____	gastrosis
1.49. stomach pain	_____	myoplasty
1.50. surgical muscle repair	_____	myorrhexis

● Term Selection

Select the correct answer and write it on the line provided.

1.51   The abnormal narrowing of an artery or arteries is called _____ .

     arteriosclerosis   arteriostenosis   arthrostenosis   atherosclerosis

1.52   Based on the word part that indicates color, the term _____ means blue coloration

       of the skin that is caused by the lack of oxygen in the blood.

     cyanosis   erythrocytes   leukocytes   melanosis

1.53.   The term _____ contains a combining vowel between two word roots.

     abdominocentesis   endoscopy   gastroenteritis   hemorrhage

1.54.   The prefix _____ means bad, difficult, or painful.

     -algia   -dynia   dys-   eu-

1.55.   A _____ is a specialist in diagnosing and treating diseases, disorders, and problems

       associated with aging.

     gerontologist   gerontology   neurologist   neurology

● Sentence Completion

Write the correct term on the line provided.

1.56.   Lower than normal blood pressure is called _____ .

1.57.   The process of recording a picture of an artery or arteries is called _____ .

1.58.   The term meaning above or outside the ribs is _____ .

1.59.   A strong dependence on a drug or substance is known as a/an _____ .

1.60.   An abnormal passage, usually between two internal organs, or leading from an organ to the surface of

       the body, is a/an _____ .

● Word Surgery

Divide each term into its component word parts. Write these word parts, in sequence, on the lines provided.

When necessary use a back slash (/) to indicate a combining vowel. (You may not need all of the lines provided.)

1.61.   **Arteriomalacia** is the abnormal softening of an artery.

_____   _____   _____   _____

1.62.   **Otorhinolaryngology** is the study of the ears, nose, and throat.

_____   _____   _____   _____

1.63.   The term **mycosis** means any disease caused by a fungus.

_____   _____   _____   _____

1.64.   The term **postnatal** describes the time and events after birth.

_____   _____   _____   _____

1.65.   A **tonsillectomy** is the surgical removal of the tonsils.

_____   _____   _____   _____

1.66.   The term **gastroenteritis** means inflammation of the stomach and small intestine.

_____   _____   _____   _____

1.67.   The term **rhinorrhea** means an excessive flow of mucus from the nose. It is also known as a runny nose.

_____   _____   _____   _____

1.68.   A **neonatologist** is a specialist in diagnosing and treating disorders of the newborn.

_____   _____   _____   _____

1.69.   The term **abdominocentesis** means the surgical puncture of the abdominal cavity to remove fluid.

_____   _____   _____   _____

1.70.   The term **appendicitis** means inflammation of the appendix.

_____   _____   _____   _____

- **Clinical Conditions**

Write the correct answer on the line provided.

1.71.   Beverly Gaston suffers from higher than normal blood pressure. This is recorded on her chart as

      _____ .

1.72.   Mrs. Tillson underwent _____ to remove excess fluid from her abdomen.

1.73.   Dr. Gusterson is trained in the treatment of the diseases and disorders associated with aging. His specialty

      is known as _____ .

1.74.   In an accident, Felipe Valladares suffered a broken toe. The medical term for this is a fractured

      _____ .

1.75.   Hal Jamison received emergency treatment for _____ , which is an inflammation

      of the appendix.

1.76.   Gina's physician explained that she had a/an _____ complication. This means that

      there was a problem pertaining to the interior or lining of an artery.

1.77.   Jennifer was interested in _____ . This is the study of disorders of the newborn.

1.78.   Joan Randolph's medication was administered by an injection into the muscle. This is called an

      _____ or IM injection.

1.79.   Andy Lewis describes that uncomfortable feeling as heartburn. The medical term for this condition is

      _____ .

1.80.   Max Greene's muscle wound required suturing. This procedure is called _____ .

- **Which Is the Correct Medical Term?**

Select the correct answer and write it on the line provided.

1.81.   The term _____ means an inflammation of a nerve or nerves.

      neuralgia   neuritis   neurology   neuroplasty

1.82.   The term _____ means loss of a large amount of blood in a short time.

      diarrhea   hemorrhage   hepatorrhagia   otorrhagia

1.83.   The term _____ means the tissue death of an artery or arteries.

   arteriomalacia   arterionecrosis   arteriosclerosis   arteriostenosis

1.84.   The term _____ describes the time and events before birth.

   neonatal   perinatal   postnatal   prenatal

1.85.   The term _____ means enlargement of the liver.

   hepatitis   hepatomegaly   nephromegaly   nephritis

● Challenge Word Building

These terms are *not* found in this chapter; however, they are made up of the following word parts. You may want

to look in the textbook glossary or use a medical dictionary to check your answers.

neo- = new	**arteri/o** = artery	**-algia** = pain and suffering
	arthr/o = joint	**-itis** = inflammation
	cardi/o = heart	**-ologist** = specialist
	nat/o = birth	**-otomy** = a surgical incision
	neur/o = nerve	**-rrhea** = flow or discharge
	rhin/o = nose	**-scopy** = visual examination

1.86.   A medical specialist concerned with the diagnosis and treatment of heart disease is a/an

   _____ .

1.87.   The term meaning a runny nose is _____ .

1.88.   The term meaning the inflammation of a joint is _____.

1.89.   A specialist in disorders of the newborn is called a/an _____ .

1.90.   The term meaning a surgical incision into a nerve is a/an _____.

1.91.   The term meaning the visual examination of the internal structure of a joint is _____ .

1.92.   The term meaning an inflammation of an artery is _____.

1.93.   The term meaning pain in a nerve or nerves is _____.

1.94.   The term meaning a surgical incision into the heart is a/an _____ .

1.95.   The term meaning an inflammation of the nose is _____.

● Labeling Exercises

Identify the numbered items in the accompanying figure.

1.96.   The combining form meaning spinal cord is

_____/ ___ .

1.97.   The combining form meaning muscle is

_____/ ___ .

1.98.   The combining form meaning bone marrow is

_____/ ___ .

1.99.   The combining form meaning nerve is

_____/ ___ .

1.100. The combining form meaning joint is

_____/ ___ .

Spinal cord
1.96

Muscle
1.97

Bone
marrow
1.98

Nerve 1.99

Joint 1.100

THE HUMAN TOUCH: CRITICAL THINKING EXERCISE

The following story and questions are designed to stimulate critical thinking through class discussion or as a brief essay response. There are right or wrong answers to these questions.

Baylie Hutchins sits at her kitchen table with her medical terminology book opened to the first chapter, highlighter in hand. Her two-year-old son, Mathias, plays with a box of Animal Crackers in his highchair, some even finding his mouth. "Arteri/o, ather/o, and arthr/o," she mutters, lips moving to shape unfamiliar sounds. "They're too much alike and they mean totally different things." Mathias sneezes loudly, and spots of Animal Cracker rain on the page, punctuating her frustration.

"Great job, Thias," she says wiping the text with her finger. "I planned on using the highlighter to mark with, not your lunch." Mathias giggles and peaks through the tunnel made by one small hand.

"Mucous and mucus," she reads aloud, each sounding the same. Then she remembers her teacher's tip for remembering the difference, "The long word's the membrane and the short one's the secretion."

Mathias picks up an Animal Cracker and excitedly shouts "Tiger, Mommy! Tiger!" "That's right, Thias. Good job!"

Turning back to the page she stares at the red words -rrhagia, -rrhaphy, -rrhea, and -rrhexis. Stumbling over the pronunciation, Baylie closes her eyes and tries to silence the voices in her head. "You can't do anything right," her ex-husband says. "Couldn't finish if your life depended on it," her mother's voice snaps.

Baylie keeps at it. "Rhin/o means nose," highlighting those three words, "and a rhinoceros has a big horn on his nose."

"Rhino!" Matthias shouts, holding up an Animal Cracker. Baylie laughs. We both have new things to learn, she realizes. And we can do it!

Suggested Discussion Topics:

1. Baylie needs to learn medical terminology if she wants a career in the medical field. What study habits would help Baylie accomplish this task?

2. A support group could help empower Baylie to accomplish her goals. What people would you suggest for this group and why?

3. How can this textbook and other resource materials help her (and you) learn medical terminology?

4. Discuss strategies the instructor could use, and has already used, to help Baylie improve her terminology skills.

5. Discuss how previous educational or learning experiences influence a student's approach to learning a new skill or subject.

2 The Human Body in Health and Disease

● Overview of the Human Body in Health and Disease

Anatomic Reference Systems	Terms used to describe the location of body planes, directions, and cavities.
Major Body Cavities	The spaces within the body that contain and protect the internal organs.
Cytology	The study of the structures of cells, chromosomes, DNA, and genetics.
Genetics	The study of how genes are transferred from the parents to their children and the role of genes in health and disease.
Congenital Disorders	Abnormal condition that exists at the time of birth.
Histology	The study of the tissues, which are composed of cells that join together to perform specific functions.
Glands	Specialized cells that secrete material used elsewhere in the body.
Organs and Body Systems	Body parts organized into systems according to function.
Pathology	The study of structural and functional changes caused by disease.

● VOCABULARY   RELATED TO THE HUMAN BODY IN HEALTH AND DISEASE

The items on this list have been identified as key word parts and terms for this chapter. However, all words in boldface in the text are also important and may be included in learning exercises and tests.

Word Parts

- ☐ -ac
- ☐ aden/o
- ☐ adip/o
- ☐ cephal/o
- ☐ coron/o
- ☐ cyt/o
- ☐ endo-
- ☐ exo-
- ☐ hist/o
- ☐ -malacia
- ☐ -ologist
- ☐ -ology
- ☐ -oma
- ☐ path/o
- ☐ -plasia

Medical Terms

- ☐ **abdominal cavity** (ab-**DOM**-ih-nal)
- ☐ **abdominopelvic cavity** (ab-**dom**-ih-noh-**PEL**-vick)
- ☐ **adenectomy** (ad-eh-**NECK**-toh-mee)
- ☐ **adenoma** (ad-eh-**NOH**-mah)
- ☐ **adenomalacia** (ad-eh-noh-mah-**LAY**-shee-ah)
- ☐ **adenosclerosis** (ad-eh-noh-skleh-**ROH**-sis)
- ☐ **adipose tissue** (**AD**-ih-pohs)
- ☐ **anaplasia** (an-ah-**PLAY**-zee-ah)
- ☐ **anomaly** (ah-**NOM**-ah-lee)
- ☐ **anterior** (an-**TEER**-ee-or)
- ☐ **aplasia** (ah-**PLAY**-zee-ah)
- ☐ **caudal** (**KAW**-dal)
- ☐ **cephalic** (seh-**FAL**-ick)
- ☐ **communicable disease** (kuh-**MEW**-nih-kuh-bul)
- ☐ **congenital disorder** (kon-**JEN**-ih-tahl)
- ☐ **coronal** (koh-**ROH**-nal)
- ☐ **cytoplasm** (**SIGH**-toh-plazm)
- ☐ **deoxyribonucleic** (dee-**ock**-see-**rye**-boh-new-**KLEE**-ick)

- ☐ **distal** (**DIS**-tal)
- ☐ **dorsal** (**DOR**-sal)
- ☐ **dysplasia** (dis-**PLAY**-see-ah)
- ☐ **endemic** (en-**DEM**-ick)
- ☐ **endocrine glands** (**EN**-doh-krin)
- ☐ **epidemic** (ep-ih-**DEM**-ick)
- ☐ **epigastric region** (ep-ih-**GAS**-trick)
- ☐ **epithelial tissue** (ep-ih-**THEE**-lee-al)
- ☐ **etiology** (ee-tee-**OL**-oh-jee)
- ☐ **exocrine glands** (**ECK**-soh-krin)
- ☐ **genome** (**JEE**-nohm)
- ☐ **hemophilia** (hee-moh-**FILL**-ee-ah)
- ☐ **histology** (hiss-**TOL**-oh-jee)
- ☐ **homeostasis** (hoh-mee-oh-**STAY**-sis)
- ☐ **hyperplasia** (high-per-**PLAY**-zee-ah)
- ☐ **hypertrophy** (high-**PER**-troh-fee)
- ☐ **hypochondriac** regions (**high**-poh-**KON**-dree-ack)
- ☐ **hypogastric region** (**high**-poh-**GAS**-trick)
- ☐ **hypoplasia** (**high**-poh-**PLAY**-zee-ah)
- ☐ **iatrogenic illness** (eye-**at**-roh-**JEN**-ick)
- ☐ **idiopathic disease** (id-ee-oh-**PATH**-ick)
- ☐ **iliac regions** (**ILL**-ee-ack)
- ☐ **infectious disease** (in-**FECK**-shus)
- ☐ **inguinal** (**ING**-gwih-nal)
- ☐ **lumbar regions** (**LUM**-bar)
- ☐ **mesentery** (**MESS**-en-**terr**-ee)
- ☐ **midsagittal plane** (mid-**SADJ**-ih-tal)
- ☐ **nosocomial infection** (nos-oh-**KOH**-mee-al)
- ☐ **nucleus** (**NEW**-klee-us)
- ☐ **pandemic** (pan-**DEM**-ick)
- ☐ **pathology** (pah-**THOL**-oh-jee)
- ☐ **pelvic cavity** (**PEL**-vick)
- ☐ **peritoneum** (pehr-ih-toh-**NEE**-um)
- ☐ **peritonitis** (pehr-ih-toh-**NIGH**-tis)
- ☐ **phenylketonuria** (fen-il-**kee**-toh-**NEW**-ree-ah)
- ☐ **physiology** (fiz-ee-**OL**-oh-jee)
- ☐ **posterior** (pos-**TEER**-ee-or)
- ☐ **proximal** (**PROCK**-sih-mal)
- ☐ **retroperitoneal** (ret-roh-**pehr**-ih-toh-**NEE**-al)
- ☐ **thoracic cavity** (thoh-**RAS**-ick)
- ☐ **transverse plane** (trans-**VERSE**)
- ☐ **ventral** (**VEN**-tral)

On completion of this chapter, you should be able to:

1. Define anatomy and physiology and use anatomic reference systems to identify the anatomic position, body planes, directions, and cavities.

2. Recognize, define, spell, and pronounce the terms related to the abdominal cavity and peritoneum.

3. Recognize, define, spell, and pronounce the terms related to the structure, function, pathology, and procedures of cells, tissues, and glands.

4. Define the terms associated with cytology and genetics including chromosomes, genes, DNA, and mutation.

5. Differentiate between genetic and congenital disorders and identify examples of each.

6. Identify the body systems in terms of their major structures and functions.

7. Recognize, define, spell, and pronounce the terms related to types of diseases and the modes of disease transmission.

ANATOMIC REFERENCE SYSTEMS

Anatomic reference systems are used to describe the location and function of body parts.

The simplest anatomic reference is the one we learn in childhood: our right hand is on the right, and our left hand on the left. In medical terminology, there are several additional ways to describe the location of different body parts. These anatomical reference systems include:

- Body planes
- Body directions
- Body cavities
- Structural units

Body parts can also be defined by their physiology, or function. Organs and tissues are grouped together into systems, such as the respiratory or circulatory system, because they work together to perform a single function.

Anatomy and Physiology Defined

- **Anatomy** (ah-**NAT**-oh-mee) is the study of the structures of the body.
- **Physiology** (**fiz**-ee-**OL**-oh-jee) is the study of the functions of these structures.

The Anatomic Position

Descriptions of the body are based on the assumption that a person is standing in the standard **anatomic position**. In this position, the individual is:

- Standing up so that the body is erect
- Facing forward
- Holding the arms at the sides
- Turning the hands with the palms toward the front

Body Planes

Body planes are imaginary vertical and horizontal lines that are used to divide the body in the anatomic position into sections for descriptive purposes.

Vertical Planes

A **vertical plane** is any up-and-down line that is at a right angle, in other words perpendicular, to the horizon. Compare with *horizontal planes*.

- A **sagittal plane** (**SADJ**-ih-tal) is any vertical plane that divides the whole body into unequal left and right portions.
- The **midsagittal plane** (mid-**SADJ**-ih-tal), also known as the **midline**, is a sagittal plane that divides the body, from top to bottom, into equal left and right halves (Figures 2.1 through 2.4).

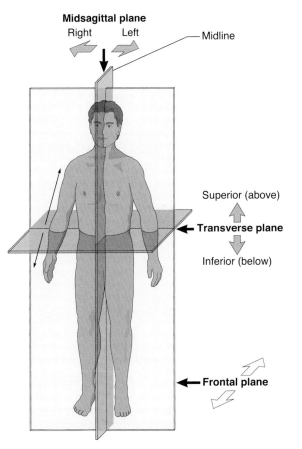

FIGURE 2.1   Body planes.

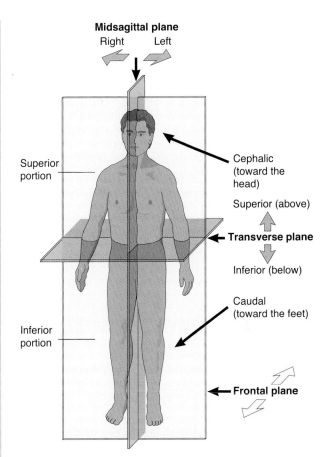

FIGURE 2.2   A transverse plane divides the body into superior and inferior portions. This division can be at the waist or at any other level across the body.

- A **coronal plane** (koh-**ROH**-nal) divides the body into anterior and posterior portions (**coron** means head or crown and **-al** means pertaining to). Also known as the **frontal plane,** this is any vertical plane located at right angles to the sagittal plane.

Horizontal Planes

A **horizontal plane** is a flat crosswise line like the horizon. Compare with *vertical planes.*

- The **transverse plane** (trans-**VERSE**) is the horizontal plane that divides the whole body into superior (upper) and inferior (lower) portions (Figures 2.1 and 2.2). The transverse plane can be at the waist level or at any other level across the body.

Body Directions

The relative location of sections of the body or of an organ can be described through the use of pairs of contrasting, or opposite, body direction terms. These terms are summarized in Table 2.1 and are illustrated in Figures 2.1 through 2.4.

MAJOR BODY CAVITIES

A **body cavity** is a space within the body that contains and protects the internal organs (Figure 2.5).

The Dorsal Cavity

The dorsal cavity, located in the skull and within the spinal column, is divided into two parts. *Dorsal* means pertaining to the back. They both protect the structures of the nervous system:

- The **cranial cavity**, which is located within the skull, protects the brain.
- The **spinal cavity**, which is located within the spinal column, protects the spinal cord.

The Ventral Cavity

The ventral cavity is located in the front of the body. It is divided into three parts, and contains many of the

Table 2.1

TERMS USED TO DESCRIBE OPPOSITE BODY DIRECTIONS

Ventral (**VEN**-tral) refers to the front or belly side of the body or organ (ventr means belly side of the body and -al means pertaining to).	**Dorsal** (**DOR**-sal) refers to the back of the body or organ (dors means back of the body and -al means pertaining to).
Anterior (an-**TEER**-ee-or) means situated in the front. It also means on the forward part of an organ (anter means front or before and -ior means pertaining to). For example, the stomach is located anterior to (in front of) the pancreas. *Anterior* is also used in reference to the ventral surface of the body.	**Posterior** (pos-**TEER**-ee-or) means situated in the back. It also means on the back part of an organ (poster means back or after and -ior means pertaining to). For example, the pancreas is located posterior to (behind) the stomach. *Posterior* is also used in reference to the dorsal surface of the body.
Superior means uppermost, above, or toward the head. For example, the lungs are located superior to (above) the diaphragm.	**Inferior** means lowermost, below, or toward the feet. For example, the stomach is located inferior to (below) the diaphragm.
Cephalic (seh-**FAL**-ick) means toward the head (cephal means head and -ic means pertaining to).	**Caudal** (**KAW**-dal) means toward the lower part of the body (caud means tail or lower part of the body and -al means pertaining to).
Proximal (**PROCK**-sih-mal) means situated nearest the midline or beginning of a body structure. For example, the proximal end of the humerus (the bone of the upper arm) forms part of the shoulder.	**Distal** (**DIS**-tal) means situated farthest from the midline or beginning of a body structure. For example, the distal end of the humerus forms part of the elbow (Figure 2.4).
Medial means the direction toward or nearer the midline. For example, the medial ligament of the knee is near the inner surface of the leg (Figure 2.4).	**Lateral** means the direction toward or nearer the side and away from the midline. For example, the lateral ligament of the knee is near the side of the leg. **Bilateral** means relating to, or having, two sides.

body organs that maintain homeostasis. **Homeostasis** (**hoh**-mee-oh-**STAY**-sis) means maintaining a constant internal environment (**home/o** means constant and **-stasis** means control).

- The **thoracic cavity** (thoh-**RAS**-ick), also known as the **chest cavity** or **thorax**, protects the heart and the lungs. The **diaphragm** is a muscle that separates the thoracic and abdominal cavities.

- The **abdominal cavity** (ab-**DOM**-ih-nal), which contains primarily the major organs of digestion, is frequently referred to simply as the **abdomen** (ab-**DOH**-men *or* **AB**-doh-men). Note that abdomen is spelled -*e*n, but the adjective abdominal is spelled -*i*nal

- The **pelvic cavity** (**PEL**-vick) is the space formed by the pelvic (hip) bones. It contains primarily the organs of the reproductive and excretory systems.

- There is no physical division between the abdominal and pelvic cavities. Together, they are referred to as the **abdominopelvic** (ab-**dom**-ih-noh-**PEL**-vick) **cavity** (**abdomin/o** means abdomen, **pelv**, means pelvis, and **-ic** means pertaining to).

Quadrants of the Abdomen

Describing where an abdominal organ or pain is located is made easier by dividing the abdomen into four imaginary quadrants (Figure 2.6). The term **quadrant** means divided into four. These quadrants are the:

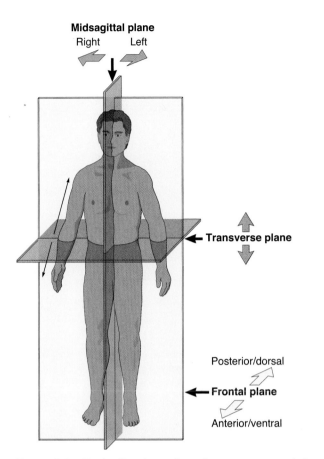

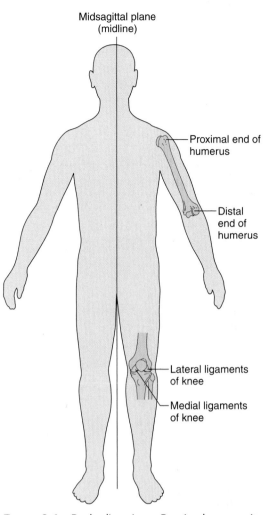

FIGURE 2.3 Body directions. *Anterior* means toward the front, and the front of the body is called the *ventral surface. Posterior* means toward the back, and the back of the body is called the *dorsal surface.*

1. Right upper quadrant (RUQ)
2. Left upper quadrant (LUQ)
3. Right lower quadrant (RLQ)
4. Left lower quadrant (LLQ)

Regions of the Thorax and Abdomen

Another descriptive system divides the abdomen and lower portion of the thorax into nine regions (Figure 2.7). These regions are:

- The **right and left hypochondriac regions** (**high-poh-KON**-dree-ack) are located on the sides and are covered by the lower ribs. As used here, *hypochondriac* means below the ribs (**hypo-** means below and **chondr/i** means cartilage and **-ac** means pertaining to). This term also means an individual with an abnormal concern about his or her health because, according to ancient lore, this region below the ribs was the seat of hypochondria.

FIGURE 2.4 Body directions. *Proximal* means situated nearest the midline, and *distal* means situated farthest from the midline. *Medial* means toward the midline, and *lateral* means toward the side.

- The **epigastric region** (**ep**-ih-**GAS**-trick) is located above the stomach.
- The **right and left lumbar regions** (**LUM**-bar) are located on the sides near the inward curve of the spine.
- The **umbilical region** (um-**BILL**-ih-kal) surrounds the **umbilicus** (um-**BILL**-ih-kus). Also known as the **belly button** or **navel**, this pit in the center of the abdominal wall marks the point where the umbilical cord was attached to the fetus.
- The **right and left iliac regions** (**ILL**-ee-ack) are located on the sides over the hipbones.
- The **hypogastric** (**high**-poh-**GAS**-trick) **region** is located below the stomach. The term **inguinal** (**ING**-gwih-nal), which means pertaining to the **groin**, refers to entire lower portion of the abdomen.

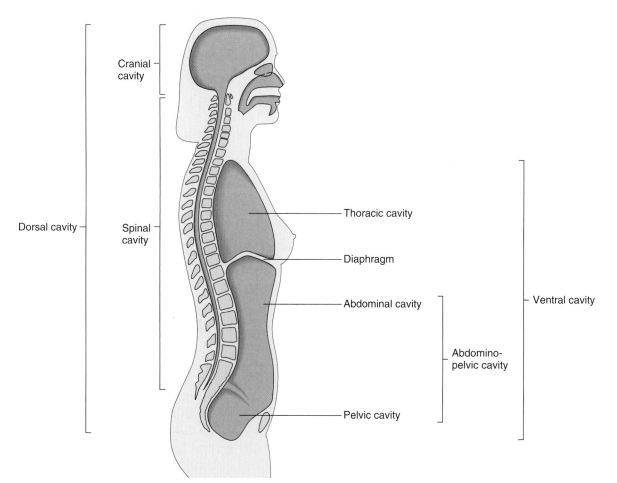

FIGURE 2.5 Major body cavities.

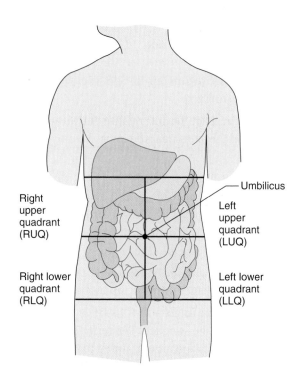

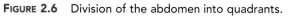

FIGURE 2.6 Division of the abdomen into quadrants.

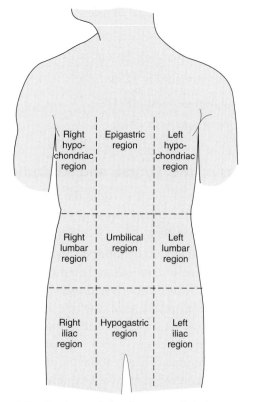

FIGURE 2.7 Regions of the thorax and abdomen.

Peritoneum

The **peritoneum** (**pehr**-ih-toh-**NEE**-um) is a multilayered membrane that protects and holds the organs in place within the abdominal cavity. A *membrane* is a thin layer of tissue that covers a surface, lines a cavity, or divides a space or organ.

- The *parietal peritoneum* (pah-**RYE**-eh-tal **pehr**-ih-toh-**NEE**-um) is the outer layer of the peritoneum, and it lines the abdominal wall. *Parietal* means cavity wall.

- The *visceral peritoneum* (**VIS**-er-al **pehr**-ih-toh-**NEE**-um) is the inner layer of the peritoneum, and it surrounds the organs of the abdominal cavity. *Visceral* means relating to the internal organs.

- The **mesentery** (**MESS**-en-**terr**-ee) is a fused double layer of the parietal peritoneum that attaches parts of the intestine to the interior abdominal wall.

- The term **retroperitoneal** (**ret**-roh-**pehr**-ih-toh-**NEE**-al) means located behind the peritoneum (**retro-** means behind, **periton** means peritoneum, and **-eal** means pertaining to).

- **Peritonitis** (**pehr**-ih-toh-**NIGH**-tis) is inflammation of the peritoneum (**periton** means peritoneum and **-itis** means inflammation).

CELLS: THE BODY'S BASIC UNIT

- **Cytology** (sigh-**TOL**-oh-jee) is the study of the formation, structure, and function of cells (**cyt** means cell and **-ology** means study of).

- Cells, which are the basic structural units of the body, are specialized and grouped together to form tissues and organs.

- When each of these cells divides, it produces an exact replica of itself. The exceptions to this rule are gametes, which are discussed under chromosomes, and stem cells.

Stem Cells

Stem cells differ from other kinds of cells in the body because of two characteristics properties:

1. Stem cells are unspecialized cells that renew themselves for long periods through cell division.

2. Under certain conditions stem cells can be induced to become cells with special functions, such as the beating cells of the heart muscle or the insulin-producing cells of the pancreas.

Stem cells are used for bone marrow transplants in the treatment of leukemia. Researchers hope they will soon become the basis for newer treatments for diseases such as diabetes, Parkinson's, and heart disease.

Sources of Stem Cells

Stem cells come from three sources: (1) a newly formed embryo, where they specialize to make all types of cells needed to form a fully developed human being; (2) the cord blood that can be harvested from the discarded umbilical cord and placenta of a newborn; and (3) in adult tissues, such as bone marrow, muscle, and the brain, where specialized populations of adult stem cells generate replacements for cells that are lost through normal wear and tear, injury, or disease.

The Structure of Cells

- The **cell membrane** (**MEM**-brain) surrounds and protects the cell by separating the cell's contents from its external environment (Figure 2.8).

- **Cytoplasm** (**SIGH**-toh-plazm) is the material within the cell membrane that is *not* part of the nucleus (**cyt/o** means cell and **-plasm** means formative material of cells).

- The **nucleus** (**NEW**-klee-us) (plural, **nuclei**), which is surrounded by the nuclear membrane, is a structure within the cell that has two important functions: (1) it controls the activities of the cell and (2) it helps the cell divide.

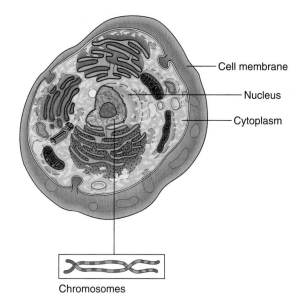

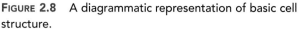

Chromosomes

FIGURE 2.8 A diagrammatic representation of basic cell structure.

Chromosomes

Chromosomes (**KROH**-moh-sohmes), which are one type of structure found in the cell nucleus, are the bearers of genes.

- Each **gene** is a functional unit of heredity. Genes control hereditary disorders and all physical traits such as hair, skin, and eye color.

- The nucleus of a **somatic cell** contains 46 chromosomes arranged into 23 pairs. *Somatic* means pertaining to the body in general. There are 22 identical pairs of chromosomes, plus an XX or XY pair that determines the sex of the individual. In a normal female, this is an XX chromosome pair. In a normal male, this is an XY chromosome pair.

- **Sex cells** (sperm and eggs), also known as **gametes** (**GAM**-eets), are the only cells that do not have 46 chromosomes. Instead, each mature sex cell has 23 single chromosomes. The female produces eggs with only X chromosomes. Males produce sperm with either an X or Y chromosome. When a sperm and ovum join to form a new life, the embryo receives half of its chromosomes from each parent.

GENETICS

Genetics is the study of how genes are transferred from the parents to their children and the role of genes in health and disease (**gene** means producing and **-tics** means pertaining to). A specialist in this field is known as a **geneticist** (jeh-**NET**-ih-sist).

- **DNA (deoxyribonucleic acid)** (dee-**ock**-see-**rye**-boh-new-**KLEE**-ick), which is the primary genetic material of all cellular organisms, is packaged in a chromosome as two strands. The strands twist together to make a *double helix*.

- A single gene makes up each segment of DNA and each gene is located in a specific site on the chromosome.

- A **genome** (**JEE**-nohm) is an entire set of genes derived from one parent. There are an estimated 30,000 or more genes on all the chromosomes in the body.

- A **clone** is an individual produced with genetic material from only one parent and is therefore an identical genetic replica of that parent.

Genetic Mutation

The term **genetic mutation** describes changes that occur within genes.

- **Somatic cell mutation** is change within the cells of the body. These changes affect the individual but cannot be transmitted to the next generation.

- **Gametic cell mutation** is change within the genes found in the gametes (sperm or ovum) that can be transmitted by parents to their children.

Dominant and Recessive Genes

- When a **dominant gene** is inherited from one parent, that offspring *will* have that genetic condition. A genetic condition, which is caused by a dominant gene, can be a physical trait (such as freckles) or a hereditary disorder (such as Huntington's disease).

- When a **recessive gene** for a genetic condition is inherited from one parent, and a normal gene is inherited from the other parent, that offspring *will not* have the condition. However, that child will carry the "trait" and can transmit that gene to his or her offspring.

- When the **recessive gene** for a genetic condition is inherited from both parents, this offspring *will have* that condition. For example, sickle cell anemia is transmitted by a recessive gene; Figure 2.9 illustrates the genetic probabilities of transmitting this condition.

Genetic Disorders

Genetic disorders, also known as **hereditary disorders**, are diseases or conditions caused by a defective gene. Although these genes are transmitted from the parents, a genetic disorder may be manifested at any time in life. The following are examples of these disorders.

- **Cystic fibrosis**, which is discussed in Chapter 7, is a genetic disorder that affects both the respiratory and digestive systems.

- **Down syndrome**, also known as **trisomy 21**, is a genetic syndrome characterized by varying degrees of mental retardation and multiple physical abnormalities. *Note:* Down's syndrome is an alternate spelling; however, Down syndrome, without the apostrophe and the *s*, is the preferred spelling.

- **Hemophilia** (hee-moh-**FILL**-ee-ah) is a group of hereditary bleeding disorders in which one of the factors needed to clot the blood is missing. Genetic transmission is usually from mother to son.

- **Huntington's disease**, also known as **Huntington's chorea**, is a hereditary disorder transmitted by a dominant gene, which means it can be passed on

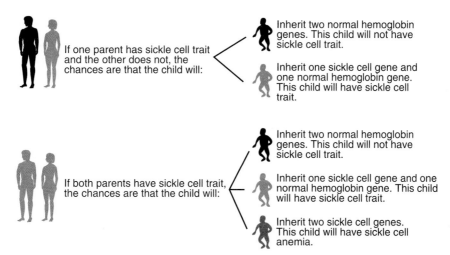

FIGURE 2.9   The genetic probabilities that parents with sickle cell trait will transmit sickle cell anemia to their children.

by just one parent. Symptoms first appear in midlife and cause the irreversible and progressive loss of muscle control and mental ability.

- **Muscular dystrophy** (**DIS**-troh-fee) is a group of genetic diseases characterized by progressive weakness of muscle fibers (see Chapter 4).

- **Phenylketonuria** (**fen**-il-**kee**-toh-**NEW**-ree-ah) is a genetic disorder in which an essential digestive enzyme is missing. PKU can be detected by the blood test given to all infants at birth. If not detected and treated early, PKU causes severe mental retardation.

- **Sickle cell anemia**, which is discussed in Chapter 5, is a group of inherited red blood cell disorders.

- **Tay-Sachs disease** is a hereditary disease in which a missing enzyme in the brain causes progressive physical degeneration, mental retardation, and early death.

CONGENITAL DISORDERS

A **congenital disorder** (kon-**JEN**-ih-tahl) is an abnormal condition that exists at the time of birth. This condition may be caused by a developmental disorder before birth, prenatal influences, premature birth, or injuries during birth.

- A *developmental disorder* may result in an anomaly or malformation such as the absence of a limb or the presence of an extra toe at birth. An **anomaly** (ah-**NOM**-ah-lee) is a deviation from what is regarded as normal.

- *Prenatal influences* are the mother's health and the care she receives before delivery. For example, maternal alcohol consumption during pregnancy can cause *fetal alcohol syndrome*, which is charac-

terized by physical and behavior traits including growth deficiencies and abnormalities, mental retardation, brain damage, and socialization difficulties.

- *Birth injuries* are congenital disorders that were not present before the events surrounding the time of birth. For example, *cerebral palsy,* which is discussed in Chapter 10, may be caused by premature birth or inadequate oxygen to the brain during birth.

TISSUE: CELLS WORKING TOGETHER

A tissue is a group or layer of similarly specialized cells that join together to perform certain specific functions.

- **Histology** (hiss-**TOL**-oh-jee) is the study of the structure, composition, and function of tissues (**hist** means tissue and **-ology** means a study of).

- A **histologist** (hiss-**TOL**-oh-jist) is a specialist in the study the organization of tissues at all levels (**hist** means tissue and **-ologist** means specialist).

Types of Tissue

The four main types of tissue are epithelial, connective, muscle, and nerve.

Epithelial Tissues

- **Epithelial tissues** (ep-ih-**THEE**-lee-al) form a protective covering for all of the internal and external surfaces of the body.

- **Epithelium** (ep-ih-**THEE**-lee-um) is the specialized epithelial tissue that forms the epidermis of the skin and the surface layer of mucous membranes. The skin is discussed in Chapter 12.

- **Endothelium** (en-doh-THEE-lee-um) is the specialized epithelial tissue that lines the blood and lymph vessels, body cavities, glands, and organs.

Glands are made up of specialized epithelial tissues that are capable of producing secretions.

Connective Tissues

- **Connective tissues** support and connect organs and other body tissues.

Bone, cartilage, and other **dense connective tissues** are discussed in Chapter 3.

- **Adipose tissue** (AD-ih-pohs), also known as **fat,** provides protective padding, insulation, and support, and acts as a nutrient reserve (**adip** means fat and **-ose** means pertaining to).

- **Loose connective tissue** surrounds various organs and supports both nerve cells and blood vessels.

- Blood and lymph, which are discussed in Chapters 5 and 6, are **liquid connective tissues.**

Muscle Tissue

Muscle tissue, which is discussed in Chapter 4, contains cells with the specialized ability to contract and relax.

Nerve Tissue

Nerve tissue, which is discussed in Chapter 10, contains cells with the specialized ability to react to stimuli and to conduct electrical impulses.

Pathology of Tissue Formation

- **Anaplasia** (an-ah-**PLAY**-zee-ah) is a change in the structure of cells and in their orientation to each other (**ana-** means excessive and **-plasia** means formation). These abnormal cells are characteristic of malignancies, which are discussed in Chapter 6.

- **Aplasia** (ah-**PLAY**-zee-ah) is the defective development, or the congenital absence, of an organ or tissue (**a-** means without and **-plasia** means formation).

- **Dysplasia** (dis-**PLAY**-see-ah) is abnormal tissue development (**dys-** means bad and **-plasia** means formation) (Figure 2.10B).

- **Hyperplasia** (high-per-**PLAY**-zee-ah) is the enlargement of an organ or tissue because of an abnormal increase in the number of cells (**hyper-** means excessive and **-plasia** means formation) (Figure 2.10C). Compare with *hypertrophy.*

- **Hypertrophy** (high-**PER**-troh-fee) is a general increase in the bulk of a part or organ, not due to tumor formation (**hyper-** means excessive and **-trophy** means development). This enlargement is due to an increase in the size, but not in the number, of cells in the tissues. Compare with *hyperplasia.*

- **Hypoplasia** (high-poh-**PLAY**-zee-ah) is the incomplete development of an organ or tissue (**hypo-** means deficient and **-plasia** means formation).

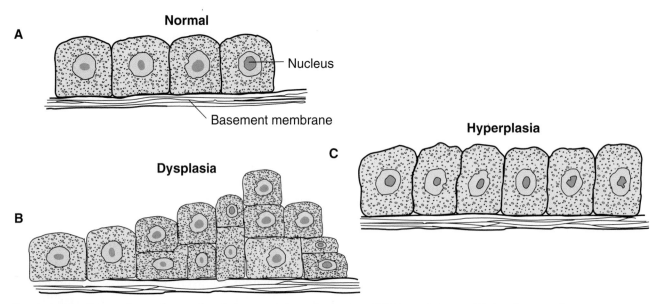

FIGURE 2.10 Comparison of normal and abnormal tissue formation. (A) Normal tissue, (B) dysplasia, and (C) hyperplasia.

GLANDS

A **gland** is a group of specialized epithelial cells that form secretions. A *secretion* is the substance produced by a gland. The two types of glands are exocrine and endocrine glands (Figure 2.11).

- **Exocrine glands** (**ECK**-soh-krin), such as sweat glands, secrete their chemical substances into ducts that lead either to other organs or out of the body (**exo-** means out of and **-crine** means to secrete).

- **Endocrine glands** (**EN**-doh-krin), which secrete hormones, do not have ducts (**endo-** means within and **-crine** means to secrete). Endocrine secretions flow directly into the bloodstream for transportation to organs and other structures throughout the body. See Chapter 13.

Pathology and Procedures of the Glands

- **Adenectomy** (**ad**-eh-**NECK**-toh-mee) is the surgical removal of a gland (**aden** means gland and **-ectomy** means surgical removal).

- **Adenitis** (**ad**-eh-**NIGH**-tis) is the inflammation of a gland (**aden** means gland and **-itis** means inflammation).

- An **adenoma** (**ad**-eh-**NOH**-mah) is a benign tumor of glandular origin and structure (**aden** means

gland and **-oma** means tumor). *Benign* means not life threatening.

- **Adenomalacia** (**ad**-eh-noh-mah-**LAY**-shee-ah) is the abnormal softening of a gland (**aden/o** means gland and **-malacia** means abnormal softening). Compare with *adenosclerosis.*

- **Adenosclerosis** (**ad**-eh-noh-skleh-**ROH**-sis) is the abnormal hardening of a gland (**aden/o** means gland and **-sclerosis** means abnormal hardening). Compare with *adenomalacia.*

- **Adenosis** (**ad**-eh-**NOH**-sis) is any disease condition of a gland (**aden** means gland and **-osis** means an abnormal condition.)

ORGANS AND BODY SYSTEMS

An **organ** is a somewhat independent part of the body that performs a special function or functions.

The tissues and organs of the body are organized into systems that perform specialized functions (Figure 2.12). These systems, with major structures and functions, are outlined in Table 2.2.

PATHOLOGY

Pathology (pah-**THOL**-oh-jee) is the study of structural and functional changes caused by disease (**path/o** and **-pathy** mean disease; however, they also mean suffering, feeling, and emotion). Pathology also means a condition caused by disease.

- A **pathologist** (pah-**THOL**-oh-jist) specializes in the laboratory analysis of tissue samples to confirm or establish a diagnosis (**path** means disease and **-ologist** means specialist). These tissue specimens may be removed as biopsies, during operations, or postmortem examinations. *Postmortem* means after death and a postmortem examination is also known as an **autopsy** (**AW**-top-see).

- **Etiology** (ee-tee-**OL**-oh-jee) is the study of the causes of diseases (**eti-** means cause and **-ology** means study of). The organisms that cause diseases are discussed further in Chapter 6.

- Terms used to describe different types of diseases are summarized in Table 2.3.

Disease Transmission

- A **communicable disease** (kuh-**MEW**-nih-kuh-bul), also known as a **contagious disease**, is any disease

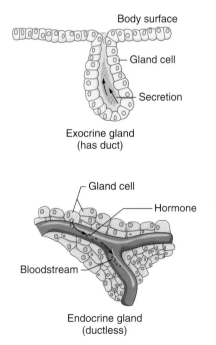

Body surface

Gland cell

Secretion

Exocrine gland
(has duct)

Gland cell

Hormone

Bloodstream

Endocrine gland
(ductless)

Figure 2.11   Exocrine glands secrete their chemical substances into ducts that lead either to other organs or out of the body. Endocrine glands pour their secretions directly into the bloodstream.

Table 2.2

MAJOR BODY SYSTEMS		
Body System	**Major Structures**	**Major Functions**
Skeletal System (Chapter 3)	bones joints cartilage	Supports and shapes the body. Protects the internal organs. Forms some blood cells and stores minerals.
Muscular System (Chapter 4)	muscles fascia tendons	Holds the body erect. Makes movement possible. Moves body fluids and generates body heat.
Cardiovascular System (Chapter 5)	heart arteries veins blood	Blood circulates throughout the body to transport oxygen and nutrients to cells, and to carry waste products to the kidneys where the waste is removed by filtration.
Lymphatic and Immune Systems (Chapter 6)	lymph, lymph vessels, and lymph nodes tonsils spleen thymus specialized blood cells	Protects the body from harmful substances. Brings oxygen and nutrients to cells. Removes waste from the cells.
Respiratory System (Chapter 7)	nose pharynx trachea larynx lungs	Brings oxygen into the body for transportation to the cells. Removes carbon dioxide and some water waste from the body.
Digestive System (Chapter 8)	mouth esophagus stomach small intestines large intestines liver pancreas	Digests ingested food so it can be absorbed into the bloodstream. Eliminates solid wastes.
Urinary System (Chapter 9)	kidneys ureters urinary bladder urethra	Filters blood to remove waste. Maintains the electrolyte and fluid balance within the body.
Nervous System (Chapter 10)	nerves brain spinal cord	Coordinates the reception of stimuli. Transmits messages throughout the body.
Special Senses (Chapter 11)	eyes ears	Receive visual and auditory information and transmit it to the brain.
Integumentary System (Chapter 12)	skin sebaceous glands sweat glands	Protects the body against invasion by bacteria. Regulates the body temperature and water content.

Table 2.2 (continued)

MAJOR BODY SYSTEMS

Body System	Major Structures	Major Functions
Endocrine System (Chapter 13)	adrenals gonads pancreas parathyroids thymus pineal pituitary thyroid	Integrates all body functions.
Reproductive Systems (Chapter 14)	**Male:** penis testicles **Female:** vagina ovaries uterus	Produces new life.

transmitted from one person to another either by direct contact or indirectly by contact with contaminated objects. *Contaminated* means a pathogen is possibly present. Contamination may occur through a lack of proper hygiene standards, such as handwashing, or by failure to take appropriate precautions.

- **Bloodborne transmission** is through contact with blood or body fluids that are contaminated with blood. Examples of bloodborne transmission are human immunodeficiency virus (HIV), hepatitis B, and most sexually transmitted diseases (STDs). These disorders are discussed in Chapters 6, 8, and 14.

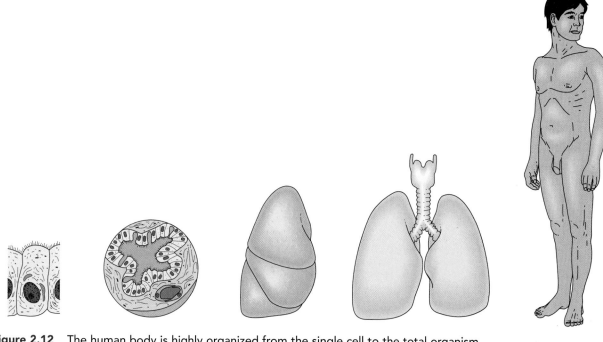

Figure 2.12   The human body is highly organized from the single cell to the total organism.

Table 2.3

TYPES OF DISEASES

An **infectious disease** (in-**FECK**-shus) is an illness caused by living pathogenic organisms such as a bacteria and viruses.	An **idiopathic disorder** (**id**-ee-oh-**PATH**-ick) is an illness without known cause (idi/o means peculiar to the individual, path means disease, and -ic means pertaining to).
In an **organic disorder** (or-**GAN**-ick), there are pathologic physical changes that explain the symptoms being experienced by the patient. For example, a gastric ulcer is an organic disorder (see Chapter 8).	In a **functional disorder** there are no detectable physical changes to explain the symptoms that are being experienced by the patient. For example, a panic attack is a functional disorder (see Chapter 10).
An **iatrogenic illness** (eye-**at**-roh-**JEN**-ick) is a problem, such as a side effect or an unfavorable response, arising from a prescribed treatment or medicine.	A **nosocomial infection** (nos-oh-**KOH**-mee-al) is an infection acquired in a hospital or clinic.

- **Airborne transmission** occurs through respiratory droplets such as contact with material from the cough or sneeze. Examples include tuberculosis, influenza, colds, and measles. These disorders are discussed in Chapter 7.

- **Foodborne and waterborne transmission,** also known as **fecal-oral transmission**, is caused by eating or drinking contaminated food or water that has not been prepared properly to kill the contamination. *Fecal-oral* refers to the transmission of bacteria from contaminated feces into the mouth due to unsanitary conditions. These disorders are discussed in Chapter 8.

Outbreaks of Diseases

- An **epidemiologist** (ep-ih-**dee**-mee-**OL**-oh-jist) specializes in the study of outbreaks of disease within a population group.

- **Endemic** (en-**DEM**-ick) refers to the ongoing presence of a disease within a population, group, or area. For example, the common cold is endemic because it is always present within the population.

- An **epidemic** (ep-ih-**DEM**-ick) is a sudden and widespread outbreak of a disease within a population group or area. For example, a sudden widespread outbreak of measles is an epidemic.

- **Pandemic** (pan-**DEM**-ick) refers to an outbreak of a disease occurring over a large geographic area, possibly worldwide. For example, AIDS is pandemic.

ABBREVIATIONS RELATED TO THE HUMAN BODY IN HEALTH AND DISEASE

Table 2.4 presents an overview of the abbreviations related to the terms introduced in this chapter. *Note:* To avoid errors or confusion, always be cautious when using abbreviations.

Table 2.4

ABBREVIATIONS RELATED TO THE HUMAN BODY IN HEALTH AND DISEASE

anterior = A	**A** = anterior
abdomen = Abd, Abdo	**Abd, Abdo** = abdomen
anatomy = anat	**anat** = anatomy
cephalic = CEPH	**CEPH** = cephalic
communicable disease = CD	**CD** = communicable disease
chromosome = CH, chr	**CH, chr** = chromosome
cystic fibrosis = CF	**CF** = cystic fibrosis
cytology, cytoplasm = cyt	**cyt** = cytology, cytoplasm
deoxyribonucleic acid = DNA	**DNA** = deoxyribonucleic acid
dorsal = D	**D** = dorsal
Down syndrome = DS	**DS** = Down syndrome
epidemic = epid	**epid** = epidemic
etiology = E	**E** = etiology
fetal alcohol syndrome = FAS	**FAS** = fetal alcohol syndrome
hemophilia = HEM, hemo	**HEM, hemo** = hemophilia
histology = HIS, Histo, histol	**HIS, Histo, histol** = histology
Huntington's disease = HD	**HD** = Huntington's disease
muscular dystrophy = MD	**MD** = muscular dystrophy
phenylketonuria = PKU	**PKU** = phenylketonuria
physiology, posterior = P	**P** = physiology, posterior
sickle cell anemia = SCA	**SCA** = sickle cell anemia
Tay-Sachs disease = TSD	**TSD** = Tay-Sachs disease
umbilical = umb	**umb** = umbilical
ventral = V, vent, ventr	**V, vent, ventr** = ventral

Learning Exercises

● Matching Word Parts 1

Write the correct answer in the middle column.

Definition	Correct Answer	Possible Answers
2.1. crown, coronary	_____	adip/o
2.2. fat	_____	aden/o
2.3. gland	_____	home/o
2.4. constant	_____	cephal/o
2.5. relating to the head	_____	coron/o

● Matching Word Parts 2

Write the correct answer in the middle column.

Definition	Correct Answer	Possible Answers
2.6. within	_____	cyt/o
2.7. above	_____	epi-
2.8. cell	_____	hist/o
2.9. out of	_____	exo-
2.10. tissue	_____	endo-

● **Matching Word Parts 3**

Write the correct answer in the middle column.

Definition	Correct Answer	Possible Answers
2.11. pertaining to	_____	**path/o**
2.12. control	_____	**retro-**
2.13. disease, suffering, and emotion	_____	**-plasm**
2.14. formative material of cells	_____	**-ac**
2.15. behind	_____	**-stasis**

● **Definitions**

Select the correct answer and write it on the line provided.

2.16.   The term describing an infection acquired in a hospital setting is _____ .

      iatrogenic   idiopathic   nosocomial   organic

2.17.   The _____ is part of the lymphatic and immune systems.

      liver   pancreas   spleen   thyroid

2.18.   The _____ cavity contains the major organs of digestion.

      abdominal   cranial   dorsal   pelvic

2.19.   The term _____ means the direction toward or nearer the midline.

      distal   lateral   medial   proximal

2.20.   The internal and external surfaces of the body are covered by _____.

      adipose tissue   endothelium   epithelium   epithelial tissue

2.21.   The genetic disorder _____ is characterized by a missing digestive enzyme.

      Huntington's disease   phenylketonuria   Tay-Sachs   trisomy 21

2.22.   The inflammation of a gland is known as _____ .

      adenectomy   adenitis   adenoma   adenosis

2.23.   The abdominal cavity is lined by the _____ .

      mesentery   parietal peritoneum   retroperitoneum   visceral peritoneum

2.24.   The functional units of heredity are known as _____ .

       cells   cytoplasm   genes   protoplasm

2.25.   The study of the structure, composition, and function of tissues is known as _____ .

       anatomy   cytology   histology   physiology

● **Matching Regions of the Thorax and Abdomen**

Write the correct answer in the middle column.

Definition	Correct Answer	Possible Answers
2.26. above the stomach	_____	epigastric
2.27. belly button	_____	hypochondriac
2.28. below the ribs	_____	hypogastric
2.29. below the stomach	_____	iliac
2.30. hipbone	_____	umbilicus

● **Which Word?**

Select the correct answer and write it on the line provided.

2.31.   The term _____ , which means pertaining to the groin, refers to the entire lower portion of the abdomen.

      inguinal   umbilical

2.32.   The study of how traits are transferred from parents to their children and the role of genes in health and disease is called _____ .

      cytology   genetics

2.33.   A specialist in the study of the outbreaks of disease is a/an _____ .

      epidemiologist   pathologist

2.34.   The _____ glands excrete their secretions through ducts.

      endocrine   exocrine

2.35.   The stomach is located _____ to the diaphragm.

      inferior   superior

● Spelling Counts

Find the misspelled word in each sentence. Then write that word, spelled correctly, on the line provided.

2.36.   The term hemiostasis means to maintain a constant internal environment. _____

2.37.   Hemaphilia is a group of hereditary bleeding disorders in which one of the factors needed to clot the

blood is missing. _____

2.38.   Hyportrophy is a general increase in the bulk of a part or organ. _____

2.39.   An idiotopathic disorder is an illness without known cause. _____

2.40.   An abnomoly is any deviation from what is regarded as normal. _____

● Matching Pathology of Tissue Formation

Write the correct answer in the middle column.

Definition	Correct Answer	Possible Answers
2.41. the abnormal development of tissues cells and cells	_____	anaplasia
2.42. a change in the structure of cells and in their orientation to each other	_____	aplasia
2.43. an abnormal increase in the number of normal cells in normal arrangement in a tissue	_____	dysplasia
2.44. incomplete development of an organ or tissue	_____	hyperplasia
2.45. the defective development or congenital absence of an organ or tissue	_____	hypoplasia

● **Term Selection**

Select the correct answer and write it on the line provided.

2.46.   The term meaning situated nearest the midline or beginning of a body structure is

_____ .

distal   lateral   medial   proximal

2.47.   The term meaning situated in the back is _____ .

anterior   posterior   superior   ventral

2.48.   The body is divided into front and back portions by the _____ plane.

coronal   horizontal   sagittal   transverse

2.49.   The body is divided vertically into equal left and right halves by the _____ plane.

frontal   midsagittal   sagittal   transverse

2.50.   Part of the elbow is formed by the _____ end of the humerus.

distal   lateral   medial   proximal

● **Sentence Completion**

Write the correct term on the line provided.

2.51.   Muscular _____ (MD) is a group of genetic diseases characterized by progressive

weakness of muscle fibers.

2.52.   The study of the functions of the structures of the body is known as _____ .

2.53.   Also known as the chest, the _____ cavity protects the heart and lungs.

2.54.   A/An _____ illness is a problem, such as a side effect or an unfavorable response,

arising from a prescribed medical treatment.

2.55.   The abdominal and pelvic cavities are referred to together as the _____ cavity.

● **Word Surgery**

Divide each term into its component word parts. Write these word parts, in sequence, on the lines provided.

When necessary use a back slash (/) to indicate a combining vowel. (You may not need all of the lines provided.)

2.56.   An **adenectomy** is the surgical removal of a gland.

_____   _____   _____   _____

2.57.   **Endocrine glands** secrete hormones directly into the bloodstream.

_____   _____   _____   _____

2.58.   A **histologist** specializes in the study of cells and microscopic tissues.

_____   _____   _____   _____

2.59.   **Retroperitoneal** means located behind the peritoneum.

_____   _____   _____   _____

2.60.   A **pathologist** specializes in the laboratory analysis of tissue samples to confirm or establish a diagnosis.

_____   _____   _____   _____

2.61.   The term **etiology** means the study of the causes of diseases.

_____   _____   _____   _____

2.62.   The term **homeostasis** means maintaining a constant internal environment.

_____   _____   _____   _____

2.63.   A **coronal plane** divides the body into anterior and posterior portions.

_____   _____   _____   _____

2.64.   The term **abdominopelvic** means pertaining to both the abdominal and pelvic cavities.

_____   _____   _____   _____

2.65.   An **idiopathic** disorder is an illness without known cause.

_____   _____   _____   _____

● **Clinical Conditions**

Write the correct answer on the line provided.

2.66.   Mr. Tseng died of cholera during a sudden and widespread outbreak of this disease in his country. Such

an outbreak is described as being a/an _____ .

2.67.   Brenda Farmer's doctor could not find any physical changes to explain her symptoms. The doctor refers

to this as a/an _____ disorder.

2.68.   Gerald Carlson inherited a bleeding disorder in which one of the clotting factors is missing. This name of

this condition is _____ .

2.69.   Wally Foster has a kidney disease. His doctor is performing tests to determine the cause or

_____ of this illness.

2.70.   Mrs. Reynolds has an inflammation of the peritoneum. The medical term for this condition is

_____ .

2.71.   Ralph Jenkins drank contaminated water while on a camping trip. Now he is very sick and his doctor says

he contracted the illness through _____ transmission.

2.72.   Jose Ortega complained of pain in the lower right area of his abdomen. Using the system that divides

the abdomen into four sections, his doctor recorded the pain as being in the lower right

_____ .

2.73.   Tracy Ames has an inflammation within the area formed by the hipbones. Her doctor describes this area

as the _____ cavity.

2.74.   In college, Gerald McClelland wants to learn more about the structure and functions of cells. To

accomplish this he has signed up for courses in _____ .

2.75.   Ashley Goldberg is fascinated by how traits and characteristics are transmitted. She wants to specialize in

this field and is studying to become a/an _____ .

● Which Is the Correct Medical Term?

Select the correct answer and write it on the line provided.

2.76.   Debbie Sanchez fell against a rock and injured her left hip and upper leg. This area is known as the left

_____ region.

| hypochondriac | iliac | lumbar | umbilical |

2.77.   Down syndrome is also known as _____ 21.

| fetal alcohol | hemophilia | Tay-Sachs | trisomy |

2.78.   The _____ are the only cells in the body that do not have 46 chromosomes.

| DNA strands | gametes | mutated | somatic |

2.79.   An example of liquid connective tissue is _____ .

| adipose tissue | blood | muscle | nerve |

2.80.   The esophagus is part of the _____ system.

| cardiovascular | digestive | respiratory | urinary |

● Challenge Word Building

This group of exercises provides an opportunity to work with the word parts you have learned in Chapters 1 and 2. To answer the question, combine the appropriate parts. While doing this, pay attention to the use of combining vowels! You may want to look in the textbook glossary or use a medical dictionary to check your answers.

gastr/o = stomach	**-algia** = pain
laryng/o = larynx	**-ectomy** = surgical removal
my/o = muscle	**-itis** = inflammation
nephr/o = kidney	**-osis** = abnormal condition
neur/o = nerve	**-plasty** = surgical repair

2.81.   The term meaning the surgical repair of a muscle is _____ .

2.82.   The term meaning pain in a nerve is _____ .

2.83.   The term meaning an abnormal condition of the stomach is _____ .

2.84.   The term meaning inflammation of the larynx is _____ .

2.85. The term meaning the surgical removal of part of a muscle is a/an _____ .

2.86. The term meaning pain in the stomach is _____ .

2.87. The term meaning surgical removal of the larynx is _____ .

2.88. The term meaning an abnormal condition of the kidney is _____ .

2.89. The medical term meaning surgical repair of a nerve is _____ .

2.90. The term meaning inflammation of the kidney is _____ .

● **Labeling Exercises**

Identify the numbered items in the accompanying figures.

2.91. This is the right _____ region.

2.92. This is the _____ region.

2.93. This is the _____ region.

2.94. This is the left _____ region.

2.95. This is the left _____ region.

2.96. This is the midline or _____ plane.

2.97. This is known as the ventral or

_____ surface.

2.98. This arrow is pointing in a/an

_____ direction.

2.99. This is known as the dorsal or

_____ surface.

2.100. This is the frontal or _____ plane.

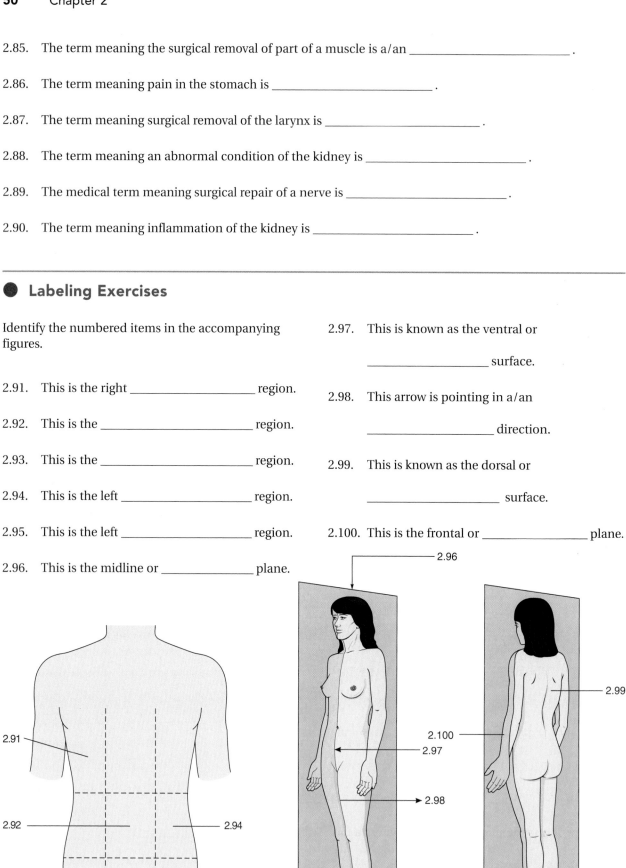

THE HUMAN TOUCH: CRITICAL THINKING EXERCISE

The following story and questions are designed to stimulate critical thinking through class discussion or as a brief essay response. There are no right or wrong answers to these questions.

Tahriah and Justise Brown have three wonderful children. The oldest is in her second year at the community college. The middle one plays third base for his high school varsity team, and the youngest is a freshman with an eye on the tennis team. The Browns are looking forward to planning weddings and spoiling grandbabies. But then, at age 44, Tahriah discovers she is pregnant.

Her obstetrician, Dr. Makay, suggests performing genetic testing using amniotic fluid gathered by a procedure called amniocentesis. He tells her, "Technical advances allow a glimpse into the womb to discover genetic anomalies. Because of your age, Tahriah, I am concerned about Down syndrome." He waits, gauging her reaction, then continues.

"This genetic disorder causes various degrees of mental retardation and physical defects. Severe cases produce a child unable to feed or care for itself. Life-threatening physical defects may require expensive, painful surgical procedures. Although they do exhibit the typical Down's facial appearance, some of these children display only marginal symptoms and function within societal norms."

Dr. Makay discusses choices the Browns would need to make if genetic testing indicates Down syndrome. Finally he says, "We can detect its presence, but not the degree or severity. Don't decide now. Go home, talk with your family, and call me soon with your decision."

Tahriah, Justise, and their children discuss the possibilities that amniocentesis presents. They talk late into the night. The decision is difficult, but in the morning Tahriah calls Dr. Makay to . . .

Suggested Discussion Topics:

1. Discuss the challenges a Down syndrome child would present to the Brown family.

2. Genetic testing can determine gender, plus certain negative and positive genetic characteristics, including a high risk of certain diseases. Discuss how this type of information could be used by parents, health care providers, and insurance companies.

3. Discuss the options available to Tahriah if the genetic test is positive for Down syndrome.

4. If you were aware that you carried a gene that gave you a 50-50 chance of having a child with a severe birth defect, would you still plan to have children? Why or why not?

5. Children with severe handicaps require expensive care whether they live at home or in an institution. Who should pay for this care and why?

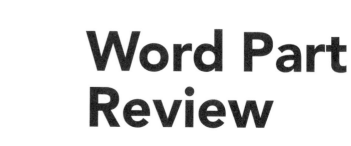

Word Part Review

In the first two chapters of your text-book you were introduced to many word parts. As you study the body system chapters, you will learn even more word parts as they relate to each system. Your study of the body systems will be much easier if you have mastered *at least* the word parts in this section.

The 50-question Word Part Practice Session gives you additional word part practice, as well as opportunities to use combining vowels correctly and build unfamiliar terms based on familiar word parts.

The 50-question Post-Test at the end of this section enables you to evaluate your mastery of these word parts.

WORD PART PRACTICE SESSION

● Matching Word Parts 1

Write the correct answer in the middle column.

Definition	**Correct Answer**	**Possible Answers**
WP.1. bad, difficult, painful	_____	**intra-**
WP.2. between, among	_____	**hyper-**
WP.3. deficient, decreased	_____	**inter-**
WP.4. excessive, increased	_____	**hypo-**
WP.5. within, inside	_____	**dys-**

● Matching Word Parts 2

Write the correct answer in the middle column.

Definition	**Correct Answer**	**Possible Answers**
WP.6. above, excessive	_____	**pre-**
WP.7. before	_____	**peri-**
WP.8. many	_____	**poly-**
WP.9. surrounding	_____	**sub-**
WP.10. under, less, below	_____	**supra-**

● Matching Word Parts 3

Write the correct answer in the middle column.

Definition	**Correct Answer**	**Possible Answers**
WP.11. inflammation	_____	**-algia**
WP.12. pain, suffering	_____	**-centesis**
WP.13. the process of producing a picture or record	_____	**-ectomy**
WP.14. surgical puncture to remove fluid	_____	**-itis**
WP.15. surgical removal	_____	**-graphy**

● Matching Word Parts 4

Write the correct answer in the middle column.

Definition	Correct Answer	Possible Answers
WP.16. surgical repair	_____	-dynia
WP.17. abnormal softening	_____	-malacia
WP.18. pain	_____	-necrosis
WP.19. tissue death	_____	-oma
WP.20. tumor or neoplasm	_____	-plasty

● Matching Word Parts 5

Write the correct answer in the middle column.

Definition	Correct Answer	Possible Answers
WP.21. abnormal condition, disease	_____	-ac
WP.22. abnormal hardening	_____	-ostomy
WP.23. cutting, surgical incision	_____	-osis
WP.24. pertaining to	_____	-otomy
WP.25. surgical creation of an opening	_____	-sclerosis

● Matching Word Parts 6

Write the correct answer in the middle column.

Definition	Correct Answer	Possible Answers
WP.26. abnormal flow, discharge	_____	-rrhagia
WP.27. abnormal tightening or narrowing	_____	-rrhaphy
WP.28. bleeding	_____	-rrhea
WP.29. rupture	_____	-rrhexis
WP.30. to suture	_____	-stenosis

● True/False

If the statement is true, write T on the line. If the statement is false, write F on the line.

WP.31. _____ **myc/o** means mucous.

WP.32. _____ **peri-** means surrounding.

WP.33. _____ **hyper-** means below, under, decreased.

WP.34. _____ **ather/o** means plaque or fatty substance.

WP.35. _____ **-gram** means an instrument for recording.

WP.36. _____ **arthr/o** means joint.

WP.37. _____ **-ologist** means study of.

WP.38. _____ **-megaly** means enlargement.

WP.39. _____ **-centesis** means to see or a visual examination.

● Word Building

Write the word you created on the line provided.

WP.40. The medical term meaning an abnormal flow commonly known as a runny nose is

_____ . (**rhin/o** means nose.)

WP.41. The term meaning the surgical removal of a kidney is a/an _____ . (**nephr/o**

means kidney.)

WP.42. The term meaning inflammation of the ear is _____ . (**ot/o** means ear.)

WP.43. The term meaning an enlarged heart is _____ . (**cardi/o** means heart.)

WP.44. The term meaning inflammation of the liver is _____ . (**hepat/o** means liver.)

WP.45. The term meaning the visual examination of the interior of a joint is _____ .

(**arthr/o** means joint.)

WP.46. A specialist in disorders of the urinary system is known as a/an _____ . (**ur/o**

means urine.)

WP.47. The study of disorders of the blood is known as _____ . (**hemat/o** means blood.)

WP.48.   The medical term meaning a surgical incision into the colon is a/an _____ .

(**col/o** means colon.)

WP.49.   The medical term meaning inflammation of a vein is _____ . (**phleb/o** means vein.)

WP.50.   The term meaning a record of the electrical activity of the heart is an ECG or a/an

_____ . (**electr/o** means electric and **cardi/o** means heart.)

WORD PART POST-TEST

Write the word part on the line provided.

PT.1.   The suffix meaning surgical removal is _____ .

PT.2.   The prefix meaning excessive, increased is _____ .

PT.3.   The suffix meaning surgical repair is _____ .

PT.4.   The suffix meaning enlargement is _____ .

PT.5.   The combining form meaning joint is _____ .

PT.6.   The combining form meaning muscle is _____ .

PT.7.   The prefix meaning between, among is _____ .

PT.8.   The combining form meaning nerve is _____ .

PT.9.   The suffix meaning to see or a visual examination is _____ .

PT.10. The suffix meaning the study of is _____ .

● Matching Word Parts 1

Write the correct answer in the middle column.

Definition	Correct Answer	Possible Answers
PT.11. tumor	_____	arteri/o
PT.12. surgical suturing	_____	-oma
PT.13. surrounding	_____	peri-
PT.14. rupture	_____	-rrhaphy
PT.15. artery	_____	-rrhexis

● Matching Word Parts 2

Write the correct answer in the middle column.

Definition	Correct Answer	Possible Answers
PT.16. abnormal hardening	_____	-itis
PT.17. bad, difficult, painful	_____	-ostomy
PT.18. inflammation	_____	-ologist
PT.19. surgical creation of an opening	_____	dys-
PT.20. specialist	_____	-sclerosis

● True/False

If the statement is true, write T on the line. If the statement is false, write F on the line.

PT.21. _____ **hem/o** means blood.

PT.22. _____ **-algia** means pain.

PT.23. _____ **oste/o** means bone.

PT.24. _____ **hyper-** means deficient or decreased.

PT.25. _____ **rhin/o** means nose.

PT.26. _____ Tonsillitis is an inflammation of the tonsils.

PT.27. _____ A myectomy is a surgical incision into a muscle.

PT.28. _____ Gastralgia is pain in the stomach.

PT.29. _____ A gerontologist specializes in the diseases of women.

PT.30. _____ **Intra-** means between or among.

● Word Building

Write the word you created on the line provided.

Regarding Nerves (**neur/o** means nerve)

PT.31.   A surgical incision into a nerve is a/an _____ .

PT.32.   A benign tumor made up of nerve tissue is a/an _____ .

PT.33.   The surgical repair of a nerve or nerves is a/an _____ .

PT.34.   The term meaning to suture the ends of a severed nerve is _____ .

PT.35.   Abnormal softening of the nerves is called _____ .

PT.36.   A specialist in diagnosing and treating disorders of the nervous system is a/an _____ .

PT.37.   The term meaning inflammation of a nerve or nerves is _____ .

Relating to Blood Vessels (**angi/o** means relating to the blood vessels)

PT.38.   The death of the walls of blood vessels is _____ .

PT.39.   The abnormal hardening of the walls of blood vessels is _____ .

PT.40.   The abnormal narrowing of a blood vessel is _____ .

PT.41.   The surgical removal of a blood vessel is a/an _____ .

PT.42.   The process of recording a picture of blood vessels is called _____ .

● **Missing Words**

Write the missing word on the line provided.

PT.43.   The surgical repair of an artery is a/an _____ . (**arteri/o** means artery.)

PT.44.   The medical term meaning inflammation of the larynx is _____ . (**laryng/o** means larynx.)

PT.45.   The surgical removal of all or part of the colon is a/an _____ . (**col/o** means colon.)

PT.46.   The abnormal softening of muscle tissue is _____ . (**my/o** means muscle.)

PT.47.   The term meaning any abnormal condition of the stomach is _____ . (**gastr/o** means stomach.)

PT.48.   The term meaning the study of the heart is _____ . (**cardi/o** means heart.)

PT.49.   The term meaning inflammation of the colon is _____ . (**col/o** means colon.)

PT.50.   The term meaning a surgical incision into a vein is _____ . (**phleb/o** means vein.)

The Skeletal System

Overview of Structures, Combining Forms, and Functions of the Skeletal System

MAJOR STRUCTURES	RELATED COMBINING FORMS	PRIMARY FUNCTIONS
Bones	oss/e, oss/i, oste/o, ost/o	Act as the framework for the body, protect the internal organs, and store the mineral calcium.
Bone Marrow	myel/o (also means spinal cord)	Red bone marrow forms some blood cells. Yellow bone marrow stores fat.
Cartilage	chondr/o	Creates a smooth surface for motion within the joints and protects the ends of the bones.
Joints	arthr/o	Work with the muscles to make a variety of motions possible.
Ligaments	ligament/o	Connect one bone to another.
Synovial Membrane	synovi/o, synov/o	Forms the lining of synovial joints and secretes synovial fluid.
Synovial Fluid	synovi/o, synov/o	Lubricant that makes smooth joint movements possible.
Bursa	burs/o	Cushions areas subject to friction during movement.

● VOCABULARY   RELATED TO THE SKELETAL SYSTEM

The items on this list have been identified as key word parts and terms for this chapter. However, all words in boldface in the text are important and may be included in the learning exercises and tests.

Word Parts

- ☐ ankyl/o
- ☐ arthr/o
- ☐ chondr/o
- ☐ cost/o
- ☐ crani/o
- ☐ -desis
- ☐ kyph/o
- ☐ lord/o
- ☐ -lysis
- ☐ myel/o
- ☐ oss/e, oss/i, ost/o, oste/o
- ☐ scoli/o
- ☐ spondyl/o
- ☐ synovi/o, synov/o
- ☐ -um

Medical Terms

- ☐ **acetabulum** (**ass**-eh-**TAB**-you-lum)
- ☐ **acetaminophen** (ah-**seet**-ah-**MIN**-oh-fen)
- ☐ **allogenic** (al-oh-**JEN**-ick)
- ☐ **ankylosing spondylitis** (**ang**-kih-**LOH**-sing spon-dih-**LYE**-tis)
- ☐ **ankylosis** (ang-kih-**LOH**-sis)
- ☐ **arthrodesis** (ar-throh-**DEE**-sis)
- ☐ **arthroplasty** (**AR**-throh-**plas**-tee)
- ☐ **arthroscopic surgery** (ar-throh-**SKOP**-ick)
- ☐ **autologous** (aw-**TOL**-uh-guss)
- ☐ **bursitis** (ber-**SIGH**-tis)
- ☐ **callus** (**KAL**-us)
- ☐ **chondroma** (kon-**DROH**-mah)
- ☐ **chondromalacia** (**kon**-droh-mah-**LAY**-shee-ah)
- ☐ **clavicle** (**KLAV**-ih-kul)
- ☐ **comminuted fracture** (**KOM**-ih-**newt**-ed)
- ☐ **craniectomy** (kray-nee-**EK**-toh-mee)
- ☐ **craniostenosis** (kray-nee-oh-steh-**NOH**-sis)
- ☐ **craniotomy** (kray-nee-**OT**-oh-mee)
- ☐ **crepitation** (krep-ih-**TAY**-shun)
- ☐ **dual x-ray absorptiometry** (ab-**sorp**-shee-**OM**-eh-tree)

- ☐ **Ewing's sarcoma** (**YOU**-ingz sar-**KOH**-mah)
- ☐ **hallux valgus** (**HAL**-ucks **VAL**-guss)
- ☐ **hemarthrosis** (hee-mahr-**THROH**-sis *or* hem-ar-**THROH**-sis)
- ☐ **kyphosis** (kye-**FOH**-sis)
- ☐ **laminectomy** (**lam**-ih-**NECK**-toh-mee)
- ☐ **lordosis** (lor-**DOH**-sis)
- ☐ **lumbago** (lum-**BAY**-goh)
- ☐ **luxation** (luck-**SAY**-shun)
- ☐ **myeloma** (**my**-eh-**LOH**-mah)
- ☐ **orthopedist** (**or**-thoh-**PEE**-dist)
- ☐ **orthotics** (or-**THOT**-icks)
- ☐ **osteitis** (**oss**-tee-**EYE**-tis)
- ☐ **osteoarthritis** (**oss**-tee-oh-ar-**THRIGH**-tis)
- ☐ **osteochondroma** (**oss**-tee-oh-kon-**DROH**-mah)
- ☐ **osteoclasis** (**oss**-tee-**OCK**-lah-sis)
- ☐ **osteomalacia** (**oss**-tee-oh-mah-**LAY**-shee-ah)
- ☐ **osteomyelitis** (**oss**-tee-oh-**my**-eh-**LYE**-tis)
- ☐ **osteopathic physician** (**oss**-tee-oh-**PATH**-ick)
- ☐ **osteopenia** (**oss**-tee-oh-**PEE**-nee-ah)
- ☐ **osteoporosis** (**oss**-tee-oh-poh-**ROH**-sis)
- ☐ **osteorrhaphy** (**oss**-tee-**OR**-ah-fee)
- ☐ **osteotomy** (**oss**-tee-**OT**-oh-mee)
- ☐ **Paget's disease** (**PAJ**-its)
- ☐ **patella** (pah-**TEL**-ah)
- ☐ **percutaneous vertebroplasty** (**per**-kyou-**TAY**-nee-us **VER**-tee-broh-**plas**-tee)
- ☐ **phalanges** (fah-**LAN**-jeez)
- ☐ **podiatrist** (poh-**DYE**-ah-trist)
- ☐ **popliteal** (pop-**LIT**-ee-al)
- ☐ **rheumatism** (**ROO**-mah-tizm)
- ☐ **rheumatoid arthritis** (**ROO**-mah-toyd ar-**THRIGH**-tis)
- ☐ **rickets** (**RICK**-ets)
- ☐ **sacroiliac** (**say**-kroh-**ILL**-ee-ack)
- ☐ **scoliosis** (skoh-lee-**OH**-sis)
- ☐ **spina bifida** (**SPY**-nah **BIF**-ih-dah)
- ☐ **spondylolisthesis** (**spon**-dih-loh-liss-**THEE**-sis)
- ☐ **subluxation** (**sub**-luck-**SAY**-shun)
- ☐ **synovectomy** (sin-oh-**VECK**-toh-mee)
- ☐ **talipes** (**TAL**-ih-peez)
- ☐ **thermal capsulorrhaphy** (**kap**-soo-**LOR**-ah-fee)
- ☐ **vertebral column** (**VER**-tee-bral *or* **VER**-teh-bral)

● OBJECTIVES

On completion of this chapter, you should be able to:

1. Identify and describe the major functions and structures of the skeletal system.

2. Describe three types of joints.

3. Differentiate between the axial and appendicular skeletons.

4. Identify the medical specialists who treat disorders of the skeletal system.

5. Recognize, define, spell, and pronounce terms related to the pathology and the diagnostic and treatment procedures of the skeletal system.

FUNCTIONS OF THE SKELETAL SYSTEM

The skeletal system has many important functions.

- Bones act as the framework of the body.
- Bones support and protect the internal organs.
- Joints working in conjunction with muscles, ligaments, and tendons make possible the wide variety of body movements. (Muscles and tendons are discussed in Chapter 4.)
- Calcium, which is required for normal nerve and muscle function, is stored in bones.
- Red bone marrow, which is located within spongy bone, has an important function in the formation of blood cells.

STRUCTURES OF THE SKELETAL SYSTEM

The structures of the skeletal system include bones, cartilage, ligaments, joints, and bursa.

THE STRUCTURE OF BONES

Bone is a form of connective tissue and is almost the hardest tissue in the human body. Only dental enamel is harder than bone.

The Tissues of Bone

Although it is very hard and dense, bone is a living structure that changes and is capable of healing itself. The tissues that make up a bone are summarized in Table 3.1 and shown in Figure 3.1.

Bone Marrow

- **Red bone marrow**, which is located within the spongy bone, is hemopoietic and manufactures red blood cells, hemoglobin, white blood cells, and thrombocytes. These types of blood cells are discussed in Chapter 5.

Table 3.1

TISSUES OF A BONE	
Periosteum (pehr-ee-OSS-tee-um)	The tough, fibrous tissue that forms the outermost covering of bone (peri- means surrounding, oste means bone, and -um is a noun ending).
Compact Bone	The hard, dense, and very strong bone that forms the outer layer of the bones.
Spongy Bone	Lighter and not as strong as compact bone, it is commonly found in the ends and inner portions of long bones such as the femur. Red bone marrow is located within this spongy bone.
Medullary Cavity (**MED**-you-**lehr**-ee)	Located in the shaft of a long bone, the medullary cavity is surrounded by compact bone and contains yellow bone marrow. *Medullary* means pertaining to the inner section.
Endosteum (en-**DOS**-tee-um)	The tissue that forms the lining of the medullary cavity.

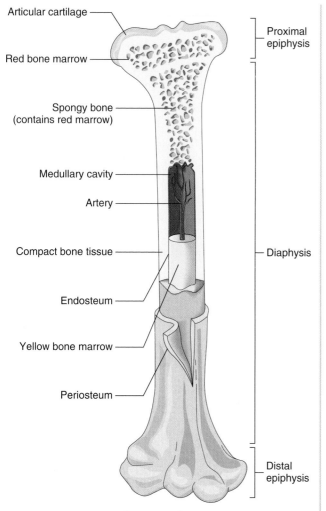

Articular cartilage

Red bone marrow

Spongy bone (contains red marrow)

Medullary cavity

Artery

Compact bone tissue

Endosteum

Yellow bone marrow

Periosteum

Proximal epiphysis

Diaphysis

Distal epiphysis

FIGURE 3.1   Anatomic features of a typical long bone.

- **Hemopoietic** (**hee**-moh poy-**ET**-ick), also known as **hematopoietic** (**hee**-mah-toh-poi-**ET**-ick), means pertaining to the formation of blood cells (**hem/o** and **hemat/o** both mean blood and **-poietic** means pertaining to formation).

- **Yellow bone marrow**, which is found in the medullary cavity, is composed chiefly of fat cells and functions as a fat storage area.

Cartilage

- **Cartilage** (**KAR**-tih-lidj) is the smooth, rubbery, blue-white connective tissue that acts as a shock absorber between bones. Cartilage, which is more elastic than bone, makes up the flexible parts of the skeleton such as the outer ear and the tip of the nose.

- **Articular cartilage** (ar-**TICK**-you-lar **KAR**-tih-lidj) covers the surfaces of bones where they form joints. This cartilage makes smooth joint movement possible and protects the bones from rubbing against each other (Figures 3.1 and 3.5).

- The **meniscus** (meh-**NIS**-kus) is the curved fibrous cartilage found in some joints, such as the knee and the temporomandibular joint of the jaw (Figure 3.4).

Anatomic Landmarks of a Bone

- The **diaphysis** (dye-**AF**-ih-sis) is the shaft of a long bone (Figure 3.1).

- The **epiphysis** (eh-**PIF**-ih-sis), which is covered with articular cartilage, is the wide end of a long bone.

- The **proximal epiphysis** is the end of the bone located nearest to the midline of the body.

- The **distal epiphysis** is the end of the bone located farthest away from the midline.

- A **foramen** (foh-**RAY**-men) is an opening in a bone through which blood vessels, nerves, and ligaments pass (plural, **foramina**). For example, the spinal cord runs through the vertebral foramen shown in Figure 3.13.

- A **process** is a normal projection on the surface of a bone that serves as an attachment for muscles and tendons. For example, the mastoid process is the bony projection located on each temporal bone just behind the ear (Figure 3.9).

JOINTS

Joints, also known as **articulations**, are connections between bones. As used here, *articulation* means to join or come together in a manner that allows motion between the parts. *Articulation* also means speaking clearly.

Types of Joints

Different types of joints make a wide range of motions possible. These types of joints include sutures, cartilaginous joints, and synovial joints.

Sutures

- A **suture** is an immovable joint. Here bones join along a jagged line to form a joint that does not move. *Suture* also means to stitch. Figure 3.2 shows the coronal and sagittal sutures across the top of the adult skull.

- The anterior and posterior **fontaneles** (**fon**-tah-**NELLS**) on a baby's head are the regions where the sutures between the bones have not yet closed. These areas, also known as the **soft spots**, disappear as the child grows and the sutures close. This is also spelled *fontanelles*.

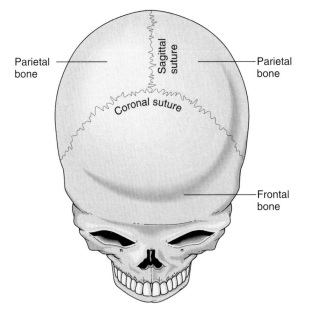
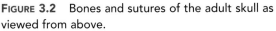

FIGURE 3.2   Bones and sutures of the adult skull as viewed from above.

Symphyses

A **symphysis** (**SIM**-fih-sis), also known as an *amphiarthrosis*, is a form of **cartilaginous joint** (**kar**-tih-**LADJ**-ih-nus) that is only slightly moveable.

- In a symphysis, two bones join and are held firmly together so that they function as one bone (plural, **symphyses**). For example, the pubic symphysis is shown in Figure 3.15.

Synovial Joints

Synovial joints (sih-**NOH**-vee-al), also known as *diarthrodial joints*, are the movable joints of the body. Although these joints are described in simple terms, they are actually very complex structures (Figure 3.3).

- **Ball and socket joints**, such as the hips and shoulders, are synovial joints that allow a wide range of movement in many directions (Figure 3.3A).
- **Hinge joints**, such as the knees and elbows, are synovial joints that allow movement primarily in one direction or plane (Figures 3.3B and 3.3C).

Structures of Synovial Joints

Ligaments

- A **ligament** (**LIG**-ah-ment) is a band of fibrous connective tissue that connects one bone to another bone. Figure 3.4 shows the complex system of ligaments that make knee movements possible.
- Be careful not to confuse ligaments and tendons. **Tendons,** which attach muscles to bones, are discussed in Chapter 4.

Synovial Membrane and Fluid

Synovial joints, which are surrounded by a fibrous capsule, are lined with synovial membrane. This specialized membrane secretes synovial fluid that acts as a lubricant to make the smooth movement of the joint possible (Figure 3.5).

Bursa

A **bursa** (**BER**-sah) is a fibrous sac that is lined with a synovial membrane and contains synovial fluid (plural, **bursae**).

- A bursa acts as a cushion to ease movement in areas that are subject to friction, such as in shoulder, elbow, and knee joints where a tendon passes over a bone (Figures 3.5 and 4.14).

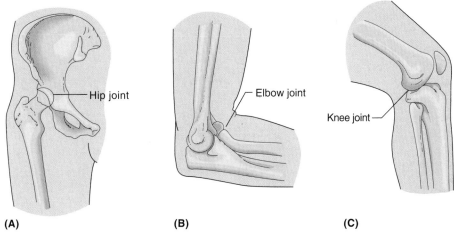

FIGURE 3.3   Examples of synovial joints. (A) Ball and socket joint of the hip. (B) Hinge joint of the elbow. (C) Hinge joint of the knee.

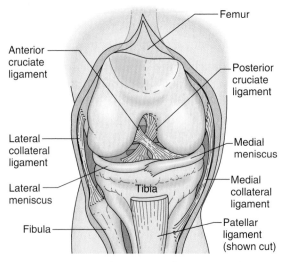

FIGURE 3.4 Major ligaments of the knee. This anterior schematic representation of the knee, with the patella removed, shows the complex system of ligaments that make knee movements possible.

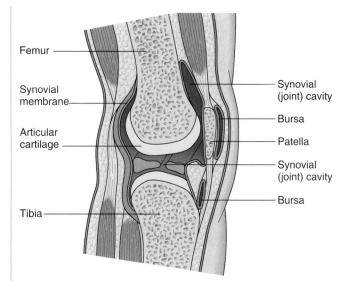

FIGURE 3.5 Structures of a synovial joint and bursa. (This is a lateral view of the knee.)

SKELETON

The 206 bones in the adult human body are shown in Figures 3.6, 3.7, and 3.8. For descriptive purposes, the skeleton is divided into the axial and appendicular skeletal systems.

Axial Skeleton

- The **axial skeleton** (80 bones) protects the major organs of the nervous, respiratory, and circulatory systems. *Axial* means pertaining to an axis. An *axis* is an imaginary line that runs lengthwise through the center of the body.

- The axial skeleton consists of the skull, spinal column, ribs, and sternum. These structures are shown in gray in Figure 3.7.

Appendicular Skeleton

- The **appendicular skeleton** (126 bones) makes body movement possible and also protects the organs of digestion, excretion, and reproduction. The term *appendicular* means referring to an appendage. An *appendage* is anything that is attached to a major part of the body.

- The appendicular skeleton is organized into the **upper extremities** (shoulders, arms, forearms, wrists, and hands) and the **lower extremities** (hips, thighs, legs, ankles, and feet). These structures are shown in blue in Figure 3.7.

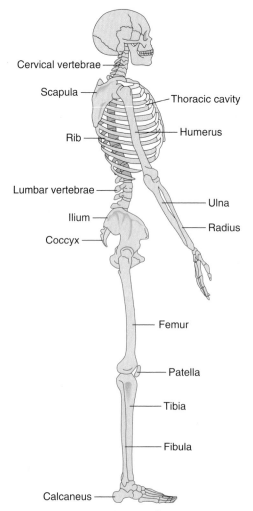

FIGURE 3.6 Lateral view of the adult human skeleton.

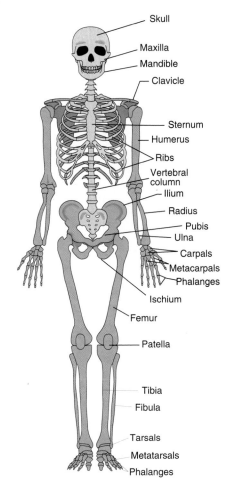

FIGURE 3.7 Anterior view of the adult human skeleton. Bones of the axial skeleton are shown in gray. The bones of the appendicular skeleton are shown in blue.

Bones of the Skull

The skull consists of eight bones that form the cranium, 14 bones that form the face, and six tiny bones in the middle ear. As you study the following bones of the skull, refer to Figures 3.9 and 3.10.

Bones of the Cranium

The **cranium** (**KRAY**-nee-um) is the portion of the skull that encloses the brain (**crani** means skull and **-um** is a noun ending). The cranium is made up of the following eight bones:

- The **frontal bone** forms the forehead.
- The two **parietal bones** (pah-**RYE**-eh-tal) form most of the roof and upper sides of the cranium.
- The **occipital bone** (ock-**SIP**-ih-tal) forms the posterior floor and walls of the cranium. The spinal cord passes through the *foramen magnum* of the occipital bone.
- The two **temporal bones** form the sides and base of the cranium.

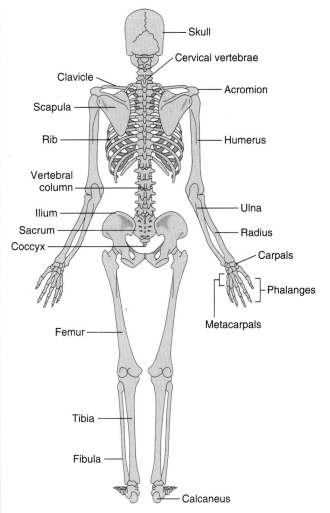

FIGURE 3.8 Posterior view of the adult human skeleton.

- The **sphenoid bone** (**SFEE**-noid) forms part of the base of the skull and parts of the floor and sides of the orbit. The *orbit* is the bony socket that surrounds and protects the eyeball.
- The **ethmoid bone** (**ETH**-moid) forms part of the nose, the orbit, and the floor of the cranium.

Auditory Ossicles

The six **auditory ossicles** (**OSS**-ih-kulz) are discussed in Chapter 11.

- The **external auditory meatus** (mee-**AY**-tus) is located in the temporal bone. A *meatus* is the external opening of a canal.

Bones of the Face

The face is made up of the following 14 bones:

- The two **nasal bones** form the upper part of the bridge of the nose.
- The two **zygomatic bones** (zye-goh-**MAT**-ick), also known as the **cheekbones**, articulate with the frontal bones.

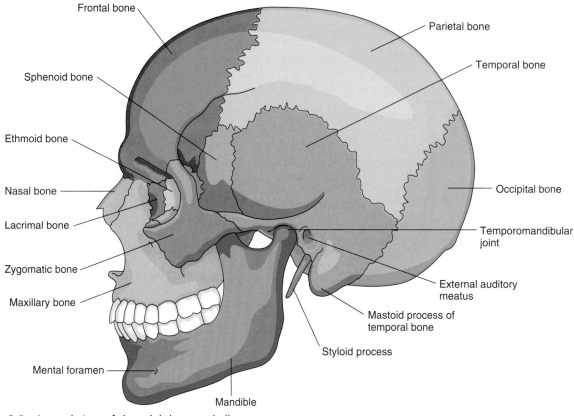

FIGURE 3.9 Lateral view of the adult human skull.

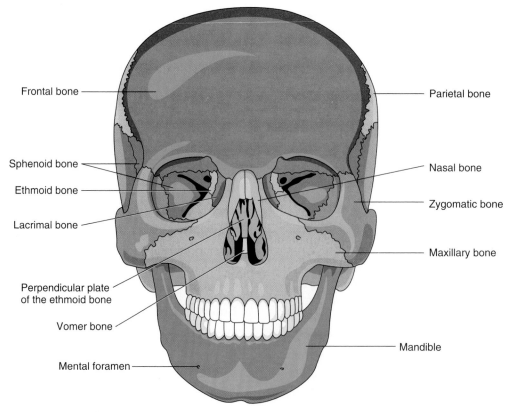

FIGURE 3.10 Anterior view of the adult human skull.

- The two **maxillary bones** (**MACK**-sih-**ler**-ee), also known as the **maxillae**, form most of the upper jaw (singular, **maxilla**).
- The two **palatine bones** (**PAL**-ah-tine) form part of the hard palate of the mouth and the floor of the nose.
- The two **lacrimal bones** (**LACK**-rih-mal) make up part of the orbit at the inner angle of the eye.
- The two **inferior conchae** (**KONG**-kee *or* **KONG**-kay) are the thin, scroll-like bones that form part of the interior of the nose (singular, **concha**).
- The **vomer bone** (**VOH**-mer) forms the base for the nasal septum. The *nasal septum* is the cartilage structure that divides the two nasal cavities.
- The **mandible** (**MAN**-dih-bul), also known as the **lower jawbone**, is the only movable bone of the skull. The mandible is attached to the skull at the **temporomandibular joint** (**tem**-poh-roh-man-**DIB**-you-lar) (**TMJ**).

Thoracic Cavity

The **thoracic cavity** (thoh-**RAS**-ick), which is part of the axial skeleton, is made up of the ribs, sternum, and thoracic vertebrae (Figure 3.6). Also known as the **rib cage**, this structure protects the heart and lungs.

Ribs

There are 12 pairs of ribs, called **costals** (**KOSS**-tulz), which attach posteriorly to the thoracic vertebrae (**cost** means rib and **-al** means pertaining to).

- The first seven pairs of ribs, called **true ribs**, are attached anteriorly to the sternum (Figure 3.11).
- The next three pairs of ribs, called **false ribs**, are attached anteriorly to cartilage that joins with the sternum.
- The last two pairs of ribs, called **floating ribs**, are not attached anteriorly.

Sternum

The **sternum** (**STER**-num), also known as the **breastbone**, forms the middle of the front of the rib cage. It is divided into three parts: the manubrium, body, and xiphoid process (Figure 3.11).

- The **manubrium** (mah-**NEW**-bree-um), which is bone, forms the upper portion of the sternum.
- The **body** of the sternum, which is bone, forms the middle portion of the sternum.
- The **xiphoid process** (**ZIF**-oid), which is cartilage, forms the lower portion of the sternum.

Shoulders

The shoulders form the **pectoral girdle** (**PECK**-toh-rahl), which supports the arms and hands; this is also known as the **shoulder girdle**. As used here, the term *girdle* means a structure that encircles the body. As you study the bones of the shoulder, refer to Figures 3.8 and 3.11.

- The **clavicle** (**KLAV**-ih-kul), also known as the **collar bone**, is a slender bone that connects the manubrium of the sternum to the scapula.
- The **scapula** (**SKAP**-you-lah) is also known as the **shoulder blade** (plural, **scapulae**).
- The **acromion** (ah-**KROH**-mee-on) is an extension of the scapula that forms the high point of the shoulder.

Arms

As you study the following bones of the arms, refer to Figures 3.11 and 3.12.

- The **humerus** (**HEW**-mer-us) is the bone of the upper arm (plural, **humeri**).
- The **radius** (**RAY**-dee-us) is the smaller bone in the forearm. The radius runs up the thumb side of the forearm.

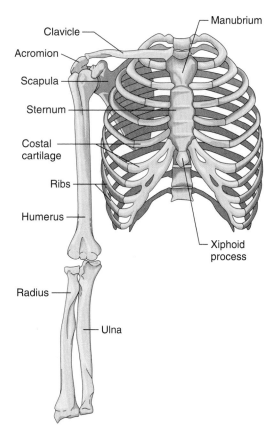

FIGURE 3.11 Anterior view of the ribs, shoulder, and arm. (Cartilage structures are shown in blue.)

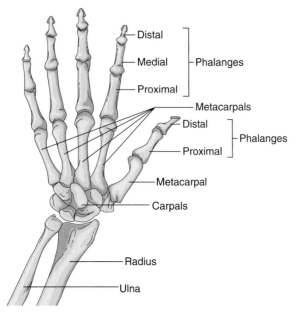

Figure 3.12   Dorsal view of the bones of the lower left arm, wrist, and hand.

- The **ulna** (**ULL**-nah) is the larger bone of the forearm. It articulates with the humerus to form the elbow joint.

- The **olecranon process** (oh-**LEK**-rah-non), commonly known as the **funny bone**, is a large projection on the upper end of the ulna that forms the point of the elbow that tingles when struck.

Wrists, Hands, and Fingers

As you study the following bones of the wrists and hands, refer to Figure 3.12.

- The 16 **carpals** (**KAR**-palz) are the bones that form the wrists.

- The 10 **metacarpals** (met-ah-**KAR**-palz) are the bones that form the palms of the hands.

- The 28 **phalanges** (fah-**LAN**-jeez) are the bones of the fingers (singular, **phalanx**). The term *phalanges* also describes the bones of the feet.

- Each finger has three bones. These are the **distal** (outermost), **medial** (middle), and **proximal** (nearest the hand) phalanges.

- The thumb has two bones. These are the **distal** and **proximal** phalanges.

Vertebral Column

The **vertebral column** (**VER**-teh-bral *or* **VER**-tee-bral), also known as the **spinal column**, consists of 26 **vertebrae** (**VER**-teh-bray) (singular, **vertebra**). The term *vertebral* means pertaining to the vertebrae.

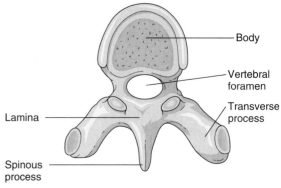

Figure 3.13   Structures of a thoracic vertebra.

- The functions of the spinal column are to support the head and body and to protect the spinal cord.

Structures of Vertebrae

As you study the following structures, refer to Figure 3.13.

- The **body** is the solid anterior portion of a vertebra.

- A **lamina** (**LAM**-ih-nah) is the posterior portion of a vertebra (plural, **laminae**). The transverse and spinous processes extend from this area.

- The **vertebral foramen** is the opening in the middle of the vertebra. The spinal cord passes through this opening.

Types of Vertebrae

As you study the types of vertebrae, refer to Figure 3.14.

- The **cervical vertebrae** (**SER**-vih-kal) are the first set of seven vertebrae that form the neck. They are also known as **C1** through **C7**. *Cervical* means pertaining to the neck.

- The **thoracic vertebrae** (thoh-**RASS**-ick) make up the second set of 12 vertebrae. They form the outward curve of the spine and are known as **T1** through **T12**.

- The **lumbar vertebrae** (**LUM**-bar) make up the third set of five vertebrae and form the inward curve of the lower spine. They are known as **L1** through **L5**. The lumbar vertebrae are the largest and strongest of the vertebrae and bear most of the body's weight.

Intervertebral Disks

The **intervertebral disks** (**in**-ter-**VER**-teh-bral), which are made of cartilage, separate and cushion the vertebrae from each other. These disks act as shock absorbers and allow for movement of the spinal column (Figure 3.21A).

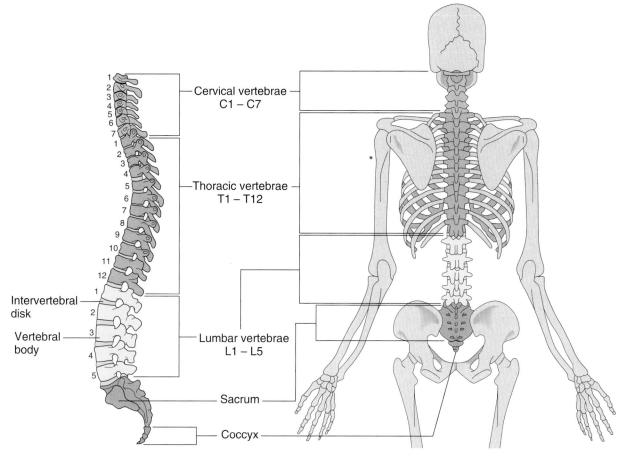

FIGURE 3.14   Lateral and posterior views of the spinal column.

Sacrum and Coccyx

As you study these structures, refer to Figures 3.14 and 3.15.

- The **sacrum** (**SAY**-krum) is the slightly curved, triangular-shaped bone near the base of the spine that forms the lower portion of the back. At birth, the sacrum is composed of five separate bones; however they fuse together in the young child to form a single bone.

- The **coccyx** (**KOCK**-sicks), also known as the **tailbone**, forms the end of the spine and is made up of four small vertebrae that are fused together.

Pelvic Girdle

The **pelvic girdle**, which protects internal organs and supports the lower extremities, is also known as the **pelvis** or **hips**. This structure consists of the ilium, ischium, and pubis (Figure 3.15).

- The **ilium** (**ILL**-ee-um) is the broad blade-shaped bone that forms the back and sides of the pubic bone. *Memory aid:* This is spelled with the letter *i* as in the word hip.

- The **sacroiliac** (**say**-kroh-**ILL**-ee-ack) is the slightly movable articulation between the sacrum and posterior portion of the ilium (**sacr/o** means sacrum, **ili** means ilium, and **-ac** means pertaining to).

- The **ischium** (**ISS**-kee-um), which forms the lower posterior portion of the pubic bone, bears the weight of the body while sitting.

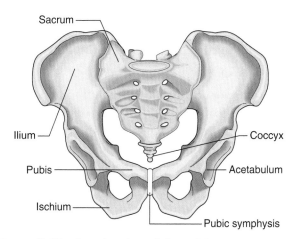

FIGURE 3.15   Anterior view of the pelvis.

- The **pubis** (**PEW**-bis), which forms the anterior portion of the pubic bone, is located just below the urinary bladder.

- The ilium, ischium, and pubis are separate at birth; however, they fuse to form the left and right **pubic bones**. These bones are held securely together by the pubic symphysis.

- The **pubic symphysis** (**PEW**-bick **SIM**-fih-sis), which is the cartilaginous joint formed at the anterior midline, holds the bones firmly together.

- The **acetabulum** (**ass**-eh-**TAB**-you-lum), also known as the **hip socket**, is the large circular cavity in each side of the pelvis that articulates with the head of the femur to form the hip joint (Figure 3.15).

Legs and Knees

As you study the following bones, refer to Figures 3.16 and 3.17.

Femur

The **femur** (**FEE**-mur) is the upper leg bone (Figure 3.16). Also known as the **thigh bone**, it is the largest bone in the body.

- The **head** of the femur articulates with the acetabulum (hip socket).

- The **femoral neck** (**FEM**-or-al) is the narrow area just below the head of the femur. *Femoral* means pertaining to the femur.

Knees

The knees are the complex joints that make possible movement between the upper and lower leg.

- The **patella** (pah-**TEL**-ah) is the bony anterior portion of the kneecap.

- The term **popliteal** (pop-**LIT**-ee-al) refers to the posterior surface of the knee and is used to describe the space, ligaments, vessels, and muscles in this area.

- The **anterior cruciate ligament (ACL)** and **posterior cruciate ligament (PCL)**, which are shown in Figure 3.4, make possible the movements of the knee. These are known as **cruciate ligaments** (**KROO**-shee-ayt) because they are shaped like a cross.

Lower Leg

The lower leg is made up of two bones: the tibia and the fibula (Figure 3.16).

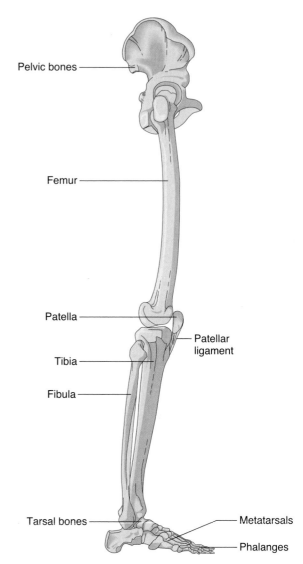

FIGURE 3.16   Lateral view of bones of the lower extremity.

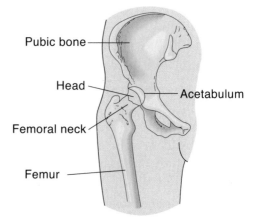

FIGURE 3.17   Structures of the proximal end of the femur and hip socket.

- The **tibia** (**TIB**-ee-ah), also known as the **shinbone**, is the larger weight-bearing bone in the anterior of the lower leg.
- The **fibula** (**FIB**-you-lah) is the smaller of the two bones of the lower leg.

The Ankles

The **tarsals** (**TAHR**-salz) are the five bones that make up each of the ankles (Figure 3.18).

- The **malleolus** (mal-**LEE**-oh-lus) is the rounded bony protuberance on each side of the ankle (plural, **malleoli**).
- The **talus** (**TAY**-luss) is the anklebone that articulates with the tibia and fibula (Figure 3.18).
- The **calcaneus** (kal-**KAY**-nee-uss), or **heel bone**, is the largest of the tarsal bones (Figure 3.18).

The Feet and Toes

- The five **metatarsals** (**met**-ah-**TAHR**-salz) form the part of the foot to which the toes are attached.
- The **phalanges** (fah-**LAN**-jeez) are the bones of the toes (singular, **phalanx**). The great toe has two phalanges. Each of the other toes has three phalanges. The term *phalanges* also means fingers.

MEDICAL SPECIALTIES RELATED TO THE SKELETAL SYSTEM

- A **chiropractor** (**KYE**-roh-**prack**-tor) holds a Doctor of Chiropractic degree and specializes in the manipulative treatment of disorders originating from misalignment of the spine.
- An **orthopedic surgeon**, also known as an **orthopedist** (**or**-thoh-**PEE**-dist), specializes in diagnosing

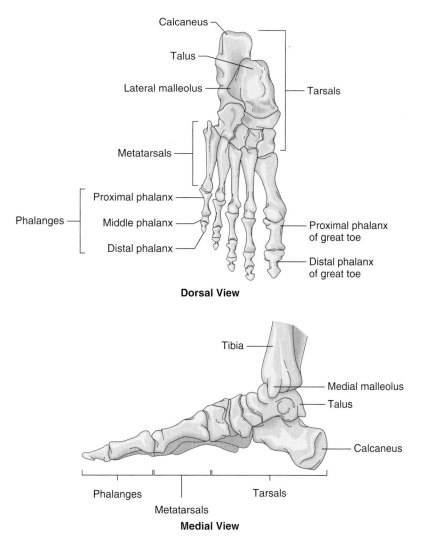

Dorsal View

Medial View

FIGURE 3.18 Superior and medial views of the bones of the right ankle and foot.

and treating diseases and disorders involving the bones, joints, and muscles.

- **Orthotics** (or-**THOT**-icks) is the field of knowledge relating to the making and fitting of orthopedic appliances, such as a brace or splint to support, align, prevent, or correct deformities or to improve the function of movable parts of the body.

- An **osteopathic physician** (**oss**-tee-oh-**PATH**-ick) holds a Doctor of Osteopathy degree and uses traditional forms of medical treatment in addition to specializing in treating health problems by spinal manipulation. This type of medical practice is known as **osteopathy** (**oss**-tee-**OP**-ah-thee); however, this term also means any bone disease (**oste/o** means bone and **-pathy** means disease). As used here, *manipulation* means changing the positions of the bones.

- A **podiatrist** (poh-**DYE**-ah-trist) holds a Doctor of Podiatry (DP) or Doctor of Podiatric Medicine (DPM) degree and specializes in diagnosing and treating disorders of the foot (**pod** mean foot and **-iatrist** means specialist).

- A **rheumatologist** (roo-mah-**TOL**-oh-jist) is a physician who specializes in the diagnosis and treatment of rheumatic diseases that are characterized by inflammation in the connective tissues.

- **Rheumatism** (**ROO**-mah-tizm) is a general term for a variety of acute and chronic conditions characterized by inflammation and deterioration of connective tissues. This group of disorders includes joint diseases such as arthritis and muscle disorders such as fibromyalgia (see Chapter 4).

PATHOLOGY OF THE SKELETAL SYSTEM

Joints

- **Ankylosis** (**ang**-kih-**LOH**-sis) is the loss, or absence, of mobility in a joint due to disease, injury, or a surgical procedure (**ankyl** means crooked, bent, or stiff and **-osis** means abnormal condition). *Mobility* means being capable of movement.

- **Arthralgia** (ar-**THRAL**-jee-ah) is pain in a joint (**arthr** means joint and **-algia** means pain).

- **Arthrosclerosis** (**ar**-throh-skleh-**ROH**-sis) is stiffness of the joints, especially in the elderly (**arthr/o** means joint and **-sclerosis** means abnormal hardening).

- **Bursitis** (ber-**SIGH**-tis) is an inflammation of a bursa (**burs** means bursa and **-itis** means inflammation).

- A **chondroma** (kon-**DROH**-mah) is a slow-growing benign tumor derived from cartilage cells (**chondr** means cartilage and **-oma** means tumor).

- **Chondromalacia** (**kon**-droh-mah-**LAY**-shee-ah) is the abnormal softening of the cartilage (**chondr/o** means cartilage and **-malacia** means abnormal softening).

- **Hallux valgus** (**HAL**-ucks **VAL**-guss), also known as a **bunion**, is an abnormal enlargement of the joint at the base of the great toe (*hallux* means big toe and *valgus* means bent).

- **Hemarthrosis** (**hee**-mahr-**THROH**-sis) or (**hem**-ar-**THROH**-sis) is blood within a joint space (**hem** means blood, **arthr** means joint, and **-osis** means abnormal condition). This condition occurs after trauma to a joint. It may also occur spontaneously in a patient who is receiving blood-thinning medications (see Chapter 5) or in individuals with a blood-clotting disorders such as hemophilia (see Chapter 2).

- **Synovitis** (sin-oh-**VYE**-tiss) is inflammation of the synovial membrane that results in swelling and pain of the affected joint (**synov** means synovial membrane and **-itis** means inflammation). This condition may be caused by an injury, infection, or irritation produced by damaged cartilage.

Dislocation

- **Dislocation**, also known as **luxation** (luck-**SAY**-shun), is the total displacement of a bone from its joint (Figure 3.19).

- **Subluxation** (**sub**-luck-**SAY**-shun) is the partial displacement of a bone from its joint.

Arthritis

Arthritis (ar-**THRIGH**-tis) is an inflammatory condition of one or more joints (**arthr** means joint and **-itis** means inflammation). There are many different forms and causes of arthritis (plural, **arthritides**).

- **Osteoarthritis** (**oss**-tee-oh-ar-**THRIGH**-tis), also known as **wear-and-tear arthritis**, is most commonly associated with aging (**oste/o** means bone, **arthr** means joint, and **-itis** means inflammation). OA is described as a *degenerative joint disease (DJD)* because it is characterized by the erosion of articular cartilage (Figure 3.20). *Erosion* means wearing away by friction or pressure.

- **Gouty arthritis** (**GOW**-tee ar-**THRIGH**-tis), also known as **gout**, is a type of arthritis caused by an

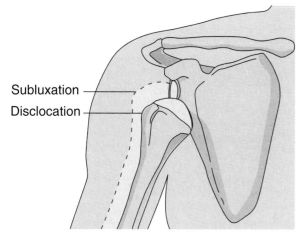

Subluxation

Dislocation

FIGURE 3.19 Subluxation and dislocation shown on a posterior view of the left shoulder.

excess of uric acid in the body. Gout occurs as episodes of sudden, severe attacks of pain and tenderness, redness, warmth, and swelling in the affected joints.

Rheumatoid Arthritis

Rheumatoid arthritis (**ROO**-mah-toyd ar-**THRIGH**-tis) is an autoimmune disorder in which the symptoms are generalized and usually more severe than those of osteoarthritis. In rheumatoid arthritis, the synovial membranes are inflamed and thickened. Other tissues are also attacked, causing the joints to become swollen, painful, and immobile.

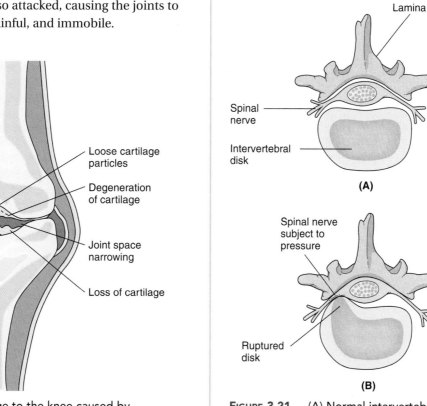

Loose cartilage particles

Degeneration of cartilage

Joint space narrowing

Loss of cartilage

FIGURE 3.20 Damage to the knee caused by osteoarthritis.

- **Ankylosing spondylitis** (**ang**-kih-**LOH**-sing **spon**-dih-**LYE**-tis) is a form of rheumatoid arthritis characterized by progressive stiffening of the spine due to the fusion of the vertebral bodies. *Ankylosing* means the progressive stiffening of a joint or joints. *Spondylitis* means the inflammation of the vertebrae (**spondyl** means vertebrae and **-itis** means inflammation).

- **Juvenile rheumatoid arthritis**, also known as juvenile idiopathic arthritis, affects children. Symptoms include pain and swelling in the joints, skin rash, fever, slowed growth, and fatigue (*idiopathic* means of unknown cause).

Spinal Column

- A **herniated disk** (**HER**-nee-**ayt**-ed), also known as a **ruptured disk**, is the breaking apart of an intervertebral disk that results in pressure on spinal nerve roots (Figure 3.21B).

- **Lumbago** (lum-**BAY**-goh), also known as **low back pain**, is pain of the lumbar region of the spine (**lumb** means lumbar and **-ago** means diseased condition) (Figure 3.14).

- **Spondylolisthesis** (**spon**-dih-loh-liss-**THEE**-sis) is the slipping forward movement of the body of one

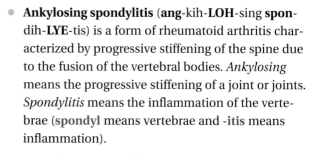

Lamina

Transverse process

Spinal nerve

Intervertebral disk

(A)

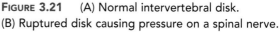

Spinal nerve subject to pressure

Ruptured disk

(B)

FIGURE 3.21 (A) Normal intervertebral disk. (B) Ruptured disk causing pressure on a spinal nerve.

of the lower lumbar vertebra on the vertebra below it, or on the sacrum (**spondyl/o** means vertebrae and **-listhesis** means slipping).

- **Spondylosis** (**spon**-dih-**LOH**-sis) is any degenerative disorder that may cause loss of normal spinal structure and function (**spondyl** means vertebrae and **-osis** means abnormal condition). The adjective *degenerative* describes the breaking down or impairment of a body part.

Spina Bifida

Spina bifida (**SPY**-nah **BIF**-ih-dah) is the congenital defect that occurs during early pregnancy in which the spinal canal fails to close around the spinal cord. (*Spina* means pertaining to the spine and *bifida* means split.) Many cases of spina bifida are due to a lack of the nutrient folic acid during the early stages of pregnancy.

Curvatures of the Spine

- **Kyphosis** (kye-**FOH**-sis) is an abnormal increase in the outward curvature of the thoracic spine as viewed from the side (**kyph** means hump and **-osis** means abnormal condition). This condition is also known as **humpback** or **dowager's hump** (Figure 3.22A).
- **Lordosis** (lor-**DOH**-sis) is an abnormal increase in the forward curvature of the lumbar spine (**lord** means bent backward and **-osis** means abnormal condition). This condition is also known as **swayback** (Figure 3.22B).
- **Scoliosis** (skoh-lee-**OH**-sis) is an abnormal lateral (sideways) curvature of the spine (**scoli** means curved and **-osis** means abnormal condition) (Figure 3.22C).

Bones

- **Craniostenosis** (kray-nee-oh-steh-**NOH**-sis) is a malformation of the skull due to the premature closure of the cranial sutures (**crani/o** means skull and **-stenosis** means abnormal narrowing).
- **Ostealgia** (oss-tee-**AL**-jee-ah), also spelled **ostalgia** or known as **osteodynia**, means pain in a bone (**ost** and **oste** both mean bone and **-algia** and **-dynia** both mean pain).
- **Osteitis** (oss-tee-**EYE**-tis), which is also spelled **ostitis**, is an inflammation of bone (**oste** means bone and **-itis** means inflammation).
- **Osteomalacia** (oss-tee-oh-mah-**LAY**-shee-ah), also known as **adult rickets**, is abnormal softening of bones in adults that is usually caused by a deficiency of vitamin D, calcium, or phosphate (**oste/o** means bone and **-malacia** means abnormal softening). Compare with *rickets*.
- **Osteomyelitis** (oss-tee-oh-**my**-eh-**LYE**-tis) is an inflammation of the bone marrow and adjacent bone (**oste/o** means bone, **myel** means bone marrow, and **-itis** means inflammation).
- **Osteonecrosis** (oss-tee-oh-neh-**KROH**-sis) is the destruction and death of bone tissue caused by an insufficient blood supply, infection, malignancy, or trauma (**oste/o** means bone and **-necrosis** means tissue death).

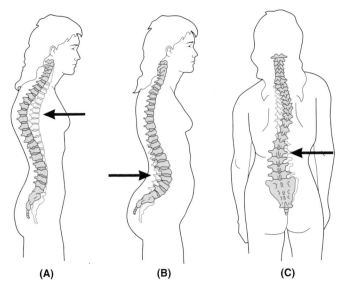

(A)   (B)   (C)

FIGURE 3.22   Abnormal curvatures of the spine. (A) Kyphosis. (B) Lordosis. (C) Scoliosis. (Normal curvatures are shown in shadow.)

- **Paget's disease** (**PAJ**-its), also known as **osteitis deformans** (**oss**-tee-**EYE**-tis dee-**FOR**-manz), is a disease of unknown cause that is characterized by extensive bone destruction followed by abnormal bone repair. As the disease progresses, the bones become deformed and weakened and may bend or break easily.
- **Periostitis** (**pehr**-ee-oss-**TYE**-tis), which is also spelled **periosteitis**, is an inflammation of the periosteum (**peri-** means surrounding, **ost** means bone, and **-itis** means inflammation).
- **Rickets** (**RICK**-ets), which occurs in children, is a disorder involving softening and weakening of the bones primarily caused by lack of vitamin D, calcium, or phosphate. Compare with *osteomalacia*.
- **Talipes** (**TAL**-ih-peez), also known as **clubfoot**, is a congenital deformity in which the foot is turned outward or inward as shown in Figure 3.23. This is so named because it involves the talus bone of the ankle.

Tumors of Bones

Malignancies and tumors are discussed further in Chapter 6.

- **Ewing's sarcoma** (**YOU**-ingz sar-**KOH**-mah), also known as **Ewing's family of tumors**, is a group of cancers that most frequently affects children or adolescents. A *sarcoma* is a malignant tumor of connective tissue, and in Ewing's sarcoma these tumors usually occur in the diaphyses of the long bones in the arms and legs. The disease may spread rapidly to other body sites.
- A **myeloma** (**my**-eh-**LOH**-mah) is a malignant tumor composed of blood-forming tissues of the bone marrow (**myel** means bone marrow and **-oma** means tumor). Myeloma may cause pathological fractures, and is often fatal.
- An **osteochondroma** (**oss**-tee-oh-kon-**DROH**-mah) is a benign bone tumor characterized by cartilage-capped bony growth that projects from the surface of the affected bone (**oste/o** means bone, **chondr** means cartilage, and **-oma** means tumor). This type of tumor is also known as an **exostosis** (**eck**-sos-**TOH**-sis) (plural, **exostoses**).

Osteoporosis

Osteoporosis (**oss**-tee-oh-poh-**ROH**-sis) is a marked loss of bone density and an increase in bone porosity that is frequently associated with aging (**oste/o** means bone, **por** means small opening, and **-osis** means abnormal condition).

- **Osteopenia** (**oss**-tee-oh-**PEE**-nee-ah) is thinner than average bone density in a young person (**oste/o** means bones and **-penia** means deficiency). This term is used to describe the condition of someone who does not yet have osteoporosis, but is at risk for developing it.

Osteoporotic Fractures

Osteoporosis is primarily responsible for three types of fractures:

- **Vertebral crush fractures**, also known as **compression fractures of the spine**, are caused by the spontaneous collapse of weakened vertebrae. This results in pain, loss of height, and development of the spinal curvature known as **dowager's hump**. These changes cause mobility problems, the crowding of the internal organs, and a reduction in lung capacity (Figure 3.24).
- **Colles' fracture**, also known as a **fractured wrist**, occurs at the lower end of the radius when a person tries to break a fall by landing on his or her hands. The impact of this fall causes the weakened bone to break (Figure 3.25).
- An **osteoporotic hip fracture** (**oss**-tee-oh-pah-**ROT**-ick), also known as a **broken hip**, can occur spontaneously or as the result of a fall. Complications from these fractures may result in the loss of function, mobility, independence, or death.

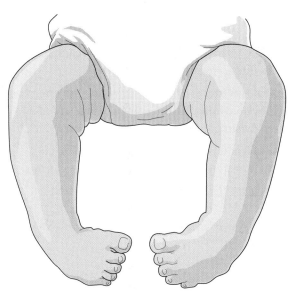

FIGURE 3.23   Talipes, also known as clubfoot, affects the ankles and causes the feet to turn inward.

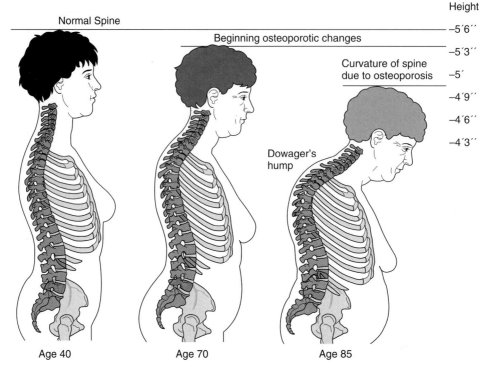

FIGURE 3.24   Curvature of the spine and related body changes caused by osteoporosis.

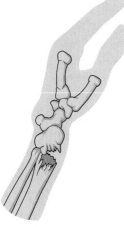

FIGURE 3.25   A Colles' fracture of the left wrist.

Fractures

A **fracture**, which is a broken bone, is described in terms of its complexity (Figure 3.26).

- A **closed fracture**, also known as a **simple** or **complete fracture**, is one in which the bone is broken but there is no open wound in the skin (see also Figure 3.27). Compare with an *open fracture*.

- An **open fracture**, also known as a **compound fracture**, is one in which the bone is broken and there is an open wound in the skin. Compare with a *closed fracture*.

- A **comminuted fracture** (**KOM**-ih-**newt**-ed) is one in which the bone is splintered or crushed. *Comminuted* means crushed into small pieces.

- A **compression fracture** occurs when the bone is pressed together (compressed) on itself (see Osteoporosis).

- A **greenstick fracture**, or **incomplete fracture**, is one in which the bone is bent and only partially broken. This type of fracture occurs primarily in children.

- An **oblique fracture** occurs at an angle across the bone.

- A **pathologic fracture** occurs when a bone, weakened due to a disease process, such as cancer, breaks under normal strain.

- A **spiral fracture** is a fracture in which the bone has been twisted apart. This occurs as the result of a severe twisting motion as in a sports injury.

- A **stress fracture**, which is an overuse injury, is a small crack in the bone that often develops from chronic, excessive impact. Overuse and sports injuries are discussed in Chapter 4.

- A **transverse fracture** occurs straight across the bone.

Additional Terms Associated with Fractures

- A **fat embolus** (**EM**-boh-lus) may form when a long bone is fractured and fat cells from yellow bone

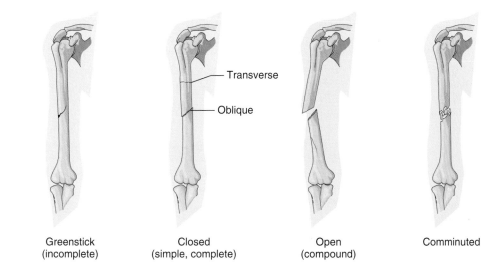

Transverse

Oblique

Greenstick
(incomplete)

Closed
(simple, complete)

Open
(compound)

Comminuted

FIGURE 3.26   Types of bone fractures.

marrow are released into the blood. An *embolus* is any foreign matter circulating in the blood that may become lodged and block the blood vessel.

- **Crepitation** (**krep**-ih-**TAY**-shun), also known as **crepitus** (**KREP**-ih-tus), is the crackling sound heard when the ends of a broken bone move together. The term *crepitation* also describes the sound heard in lungs affected with pneumonia and with the noisy discharge of gas from the intestine.

- As the bone heals, a **callus** (**KAL**-us) forms a bulging deposit around the area of the break. This tissue eventually becomes bone. A *callus* is also a thickening of the skin that is caused by repeated rubbing.

DIAGNOSTIC PROCEDURES OF THE SKELETAL SYSTEM

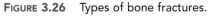

- **Radiographs**, also known as **x-rays**, are used to visualize bone fractures and other abnormalities (Figure 3.27).

- **Arthroscopy** (ar-**THROS**-koh-pee) is the visual examination of the internal structure of a joint (**arthr/o** means joint and **-scopy** means visual examination) using an **arthroscope** (Figure 3.28).

- A **bone marrow biopsy** is a diagnostic test to determine why blood cells are abnormal or to find a donor match for a bone marrow transplant. This test is performed by inserting a sharp needle into the hipbone or sternum and removing bone marrow cells.

- **Magnetic resonance imaging** is used to image soft tissue structures such as the interior of complex

joints. It is not the most effective method of imaging hard tissues such as bone.

- **Bone scans**, a form of nuclear medicine, and **arthrocentesis** are discussed in Chapter 15.

Bone Density Testing

Bone density testing is used to determine losses or changes in bone density. These tests are indicated for conditions such as osteoporosis, osteomalacia, and Paget's disease.

- **Ultrasonic bone density testing** is a screening test for osteoposoris or other conditions that cause a loss of bone mass. In this procedure sound waves are used to take measurements of the calcaneus (heel) bone. If the results indicate risks, more definitive testing is indicated.

- **Dual x-ray absorptiometry** (ab-**sorp**-shee-**OM**-eh-tree) produces more definitive results than ultrasonic bone density testing. DXA is a low-exposure radiographic measurement of the spine and hips that is able to detect early signs of osteoporosis.

TREATMENT PROCEDURES OF THE SKELETAL SYSTEM

Medications

- **Nonsteroidal anti-inflammatory drugs**, also known as **NSAIDs**, are administered to control pain and to reduce inflammation and swelling. Medications in this group may also thin the blood and attack the stomach lining. Examples of over-the-counter NSAIDs include aspirin, ibuprofen

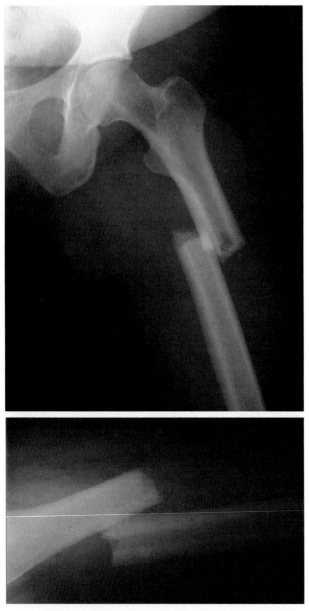

Figure 3.27   Radiographs of a closed (simple) fracture of the femur. Top: an anterior posterior (AP) view. Bottom: A lateral view of the same fracture. This view more exactly locates the ends of the fracture.

(Advil), and naproxen (Aleve and Naprosyn). Additional NSAIDs are available by prescription.

- **Acetaminophen** (ah-**seet**-ah-**MIN**-oh-fen), which is also known by the brand name Tylenol, controls pain without the side effects as NSAIDs; however, it does not have their ability to reduce inflammation and swelling.

- Aspirin and acetaminophen are also used as antipyretics. An **antipyretic** (**an**-tih-pye-**RET**-ick) is administered to reduce fever (**anti-** means against, **pyret** means fever, and **-ic** means pertaining to).

- **COX-2 inhibitors** control the pain and inflammation of osteoarthritis and rheumatoid arthritis with fewer side effects than with NSAIDs. These medications are named for the two *cyclooxygenase* (COX) enzymes that are associated with arthritic pain and inflammation.

Bone Marrow Transplants

A **bone marrow transplant**, also known as a **stem cell transplant**, is used to treat certain types of cancers, such as leukemia and lymphomas, that affect bone marrow. Stem cells are discussed in Chapter 2, leukemia is discussed in Chapter 5, and lymphomas are discussed in Chapter 6.

- In this treatment, both the cancer and the patient's bone marrow are destroyed with high-intensity radiation and chemotherapy.

- Next, healthy stem cells are transfused into the recipient's blood. These cells migrate to the spongy bone, where they grow into cancer-free red bone marrow.

Autologous Bone Marrow Transplant

In an **autologous** (aw-**TOL**-uh-guss) **bone marrow transplant**, the patient receives his own bone marrow, which was harvested before treatment began. *Autologous* means originating within an individual.

Allogenic Bone Marrow Transplant

An **allogenic** (**al**-oh-**JEN**-ick) **bone marrow transplant** may be a possibility if the patient's bone marrow cannot be utilized. In this type of transplant, the recipient (patient) receives bone marrow from a donor. However, unless this is a perfect match, there is the danger that the recipient's body will reject the transplant. *Allogenic* means originating within another.

Joints

- **Arthrodesis** (**ar**-throh-**DEE**-sis), also known as **fusion** or **surgical ankylosis**, is a surgical procedure to stiffen a joint, such as an ankle, elbow, or shoulder (**arthr/o** means joint and **-desis** means surgical fixation of bone or joint). This procedure is performed to treat severe arthritis or a damaged joint. Compare with *arthrolysis*.

- **Arthrolysis** (ar-**THROL**-ih-sis) is the surgical loosening of an ankylosed joint (**arthr/o** means joint and **-lysis** means loosening or setting free). *Note:* The suffix **-lysis** also means breaking down or destruction and may indicate either a pathologic state or a therapeutic procedure. Compare with *arthrodesis*.

- **Arthroscopic surgery** (**ar**-throh-**SKOP**-ick) is a minimally invasive procedure for the treatment of the interior of a joint. For example, torn cartilage may be removed with the use of an arthroscope and instruments inserted through small incisions (Figure 3.28).

- A **bursectomy** (ber-**SECK**-toh-mee) is the surgical removal of a bursa (**burs** means the bursa and **-ectomy** means surgical removal).

- **Chondroplasty** (**KON**-droh-**plas**-tee) is the surgical repair of damaged cartilage (**chondr/o** means cartilage and **-plasty** means surgical repair).

- A **synovectomy** (sin-oh-**VECK**-toh-mee) is the surgical removal of a synovial membrane from a joint (**synov** means synovial membrane and **-ectomy** means surgical removal). This procedure is performed to repair joint damage caused by rheumatoid arthritis.

- A **thermal capsulorrhaphy** (**kap**-soo-**LOR**-ah-fee) is an arthroscopic technique in which heat is used to shrink and tighten the tissues involved in shoulder instability disorders.

Joint Replacement

Based on its word parts, the term **arthroplasty** (**AR**-throh-**plas**-tee) means the surgical repair of a damaged joint (**arthr/o** means joint and **-plasty** means surgical repair); however, this term also has come to mean the surgical replacement of a joint with an artificial joint. These procedures are named for the involved joint and the amount of the joint that is replaced.

- The replacement part is a **prosthesis** (pros-**THEE**-sis), which is also known as an **implant** (Figure 3.29). The broader definition of *prosthesis* is a substitute for a diseased or missing part of the body (plural, **prostheses**).

- A **total knee replacement** means that all of the parts of the knee were replaced. This procedure is also known as a **total knee arthroplasty** (Figure 3.30).

- A **partial knee replacement** (**PKR**) means that only part of the knee was replaced.

- A **total hip replacement**, also known as a **total hip arthroplasty**, consists of a metal shaft with a ball at the top and a plastic lined cup. The metal shaft is fitted into the femur. The metal ball fits into the plastic lined cup that replaces the acetabulum within the hipbone (see Figure 3.29).

- **Revision surgery** is the replacement of a worn or failed implant.

Spinal Column

- A **percutaneous diskectomy** (per-kyou-**TAY**-nee-us dis-**KECK**-toh-mee) is performed to treat a herniat-

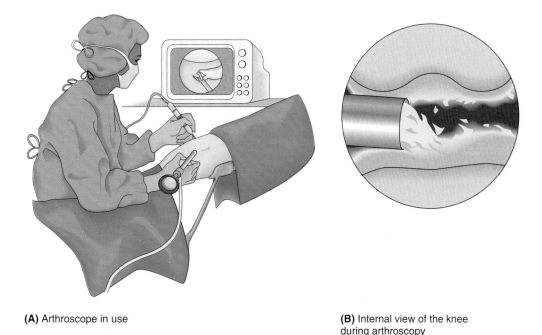

(A) Arthroscope in use

(B) Internal view of the knee during arthroscopy

FIGURE 3.28   Arthroscopic surgery. (A) The physician views progress on a monitor. (B) Internal view as diseased tissue is removed during surgery.

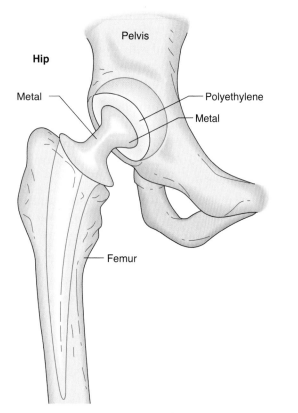

FIGURE 3.29 Components of a total hip replacement. Polyethylene, a smooth tough plastic, makes smooth movement possible.

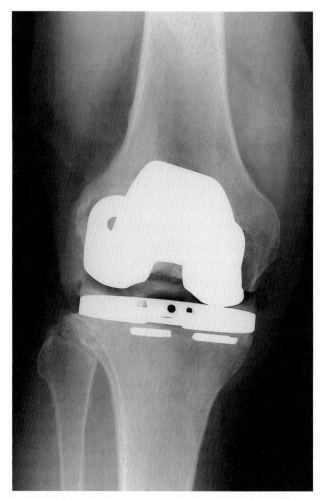

FIGURE 3.30 Radiograph (x-ray) of a total knee replacement. On the film, the metallic components appear brighter than the bone.

ed disk. In this procedure a thin tube is inserted through the skin of the back to suction out the ruptured disk or to vaporize it with a laser. *Percutaneous* means performed through the skin.

- A **percutaneous vertebroplasty** (**per**-kyou-**TAY**-nee-us **VER**-tee-broh-**plas**-tee) is performed to treat osteoporosis-related compression fractures (**vertebr/o** means vertebra and **-plasty** means surgical repair). In this minimally invasive procedure, bone cement is injected to stabilize compression fractures within the spinal column.

- A **laminectomy** (**lam**-ih-**NECK**-toh-mee) is the surgical removal of a lamina from a vertebra (**lamin** means lamina and **-ectomy** means surgical removal).

- **Spinal fusion** is a technique to immobilize part of the spine by joining together (fusing) two or more vertebrae. *Fusion* means to join together.

Bones

- A **craniectomy** (**kray**-nee-**EK**-toh-mee) is the surgical removal of a portion of the skull (**crani** means skull and **-ectomy** means surgical removal). This procedure is performed to treat craniostenosis.

- A **craniotomy** (**kray**-nee-**OT**-oh-mee), also known as a **bone flap**, is a surgical incision or opening into the skull (**crani** means skull and **-otomy** means a surgical incision). This procedure is performed to gain access to the brain to remove a tumor or to relieve intracranial pressure (Figure 3.31). Intracranial pressure is discussed in Chapter 10.

- A **cranioplasty** (**KRAY**-nee-oh-**plas**-tee) is the surgical repair of the skull (**crani/o** means skull and **-plasty** means surgical repair).

- **Osteoclasis** (**oss**-tee-**OCK**-lah-sis) is the surgical fracture of a bone to correct a deformity (**oste/o** means bone and **-clasis** means to break).

- An **ostectomy** (oss-**TECK**-toh-mee) is the surgical removal of bone (**ost** means bone and **-ectomy** means the surgical removal).

- **Osteoplasty** (**OSS**-tee-oh-**plas**-tee) is the surgical repair of a bone or bones (**oste/o** means bone and **-plasty** means surgical repair).

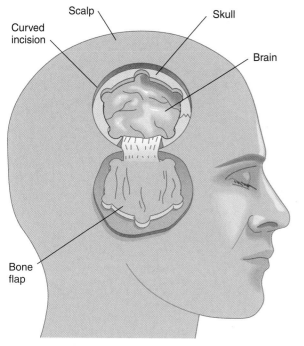

FIGURE **3.31** A craniotomy is performed to gain access to a portion of the brain.

- **Osteorrhaphy** (**oss**-tee-**OR**-ah-fee) is the surgical suturing, or wiring together, of bones (**oste/o** means bone and **-rrhaphy** means surgical suturing).

- **Osteotomy** (**oss**-tee-**OT**-oh-mee) is a surgical incision or sectioning of a bone (**oste** means bone and **-otomy** means a surgical incision).

- A **periosteotomy** (**pehr**-ee-**oss**-tee-**OT**-oh-mee) is an incision through the periosteum to the bone (**peri-** means surrounding, **oste** means bone, and **-otomy** means surgical incision).

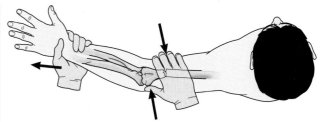

FIGURE **3.32** Closed reduction of a fractured left humerus.

Treatment of Fractures

- **Manipulation**, also known as **closed reduction**, is the attempted realignment of the bone involved in a fracture or joint dislocation. The affected bone is returned to its normal anatomic alignment by manually applied forces and then is usually immobilized to maintain the realigned position during healing (Figure 3.32).

- **Traction** is a pulling force exerted on a limb in a distal direction in an effort to return the bone or joint to normal alignment.

- **Immobilization**, also known as **stabilization**, is the act of holding, suturing, or fastening the bone in a fixed position with strapping or a cast.

External and Internal Fixation

- **External fixation** is a fracture treatment procedure in which pins are placed through the soft tissues and bone so that an external appliance can be used to hold the pieces of bone firmly in place during healing. When healing is complete, the appliance is removed (Figure 3.33).

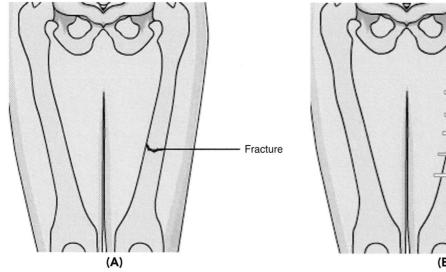
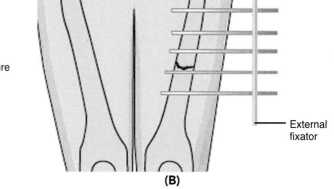

FIGURE **3.33** External fixation. (A) Fracture of the epiphysis of a femur. (B) External fixation stabilizes the bone and is removed after the bone has healed.

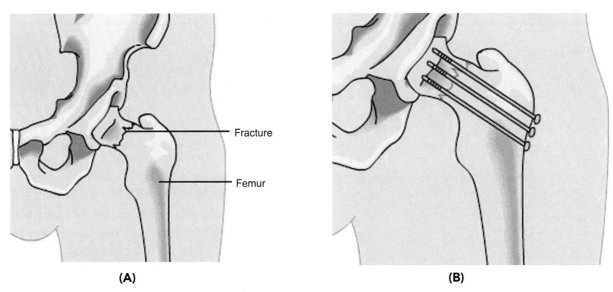

(A)   **(B)**

FIGURE 3.34   Internal fixation. (A) Fracture of the femoral neck. (B) Internal fixation pins are placed to stabilize the bone. These are not removed.

- **Internal fixation**, which is also known as **open reduction internal fixation (ORIF)**, is a fracture treatment in which pins or a plate are placed directly into the bone to hold the broken pieces in place. This form of fixation is *not* usually removed after the fracture has healed (Figure 3.34).

ABBREVIATIONS RELATED TO THE SKELETAL SYSTEM

Table 3.2 presents an overview of the abbreviations related to the terms introduced in this chapter. *Note:* To avoid errors or confusion, always be cautious when using abbreviations.

Table 3.2

ABBREVIATIONS RELATED TO THE SKELETAL SYSTEM

acetaminophen = APAP	**APAP** = acetaminophen
bone density testing = BDT	**BDT** = bone density testing
bone marrow biopsy = BMB	**BMB** = bone marrow biopsy
bone marrow transplant = BMT	**BMT** = bone marrow transplant
closed reduction = CR	**CR** = closed reduction
craniostenosis = CSO	**CSO** = craniostenosis
dual x-ray absorptiometry = DXA	**DXA** = dual x-ray absorptiometry
fracture = Fx	**Fx** = fracture
hallux valgus = HV	**HV** = hallux valgus
juvenile rheumatoid arthritis = JRA	**JRA** = juvenile rheumatoid arthritis
magnetic resonance imaging = MRI	**MRI** = magnetic resonance imaging

Table 3.2 (continued)

ABBREVIATIONS RELATED TO THE SKELETAL SYSTEM

nonsteroidal anti-inflammatory drug = NSAID	**NSAID** = nonsteroidal anti-inflammatory drug
osteoarthritis = OA	**OA** = osteoarthritis
osteoporosis = OP	**OP** = osteoporosis
open reduction internal fixation = ORIF	**ORIF** = open reduction internal fixation
partial knee replacement = PKR	**PKR** = partial knee replacement
rheumatoid arthritis = RA	**RA** = rheumatoid arthritis
spina bifida = SB	**SB** = spina bifida
total hip arthroplasty = THA	**THA** = total hip arthroplasty
total hip replacement = THR	**THR** = total hip replacement
total joint arthroplasty = TJA	**TJA** = total joint arthroplasty
total knee arthroplasty = TKA	**TKA** = total knee arthroplasty
total knee replacement = TKR	**TKR** = total knee replacement

Learning Exercises

● Matching Word Parts 1

Write the correct answer in the middle column.

Definition	Correct Answer	Possible Answers
3.1. hump	_____	ankyl/o
3.2. cartilage	_____	arthr/o
3.3. crooked, bent, or stiff	_____	-um
3.4. joint	_____	kyph/o
3.5. noun ending	_____	chondr/o

● Matching Word Parts 2

Write the correct answer in the middle column.

Definition	Correct Answer	Possible Answers
3.6. cranium, skull	_____	cost/o
3.7. rib	_____	crani/o
3.8. setting free, loosening	_____	-desis
3.9. spinal cord, bone marrow	_____	-lysis
3.10. surgical fixation of bone or joint	_____	myel/o

● **Matching Word Parts 3**

Write the correct answer in the middle column.

Definition	Correct Answer	Possible Answers
3.11. vertebra, vertebrae	_____	**oste/o**
3.12. curved	_____	**spondyl/o**
3.13. bent backward	_____	**lord/o**
3.14. synovial membrane	_____	**synovi/o, synov/o**
3.15. bone	_____	**scoli/o**

● **Definitions**

Select the correct answer and write it on the line provided.

3.16.   The shaft of a long bone is known as the _____ .

     diaphysis   distal epiphysis   endosteum   proximal epiphysis

3.17.   The ankles are made up of the _____ .

     carpals   metatarsals   phalanges   tarsals

3.18.   The upper portion of the sternum is the _____ .

     clavicle   mandible   manubrium   xiphoid process

3.19.   The _____ joints are movable.

     cartilaginous   fibrous   suture   synovial

3.20.   The _____ is the anterior portion of the pelvic girdle.

     ilium   ischium   pubis   sacrum

3.21.   The opening in a bone through which the blood vessels, nerves, and ligaments pass is a

     _____ .

     foramen   process   suture   symphysis

3.22.   The tissue that connects one bone to another bone is known as a/an _____ .

     articular cartilage   ligament   synovial membrane   tendon

3.23.   The hip socket is known as the _____ .

     acetabulum   malleolus   patella   trochanter

3.24.   The _____ are the bones of the fingers and toes.

        carpals   metatarsals   tarsals   phalanges

3.25.   A normal projection on the surface of a bone is a/an _____ .

        cruciate   exostosis   popliteal   process

● Matching Structures

Write the correct answer in the middle column.

Definition	Correct Answer	Possible Answers
3.26. breastbone	_____	clavicle
3.27. cheek bones	_____	olecranon
3.28. collar bone	_____	sternum
3.29. kneecap	_____	patella
3.30. point of the elbow	_____	zygomatic

● Which Word?

Select the correct answer and write it on the line provided.

3.31.   The surgical procedure to loosen an ankylosed joint is called _____ .

        arthrodesis   arthrolysis

3.32.   A physician who specializes in the diagnosis and treatment of diseases characterized by inflammation in the connective tissues is a/an _____ .

        orthopedist   rheumatologist

3.33.   An _____ transplant uses bone marrow from a donor.

        allogenic   autologous

3.34.   A percutaneous _____ is performed to treat osteoporosis related compression fractures.

        diskectomy   vertebroplasty

3.35.   The type of arthritis that is commonly known as wear-and-tear arthritis is _____ .

        osteoarthritis   rheumatoid arthritis

● Spelling Counts

Find the misspelled word in each sentence. Then write that word, spelled correctly, on the line provided.

3.36.   The medical term for the condition commonly known as low back pain is lumbaego. _____

3.37.   The surgical fracture of a bone to correct a deformity is known as osteclasis. _____

3.38.   Ankylosing spondilitis is a form of rheumatoid arthritis characterized by progressive stiffening of the

 spine. _____

3.39.   An osterrhaphy is the surgical suturing, or wiring together, of bones. _____

3.40.   Crepetation is the sound that is heard when the ends of a broken bone move together.

 _____

● Spelling Out Abbreviations

Write the correct answer on the line provided.

3.41.   **BMT** _____

3.42.   **Fx** _____

3.43.   **NSAID** _____

3.44.   **ORIF** _____

3.45.   **RA** _____

● Term Selection

Select the correct answer and write it on the line provided.

3.46.   The term meaning the death of bone tissue is _____.

 osteitis deformans   osteomyelitis   osteonecrosis   osteoporosis

3.47.   An abnormal increase in the forward curvature of the lower or lumbar spine is known as

 _____ .

 kyphosis   lordosis   scoliosis   spondylosis

3.48. The condition known as _____ is a congenital defect.

   juvenile arthritis   osteoarthritis   rheumatoid arthritis   spina bifida

3.49. A malignant tumor composed of cells derived from blood-forming tissues of the bone marrow is known

   as a/an _____ .

   chondroma   Ewing's sarcoma   myeloma   osteochondroma

3.50. The bulging deposit that forms around the area of the break during the healing of a fractured bone is a

   _____ .

   callus   crepitation   crepitus   luxation

● Sentence Completion

Write the correct term on the line provided.

3.51. A/An _____ is performed to treat a patient with craniostenosis.

3.52. The partial displacement of a bone from its joint is known as _____ .

3.53. The procedure, also known as fusion, that stiffens a joint or joins several vertebrae is a/an

   _____ .

3.54. The surgical procedure to replace a joint with an artificial joint is known as _____ .

3.55. A medical term for the condition commonly known as a bunion is _____ .

● Word Surgery

Divide each term into its component word parts. Write these word parts, in sequence, on the lines provided.

When necessary use a back slash (/) to indicate a combining vowel. (You may not need all of the lines provided.)

3.56. A **bursectomy** is the surgical removal of a bursa.

   _____   _____   _____   _____

3.57. An **osteochondroma** is the most common benign bone tumor.

   _____   _____   _____   _____

3.58. **Osteomalacia**, also known as adult rickets, is abnormal softening of bones in adults.

   _____   _____   _____   _____

3.59. **Periostitis** is an inflammation of the periosteum.

_____   _____   _____   _____

3.60. **Spondylolisthesis** is the forward movement of the body of one of the lower lumbar vertebra on the

vertebra below it.

_____   _____   _____   _____

● True/False

If the statement is true, write **T** on the line. If the statement is false, write **F** on the line.

3.61. _____ Osteopenia is thinner than average bone density in a young person.

3.62. _____ Paget's disease is caused by a deficiency of calcium and vitamin D in early childhood.

3.63. _____ A thermal capsulorrhaphy uses heat to shrink and tighten tissues involved in shoulder instability

disorders such as dislocation.

3.64. _____ Luxation is the partial displacement of a bone from its joint.

3.65. _____ Arthroscopic surgery is a minimally invasive procedure for the treatment of the interior of a joint.

● Clinical Conditions

Write the correct answer on the line provided.

3.66. When Bobby Kuhn fell out of a tree, the bone in his arm was partially bent and partially broken. Dr.

Parker described this as _____ fracture and told the family that this type of frac-

ture occurs primarily in children.

3.67. Eduardo Sanchez has an inflammation of the bone and bone marrow. The medical term for this condi-

tion is _____ .

3.68. Brent Hargraves, who is 16, was diagnosed as having _____ sarcoma. This is a

group of cancers that most frequently affect children or adolescents.

3.69. Mrs. Morton suffers from dowager's hump. The medical term for this abnormal curvature of the spine is

_____ .

3.70. Henry Turner specializes in creating _____ . These are orthopedic appliances to

align, prevent, or correct deformities or to improve the function of movable parts of the body.

3.71. After an auto accident, Tiffany required a/an _____ to relieve the intracranial pressure on her brain.

3.72. Mrs. Gilmer's leukemia is being treated with a bone marrow transplant. Some of her bone marrow was harvested so that she will be able to receive a/an _____ bone marrow transplant.

3.73. Betty Greene has been running for several years; however, now her knees hurt. Dr. Baskin diagnosed her condition as _____ , which is an abnormal softening of the cartilage in these joints.

3.74. Patty Turner (age 7) has symptoms that include a skin rash, fever, slowed growth, fatigue, and swelling in the joints. She was diagnosed as having juvenile _____ arthritis.

3.75. Robert Young has a very sore shoulder. Dr. Wilson diagnosed it as an inflammation of the bursa and called it _____ .

● Which Is the Correct Medical Term?

Select the correct answer and write it on the line provided.

3.76. Rodney Horner is being treated for a _____ fracture, in which the ends of the bones were crushed together.

    Colles'   comminuted   compound   spiral

3.77. Alex Jordon's doctor performed a/an _____ to surgically repair the cartilage that Alex damaged when she fell.

    arthroplasty   chondritis   chondroplasty   osteoplasty

3.78. Jane Parker is at high risk for osteoporosis. To obtain a definitive evaluation of her condition, Jane's doctor ordered a/an _____ test.

    blood calcium   DXA   MRI   ultrasonic bone density testing

3.79. In an effort to return a fractured bone to normal alignment, Dr. Wong ordered _____ . This procedure exerts a pulling force on the distal end of the affected limb.

    external fixation   immobilization   internal fixation   traction

3.80. Baby Juanita was treated for a congenital deformity in which her foot turned inward. Her family called this clubfoot; however the medical term for this condition is _____ .

    hallux valgus   rickets   scoliosis   talipes

● Challenge Word Building

These terms are *not* found in this chapter; however, they are made up of the following familiar word parts. You may want to look in the textbook glossary or use a medical dictionary to check your answers.

poly-	arthr/o	-ectomy
	chondr/o	-itis
	cost/o	-malacia
	crani/o	-otomy
	oste/o	-pathy
		-sclerosis

3.81. Abnormal hardening of bone is called _____ .

3.82. The surgical removal of a rib is a/an _____ .

3.83. The term meaning a disease of the cartilage is _____ .

3.84. A surgical incision into a joint is a/an _____ .

3.85. The term meaning inflammation of cartilage is _____ .

3.86. The surgical removal of a joint is a/an _____ .

3.87. The term meaning inflammation of more than one joint is _____ .

3.88. The term meaning any disease involving the bones and joints is _____ .

3.89. A surgical incision or division of a rib is a/an _____ .

3.90. The term meaning abnormal softening of the skull is _____ .

● **Labeling Exercises**

Identify the numbered items on the accompanying figures.

3.91. _____ vertebrae

3.92. _____

3.93. _____

3.94. _____

3.95. _____

3.96. _____

3.97. _____

3.98. _____

3.99. _____

3.100. _____

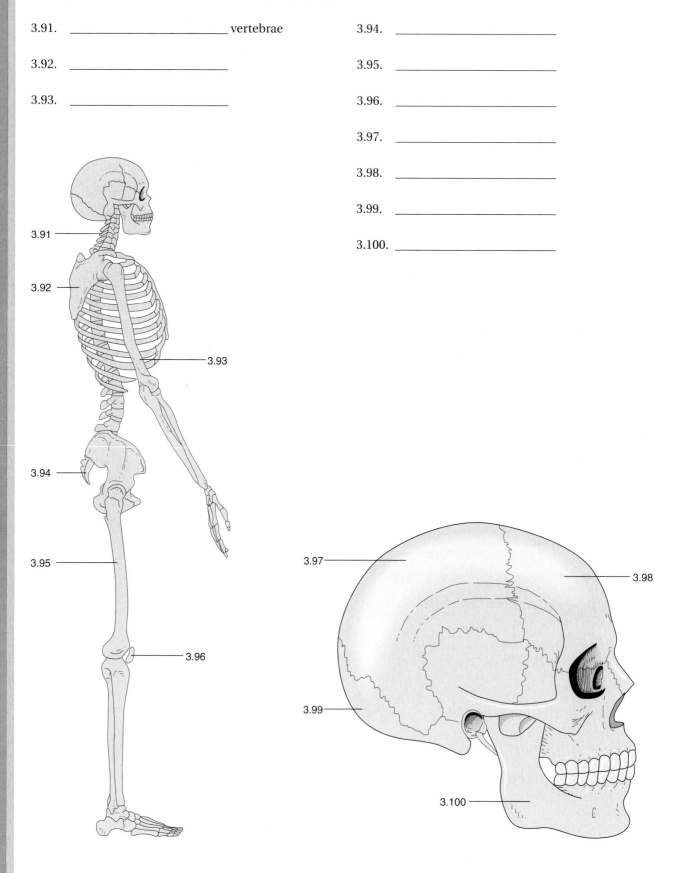

THE HUMAN TOUCH: CRITICAL THINKING EXERCISE

The following story and questions are designed to stimulate critical thinking through class discussion or as a brief essay response. There are no right or wrong answers to these questions.

Dr. Johnstone didn't like what he saw. The x-rays of Gladys Gwynn's hip showed a fracture of the femoral neck and severe osteoporosis of the hip. Mrs. Gwynn had been admitted to the orthopedic ward of Hamilton Hospital after a fall that morning at Sunny Meadows, an assisted-living facility. The accident had occurred when Sheri Smith, a new aide, lost her grip while helping Mrs. Gwynn in the shower.

A frail but alert and cheerful woman of 85, Gladys Gwynn has osteoarthritis and osteoporosis that have forced her to rely on a walker. She has been living at Sunny Meadows since her husband's death four years ago. Dr. Johnstone knew that she didn't have any relatives in the area, and he did not think that she had signed a health care power of attorney designating someone to help with medical decisions like this.

A total hip replacement (THP) would be the logical treatment for a younger patient because it could restore some of her lost mobility. However, for a frail patient like Mrs. Gwynn, internal fixation of the fracture might be the treatment of choice. This would repair the break but not improve her mobility.

Dr. Johnstone needed to make a decision soon, but Mrs. Gwynn was still groggy from the pain medication. With one more look at the x-ray, Dr. Johnstone sighed and walked toward Mrs. Gwynn's room.

Suggested Discussion Topics:

1. Gladys Gwynn has no children or other relatives in the area and is unable to speak for herself. Who should decide which surgery should be performed?

2. Do you think Sheri Smith or Sunny Meadows should be held responsible for Mrs. Gwynn's accident? If so, who should be held responsible?

3. A total hip replacement is more expensive than the internal fixation procedure and has a longer, more strenuous recovery period. Given the patient's condition and the limited dollars available for health care, which procedure should be performed?

4. Would you have answered Question 3 differently if Mrs. Gwynn were your mother?

5. If Mrs. Gwynn's recovery does not go well and she is no longer able to get around by herself, will she be allowed to continue living at Sunny Meadows?

4 The Muscular System

● Overview of Structures, Combining Forms, and Functions of the Muscular System

MAJOR STRUCTURES	RELATED COMBINING FORMS	PRIMARY FUNCTIONS
Muscles	my/o, myos/o	Make body movement possible, hold body erect, move body fluids, and produce body heat.
Fascia	fasci/o	Cover, support, and separate muscles.
Tendons	ten/o, tend/o, tendin/o	Attach muscles to bones.

● **VOCABULARY**   **RELATED TO THE MUSCULAR SYSTEM**

The items on this list have been identified as key word parts and terms for this chapter. However, all words in boldface in the text are important and may be included in the learning exercises and tests.

Word Parts

- [ ] bi-
- [ ] -cele
- [ ] dys-
- [ ] fasci/o
- [ ] -ia
- [ ] -ic
- [ ] kinesi/o
- [ ] fibr/o
- [ ] my/o
- [ ] -plegia
- [ ] -rrhexis
- [ ] tax/o
- [ ] ten/o, tend/o, tendin/o
- [ ] ton/o
- [ ] tri-

Medical Terms

- [ ] **abduction** (ab-**DUCK**-shun)
- [ ] **Achilles tendinitis** (**ten**-dih-**NIGH**-tis)
- [ ] **adduction** (ah-**DUCK**-shun)
- [ ] **adhesion** (ad-**HEE**-zhun)
- [ ] **anticholinergic** (**an**-tih-**koh**-lin-**ER**-jik)
- [ ] **ataxia** (ah-**TACK**-see-ah)
- [ ] **atonic** (ah-**TON**-ick)
- [ ] **atrophy** (**AT**-roh-fee)
- [ ] **atropine** (**AT**-roh-peen)
- [ ] **bradykinesia** (**brad**-ee-kih-**NEE**-zee-ah *or* **brad**-ee-kih-**NEE**-zhuh)
- [ ] **carpal tunnel syndrome** (**KAR**-pul)
- [ ] **circumduction** (**ser**-kum-**DUCK**-shun)
- [ ] **contracture** (kon-**TRACK**-chur)
- [ ] **dorsiflexion** (**dor**-sih-**FLECK**-shun)
- [ ] **dyskinesia** (**dis**-kih-**NEE**-zee-ah)
- [ ] **dystaxia** (dis-**TACK**-see-ah)
- [ ] **dystonia** (dis-**TOH**-nee-ah)
- [ ] **electromyography** (ee-**leck**-troh-my-**OG**-rah-fee)
- [ ] **electroneuromyography** (ee-**leck**-troh-**new**-roh-my-**OG**-rah-fee)
- [ ] **epicondylitis** (ep-ih-**kon**-dih-**LYE**-tis)

- [ ] **ergonomics** (er-goh-**NOM**-icks)
- [ ] **fasciitis** (**fas**-ee-**EYE**-tis)
- [ ] **fascioplasty** (**FASH**-ee-oh-**plas**-tee)
- [ ] **fibromyalgia syndrome** (**figh**-broh-my-**AL**-jee-ah)
- [ ] **ganglion cyst** (**GANG**-glee-on **SIST**)
- [ ] **hemiparesis** (**hem**-ee-pah-**REE**-sis)
- [ ] **hemiplegia** (**hem**-ee-**PLEE**-jee-ah)
- [ ] **hyperkinesia** (**high**-per-kye-**NEE**-zee-ah)
- [ ] **hypertonia** (**high**-per-**TOH**-nee-ah)
- [ ] **hypokinesia** (**high**-poh-kye-**NEE**-zee-ah)
- [ ] **hypotonia** (**high**-poh-**TOH**-nee-ah)
- [ ] **impingement syndrome** (im-**PINJ**-ment **SIN**-drohm)
- [ ] **intermittent claudication** (klaw-dih-**KAY**-shun)
- [ ] **kinesiology** (kih-**nee**-see-**OL**-oh-jee)
- [ ] **muscular dystrophy** (**DIS**-troh-fee)
- [ ] **myalgia** (my-**AL**-jee-ah)
- [ ] **myasthenia gravis** (**my**-as-**THEE**-nee-ah **GRAH**-vis)
- [ ] **myocele** (**MY**-oh-seel)
- [ ] **myoclonus** (**my**-oh-**KLOH**-nus *or* my-**OCK**-loh-nus)
- [ ] **myofascial damage** (**my**-oh-**FASH**-ee-ahl)
- [ ] **myolysis** (my-**OL**-ih-sis)
- [ ] **myoparesis** (**my**-oh-**PAR**-eh-sis)
- [ ] **myorrhaphy** (my-**OR**-ah-fee)
- [ ] **myositis** (**my**-oh-**SIGH**-tis)
- [ ] **myotonia** (**my**-oh-**TOH**-nee-ah)
- [ ] **paraplegia** (**par**-ah-**PLEE**-jee-ah)
- [ ] **physiatrist** (**fiz**-ee-**AT**-rist)
- [ ] **plantar fasciitis** (**PLAN**-tar **fas**-ee-**EYE**-tis)
- [ ] **polymyositis** (**pol**-ee-**my**-oh-**SIGH**-tis)
- [ ] **pronation** (proh-**NAY**-shun)
- [ ] **quadriplegia** (**kwad**-rih-**PLEE**-jee-ah)
- [ ] **sarcopenia** (**sar**-koh-**PEE**-nee-ah)
- [ ] **singultus** (sing-**GUL**-tus)
- [ ] **spasmodic torticollis** (spaz-**MOD**-ick **tor**-tih-**KOL**-is)
- [ ] **sphincter** (**SFINK**-ter)
- [ ] **supination** (**soo**-pih-**NAY**-shun)
- [ ] **tenodesis** (ten-**ODD**-eh-sis)
- [ ] **tenodynia** (**ten**-oh-**DIN**-ee-ah)
- [ ] **tenolysis** (ten-**OL**-ih-sis)
- [ ] **tenorrhaphy** (ten-**OR**-ah-fee)

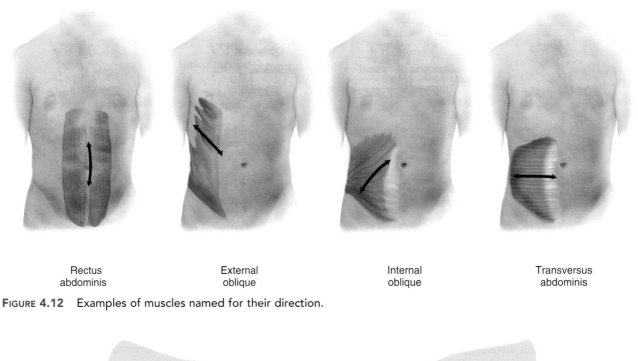

| Rectus abdominis | External oblique | Internal oblique | Transversus abdominis |

FIGURE 4.12 Examples of muscles named for their direction.

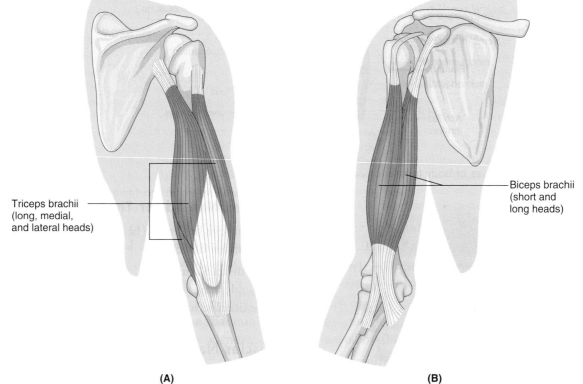

FIGURE 4.13 Muscles named for the number of divisions. (A) Posterior view. (B) Anterior view.

MEDICAL SPECIALTIES RELATED TO THE MUSCULAR SYSTEM

Specialists Treating Skeletal Muscle Disorders

- An **orthopedic surgeon** treats injuries and disorders involving bones, joints, muscles, and tendons.

- A **rheumatologist** (roo-mah-**TOL**-oh-jist) treats disorders that involve the inflammation of connective tissues, including muscles.

- A **neurologist** (new-**ROL**-oh-jist) treats the cause of paralysis and similar muscular disorders in which there is a loss of function.

- A **physiatrist** (fiz-ee-**AT**-rist) is a physician who specializes in physical medicine and rehabilitation. This specialty includes treating problems ranging from sore shoulders to spinal cord injuries, with the focus on restoring function.
- A **sports medicine physician** is a specialist who treats sports-related injuries of the bones, joints, and muscles.

Specialists Treating Smooth Muscle Disorders

Smooth muscles are a key component in most body systems. The specialist who treats the involved body system also cares for any muscle disorders within that body system.

Specialists Treating Myocardial Muscle Disorders

- A **cardiologist** treats disorders of the myocardial muscle; these are discussed in Chapter 5.

PATHOLOGY OF THE MUSCULAR SYSTEM

Fibers, Fascia, and Tendons

- **Fasciitis** (fas-ee-**EYE**-tis) is inflammation of a fascia (**fasci** means fascia and **-itis** means inflammation). *Note:* This term is spelled correctly with a double *i*; however, *fascitis* is also an acceptable spelling.
- **Tenodynia** (ten-oh-**DIN**-ee-ah) is pain in a tendon (**ten/o** means tendon and **-dynia** means pain).
- **Tendonitis** (ten-doh-**NIGH**-itis) is an inflammation of the tendons caused by excessive or unusual use of the joint (**tendon** means tendon and **-itis** means inflammation). The terms *tendinitis, tenonitis,* and *tenontitis* all have the same meaning.

Muscles

- An **adhesion** (ad-**HEE**-zhun) is a band of fibrous tissue that holds structures together abnormally. Adhesions can form in muscles or internal organs as the result of an injury or surgery.
- **Atrophy** (**AT**-roh-fee) means weakness or wearing away of body tissues and structures. **Muscle atrophy** can be caused by pathology or by disuse of the muscle over a long period of time.
- **Myalgia** (my-**AL**-jee-ah) is muscle tenderness or pain (**my** means muscle and **-algia** means pain).

- **Myolysis** (my-**OL**-ih-sis) is the degeneration of muscle tissue (**my/o** means muscle and **-lysis** means destruction or breaking down in disease). *Degeneration* means deterioration or breaking down.
- **Myomalacia** (my-oh-mah-**LAY**-shee-ah) is abnormal softening of muscle tissue (**my/o** means muscle and **-malacia** means abnormal softening). Compare with *myosclerosis.*
- **Myorrhexis** (my-oh-**RECK**-sis) is the rupture of a muscle (**my/o** means muscle and **-rrhexis** means rupture).
- **Myosclerosis** (my-oh-skleh-**ROH**-sis) is abnormal hardening of muscle tissue (**my/o** means muscle and **-sclerosis** means abnormal hardening). Compare with *myomalacia.*
- **Myositis** (my-oh-**SIGH**-tis) is the inflammation of a skeletal muscle (**myos** means muscle and **-itis** means inflammation).
- **Polymyositis** (pol-ee-my-oh-**SIGH**-tis) is the inflammation of several skeletal muscles at the same time (**poly-** means many, **myos** means muscle, and **-itis** means inflammation).
- **Sarcopenia** (sar-koh-**PEE**-nee-ah) is the age-related reduction in skeletal muscle mass in the elderly (**sarc/o** means flesh and **-penia** means deficiency). A weight or resistance training program can significantly improve muscle mass and slow, but not stop, this process.

Hernias

- A **hernia** (**HER**-nee-ah) is the protrusion of a part or structure through the tissues normally containing it.
- A **myocele** (**MY**-oh-seel) is the protrusion of a muscle through its ruptured sheath or fascia (**my/o** means muscle and **-cele** means a hernia).

Muscle Tone

- **Atonic** (ah-**TON**-ick) means lacking normal tone or strength (**a-** means without, **ton** means tone, and **-ic** means pertaining to).
- **Dystonia** (dis-**TOH**-nee-ah) is a condition of abnormal muscle tone (**dys-** means bad, **ton** means tone, and **-ia** means condition).
- **Hypertonia** (high-per-**TOH**-nee-ah) is a condition of excessive tone of the skeletal muscles (**hyper-** means excessive, **ton** means tone, and **-ia** means condition). Compare with *hypotonia.*

- **Hypotonia** (**high**-poh-**TOH**-nee-ah) is a condition in which there is diminished tone of the skeletal muscles (**hypo-** means deficient, **ton** means tone, and **-ia** means condition). Compare with *hypertonia*.

- **Myotonia** (**my**-oh-**TOH**-nee-ah) is the delayed relaxation of a muscle after a strong contraction (**my/o** means muscle, **ton** means tone, and **-ia** means condition).

Voluntary Muscle Movement

- **Ataxia** (ah-**TACK**-see-ah) is the inability to coordinate muscle activity during voluntary movement (**a-** means without, **tax** means coordination, and **-ia** means condition).

- **Dystaxia** (dis-**TACK**-see-ah), also known as **partial ataxia**, is difficulty in controlling voluntary movement (**dys-** means bad, **tax** means coordination, and **-ia** means condition).

- A **contracture** (kon-**TRACK**-chur) is the permanent tightening of fascia, muscles, tendons, ligaments, or skin that occurs when normally elastic connective tissues are replaced with nonelastic fibrous tissues. The most common cause of contractures are scarring and the lack of use due to immobilization or inactivity.

- **Intermittent claudication** (klaw-dih-**KAY**-shun) is pain in the leg muscles that occurs in the legs during exercise and is relieved by rest. *Intermittent* means coming and going at intervals and *claudication* means limping. This condition is caused by poor circulation in the legs.

- A **spasm** is a sudden, violent, involuntary contraction of one or more muscles.

- A **cramp** is a localized muscle spasm named for its cause such as a heat cramp or writer's cramp.

- **Spasmodic torticollis** (spaz-**MOD**-ick **tor**-tih-**KOL**-is), also known as **wryneck**, is a stiff neck due to spasmodic contraction of the neck muscles that pull the head toward the affected side. *Spasmodic* means relating to a spasm and *torticollis* means a contraction, or shortening, of the muscles of the neck.

Muscle Function

- **Bradykinesia** (**brad**-ee-kih-**NEE**-zee-ah *or* **brad**-ee-kih-**NEE**-zhuh) is extreme slowness in movement (**brady-** means slow, **kines** means movement, and **-ia** means condition).

- **Dyskinesia** (**dis**-kih-**NEE**-zee-ah) is the distortion or impairment of voluntary movement as in a tic or spasm (**dys-** means bad, **kines** means movement, and **-ia** means condition). A *tic* is a spasmodic muscular contraction that often involves parts of the face. Although these movements appear purposeful, they are not under voluntary control.

- **Hyperkinesia** (**high**-per-kye-**NEE**-zee-ah), also known as **hyperactivity**, is abnormally increased motor function or activity (**hyper-** means excessive, **kines** means movement, and **-ia** means condition). Compare with *hypokinesia*.

- **Hypokinesia** (**high**-poh-kye-**NEE**-zee-ah) is abnormally decreased motor function or activity (**hypo-** means deficient, **kines** means movement, and **-ia** means condition). Compare with *hyperkinesia*.

Myoclonus

Myoclonus (**my**-oh-**KLOH**-nus *or* my-**OCK**-loh-nus) is a spasm or twitching of a muscle or group of muscles (**my/o** means muscle, **clon** mean violent action, and **-us** is a singular noun ending).

- **Nocturnal myoclonus** (nock-**TER**-nal **my**-oh-**KLOH**-nus *or* my-**OCK**-loh-nus) is jerking of the limbs that can occur normally as a person is falling asleep. *Nocturnal* means pertaining to night.

- **Singultus** (sing-**GUL**-tus), also known as **hiccups**, is myoclonus of the diaphragm that causes the characteristic hiccup sound with each spasm.

Myasthenia Gravis

Myasthenia gravis (**my**-as-**THEE**-nee-ah **GRAH**-vis) is a chronic autoimmune disease that affects the neuromuscular junction and produces serious weakness of voluntary muscles. *Myasthenia* means muscle weakness (**my** means muscle and **-asthenia** means weakness or lack of strength). *Gravis* comes from the Latin meaning grave or serious.

Muscular Dystrophy

Muscular dystrophy (**DIS**-troh-fee) is a group of inherited muscle disorders that cause muscle weakness without affecting the nervous system. There are more than 20 specific genetic disorders considered to be MD. The two most common forms are Duchenne's muscular dystrophy and Becker's muscular dystrophy.

- **Duchenne's muscular dystrophy** (doo-**SHENZ**), which affects only males, appears between 2 and 6 years of age and progresses slowly. Survival is rare beyond the late twenties.

- **Becker's muscular dystrophy** (**BECK**-urz), which also affects only males, is a less severe illness than DMD. BMD does not appear until early adolescence or adulthood and the progression is slower with survival usually well into middle to late adulthood.

Fibromyalgia Syndrome

Fibromyalgia syndrome (**figh**-broh-my-**AL**-jee-ah) is a chronic, often disabling, condition of unknown cause characterized by uncontrollable fatigue and widespread pain in the muscles, ligaments, and tendons (**fibr/o** means fibrous connective tissue, **my** means muscle, and **-algia** means pain).

Repetitive Motion Disorders

Repetitive motion disorders, also known as **repetitive stress disorders**, are a variety of muscular conditions that result from repeated motions performed in the course of normal work, daily activities, or recreation such as sports. The symptoms caused by these repetitive motions involve muscles, tendons, nerves, and joints.

- **Overuse injuries** are minor tissue injuries that have not been given time to heal. Such injuries can be caused by spending hours at the keyboard or by lengthy sports training sessions. For example, **overuse tendinitis**, also known as **overuse tendinosis**, is inflammation of tendons caused by excessive or unusual use of a joint.

- **Stress fractures**, which are also overuse injuries, are discussed in Chapter 3.

- The term **ergonomics** (er-goh-**NOM**-icks) describes the study of human factors that affect the design and operation of tools and the work environment. This term is usually applied to the design of equipment and workspaces.

Myofascial Damage

Myofascial damage (**my**-oh-**FASH**-ee-ahl), which can be caused by overworking the muscles, results in tenderness and swelling of the muscles and their surrounding fascia (**my/o** means muscle, **fasci** means fascia, and **-al** means pertaining to).

Rotator Cuff Injuries

- **Rotator cuff tendinitis** (ten-dih-**NIGH**-tis) is an inflammation of the tendons of the rotator cuff (Figure 4.14). This condition is often named for the cause, such as **tennis shoulder** or **pitcher's shoulder**.

- If rotator cuff tendinitis is left untreated, or if the overuse continues, the irritated tendon can weaken and tear, becoming a **torn tendon**. A torn tendon can also be caused by an injury.

- **Impingement syndrome** (im-**PINJ**-ment) occurs when inflamed and swollen tendons are caught in the narrow space between the bones within the shoulder joint.

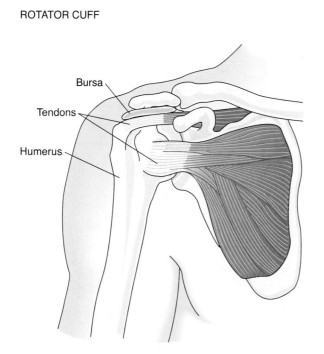
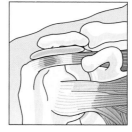
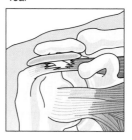

FIGURE 4.14 The rotator cuff in health (left) and with injuries (right).

Carpal Tunnel Syndrome

- The **carpal tunnel** (**KAR**-pul) is a narrow bony passage under the carpal ligament located 1/4 inch below the inner surface of the wrist. The median nerve and the nine tendons that bend the fingers pass through this tunnel. *Carpal* means pertaining to the wrist.

- **Carpal tunnel syndrome** symptoms occur when the tendons passing through the carpal tunnel are chronically overused and become inflamed and swollen (Figure 4.15). This swelling creates pressure on the median nerve as it passes through the carpal tunnel. This causes pain, burning, and paresthesia in the fingers and hand. *Paresthesia* is an abnormal sensation, such as burning, tingling, or numbness.

- **Carpal tunnel release** is the surgical enlargement of the carpal tunnel or cutting of the carpal ligament to relieve nerve pressure. This treatment is used to relieve the pressure on tendons and nerves in severe cases of carpal tunnel syndrome.

- A **ganglion cyst** (**GANG**-glee-on **SIST**) is a harmless fluid-filled swelling that occurs most commonly on the outer surface of the wrist. This condition, which can be caused by repeated minor injuries, is usually painless and does not require treatment. (Do not confuse this use of the term *ganglion* here with the nerve ganglions described in Chapter 10.)

Epicondylitis

Epicondylitis (**ep**-ih-**kon**-dih-**LYE**-tis) is inflammation of the tissues surrounding the elbow (**epi-** means on, **condyl-** means condyle, and **-itis** means inflammation).

- *Lateral epicondylitis*, with pain on the outer side of the arm of the forearm, is also known as *tennis elbow.*

- *Medial epicondylitis*, with pain on the palm-side of the forearm, is also known as *golfer's elbow.*

Plantar Fasciitis and Heel Spurs

- **Plantar fasciitis** (**PLAN**-tar **fas**-ee-**EYE**-tis) is an inflammation of the plantar fascia causing foot or heel pain when walking or running.

- **Heel spurs**, which are hardened deposits in the plantar fascia near its attachment to the heel, usually result from repetitive stresses and inflammation in the plantar fascia (Figure 4.16).

Sports Injuries

The following injuries are frequently associated with sports overuse; however, some can also be caused by other forms of trauma.

- A **sprain** is an injury to a joint, such as ankle, knee, or wrist, that usually involves a stretched or torn ligament.

- A **strain** is an injury to the body of the muscle or the attachment of a tendon. Strains usually are associated with overuse injuries that involve a stretched or torn muscle or tendon attachment.

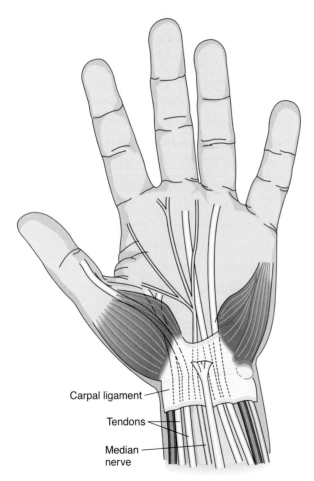

Carpal ligament

Tendons

Median nerve

FIGURE 4.15 Carpal tunnel syndrome.

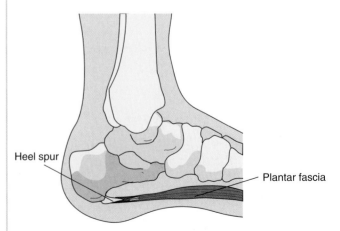

Heel spur

Plantar fascia

FIGURE 4.16 Plantar fasciitis and heel spur.

- A **shin splint** is a painful condition caused by the muscle tearing away from the tibia, which is also known as the **shinbone**. Shin splints can develop in the anterolateral (front and side) muscles or in the posteromedial (back and side) muscles of the lower leg (Figures 4.9 and 4.10). This type of injury is usually caused by repeated stress to the lower leg, such as playing soccer.

- A **hamstring injury** may be a strain or tear on any of the three hamstring muscles that straighten the hip and bend the knee. If these muscles contract too quickly it can cause an injury characterized by sudden and severe pain in the back of the thigh.

- **Achilles tendinitis** (**ten**-dih-**NIGH**-tis) is a painful inflammation of the Achilles tendon caused by excessive stress being placed on that tendon.

Paralysis

Paralysis (pah-**RAL**-ih-sis) is the loss of sensation and voluntary muscle movements in a muscle through disease or injury to its nerve supply. Damage may be either temporary or permanent (plural, **paralyses**).

- **Myoparesis** (**my**-oh-**PAR**-eh-sis) is a weakness or slight paralysis of a muscle (**my/o** means muscle and **-paresis** means partial or incomplete paralysis).

- **Hemiparesis** (**hem**-ee-pah-**REE**-sis) is slight paralysis of one side of the body (**hemi-** means half and **-paresis** means partial or incomplete paralysis). Compare with *hemiplegia*.

- **Hemiplegia** (**hem**-ee-**PLEE**-jee-ah) is the total paralysis of one side of the body (**hemi-** means half and **-plegia** means paralysis). This form of paralysis is usually associated with a stroke or brain damage. Damage to one side of the brain causes paralysis on the opposite side of the body. An individual affected with hemiplegia is known as a *hemiplegic*. Compare with *hemiparesis*.

- **Cardioplegia** (**kar**-dee-oh-**PLEE**-jee-ah) is paralysis of the muscles of the heart (**cardi/o** means heart and **-plegia** means paralysis).

Paralysis Due to Spinal Cord Injuries

A **spinal cord injury (SCI)** causes paralysis when the damage prevents nerve impulses from being transmitted below the level of the injury (Figure 4.17).

- **Paraplegia** (**par**-ah-**PLEE**-jee-ah) is the paralysis of both legs and the lower part of the body. An SCI below the cervical vertebrae results in paraplegia.

An individual affected with paraplegia is known as a *paraplegic*.

- **Quadriplegia** (**kwad**-rih-**PLEE**-jee-ah) is the paralysis of all four extremities (**quadri** means four and **-plegia** means paralysis). An SCI involving the cervical vertebrae causes quadriplegia. If the injury is above C5, it also affects respiration. An individual affected with quadriplegia is known as a *quadriplegic*.

DIAGNOSTIC PROCEDURES OF THE MUSCULAR SYSTEM

- **Deep tendon reflexes** are tested with a reflex hammer used to strike a tendon. Figure 4.18 shows reflex testing on the kneecap (patellar reflex) and Achilles tendon (calcaneus reflex). No response, or an abnormal response, may indicate a disruption of the nerve supply to the involved muscles. Reflexes also are lost in deep coma or because of medication such as heavy sedation.

- **Electromyography** (ee-**leck**-troh-my-**OG**-rah-fee) is a diagnostic test that measures the electrical activity within muscle fibers in response to nerve stimulation (**electr/o** means electricity, **my/o** means muscle, and **-graphy** means the process of producing a picture or record). The resulting record is called an *electromyogram*. Electromyography is most frequently used when people have symptoms of weakness and examination shows impaired muscle strength.

- **Electroneuromyography** (ee-**leck**-troh-new-roh-my-**OG**-rah-fee), also known as **nerve conduction studies**, is a diagnostic procedure for testing and recording neuromuscular activity by the electric stimulation of the nerve trunk that carries fibers to and from the muscle (**electr/o** means electricity, **neur/o** means nerve, **my/o** means muscle, and **-graphy** means the process of producing a picture or record). The primary goal of this examination is to determine the site of a nerve lesion or muscle pathology.

- **Range of motion testing** is a diagnostic procedure to evaluate joint mobility and muscle strength (Figure 4.19).

TREATMENT PROCEDURES OF THE MUSCULAR SYSTEM

Medications

- An **anti-inflammatory**, such as ibuprofen (Motrin) relieves inflammation. It also acts as an analgesic.

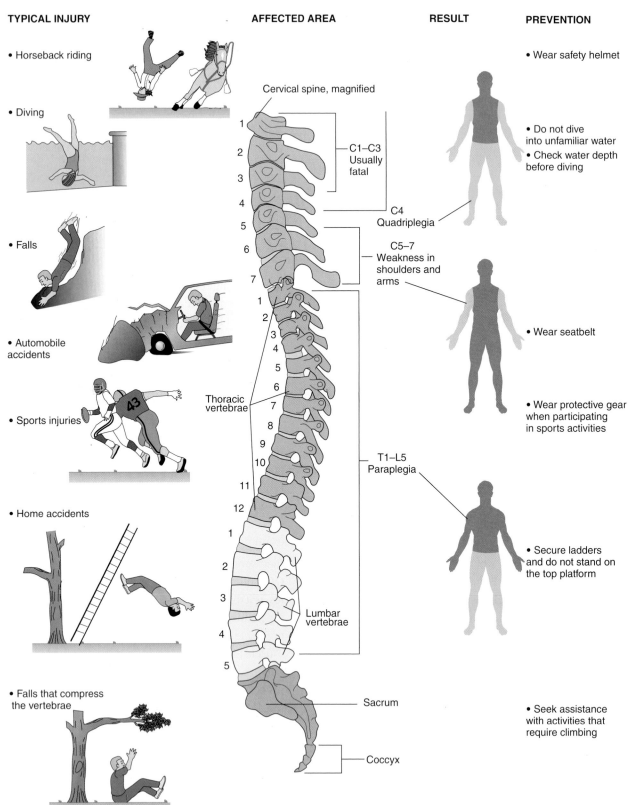

TYPICAL INJURY

- Horseback riding
- Diving
- Falls
- Automobile accidents
- Sports injuries
- Home accidents
- Falls that compress the vertebrae

AFFECTED AREA

Cervical spine, magnified

C1–C3 Usually fatal

C4 Quadriplegia

C5–7 Weakness in shoulders and arms

Thoracic vertebrae

T1–L5 Paraplegia

Lumbar vertebrae

Sacrum

Coccyx

RESULT

PREVENTION

- Wear safety helmet
- Do not dive into unfamiliar water
- Check water depth before diving
- Wear seatbelt
- Wear protective gear when participating in sports activities
- Secure ladders and do not stand on the top platform
- Seek assistance with activities that require climbing

FIGURE 4.17   Spinal cord injuries.

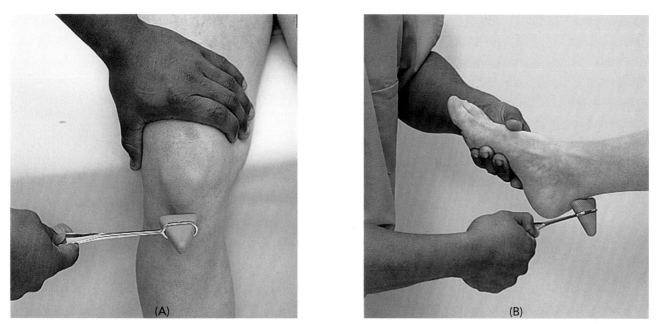

FIGURE 4.18 Assessment of deep tendon reflexes. (A) Testing the patellar reflex. (B) Testing the Achilles tendon reflex.

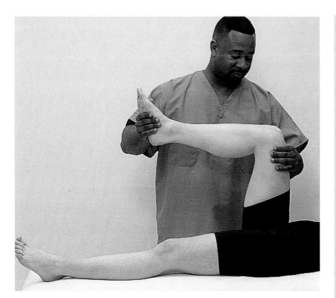

FIGURE 4.19 Range of motion (ROM) exercises aid in restoring joint mobility and muscle strength.

An *analgesic* relieves pain without affecting consciousness.

- An **anticholinergic drug** (**an**-tih-**koh**-lin-**ER**-jik), also known as an **antispasmodic**, is administered to control spasmodic activity of smooth muscles such as those of the intestine.

- **Atropine** (**AT**-roh-peen) is an antispasmodic that may be administered preoperatively to relax smooth muscles.

- A **muscle relaxant**, such as diazepam (Valium), acts on the central nervous system to relax the muscle tone and relieve spasms of skeletal muscles. Many of these medications also relieve anxiety and tension.

- A **neuromuscular blocker**, also known as a **neuromuscular blocking agent**, is a drug that causes temporary paralysis by blocking the transmission of nerve stimuli to the muscles. These drugs are used as an adjunct to anesthesia during surgery to cause skeletal muscles to relax. As used here, *adjunct* means in addition to.

Physical Therapy

Physical therapy (PT) is treatment to prevent disability or to restore functioning through the use of exercise, heat, massage, and other methods to improve circulation, flexibility, and muscle strength.

- **Range of motion exercises** are one form of PT. The goal of these therapeutic measures is to increase strength, flexibility, and mobility (Figure 4.19).

Therapeutic Ultrasound

Therapeutic ultrasound utilizes high-frequency sound waves to treat muscle injuries by generating heat deep within muscle tissue. This heat eases pain, reduces muscle spasms, and accelerates healing by increasing the flow of blood into the target tissues.

Activities of Daily Living

The minimum goal of therapy is to restore the individual to the level of self-help known as **activities of daily living.** These activities include personal hygiene, dressing, grooming, eating, and toileting.

Fascia

- A **fasciotomy** (**fash**-ee-**OT**-oh-mee) is a surgical incision through a fascia to relieve tension or pressure (**fasci** means fascia and **-otomy** means a surgical incision).

- **Fascioplasty** (**FASH**-ee-oh-**plas**-tee) is the surgical repair of a fascia (**fasci/o** means fascia and **-plasty** means surgical repair).

Tendons

- **Tenodesis** (ten-**ODD**-eh-sis) is the surgical suturing of the end of a tendon to bone (**ten/o** means tendon and **-desis** means to bind or tie together). Compare with *tenolysis.*

- **Tenolysis** (ten-**OL**-ih-sis) means to free a tendon from adhesions (**ten/o** means tendon and **-lysis** means to set free). Compare with *tenodesis.*

- A **tenectomy** (teh-**NECK**-toh-mee), also known as a **tenonectomy** (ten-oh-**NECK**-toh-mee), is the surgical removal of a portion of a tendon or tendon sheath (**ten** means tendon and **-ectomy** means surgical removal).

- A **tenotomy** (teh-**NOT**-oh-mee), also known as a **tendotomy**, is the surgical division of a tendon for relief of a deformity caused by the abnormal shortening of a muscle, such as strabismus (**ten** means tendon and **-otomy** means surgical incision). *Strabismus* is discussed in Chapter 11.

- **Tenoplasty** (**TEN**-oh-**plas**-tee), also known as **tendinoplasty**, is the surgical repair of a tendon (**ten/o** means tendon and **-plasty** means surgical repair).

- **Tenorrhaphy** (ten-**OR**-ah-fee) is the surgical suturing of a divided tendon (**ten/o** means tendon and **-rrhaphy** means surgical suturing).

Muscles

- A **myectomy** (my-**ECK**-toh-mee) is the surgical removal of a portion of a muscle (**my** means muscle and **-ectomy** means surgical removal).

- **Myoplasty** (**MY**-oh-**plas**-tee) is the surgical repair of a muscle (**my/o** means muscle and **-plasty** means surgical repair).

- **Myorrhaphy** (my-**OR**-ah-fee) is the surgical suturing of a muscle wound (**my/o** means muscle and **-rrhaphy** means surgical suturing).

- A **myotomy** (my-**OT**-oh-mee) is a surgical incision into a muscle (**my** means muscle and **-otomy** means surgical incision).

ABBREVIATIONS RELATED TO THE MUSCULAR SYSTEM

Table 4.2 presents an overview of the abbreviations related to the terms introduced in this chapter. *Note:* To avoid errors or confusion, always be cautious when using abbreviations.

Table 4.2

ABBREVIATIONS RELATED TO THE MUSCULAR SYSTEM

Achilles tendon = AT	**AT** = Achilles tendon
activities of daily living = ADL	**ADL** = activities of daily living
adhesion = ADH	**ADH** = adhesion
atrophy = atr	**atr** = atrophy
Becker's muscular dystrophy = BMD	**BMD** = Becker's muscular dystrophy
carpal tunnel release = CTR	**CTR** = carpal tunnel release
carpal tunnel syndrome = CTS	**CTS** = carpal tunnel syndrome
deep tendon reflexes = DTR	**DTR** = deep tendon reflexes
dorsiflexion = DF	**DF** = dorsiflexion
Duchenne's muscular dystrophy = DMD	**DMD** = Duchenne's muscular dystrophy
electromyography = EMG	**EMG** = electromyography
fibromyalgia syndrome = FMS	**FMS** = fibromyalgia syndrome
hyperextension = HE	**HE** = hyperextension
hemiplegia = hemi	**hemi** = hemiplegia
impingement syndrome = IS	**IS** = impingement syndrome
intermittent claudication = IC	**IC** = intermittent claudication
muscular dystrophy = MD	**MD** = muscular dystrophy
myasthenia gravis = MG	**MG** = myasthenia gravis
neuromuscular = nm	**nm** = neuromuscular
physical therapy = PT	**PT** = physical therapy
polymyositis = PM	**PM** = polymyositis
quadriplegia, quadriplegic = quad	**quad** = quadriplegia, quadriplegic
range of motion = ROM	**ROM** = range of motion
repetitive motion disorder = RMD	**RMD** = repetitive motion disorder
repetitive stress disorder = RSD	**RSD** = repetitive stress disorder
spinal cord injury = SCI	**SCI** = spinal cord injury

Learning Exercises

● Matching Word Parts 1

Write the correct answer in the middle column.

Definition	Correct Answer	Possible Answers
4.1. movement, motion	_____	-cele
4.2. hernia, swelling	_____	fasci/o
4.3. fibrous connective tissue	_____	fibr/o
4.4. fascia	_____	-ia
4.5. condition, state of	_____	kinesi/o

● Matching Word Parts 2

Write the correct answer in the middle column.

Definition	Correct Answer	Possible Answers
4.6. tone, tension, stretching	_____	my/o
4.7. tendon	_____	-rrhexis
4.8. rupture	_____	tax/o
4.9. muscle	_____	tend/o
4.10. coordination	_____	ton/o

Matching Muscle Directions and Positions

Write the correct answer in the middle column.

Definition	Correct Answer	Possible Answers
4.11. cross-wise	_____	lateralis
4.12. ring-like	_____	oblique
4.13. slanted at an angle	_____	rectus
4.14. straight	_____	sphincter
4.15. toward the side	_____	transverse

Definitions

Select the correct answer and write it on the line provided.

4.16. Muscles under voluntary control are known as _____ .

    involuntary   nonstriated   skeletal   visceral

4.17. A thickening on the surface of the calcaneus bone that causes severe pain when standing is known as a/an _____ .

    heel spur   impingement syndrome   overuse injury   shin splint

4.18. Turning the hand so the palm is upward is called _____ .

    extension   flexion   pronation   supination

4.19. The term meaning extreme slowness of movement is _____ .

    bradykinesia   dyskinesia   hypotonia   myotonia

4.20. The _____ muscle inserts into the mastoid process.

    extensor carpi   pectoralis major   rectus abdominus   sternocleidomastoid

4.21. The term meaning pertaining to muscle tissue and fascia is _____ .

    aponeurosis   fibrous sheath   myocardium   myofascial

4.22. A narrow band of nonelastic, fibrous tissue that attaches a muscle to bone is a/an _____ .

    aponeurosis   fascia   ligament   tendon

4.23.   The term meaning a band of fibers that hold structures together abnormally is _____.

adhesion   aponeurosis   atrophy   contracture

4.24.   The bending motion of the wrist is made possible by the _____ muscle.

extensor carpi   flexor carpi   vastus lateralis   vastus medialis

4.25.   The term meaning pain in a tendon is _____.

tenodesis   tenodynia   tendinosis   tenolysis

● Abbreviation Identification

Write the correct answer on the line provided.

4.26.   **BMD**   _____

4.27.   **CTS**   _____

4.28.   **MG**   _____

4.29.   **RSD**   _____

4.30.   **SCI**   _____

● Which Word?

Select the correct answer and write it on the line provided.

4.31.   An injury to the body of the muscle or attachment of the tendon is known as a _____.

sprain   strain

4.32.   A/An _____ is a drug that causes temporary muscle paralysis by blocking the transmission of nerve stimuli to the muscles.

anticholinergic   neuromuscular blocker

4.33.   The term meaning a condition of abnormal muscle tone is _____.

dystaxia   dystonia

4.34.   The form of muscular dystrophy in which survival is rarely beyond the late twenties is _____ dystrophy.

Becker's   Duchenne's

4.35.   The term meaning the study of human factors that affect the work environment is _____ .

ergonomics   kinesiology

● Spelling Counts

Find the misspelled word in each sentence. Then write that word, spelled correctly, on the line provided.

4.36.   The tricips brachii is the muscle of the posterior upper arm. _____

4.37.   The medical term for hiccups is singulutas. _____

4.38.   Muscle tone, which is also known as tonis, is the normal state of balanced tension that is present in

the body. _____

4.39.   Jamie Vaughn suffers from a lack of muscle coordination that is known as ataxis. _____

4.40.   The gleoteus maximus is the largest muscle of the buttock. _____

● Term Selection

Select the correct answer and write it on the line provided.

4.41.   The term meaning the rupture of a muscle is _____ .

myocele   myorrhaphy   myorrhexis   myotomy

4.42.   The term meaning the breaking down of muscle tissue is _____ .

myoclonus   myolysis   myomalacia   myoparesis

4.43.   The term meaning abnormally decreased motor function or activity is _____ .

hyperkinesia   hypertonia   hypokinesia   hypotonia

4.44.   A tear or strain of the posterior femoral muscles is known as a/an _____ injury.

Achilles tendon   hamstring   myofascial   shin splint

4.45.   The treatment of carpal tunnel syndrome is known as a/an _____ .

carpal tunnel release   tenectomy   tenodesis   tenotomy

● Sentence Completion

Write the correct term on the line provided.

4.46. The process of recording the strength of muscle contractions as the result of electrical stimulation is

called _____ (EMG).

4.47. An inflammation of the tissues surrounding the elbow is known as _____ .

4.48. The group of muscles that hold the head of the humerus securely in place as it rotates within the shoul-

der joint form the _____ cuff.

4.49. When tendons become inflamed and get caught in the narrow space between the bones within the

shoulder joint, this is known as the _____ syndrome.

4.50. An inflammation of the plantar causing foot or heel pain when walking or running is known as

plantar _____ .

4.51. The term meaning difficulty in controlling voluntary movement is _____ .

4.52. The term meaning to suture the end of a tendon to bone is _____ .

4.53. Ibuprofen (Motrin) is a/an _____ medication.

4.54. Inflammation of a tendon caused by excessive or unusual use of the joint is called _____ .

4.55. A/An _____ drug acts to control spasmodic activity of the smooth muscles. It is

also known as an antispasmodic.

● Word Surgery

Divide each term into its component word parts. Write these word parts, in sequence, on the lines provided.

When necessary use a back slash (/) to indicate a combining vowel. (You may not need all of the lines provided.)

4.56. **Electroneuromyography** is a procedure for testing and recording neuromuscular activity by the electric

stimulation of the nerve trunk.

_____   _____   _____   _____

4.57. **Hyperkinesia** means abnormally increased motor function or activity.

_____   _____   _____   _____

4.58. **Myoclonus** is a spasm or twitching of a muscle or group of muscles.

_____   _____   _____   _____

4.59. **Polymyositis** is the inflammation of several skeletal muscles at the same time.

_____   _____   _____   _____

4.60. **Sarcopenia** is the age-related reduction in skeletal muscle mass in the elderly.

_____   _____   _____   _____

● True/False

If the statement is true, write **T** on the line. If the statement is false, write **F** on the line.

4.61. ____ Overuse injuries are minor tissue injuries that have not been given time to heal.

4.62. ____ Hemiplegia is the total paralysis of the lower half of the body.

4.63. ____ A spasm is a sudden, violent, involuntary contraction of one or more muscles.

4.64. ____ Claudication means limping.

4.65. ____ Cardiac muscle is a specialized type of muscle found only in the heart.

● Clinical Conditions

Write the correct answer on the line provided.

4.66. George Quinton has a/an _____ _____on his wrist. This fluid-filled swelling is harmless and does not cause pain.

4.67. Jeff Burleson has a protrusion of a muscle through its ruptured sheath. This condition is known as a/an

_____.

4.68. Due to the lack of exercise while she was confined to bed, Louisa Hastings experienced muscle

_____ .

4.69. Jill Franklin has abnormal hardening of muscle tissue. This condition is called _____ .

4.70. Allison Cox was diagnosed as having _____ syndrome (FMS). Her condition is characterized by widespread body pain and uncontrollable fatigue.

4.71.   While running, Chuan Lee fell and injured his Achilles tendon. This condition is called Achilles

   _____ .

4.72.   For the first several days after her accident, Beth Hill suffered severe muscle pain. The medical term for

   this condition is _____ .

4.73.   Several months after an accident, Jackson Brooks underwent _____ to free the

   tendons in his arm from the adhesions caused by his injury.

4.74.   Steve Giannati suffered paralysis of all four limbs caused by a spinal injury. This condition is called

   _____ .

4.75.   After suffering a stroke, Juan Hernandez has slight paralysis on one side of his body. His doctor describes

   this as _____ .

● Which Is the Correct Medical Term?

Select the correct answer and write it on the line provided.

4.76.   The term meaning delayed relaxation of a muscle after a strong contraction is _____ .

atonic	dystaxia	dystonia	myotonia

4.77.   The surgical repair of a tendon is known as _____ .

tenectomy	tenodesis	tenolysis	tenoplasty

4.78.   The term meaning movement toward the midline of the body is _____ .

abduction	adduction	circumduction	rotation

4.79.   Abnormal softening of a muscle is known as _____ .

myomalacia	myorrhexis	myosclerosis	myositis

4.80.   The term _____ means bending the foot upward at the ankle.

abduction	dorsiflexion	elevation	plantar flexion

● Challenge Word Building

These terms are *not* found in this chapter; however, they are made up of the following familiar word parts. You

may want to look in the textbook glossary or use a medical dictionary to check your answers.

poly-	card/o	-algia
	fasci/o	-desis
	herni/o	-ectomy
	my/o	-itis
	sphincter/o	-necrosis
		-otomy
		-pathy
		-rrhaphy

4.81.   The term meaning any abnormal condition of skeletal muscles is _____ .

4.82.   The term meaning pain in several muscle groups is _____ .

4.83.   The term meaning the death of individual muscle fibers is _____ .

4.84.   The term meaning the surgical suturing of torn fascia is _____ .

4.85.   The term meaning a surgical incision into a muscle is a/an _____ .

4.86.   The term meaning suturing fascia to a skeletal attachment is _____ .

4.87.   The term meaning inflammation of the muscle of the heart is _____ .

4.88.   The term meaning the surgical removal of fascia is a/an _____ .

4.89.   The term meaning the surgical suturing of a defect in a muscular wall, such as the repair of a hernia, is

a/an_____ .

4.90.   The term meaning an incision into a sphincter muscle is a/an _____ .

to the myocardium. These episodes are due to ischemia of the heart muscle.

- A **myocardial infarction** (**my**-oh-**KAR**-dee-al in-**FARK**-shun), also known as a **heart attack**, is the occlusion (blockage) of one or more coronary arteries resulting in an infarct of the affected myocardium. This damage to the myocardium impairs the heart's ability to pump blood throughout the body.

An *infarction* is a sudden insufficiency of blood that causes necrosis (tissue death). An **infarct** (**IN**-farkt) is the resulting localized area of necrosis (Figures 5.13).

Congestive Heart Failure

Congestive heart failure (CHF) is a syndrome in which the heart is unable to pump enough blood to meet the body's needs for oxygen and nutrients. In response to the reduced blood flow, the kidneys retain more fluid within the body, and this fluid accumulates in the legs, ankles, and lungs. The term *congestive* is an adjective that describes fluid buildup (Figure 5.15).

- **Cardiomegaly** (**kar**-dee-oh-**MEG**-ah-lee) is the abnormal enlargement of the heart (**cardi/o** means heart, and **-megaly** means abnormal enlargement).

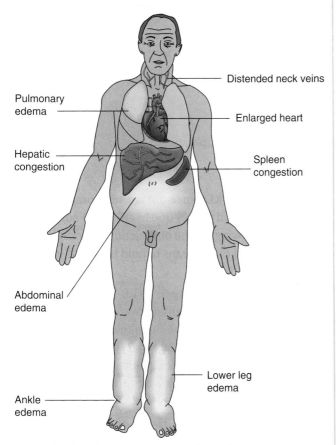

Pulmonary edema

Hepatic congestion

Abdominal edema

Ankle edema

Distended neck veins

Enlarged heart

Spleen congestion

Lower leg edema

FIGURE 5.15 Signs of congestive heart failure.

This condition is frequently associated with CHF when the heart enlarges in order to compensate for losses in its pumping ability.

Carditis

Carditis (kar-**DYE**-tis) is an inflammation of the heart (**card** means heart and **-itis** means inflammation). *Note the spelling of carditis:* In this term, the word root **card/o** is used to avoid having a double *i* when it is joined with the suffix **-itis**.

- **Endocarditis** (**en**-doh-kar-**DYE**-tis) is an inflammation of the inner lining of the heart (**endo-** means within, **card** means heart, and **-itis** means inflammation).
- **Bacterial endocarditis** is an inflammation of the lining or valves of the heart caused by bacteria that are present in the bloodstream.
- **Myocarditis** (**my**-oh-kar-**DYE**-tis) is an inflammation of the myocardium (**my/o** means muscle, **card** means heart, and **-itis** means inflammation).
- **Pericarditis** (**pehr**-ih-kar-**DYE**-tis) is an inflammation of the pericardium (**peri-** means surrounding, **card** means heart, and **-itis** means inflammation).

Heart Valves

Valvulitis (**val**-view-**LYE**-tis) is an inflammation of a heart valve (**valvul** means valve and **-itis** means inflammation).

- A **valvular prolapse** is the abnormal protrusion of the value that results in the inability of the valve to close completely. *Prolapse* means the falling or dropping down of an organ or internal part. This condition is named for the affected valve, such as a mitral valve prolapse.
- **Stenosis** (steh-**NOH**-sis) is the abnormal narrowing of the opening of a valve. This condition is named for the affected valve, such as aortic stenosis, mitral stenosis, and tricuspid stenosis.

Cardiac Arrhythmia and Fibrillation

- **Cardiac arrhythmia** (ah-**RITH**-mee-ah), also known as **dysrhythmia** (dis-**RITH**-mee-ah), is a change in the rhythm of the heartbeat.
- **Fibrillation** (fih-brih-**LAY**-shun) describes rapid, random, quivering, and ineffective contractions of the heart.

Altered Heartbeat Rates

- **Bradycardia** (**brad**-ee-**KAR**-dee-ah) is an abnormally slow heartbeat (**brady-** means slow, **card** means heart, and **-ia** means abnormal condition). This term is usually applied to rates less than 60 beats per minute. Compare with *tachycardia*.

- **Tachycardia** (**tack**-ee-**KAR**-dee-ah) is an abnormally rapid heartbeat (**tachy-** means rapid, **card** means heart, and **-ia** means abnormal condition). This term is usually applied to rates greater than 100 beats per minute. Compare with *bradycardia*.

- **Palpitation** (**pal**-pih-**TAY**-shun) is a pounding or racing heart with or without irregularity in rhythm. This is associated with certain heart disorders; however, it also may be a response accompanying a panic attack. (See Chapter 10.)

Atrial Disorders

- **Paroxysmal atrial tachycardia** (**par**-ock-**SIZ**-mal **tack**-ee-**KAR**-dee-ah), also known as **PAT**, is an episode that begins and ends abruptly during which there are very rapid and regular heartbeats that originate in the atrium. PAT is caused by an abnormality in the electrical system. *Paroxysmal* means pertaining to sudden occurrence (Figure 5.16A).

- In **atrial fibrillation**, also known as **A fib**, the normal rhythmic contractions of the atria are replaced by rapid irregular twitching of the muscular wall.

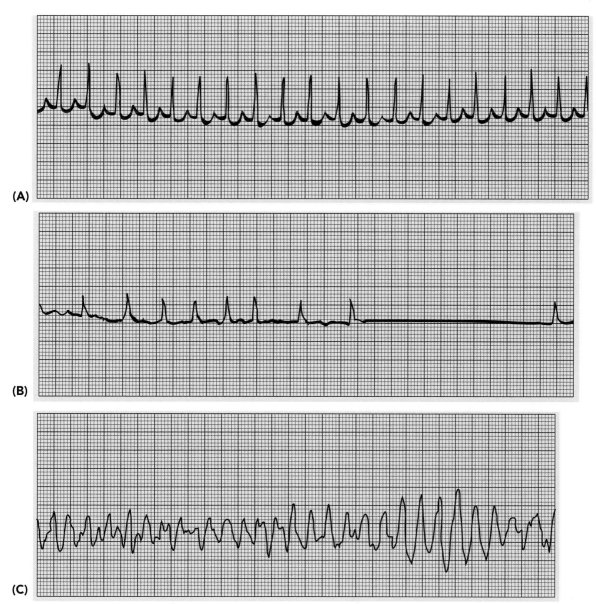

(A)

(B)

(C)

FIGURE 5.16 ECGs showing disruptions of heart rhythms. (A) Paroxysmal atrial tachycardia (PAT). (B) Atrial fibrillation. (C) Ventricular fibrillation.

AF causes an irregular and quivering action of the atria (Figure 5.16B).

Ventricular Disorders

- **Ventricular fibrillation** (ven-**TRICK**-you-ler fih-brih-**LAY**-shun), also known as **V fib**, is the rapid, irregular, and useless contractions of the ventricles. This condition is usually fatal unless reversed by electric defibrillation (Figure 5.16C).

Blood Vessels

- **Angiitis** (**an**-jee-**EYE**-tis), also known as **vasculitis** (**vas**-kyou-**LYE**-tis), is the inflammation of a blood or lymph vessel (**angi** means vessel and **-itis** means inflammation). *Note:* This term is also spelled as *angitis*.
- An **angiospasm** (**AN**-jee-oh-**spazm**) is a spasmodic contraction of the blood vessels (**angi/o** means vessel and **-spasm** means tightening or cramping).
- **Angiostenosis** (**AN**-jee-oh-steh-**NOH**-sis) is the narrowing of a blood vessel (**angi/o** means vessel and **-stenosis** means abnormal narrowing).
- A **hemangioma** (hee-**man**-jee-**OH**-mah) is a benign tumor made up of newly formed blood vessels (**hemangi** means blood vessel and **-oma** means tumor). (See also Chapter 12.)
- **Hypoperfusion** (**high**-poh-per-**FYOU**-zhun) is a deficiency of blood passing through an organ or body part. **Perfusion** (per-**FYOU**-zuhn) is the flow of blood through the vessels of an organ.
- The term **peripheral vascular disease** refers to disorders of blood vessels outside the heart and brain. Most commonly, this term describes the narrowing of vessels that carry blood to and from the leg and arm muscles.

Arteries

- An **aneurysm** (**AN**-you-rizm) is a localized weak spot, or balloon-like enlargement, of the wall of an artery. The rupture of an aneurysm may be fatal because of the rapid loss of blood.
- **Arteriosclerosis** (ar-**tee**-ree-oh-skleh-**ROH**-sis) is any of a group of diseases that are characterized by thickening and the loss of elasticity of arterial walls (**arteri/o** means artery and **-sclerosis** mean abnormal hardening).
- **Polyarteritis** (**pol**-ee-**ar**-teh-**RYE**-tis) is an inflammation involving several arteries at the same time

(**poly-** means many, **arter** means artery, and **-itis** mean inflammation).

- **Raynaud's phenomenon** (ray-**NOHZ**) consists of intermittent attacks of pallor (paleness), cyanosis (blue color), and redness of the fingers and toes. These symptoms are due to arterial contraction that may be due to cold or emotion.

Veins

- **Phlebitis** (fleh-**BYE**-tis) is the inflammation of a vein (**phleb** means vein and **-itis** means inflammation). This usually occurs in a superficial vein (Figure 5.17).
- **Varicose veins** (**VAR**-ih-kohs **VAYNS**) are abnormally swollen veins, usually occurring in the legs.

Thromboses and Embolisms

Thromboses and embolisms are both conditions that can result in the fatal blockage of a blood vessel.

Thrombosis

A **thrombosis** (throm-**BOH**-sis) is the abnormal condition of having a thrombus (**thromb** means clot and **-osis** means abnormal condition) (plural, **thromboses**).

- A **thrombus** (**THROM**-bus) is a blood clot attached to the interior wall of an artery or vein (**thromb** means clot and **-us** is a singular noun ending) (plural, **thrombi**).
- A **thrombotic occlusion** (throm-**BOT**-ick ah-**KLOO**-zhun) is the blocking of an artery by a thrombus (**thromb/o** means clot and **-tic** means pertaining to). *Thrombotic* means caused by a thrombus. As used here, *occlusion* means a blockage.
- A **coronary thrombosis** (**KOR**-uh-**nerr**-ee throm-**BOH**-sis) is damage to the heart muscle caused by a thrombus blocking a coronary artery.
- A **deep vein thrombosis** is the condition of having a thrombus attached to the wall of a deep vein. When a patient is bedridden, these sometimes form in the legs. The danger is that the thrombus will break loose and travel to a lung where it can be fatal (Figure 5.17).

Embolism

An **embolism** (**EM**-boh-lizm) is the sudden blockage of a blood vessel by an embolus (**embol** means something inserted and **-ism** means condition). The embolism is often named for the causative factor, such as an air embolism or a fat embolism.

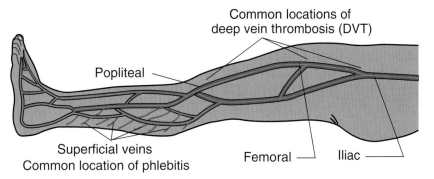

Common locations of
deep vein thrombosis (DVT)

Popliteal

Superficial veins
Common location of phlebitis

Femoral   Iliac

FIGURE 5.17   Common sites for the development of phlebitis and deep vein thrombosis.

- An **embolus** (**EM**-boh-lus) is a foreign object, such as a blood clot, quantity of air or gas, or a bit of tissue or tumor that is circulating in the blood (**embol** means something inserted and **-us** is a singular noun ending) (plural, **emboli**).

Blood Disorders

- **Dyscrasia** (dis-**KRAY**-zee-ah) is any pathologic condition of the cellular elements of the blood (**dys-** means bad and **-crasia** means a mixture or blending).

- **Hemochromatosis** (**hee**-moh-**kroh**-mah-**TOH**-sis) is a genetic disorder in which the intestines absorb too much iron (**hem/o** means blood, **chromat** means color, and **-osis** means abnormal condition). Also known as **iron overload disease**, the excess iron that is absorbed enters the bloodstream and accumulates in organs where it causes damage.

- **Septicemia** (**sep**-tih-**SEE**-mee-ah), also known as **blood poisoning**, is a systemic disease caused by the spread of microorganisms and their toxins via the circulating blood.

- **Hemolytic reaction** (**hee**-moh-**LIT**-ick), also known as a **transfusion reaction**, is the destruction of erythrocytes that occurs when a patient receives a transfusion of mismatched blood. *Hemolytic* means pertaining to breaking down of red blood cells (**hem/o** means relating to blood and **-lytic** means to destroy).

Cholesterol

Cholesterol (koh-**LES**-ter-ol) is a waxy fat like substance that travels in the blood in packages called lipoproteins. Some cholesterol in the blood is necessary; however, excessively high levels can lead to heart disease.

- **Low-density lipoprotein cholesterol**, also known as **LDL**, is called **bad cholesterol** because excess quantities contribute to plaque buildup in the arteries. *Memory aid:* LDL is bad.

- **High-density lipoprotein cholesterol**, is also known as **HDL** or **good cholesterol** because it carries unneeded cholesterol back to the liver for processing and does not contribute to plaque buildup. *Memory aid:* HDL is good.

- **Triglycerides** (try-**GLIS**-er-eyeds) are combinations of fatty acids attached to glycerol that are also found normally in the blood in limited quantities.

- **Homocysteine** (**hoh**-moh-**SIS**-teen) is an amino acid normally found in the blood and used by the body to build and maintain tissues. However, when present in elevated levels, homocysteine can damage arterial walls and increase the risk of coronary artery disease. Such increases may be caused by a diet severely lacking in several B vitamins.

- **Hyperlipidemia** (**high**-per-**lip**-ih-**DEE**-mee-ah), also known as **hyperlipemia** (**high**-per-lye-**PEE**-mee-ah), is a general term for the condition of elevated plasma concentrations of cholesterol, triglycerides, and lipoproteins (**hyper-** means excessive, **lipid** means fat, and **-emia** means blood condition).

Leukemia

- **Myelodysplastic syndrome** (**my**-eh-loh-dis-**PLAS**-tick), also known as **preleukemia**, is a progressive condition of dysfunctional bone marrow that may eventually develop into leukemia. This condition is usually treated with blood transfusions.

- **Leukemia** (loo-**KEE**-mee-ah) is a malignancy characterized by a progressive increase in the number of abnormal leukocytes (white blood cells) found in hemopoietic tissues, other organs, and in the circulating blood (**leuk** means white and **-emia** means blood condition). This condition is usually treated with bone marrow transplants, which are discussed in Chapter 3.

Anemias

Anemia (ah-**NEE**-mee-ah) is a disorder characterized by lower than normal levels of red blood cells in the blood (**an-** means without or less than and **-emia** means blood condition).

- **Aplastic anemia** (ay-**PLAS**-tick ah-**NEE**-mee-ah) is characterized by an absence of *all* formed blood elements (**a-** means without, **plast** means growth, and **-ic** means pertaining to). This condition is caused by the failure of blood cell production in the bone marrow.

- In **hemolytic anemia** (hee-moh-**LIT**-ick ah-**NEE**-mee-ah) red blood cells are destroyed more rapidly than the bone marrow can replace them. *Hemolytic* means pertaining to breaking down of red blood cells (**hem/o** means relating to blood and **-lytic** means to destroy).

- **Iron-deficiency anemia** is a decrease in the red cells of the blood that is caused by too little iron. This may be caused by inadequate iron intake, malabsorption of iron, pregnancy and lactation, or chronic blood loss.

- **Megaloblastic anemia** (**MEG**-ah-loh-**blas**-tick ah-**NEE**-mee-ah) is a blood disorder in which red blood cells are larger than normal. This condition is usually caused by a deficiency of folic acid, or vitamin B_{12}.

- **Pernicious anemia** (per-**NISH**-us ah-**NEE**-mee-ah) is an autoimmune disorder in which the red blood cells are abnormally formed, due to an inability to absorb vitamin B_{12}. *Pernicious* means destructive, fatal, or harmful.

- **Sickle cell anemia** is a genetic disorder that causes abnormal hemoglobin, resulting in red blood cells that assume an abnormal sickle shape (Figure 5.18). This abnormal shape interferes with normal blood flow, resulting in damage to most of the body systems. The genetic transmission of sickle cell anemia is discussed in Chapter 2.

- **Thalassemia** (thal-ah-**SEE**-mee-ah), also known as **Cooley's anemia**, is a diverse group of genetic blood diseases that are characterized by absent or decreased production of normal hemoglobin.

Hypertension

- **Essential hypertension**, also known as **primary** or **idiopathic hypertension**, is consistently elevated blood pressure of unknown cause. *Idiopathic* means of unknown cause. The classifications of blood pressure for adults are summarized in Table 5.2.

FIGURE 5.18 Normal and sickle-shaped red blood cells magnified through a scanning electron microscope. (Courtesy of Philips Electronic Instruments Company.)

Table 5.2

BLOOD PRESSURE CLASSIFICATIONS FOR ADULTS

Category	Systolic (mm Hg)	Diastolic (mm Hg)
Normal blood pressure	less than 120	less than 80
Prehypertension	120 to 139	80 to 89
Stage 1 Hypertension	140 to 159	90 to 99
Stage 2 Hypertension	160 and higher	100 and higher

Source: Seventh Report of the Joint National Committee on Prevention, Detection, Evaluation, and Treatment of High Blood Pressure, May 2003.

- **Secondary hypertension** is caused by a different medical problem, such as a kidney disorder or a tumor on the adrenal glands. When the other problem is cured, the secondary hypertension should be resolved.

- **Malignant hypertension** is characterized by the sudden onset of severely elevated blood pressure. It can be life-threatening and commonly damages small vessels in the brain, retina, heart, and kidneys.

Hypotension

Hypotension (**high**-poh-**TEN**-shun) is lower than normal arterial blood pressure. Symptoms may include dizziness, lightheadedness, or fainting.

- **Orthostatic hypotension** (**or**-thoh-**STAT**-ick **high**-poh-**TEN**-shun), also known as **postural hypotension**, is low blood pressure that occurs in a standing posture. *Orthostatic* means relating to an upright or standing position.

DIAGNOSTIC PROCEDURES OF THE CARDIOVASCULAR SYSTEM

- **Blood tests** and **ultrasonic diagnostic procedures** are discussed in Chapter 15.

- **Angiography** (**an**-jee-**OG**-rah-fee) is a radiographic (x-ray) study of the blood vessels after the injection of a contrast medium (**angi/o** means blood vessel and **-graphy** means the process of recording). The resulting film is an **angiogram** (Figure 5.19).

- **Digital subtraction angiography** is a diagnostic technique that combines video with computer-assisted enhancement of images obtained by conventional angiography. This technology makes it possible to view vascular structures without superimposed bone and soft tissue densities.

- **Cardiac catheterization** (**KAR**-dee-ack **kath**-eh-ter-eye-**ZAY**-shun) is a diagnostic procedure in which a catheter is passed into a vein or artery and then guided into the heart (Figure 5.20). When the catheter is in place, a contrast medium is introduced to produce an angiogram to determine how well the heart is working. This procedure is also used for treatment purposes. See the section on clearing blocked arteries later in this chapter.

- **Phlebography** (fleh-**BOG**-rah-fee), also known as **venography**, is the technique of preparing an x-ray image of veins injected with a contrast medium (**phleb/o** means vein and **-graphy** means the process of recording). The resulting film is a *phlebogram.*

- **Coronary calcium screening**, which utilizes computerized tomography (CT), identifies the presence and quantity of coronary artery calcium deposits. Although this is not a diagnostic test, the resulting figures may be of value in assessing and predicting the risk for future coronary heart disease.

Electrocardiography

- **Electrocardiography** (ee-**leck**-troh-kar-dee-**OG**-rah-fee) is the process of recording the electrical activity of the myocardium (**electr/o** means electric, **cardi/o** means heart, and **-graphy** means the process of recording). An **electrocardiogram** (ee-**leck**-troh-**KAR**-dee-oh-**gram**) is the record produced by this process (Figure 5.16).

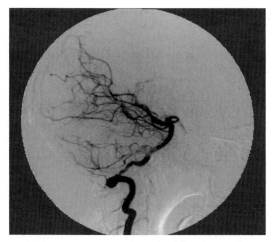

FIGURE 5.19   In an angiogram, the blood vessels (in black) are made visible by a contrast medium.

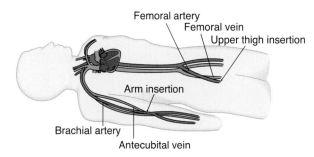

FIGURE 5.20   In cardiac catheterization, after the catheter has been threaded into place in the heart, a contrast medium is injected.

- A **Holter monitor** is a portable electrocardiograph that is worn by an ambulatory patient to continuously monitor the heart rates and rhythms over a 24-hour period.
- **Stress tests** are electrocardiography used to assess cardiovascular health and function during and after stress such as exercise on a treadmill.

In a **thallium stress test** (**THAL**-ee-um), the flow of blood through the heart during activity is assessed through the use of the radionuclide thallium during a stress test. Radionuclides are discussed in Chapter 15.

TREATMENT PROCEDURES OF THE CARDIOVASCULAR SYSTEM

Antihypertensive Medications

An **antihypertensive drug** (**an**-tih-**high**-per-**TEN**-siv) is administered to lower blood pressure. The following are medications used for this purpose:

- **ACE inhibitors** (angiotensin converting enzyme) are administered to treat hypertension and congestive heart failure. ACE inhibitors act by interfering with the action of the kidney enzyme renin that causes the heart muscles to contract.
- **Beta-blockers** reduce blood pressure by slowing the heartbeat.
- **Calcium channel blockers** reduce the contraction of the muscles that squeeze blood vessels tight. These medications are used to treat hypertension, angina, and arrhythmia.
- **Diuretics** (**dye**-you-**RET**-icks), which increase urine secretion to rid the body of excess sodium and water, are administered to treat hypertension and congestive heart failure (CHF).

Additional Medications

- **Cholesterol-lowering drugs**, such as **statins**, are used to combat hyperlipidemia by reducing the undesirable cholesterol levels in the blood.
- **Digoxin** (dih-**JOCK**-sin), also known as **digitalis** (**dij**-ih-**TAL**-is), slows and strengthens the heart muscle contractions and is used in the treatment of atrial fibrillation and CHF.
- **Nitroglycerin** is a vasodilator that is prescribed to relieve the pain of angina pectoris. It may be administered sublingually (under the tongue), through the skin (by a patch), or orally as a spray.

- An **anticoagulant** (**an**-tih-koh-**AG**-you-lant), slows coagulation and prevents new clots from forming. *Coagulation* is the formation of blood clots.
- A **thrombolytic** (**throm**-boh-**LIT**-ick), also known as a clot-busting drug, causes the dissolving or breaking up of a thrombus (**thromb/o** means clot and **-lytic** means to destroy).
- An **antiarrhythmic** (**an**-tih-ah-**RITH**-mick) is administered to control irregularities of the heartbeat.
- **Tissue plasminogen activator** (**TISH**-you plaz-**MIN**-oh-jen **ACK**-tih-**vay**-tor) is a thrombolytic that is administered to certain patients having a heart attack or stroke. If administered within a few hours after symptoms begin, tPA can dissolve the damaging blood clots.
- A **vasoconstrictor** (**vas**-oh-kon-**STRICK**-tor) constricts (narrows) the blood vessels. Compare with a *vasodilator*.
- A **vasodilator** (**vas**-oh-dye-**LAYT**-or) dilates (expands) the blood vessels. Compare with a *vasoconstrictor*.

Clearing Blocked Arteries

- **Percutaneous** (**per**-kyou-**TAY**-nee-us) **transluminal coronary angioplasty** is also called **balloon angioplasty** (**AN**-jee-oh-**plas**-tee) (Figure 5.21). In this procedure, a small balloon on the end of a catheter is used to open a partially blocked coronary artery by flattening the plaque deposit and stretching the lumen. After the plaque has been flattened, the balloon is deflated and the catheter and balloon are removed. *Percutaneous* means through the skin and *transluminal* means within the lumen of an artery.
- In a similar technique, a **stent** (a wire-mesh tube) is implanted in a coronary artery to provide support to the arterial wall to prevent restenosis (Figure 5.22). *Restenosis* describes the condition when an artery that has been opened by angioplasty closes again (**re-** means again and **-stenosis** means narrowing).
- An **atherectomy** (**ath**-er-**ECK**-toh-mee) is the surgical removal of plaque from the interior lining of an artery (**ather** means plaque and **-ectomy** means surgical removal). This procedure involves the use of a cutting tool that shaves off pieces of the plaque buildup (Figure 5.23).

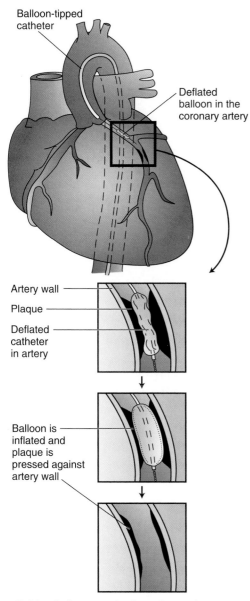

FIGURE 5.21   Balloon angioplasty is used to reopen a blocked coronary artery.

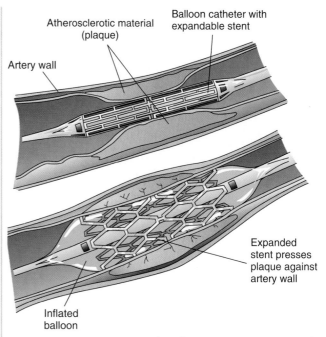

FIGURE 5.22   A stent is placed to prevent restenosis of the treated artery.

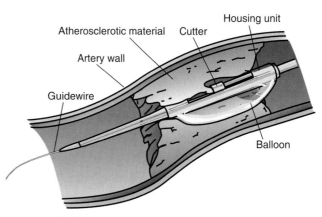

FIGURE 5.23   A cutting instrument is used to remove plaque from the artery wall.

- An **endarterectomy** (**end**-ar-ter-**ECK**-toh-mee) is the surgical removal of the lining of an artery that is clogged with plaque (**end-** means within, **arter** means artery, and **-ectomy** means surgical removal).

- A **carotid endarterectomy** is the surgical removal of the lining of a portion of a clogged carotid artery leading to the brain. This procedure is performed to reduce the risk of stroke that might be caused by a disruption of the blood flow to the brain. Strokes are discussed in Chapter 10.

Coronary Artery Bypass Graft

- **Coronary artery bypass graft** is also known as **bypass surgery** (Figure 5.24). In this surgery, which requires opening the chest, a piece of vein from the leg or chest is implanted on the heart to replace a blocked coronary artery and to improve the flow of blood to the heart.

- A **minimally invasive direct coronary artery bypass,** also known as a **keyhole** or **buttonhole bypass,** is an alternative technique for some bypass cases. This procedure is performed with the aid of a fiberoptic camera through small openings between the ribs.

Cardiac Dysrhythmias

- **Defibrillation** (dee-**fib**-rih-**LAY**-shun), also known as **cardioversion** (**kar**-dee-oh-**VER**-zhun), is the use

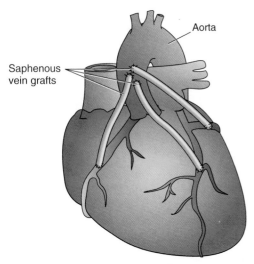

FIGURE 5.24 Coronary artery bypass surgery.

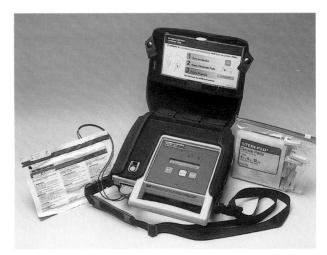

FIGURE 5.25 An automated external defibrillator (AED).

of electrical shock to restore the heart's normal rhythm. This shock is provided by a **defibrillator** (dee-**fib**-rih-**LAY**-ter).

- An **automated external defibrillator (AED)**, which is designed for use by nonprofessionals, automatically samples the electrical rhythms of the heart. If necessary, the AED externally shocks the heart to restore a normal cardiac rhythm (Figure 5.25).

- A **pacemaker** is an electronic device that may be attached externally or implanted under the skin, with connections leading into the heart to regulate the heartbeat. Pacemakers are used primarily as treatment for bradycardia or atrial fibrillation.

- An **implantable cardioverter defibrillator** (**KAR**-dee-oh-**ver**-ter dee-**fib**-rih-**LAY**-ter) is a double-action pacemaker. (1) It constantly regulates the heartbeat to ensure that the heart does not beat too slowly. (2) If a dangerous dysrhythmia, such as tachycardia, occurs it acts as an automatic defibrillator (Figure 5.26).

- **Valvoplasty** (**VAL**-voh-**plas**-tee), also known as **valvuloplasty** (**VAL**-view-loh-**plas**-tee), is the surgical repair or replacement of a heart valve (**valv/o** means valve and **-plasty** means surgical repair).

- **Cardiopulmonary resuscitation** is an emergency procedure for life support consisting of artificial respiration and manual external cardiac compression.

Blood Vessels, Blood, and Bleeding

- An **aneurysmectomy** (**an**-you-riz-**MECK**-toh-mee) is the surgical removal of an aneurysm (**aneurysm** means aneurysm and **-ectomy** means surgical removal).

- An **aneurysmorrhaphy** (**an**-you-riz-**MOR**-ah-fee) is the surgical suturing of an aneurysm (**aneurysm/o** means aneurysm and **-rrhaphy** means surgical suturing).

- An **arteriectomy** (**ar**-teh-ree-**ECK**-toh-mee) is the surgical removal of part of an artery (**arteri** means artery and **-ectomy** means surgical removal).

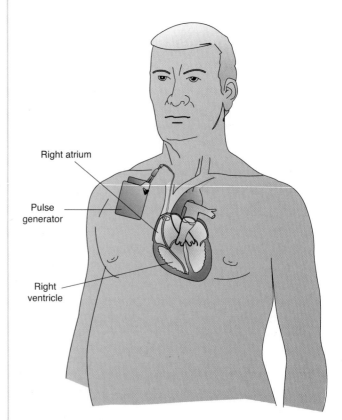

Right atrium

Pulse generator

Right ventricle

FIGURE 5.26 An implantable cardioverter defibrillator.

- **Hemostasis** (**hee**-moh-**STAY**-sis) means to stop or control bleeding (**hem/o** means blood and **-stasis** means stopping or controlling).
- **Plasmapheresis** (**plaz**-mah-feh-**REE**-sis) is the removal of whole blood from the body, separation of its cellular elements, and reinfusion of these cellular elements suspended in saline or a plasma substitute.

ABBREVIATIONS RELATED TO THE CARDIOVASCULAR SYSTEM

Table 5.3 presents an overview of the abbreviations related to the terms introduced in this chapter. *Note:* To avoid errors or confusion, always be cautious when using abbreviations.

Table 5.3

ABBREVIATIONS RELATED TO THE CARDIOVASCULAR SYSTEM	
anticoagulant = AC	**AC** = anticoagulant
aneurysm = AN	**AN** = aneurysm
angina pectoris = AP	**AP** = angina pectoris
antihypertensive drug = AHD	**AHD** = antihypertensive drug
atrial fibrillation = AF	**AF** = atrial fibrillation
automated external defibrillator = AED	**AED** = automated external defibrillator
blood pressure = BP	**BP** = blood pressure
cardiac catheterization = card cath, CC	**card cath, CC** = cardiac catheterization
cholesterol = C	**C** = cholesterol
cardiopulmonary resuscitation = CPR	**CPR** = cardiopulmonary resuscitation
congestive heart failure = CHF	**CHF** = congestive heart failure
coronary artery bypass graft = CABG	**CABG** = coronary artery bypass graft
coronary artery disease = CAD	**CAD** = coronary artery disease
digital subtraction angiography = DSA	**DSA** = digital subtraction angiography
deep vein thrombosis = DVT	**DVT** = deep vein thrombosis
electrocardiogram = ECG, EKG	**ECG, EKG** = electrocardiogram
embolism = emb	**emb** = embolism
hemoglobin = Hb or HB	**Hb or HB** = hemoglobin
hemolytic anemia = HA	**HA** = hemolytic anemia
high-density lipoprotein = HDL	**HDL** = high-density lipoprotein
Holter monitor = HM	**HM** = Holter monitor
implantable cardioverter defibrillator = ICD	**ICD** = implantable cardioverter defibrillator
ischemic heart disease = IHD	**IHD** = ischemic heart disease

(continues)

Table 5.3 (continued)

ABBREVIATIONS RELATED TO THE CARDIOVASCULAR SYSTEM	
low-density lipoprotein = LDL	**LDL** = low-density lipoprotein
minimally invasive direct coronary artery bypass = MIDCAB	**MIDCAB** = minimally invasive direct coronary artery bypass
myelodysplastic syndrome = MDS	**MDS** = myelodysplastic syndrome
myocardial infarction = MI	**MI** = myocardial infarction
percutaneous transluminal coronary angioplasty = PTCA	**PTCA** = percutaneous transluminal coronary angioplasty
peripheral vascular disease = PVD	**PVD** = peripheral vascular disease
polyarteritis = PA	**PA** = polyarteritis
Raynaud's phenomenon = RP	**RP** = Raynaud's phenomenon
thallium stress test = TST	**TST** = thallium stress test
thrombosis = T	**T** = thrombosis
tissue plasminogen activator = tPA	**tPA** = tissue plasminogen activator
varicose veins = VV	**VV** = varicose veins

Learning Exercises

● Matching Word Parts 1

Write the correct answer in the middle column.

Definition	Correct Answer	Possible Answers
5.1. aorta	_____	angi/o
5.2. artery	_____	aort/o
5.3. plaque, fatty substance	_____	arteri/o
5.4. relating to blood or lymph vessels	_____	ather/o
5.5. slow	_____	brady-

● Matching Word Parts 2

Write the correct answer in the middle column.

Definition	Correct Answer	Possible Answers
5.6. blood or blood condition	_____	cardi/o
5.7. crown, coronary	_____	coron/o
5.8. heart	_____	ven/o
5.9. red	_____	-emia
5.10. vein	_____	erythr/o

● Matching Word Parts 3

Write the correct answer in the middle column.

Definition	Correct Answer	Possible Answers
5.11. white	_____	**hem/o**
5.12. vein	_____	**leuk/o**
5.13. fast, rapid	_____	**phleb/o**
5.14. clot	_____	**tachy-**
5.15. blood, relating to blood	_____	**thromb/o**

● Definitions

Select the correct answer and write it on the line provided.

5.16.   The term meaning white blood cells is _____ .

   erythrocytes   leukocytes   platelets   thrombocytes

5.17.   Commonly known as the natural pacemaker, the proper name of the structure is/are the

   _____ .

 atrioventricular (A-V) node   bundle of His   Purkinje fibers   sinoatrial (S-A) node

5.18.   The myocardium receives its blood supply from the _____ .

   aorta   coronary arteries   inferior vena cava   superior vena cava

5.19.   An elevated _____count usually indicates a chronic infection.

   basophil   eosinophil   erythrocyte   monocyte

5.20.   The bicuspid heart valve is also known as the _____ valve.

   aortic   mitral   pulmonary   tricuspid

5.21.   The heart chamber that pumps blood to the lungs is the _____ .

   left atrium   left ventricle   right atrium   right ventricle

5.22.   The smallest formed elements in the blood are the _____ .

   erythrocytes   leukocytes   monocytes   thrombocytes

5.23. The term that describes a foreign object circulating in the blood is _____.

      embolism   embolus   thrombosis   thrombus

5.24. Blood flows from the right ventricle to the _____.

      body   left atrium   lungs   right atrium

5.25. The white blood cells that fight infection by phagocytosis are _____.

      erythrocytes   leukocytes   neutrophils   thrombocytes

● Matching Structures

Write the correct answer in the middle column.

Definition	Correct Answer	Possible Answers
5.26. a hollow muscular organ	_____	endocardium
5.27. cardiac muscle	_____	epicardium
5.28. external layer of the heart	_____	heart
5.29. inner lining of the heart	_____	myocardium
5.30. sac enclosing the heart	_____	pericardium

● Which Word?

Select the correct answer and write it on the line provided.

5.31. The substance also known as good cholesterol is _____ lipoprotein.

      high-density   low-density

5.32. An abnormally slow heartbeat is described as _____.

      bradycardia   tachycardia

5.33. Rapid, random, and ineffective contractions of the heart are described as _____.

      dysrhythmia   fibrillation

5.34. When the ventricles of the heart contract, _____ pressure occurs.

      diastolic   systolic

5.35. A/An _____ occurs when a patient receives a transfusion of mismatched blood.

      hemolytic anemia   hemolytic reaction

● Spelling Counts

Find the misspelled word in each sentence. Then write that word, spelled correctly, on the line provided.

5.36.   The autopsy indicated that the cause of death was a ruptured aneuryism. _____

5.37.   A bedridden patient may form a deep vein thombis in the leg. _____

5.38.   A change in the rhythm of the heartbeat is known as a cardiac arrhythemia. _____

5.39.   Thallassemia is a genetic disorder characterized by short-lived red blood cells. _____

5.40.   Cholestarol is a fatty substance that circulates in the blood. _____

● Abbreviation Identification

In the space provided, write the words that each abbreviation stands for.

5.41.   **CAD**   _____

5.42.   **CHF**   _____

5.43.   **Hb** or **HB**   _____

5.44.   **MI**   _____

5.45.   **VF**   _____

● Term Selection

Select the correct answer and write it on the line provided.

5.46.   The systemic disease caused by the spread of microorganisms and their toxins via the circulating blood is

known as _____ .

dyscrasia   endocarditis   pericarditis   septicemia

5.47.   Chronic hypertension, which is caused by a different medical problem, is known as

_____ hypertension.

essential   primary   malignant   secondary

5.48.   The blood disorder in which red blood cells are larger than normal, and which is usually caused by a deficiency of folic acid or vitamin B_{12}, is _____ anemia.

      aplastic   hemolytic   megaloblastic   pernicious

5.49.   Medications administered to lower high blood pressure are known as _____ .

      antiarrhythmics   antihypertensives   digitalis   statins

5.50.   A bacterial infection of the lining or valves of the heart is known as bacterial _____ .

      endocarditis   myocarditis   pericarditis   valvulitis

● Sentence Completion

Write the correct term on the line provided.

5.51.   Plasma with the clotting proteins removed is called _____ .

5.52.   An abnormal increase in the number of platelets in the circulating blood is known as

_____ .

5.53.   The term meaning the surgical removal of the lining of an artery is a/an _____ .

5.54.   Digital _____ angiography (DSA) uses video and computer-assisted enhancement of images obtained with conventional angiography.

5.55.   When present in the blood in elevated levels, the amino acid _____ can damage arterial walls and increase the risk of coronary artery disease.

● Word Surgery

Divide each term into its component word parts. Write these word parts, in sequence, on the lines provided.

When necessary use a back slash (/) to indicate a combining vowel. (You may not need all of the lines provided.)

5.56.   **Aneurysmorrhaphy** means the surgical suturing an aneurysm.

    _____   _____   _____   _____

5.57.   **Aplastic** anemia is characterized by an absence of *all* formed blood elements.

    _____   _____   _____   _____

5.58.   **Electrocardiography** is the process of recording the electrical activity of the myocardium.

_____   _____   _____   _____

5.59   **Polyarteritis** is an inflammation involving several arteries at the same time.

_____   _____   _____   _____

5.60.   **Valvoplasty** is the surgical repair or replacement of a heart valve.

_____   _____   _____   _____

● True/False

If the statement is true, write **T** on the line. If the statement is false, write **F** on the line.

5.61.   _____ A thrombus is a clot or piece of tissue circulating in the blood.

5.62.   _____ Hemochromatosis is also known as iron overload disease.

5.63.   _____ Plasmapheresis is the removal of whole blood from the body, separation of its cellular elements,

and reinfusion of these cellular elements suspended in saline or a plasma substitute.

5.64.   _____ A vasoconstrictor is a drug that enlarges the blood vessels.

5.65.   _____ The term peripheral vascular disease (PVD) is most commonly used to describes the narrowing of

vessels that carry blood to leg and arm muscles.

● Clinical Conditions

Write the correct answer on the line provided.

5.66.   Allen Franklin has a/an _____ . This condition is a benign tumor made up of

newly formed blood vessels.

5.67.   After his surgery, Ramon Martinez developed a deep vein _____ (DVT) in his leg.

5.68.   During her pregnancy, Polly Olson suffered from abnormally swollen veins in her legs. The medical term

for this condition is _____ veins.

5.69.   Thomas Willis suffers from spasmodic choking or suffocating pain caused by a lack of oxygen to his heart

muscle. The condition is known as _____ _____ .

5.70. When Mr. Klein stands up too quickly, his blood pressure drops. His physician describes this as postural

or _____ hypotension.

5.71. Helen Grovenor had a/an _____ implanted as treatment to control atrial fibrillation.

5.72. Dr. Lawson read the patient's _____ . This is also known as an ECG or EKG.

5.73. Jason Turner suffered from cardiac arrest. The paramedics saved his life by using _____

_____ (CPR).

5.74. Darlene Nolan has _____ _____ . This is an obstructive

lesion in the mitral valve of the heart.

5.75. Hamilton Edwards Sr. suffers from _____ heart disease (IHD). This is a group of

cardiac disabilities resulting from an insufficient supply of oxygenated blood to the heart.

___

● Which Is the Correct Medical Term?

Select the correct answer and write it on the line provided.

5.76. A fatty plaque deposit within an artery is called an _____ . This condition is char-

acteristic of atherosclerosis.

| angiitis | angiostenosis | arteriosclerosis | atheroma |

5.77. A fast heartbeat of sudden onset is known as _____.

| atrial fibrillation | bradycardia | palpitation | paroxysmal atrial tachycardia |

5.78. Inflammation of a vein is known as _____ .

| angiitis | arteritis | phlebitis | phlebostenosis |

5.79. The term meaning any abnormal or pathologic condition of the blood is _____ .

| anemia | dyscrasia | hemochromatosis | septicemia |

5.80. The term meaning the surgical removal of an aneurysm is a/an _____ .

| aneurysmectomy | aneurysmoplasty | aneurysmorrhaphy | aneurysmotomy |

● Challenge Word Building

These terms are *not* found in this chapter; however, they are made up of the following familiar word parts. You may want to look in the textbook glossary or use a medical dictionary to check your answers.

peri-	angi/o	-ectomy
	arter/o	-itis
	cardi/o	-necrosis
	phleb/o	-rrhaphy
		-rrhexis
		-stenosis

5.81. The term meaning inflammation of an artery is _____ .

5.82. The surgical removal of a portion of a blood vessel is a/an _____ .

5.83. The abnormal narrowing of the lumen of a vein is called _____ .

5.84. The surgical removal of a portion of the tissue surrounding the heart is a/an _____ .

5.85. The procedure to surgically suture the wall of the heart is a/an _____ .

5.86. The term meaning the rupture of a vein is _____ .

5.87. The suture repair of any vessel, especially a blood vessel, is called a/an _____ .

5.88. The term meaning rupture of the heart is _____ .

5.89. The procedure to suture the tissue surrounding the heart is a/an _____ .

5.90. The term meaning tissue death of the walls of the blood vessels is _____ .

● Labeling Exercises

Identify the numbered items in the accompanying figures.

5.91. Superior _____ _____

5.92. Right _____

5.93. Right _____

5.94. Left pulmonary _____

5.95. Left pulmonary _____

5.96. Pulmonary _____ valve

5.97. _____ valve

5.98. _____

5.99. _____ semilunar valve

5.100. _____ valve

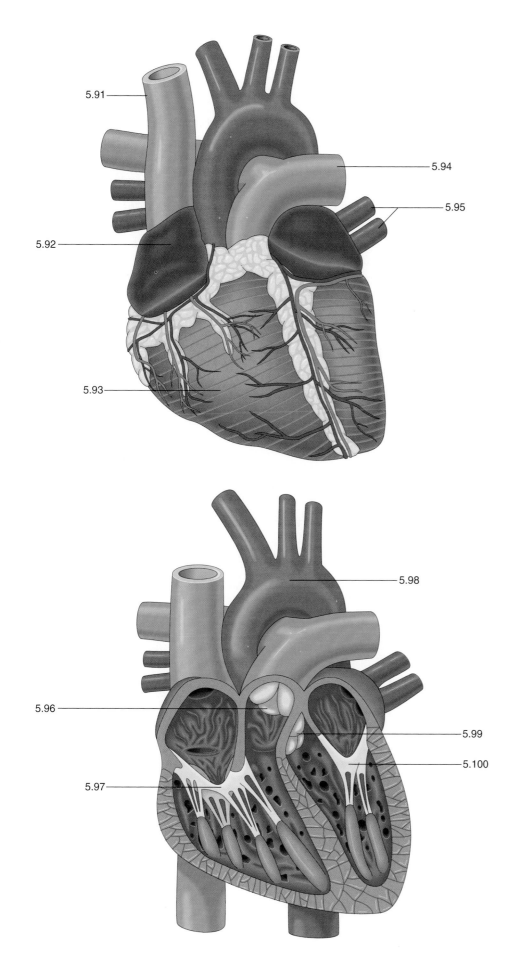

5.91

5.94

5.95

5.92

5.93

5.98

5.96

5.99

5.100

5.97

THE HUMAN TOUCH: CRITICAL THINKING EXERCISE

The following story and questions are designed to stimulate critical thinking through class discussion or as a brief essay response. There are no right or wrong answers to these questions.

Randi Marchant, a 42-year-old waitress, was vacuuming the family room when she felt that painful squeezing in her chest again. Third time today, but this one really hurt. She sat down to catch her breath and stubbed out the cigarette smoldering in the half-filled ashtray by the couch. Her husband, Jimmy, and stepdaughter Melonie had pestered her until she finally had taken time off work to see her doctor. Dr. Harris found that her blood pressure was 158/88—probably owing to the noon rush stress at work, she rationalized. At least her cholesterol test was only 30 points above average this time. It had been slowly coming down, even though she cheated on her diet.

Another wave of pain tightened its icy fingers around her heart, and the pain moved up into both sides of her jaw. Randi thought, "Probably just a little heartburn. Since the pain doesn't radiate down my left arm it couldn't be my heart, could it?"

"Don't think about the pain," she told herself. "Think of something else. Melonie's prom dress needs altering." Randi fell to the floor, clutching her chest, just as Melonie walked in. She saw her stepmother slumped on the floor and screamed, "Oh my God! Help, somebody help!"

Suggested Discussion Topics:

1. What information in the story indicates that Randi might be a candidate for heart disease?

2. Discuss why Randi thought this was not a heart attack because there was no pain in her left arm.

3. What can Melonie do immediately to save Randi's life?

4. Assuming that Randi is having a heart attack, discuss why it is important that she receive appropriate treatment quickly.

5. What steps should someone at risk for heart disease take to help prevent the problem from becoming more serious?

CHAPTER

6

The Lymphatic and Immune Systems

Overview of Structures, Combining Forms, and Functions of the Lymphatic and Immune Systems

MAJOR STRUCTURES	RELATED COMBINING FORMS	PRIMARY FUNCTIONS
Lymph	lymph/o	Removes cellular waste products, pathogens, and dead blood cells from the tissues.
Lymph Vessels	lymphangi/o	Returns lymph to the circulatory system.
Lymph Nodes	lymphaden/o	Produce lymphocytes and filter harmful substances from lymph.
Tonsils and Adenoids	tonsill/o, adenoid/o	Protect the entry into the respiratory system.
Spleen	splen/o (Notice that this combining form is spelled with only one *e*.)	Filters foreign materials from the blood. Maintains the appropriate balance between cells and plasma in the blood. Destroys old worn-out blood cells, acts as a blood reservoir, and stores platelets.
Bone Marrow	myel/o	Produces blood cells (see Chapter 3).
Lymphocytes	lymphocyt/o	Play an important role in immune reactions.
Thymus	thym/o	Produces T lymphocytes and secretes thymosin for the immune system.
Immune System	immun/o	Defends the body against harmful substances, such as pathogenic microorganisms, allergens, toxins, and malignant cells.

● VOCABULARY   RELATED TO THE LYMPHATIC AND IMMUNE SYSTEMS

The items on this list have been identified as key word parts and terms for this chapter. However, all words in boldface in the text are important and may be included in the learning exercises and tests.

Word Parts

- [ ] carcin/o
- [ ] cervic/o
- [ ] immun/o
- [ ] lymph/o
- [ ] lymphaden/o
- [ ] lymphangi/o
- [ ] neo-
- [ ] -oma
- [ ] onc/o
- [ ] phag/o
- [ ] -plasm
- [ ] sarc/o
- [ ] splen/o
- [ ] -tic
- [ ] tox/o

Medical Terms

- [ ] **allergen** (**AL**-er-jen)
- [ ] **anaphylaxis** (**an**-ah-fih-**LACK**-sis)
- [ ] **antibody** (**AN**-tih-**bod**-ee)
- [ ] **antigen** (**AN**-tih-jen)
- [ ] **aspergillosis** (**ass**-per-jil-**OH**-sis)
- [ ] **autoimmune disorder** (**aw**-toh-ih-**MYOUN**)
- [ ] **bacilli** (bah-**SILL**-eye)
- [ ] **bacteria** (back-**TEER**-ree-ah)
- [ ] **bactericide** (back-**TEER**-ih-sighd)
- [ ] **bacteriostatic** (bac-**tee**-ree-oh-**STAT**-ick)
- [ ] **brachytherapy** (**brack**-ee-**THER**-ah-pee)
- [ ] **carcinoma** (**kar**-sih-**NOH**-mah)
- [ ] **complement** (**KOM**-pleh-ment)
- [ ] **cytomegalovirus** (**sigh**-toh-**meg**-ah-loh-**VYE**-rus)
- [ ] **cytotoxic** (**sigh**-toh-**TOK**-sick)
- [ ] **ductal carcinoma in situ**
- [ ] **hemolytic** (**hee**-moh-**LIT**-ick)
- [ ] **herpes zoster** (**HER**-peez **ZOS**-ter)
- [ ] **Hodgkin's lymphoma** (**HODJ**-kinz lim-**FOH**-mah)
- [ ] **immunodeficiency disorder** (**im**-you-noh-deh-**FISH**-en-see)

- [ ] **immunoglobulins** (**im**-you-noh-**GLOB**-you-lins)
- [ ] **immunologist** (**im**-you-**NOL**-oh-jist)
- [ ] **immunosuppressant** (**im**-you-noh-soo-**PRES**-ant)
- [ ] **immunotherapy** (ih-**myou**-noh-**THER**-ah-pee)
- [ ] **infectious mononucleosis** (**mon**-oh-**new**-klee-**OH**-sis)
- [ ] **infiltrating ductal carcinoma**
- [ ] **interferon** (**in**-ter-**FEAR**-on)
- [ ] **lymphadenitis** (lim-**fad**-eh-**NIGH**-tis)
- [ ] **lymphadenopathy** (lim-**fad**-eh-**NOP**-ah-thee)
- [ ] **lymphangiography** (lim-**fan**-jee-**OG**-rah-fee)
- [ ] **lymphangioma** (lim-**fan**-jee-**OH**-mah)
- [ ] **lymphedema** (**lim**-feh-**DEE**-mah)
- [ ] **lymphocytes** (**LIM**-foh-sights)
- [ ] **lymphokines** (**LIM**-foh-kyens)
- [ ] **lymphoma** (lim-**FOH**-mah)
- [ ] **macrophage** (**MACK**-roh-fayj)
- [ ] **metastasis** (meh-**TAS**-tah-sis)
- [ ] **metastasize** (meh-**TAS**-tah-sighz)
- [ ] **moniliasis** (mon-ih-**LYE**-ah-sis)
- [ ] **myoma** (my-**OH**-mah)
- [ ] **myosarcoma** (**my**-oh-sahr-**KOH**-mah)
- [ ] **neoplasm** (**NEE**-oh-plazm)
- [ ] **non-Hodgkin's lymphoma** (non-**HODJ**-kinz lim-**FOH**-mah)
- [ ] **oncologist** (ong-**KOL**-oh-jist)
- [ ] **oncology** (ong-**KOL**-oh-jee)
- [ ] **opportunistic infection** (**op**-ur-too-**NIHS**-tick)
- [ ] **osteosarcoma** (**oss**-tee-oh-sar-**KOH**-mah)
- [ ] **parasite** (**PAR**-ah-sight)
- [ ] **pathogen** (**PATH**-oh-jen)
- [ ] **phagocytosis** (**fag**-oh-sigh-**TOH**-sis)
- [ ] **rabies** (**RAY**-beez)
- [ ] **rickettsia** (rih-**KET**-see-ah)
- [ ] **rubella** (roo-**BELL**-ah)
- [ ] **sarcoma** (sar-**KOH**-mah)
- [ ] **spirochetes** (**SPY**-roh-keets)
- [ ] **splenomegaly** (**splee**-noh-**MEG**-ah-lee)
- [ ] **splenorrhagia** (**splee**-noh-**RAY**-jee-ah)
- [ ] **staphylococci** (**staf**-ih-loh-**KOCK**-sigh)
- [ ] **streptococci** (**strep**-toh-**KOCK**-sigh)
- [ ] **teletherapy** (**tel**-eh-**THER**-ah-pee)

On completion of this chapter, you should be able to:

1. Describe the major functions and structures of the lymphatic and immune systems.

2. Recognize, define, spell, and pronounce the major terms related to the pathology and the diagnostic and treatment procedures of the lymphatic and immune systems.

3. Recognize, define, spell, and pronounce terms related to oncology.

MEDICAL SPECIALTIES RELATED TO THE LYMPHATIC AND IMMUNE SYSTEMS

- An **allergist** (**AL**-er-jist) specializes in diagnosing and treating conditions of altered immunologic reactivity, such as allergic reactions.

- A **hematologist** (**hee**-mah-**TOL**-oh-jist) specializes in diagnosing and treating diseases and disorders of the blood and blood-forming tissues (**hemat** means blood and -**ologist** means specialist).

- An **immunologist** (**im**-you-**NOL**-oh-jist) specializes in diagnosing and treating disorders of the immune system (**immun** means protected and -**ologist** means specialist).

- An **oncologist** (ong-**KOL**-oh-jist) specializes in diagnosing and treating malignant disorders such as tumors and cancer (**onc** means tumor and -**ologist** means specialist).

FUNCTIONS AND STRUCTURES OF THE LYMPHATIC SYSTEM

Functions of the Lymphatic System

The lymphatic system has three primary functions. These are to:

- Absorb fats and fat-soluble vitamins from the digestive system and transport them to the cells.

- Remove cellular waste products from the tissues, then to filter and return this excess tissue fluid to the circulatory system.

- Fill important roles as part of the immune system.

Structures of the Lymphatic System

The major structures of the lymphatic system are **lymph**, **lymphatic vessels**, **lymph nodes**, **tonsils**, **spleen**, and the **thymus**. **Lymphocytes**, which are spe-

cialized white blood cells (WBCs) that have roles in both the lymphatic and immune systems, are discussed later in this chapter under specialized cells of the immune reaction.

Lymph

- **Interstitial fluid** (**in**-ter-**STISH**-al), also known as **intercellular fluid** or **tissue fluid**, is plasma that flows out of the capillaries into the spaces between the cells. This fluid carries food, oxygen, and hormones to the cells (Figure 6.1).

- Ninety percent of the intercellular fluid is resorbed by the capillaries and returns to the circulatory system. *Resorb* means taken up again.

- **Lymph** is the remaining intercellular fluid that has not been resorbed. Lymph removes cellular waste products, pathogens, and dead blood cells from the tissues. Lymph must be filtered by the lymph nodes to remove this contamination before it reenters the bloodstream.

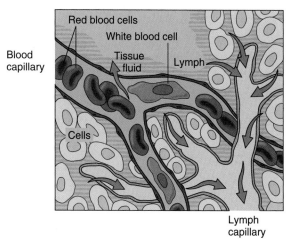
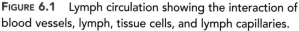

FIGURE 6.1 Lymph circulation showing the interaction of blood vessels, lymph, tissue cells, and lymph capillaries.

Lymphatic Vessels

- **Lymph capillaries** which are microscopic thin-walled tubes located just under the skin, carry lymph from the tissues to the deeper and larger **lymphatic vessels** and **ducts** (Figure 6.2).

- The right side of the head and neck, and the upper right quadrant of the body drain into the **right lymphatic duct**. This duct returns lymph to the bloodstream by emptying into the lymph to the right subclavian vein (Figure 6.3). The subclavian vein is located below the clavicle (collar bone).

- All other areas of the body drain into the **thoracic duct**, which is the largest lymph vessel in the body. This duct returns lymph to the bloodstream by emptying into to the left subclavian vein.

- **Lacteals** (**LACK**-tee-ahls) are specialized lymph capillaries located in the villi that line the walls of the small intestine. Fats and fat-soluble vitamins are absorbed by the lacteals and carried into the bloodstream.

Lymph Nodes

Lymph nodes are small bean-shaped structures located in lymph vessels (Figures 6.2 and 6.3 and Table 6.1).

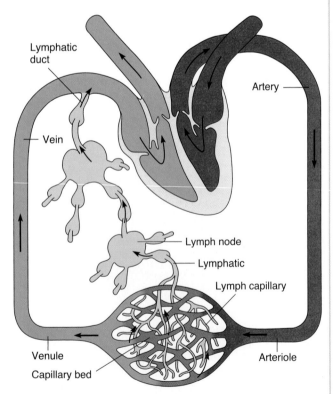

Figure 6.2   Lymph is filtered by lymph nodes before it is transported by the lymphatic ducts to be returned to the venous circulation.

- Lymph nodes filter harmful substances such as bacteria, viruses, and malignant cells out of the lymph before the lymph is returned to the circulatory system. Because of this function, swollen lymph nodes are often an indication of a disease process.

The Tonsils

The **tonsils** (**TON**-sils) are masses of lymphatic tissue that form a protective ring around the nose and upper throat (Figure 6.4). These lymphatic tissues play an important role in the immune system.

- The **adenoids** (**AD**-eh-noids), also known as the **nasopharyngeal tonsils** (**nay**-zoh-fah-**RIN**-jee-al), are located in the nasopharynx. The nasopharynx is discussed in Chapter 7.

- The **palatine tonsils** (**PAL**-ah-tine) are located on the left and right sides of the portion of the throat that is visible through the mouth. *Palatine* means referring to the hard and soft palates.

- The **lingual tonsils** (**LING**-gwal) are located at the base of the tongue. *Lingual* means pertaining to the tongue.

The Vermiform Appendix and Peyer's Patches

The **vermiform appendix** and **Peyer's patches** protect against the entry of invaders through the digestive system (Figure 6.6).

- The **vermiform appendix** is lymphatic tissue that hangs from the lower portion of the cecum of the large intestine.

- **Peyer's patches** are small bundles of lymphatic tissue located on the walls of the ileum. The *ileum* is the final portion of the small intestine.

The Spleen

The **spleen** is a saclike mass of lymphatic tissue located in the left upper quadrant of the abdomen, just inferior to (below) the diaphragm and posterior to (behind) the stomach (Figure 6.5).

- The spleen filters microorganisms and other foreign material from the blood.

- The spleen forms lymphocytes and monocytes, which are specialized white blood cells (WBCs) with roles in the immune system.

- The spleen is **hemolytic** (**hee**-moh-**LIT**-ick), which means that it destroys worn-out red blood cells and liberates hemoglobin (**hem/o** means blood and **-lytic** means to destroy).

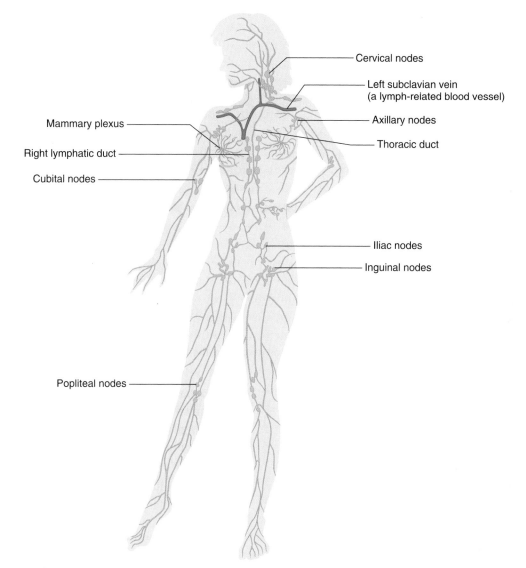

Cervical nodes

Left subclavian vein
(a lymph-related blood vessel)

Mammary plexus

Axillary nodes

Thoracic duct

Right lymphatic duct

Cubital nodes

Iliac nodes

Inguinal nodes

Popliteal nodes

FIGURE 6.3 Lymphatic circulation and major lymph node locations.

Table 6.1

MAJOR LYMPH NODE SITES

Cervical lymph nodes (**SER**-vih-kal) are located in the neck (**cervic** means neck and **-al** means pertaining to).

Axillary lymph nodes (**AK**-sih-**lar**-ee) are located under the arms (**axill** means armpit and **-ary** means pertaining to).

Inguinal lymph nodes (**ING**-gwih-nal) are located in the inguinal (groin) area of the lower abdomen (**inguin** means groin and **-al** means pertaining to).

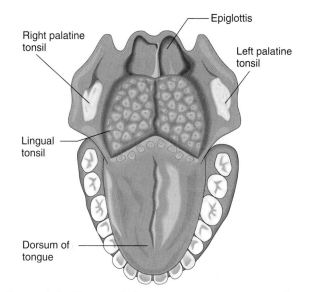

Epiglottis

Right palatine tonsil

Left palatine tonsil

Lingual tonsil

Dorsum of tongue

FIGURE 6.4 The tonsils form a protective ring around the entrance to the respiratory system.

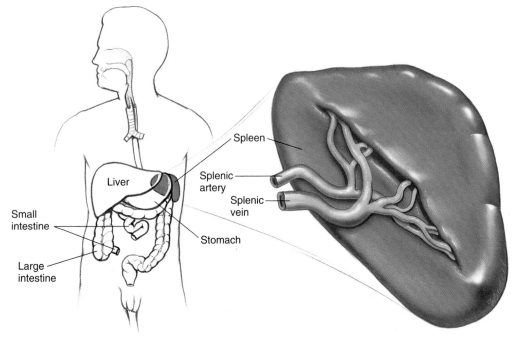

FIGURE 6.5   The spleen performs many important functions related to the immune system.

● The spleen also stores extra erythrocytes and maintains the appropriate balance between the circulating red blood cells (RBCs) and plasma.

The Thymus

The **thymus** (**THIGH**-mus) is located superior to (above) the heart and is composed largely of lymphatic tissue (Figure 6.6). The thymus, which reaches its maximum development during puberty, becomes gradually smaller with reduced function. The thymus plays roles in both the immune and endocrine systems. (See Chapter 13.)

Pathology and Diagnostic Procedures of the Lymphatic System

● **Lymphadenitis** (lim-**fad**-eh-**NIGH**-tis), also known as **swollen glands**, is an inflammation of the lymph nodes (**lymphaden** means lymph node and **-itis** means inflammation).

● **Lymphadenopathy** (lim-**fad**-eh-**NOP**-ah-thee) is any disease process usually involving enlargement of the lymph nodes (**lymphaden/o** means lymph node and **-pathy** means disease).

● **Persistent generalized lymphadenopathy (PGL)** is the continued presence of enlarged lymph nodes. PGL is often an indication of the presence of a malignancy or a deficiency in immune system function.

● A **lymphangioma** (lim-**fan**-jee-**OH**-mah), which is a congenital malformation of the lymphatic system, is a benign tumor formed by an abnormal collection of lymphatic vessels (**lymphangi** means lymph vessel and **-oma** means tumor).

● **Splenomegaly** (**splee**-noh-**MEG**-ah-lee) is an abnormal enlargement of the spleen (**splen/o** means spleen and **-megaly** means abnormal enlargement). This condition may be due to bleeding caused by an injury, an infectious disease such as mononucleosis, or abnormal functioning of the immune system.

● **Splenorrhagia** (**splee**-noh-**RAY**-jee-ah) is bleeding from the spleen (**splen/o** means spleen and **-rrhagia** means bleeding).

● **Lymphangiography** (lim-**fan**-jee-**OG**-rah-fee) is the radiographic examination of the lymphatic vessels after the injection of a contrast medium (**lymphangi/o** means lymph vessel and **-graphy** means process of recording). The resulting **lymphangiogram** (lim-**FAN**-jee-oh-**gram**) is used primarily to diagnose and monitor treatment of lymphomas, (**lymphangi/o** means lymph vessel and **-gram** means resulting record).

Lymphedema

Lymphedema (**lim**-feh-**DEE**-mah) is swelling due to an abnormal accumulation of lymph within the tissues (**lymph** means lymph and **-edema** means swelling).

- **Primary lymphedema** is a hereditary disorder that may appear at any time in life and most commonly affects the legs.
- **Secondary lymphedema** is caused by cancer treatment (lymph node removal, chemotherapy, and/or radiation therapy), burns, or trauma. This condition usually affects the limb or body area nearest the missing lymph nodes.

FUNCTION AND STRUCTURES OF THE IMMUNE SYSTEM

Function of the Immune System

The primary function of the immune system is to protect the body from harmful substances such as **pathogens**, **allergens**, **toxins**, and **malignant cells**. If these substances gain entry to the body, the immune system immediately begins working to destroy them. *Pathogens* are disease-producing microorganisms, *allergens* are substances that produce an allergic reaction, and *toxins* are poisons.

Structures of the Immune System

Unlike other body systems, the immune system is not contained within a single set of organs or vessels. Instead, its functions depend on structures from several other body systems (Figure 6.6).

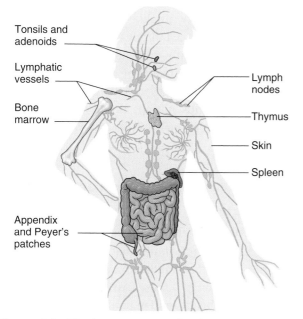

Tonsils and adenoids

Lymphatic vessels

Bone marrow

Lymph nodes

Thymus

Skin

Spleen

Appendix and Peyer's patches

FIGURE 6.6 The immune system involves structures from many body systems.

The First Lines of Defense

The immune system prevents foreign substances from entering the body by using parts of other body systems as the first line of defense.

- **Intact skin** wraps the body in a physical barrier that prevents invading organisms from entering the body. *Intact* means there are no cuts, scrapes, open sores, or breaks in the skin.
- The **respiratory system** traps breathed-in foreign matter with nose hairs and the moist mucous membrane lining of the respiratory system. Coughing and sneezing help expel foreign matter from the respiratory system.
- The **digestive system** uses the acids and enzymes produced by the stomach to destroy invaders that are swallowed or consumed with food.
- The **lymphatic system** provides lymph nodes that fight invaders by filtering lymph and destroying pathogens that have entered the tissues of the body.

The Immune Reaction

The **immune reaction**, also known as the **antigen-antibody reaction**, is one way in which the immune system destroys pathogens that have entered the body.

- An **antigen** (**AN**-tih-jen) is any substance that the body regards as being foreign. Substances that the body recognizes as antigens include viruses, bacteria, toxins, and transplanted tissues. The immune system immediately responds to the presence of any antigen.
- An **antibody** (**AN**-tih-**bod**-ee) is a disease-fighting protein created by the immune system in response to the presence of a specific antigen. Antibodies are discussed further under immunoglobulins.
- The **antigen-antibody reaction** involves binding antigens to antibodies to form antigen-antibody complexes. This action tags the potentially dangerous antigen so that it can be recognized and destroyed by other cells of the immune system.

Specialized Cells of the Immune Reactions

The immune response requires the actions of many specialized cells.

Lymphocytes

- **Lymphocytes** (**LIM**-foh-sights), which are formed in bone marrow as stem cells, are white blood cells that specialize to act as antibodies so they can attack specific antigens (**lymph/o** means lymph and **-cytes** means cells). (See Chapter 2.)

- These lymphocytes undergo further maturation and differentiation in lymphatic tissues throughout the body. *Maturation* means the process of becoming mature. *Differentiation* means to be modified to perform a specific function.

B Cells

B cells, also known as **B lymphocytes**, are specialized lymphocytes that produce and secrete antibodies. Each lymphocyte makes a specific antibody that is capable of destroying a specific antigen. B cells are most effective against viruses and bacteria circulating in the blood.

- When a B cell is confronted with the antigen that it is coded to destroy, that B cell is transformed into a plasma cell. A *plasma cell* is capable of producing and secreting antibodies that are coded to destroy the antigen.

T Cells

T cells, also known as **T lymphocytes**, are small lymphocytes that have matured in the thymus as a result of their exposure to thymosin. *Thymosin* is the hormone secreted by the thymus.

- T cells contribute to the immune defense by coordinating immune defenses and by killing infected cells on contact.
- **Interferon** (**in**-ter-**FEAR**-on), which is produced by the T cells, is a family of proteins whose specialty is fighting viruses by slowing or stopping their multiplication.
- **Lymphokines** (**LIM**-foh-kyens), which are produced by the T cells, direct the immune response by signaling between the cells of the immune system. Lymphokines attract macrophages to the infected site and prepare them to attack the invaders.
- A **macrophage** (**MACK**-roh-fayj) protects the body by eating invading cells and by interacting with the other cells of the immune system (**macro-** means large and **-phage** means a cell that eats).
- A **phagocyte** (**FAG**-oh-sight) is a large white blood cell that can eat and destroy substances such as cell debris, dust, pollen, and pathogens (**phag/o** means to eat or swallow and **-cyte** means cell).
  Phagocytosis (**fag**-oh-sigh-**TOH**-sis) is the process by which phagocytes eat and destroy substances.

Immunoglobulins

Immunoglobulins (**im**-you-noh-**GLOB**-you-lins) (**Ig**), which are secreted by B cells, are also known as **antibodies**. The five major classes of immunoglobulins are: immunoglobulin A (IgA), immunoglobulin D (IgD), immunoglobulin E (IgE), immunoglobulin G (IgG), and immunoglobulin M (IgM). Each type of immunoglobulin has specific functions in the antigen-antibody reaction.

Complement

Complement (**KOM**-pleh-ment) is a series of more than 25 complex proteins that normally circulate in the blood in an inactive form. They are activated by contact with an antigen and when activated, they puncture the antigen's cell membrane. *Memory aid:* These proteins "complement" the work of antibodies in destroying bacteria.

Immunity

Immunity is the state of being resistant to a specific disease.

- **Natural immunity** is passed from the mother to her developing child before birth. Immediately after birth additional immunity is passed from mother to child through breast milk.
- **Acquired immunity**, also known as **active immunity**, is obtained by the development of antibodies during an attack of an infectious disease such as chickenpox.
- **Artificial immunity**, also known as **acquired immunity**, is obtained through **immunization** or **vaccination**. Currently, artificial immunity is available against diseases including chickenpox, diphtheria, hepatitis B, some types of influenza, measles, meningitis, mumps, pertussis, some types of pneumonia, poliomyelitis, smallpox, tetanus, and typhoid.

Immune System Response Factors

Important factors that influence the immune system's ability to respond are health, age, and heredity.

- **Health** The better the individual's general health, the more likely it is that the immune system can respond effectively. Disease strikes more easily when general health, and in particular the functioning of the immune system, is compromised and not functioning properly.

- **Age** Older individuals usually have more acquired immunity; however, their immune systems tend to respond less quickly and effectively to new challenges.

- **Heredity** Genes and genetic disorders shape the makeup of antibodies and other immune cells that influence the body's ability to respond to invaders. Genetic disorders are discussed in Chapter 2.

- An **opportunistic infection** (**op**-ur-too-**NIHS**-tick) is a pathogen that normally does not cause disease; however, if the host is debilitated (weakened) by another condition, the pathogen is able to cause illness in a weakened host.

Pathology and Diagnostic Procedures of the Immune System

Allergic Reactions

- An **allergy**, also known as **hypersensitivity**, is an overreaction by the body to a particular antigen.

- An allergic reaction occurs when the body's immune system reacts to a harmless allergen, such as pollen, food, or animal dander, as if it were a dangerous invader. An **allergen** (**AL**-er-jen) is an antigen that is capable of causing an allergic response.

- In a **cellular response**, also known as a **localized** or **delayed allergic response**, the body does not react the first time it is exposed to the allergen. However, sensitivity is established and future contacts cause symptoms that include itching, redness of the skin, and large hives. For example, contact dermatitis is a skin reaction caused by a localized allergic response. (See Chapter 12.)

- A **systemic reaction**, also described as **anaphylaxis** (**an**-ah-fih-**LACK**-sis), is a severe response to a foreign substance, such as a drug, food, insect venom, or chemical. Symptoms develop very quickly and include swelling, blockage of air passages, and a drop in blood pressure. Without appropriate care, the patient may die within minutes.

- A **scratch test** is a diagnostic test to identify commonly troublesome allergens, such as tree pollen and ragweed. Swelling and itching indicate an allergic reaction (Figure 6.7).

- **Antihistamines** are medications that are administered to block and control allergic reactions.

Autoimmune Disorders

An **autoimmune disorder** (**aw**-toh-ih-**MYOUN**) is a condition in which the immune system reacts incor-

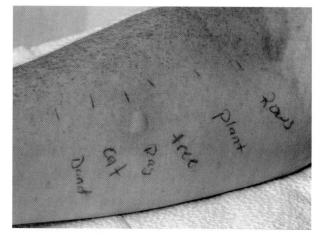

FIGURE 6.7   In scratch tests, allergens are placed on the skin, the skin is scratched, and the allergen is labeled. Reactions usually occur within 20 minutes. Pictured is a reaction to ragweed.

rectly to normal antigens and creates antibodies against the body's own tissues. These disorders, which appear to be genetically transmitted, can affect most body systems (Table 6.2). For reasons that are not understood, 75 percent of these diseases occur in women during the childbearing years.

Immunodeficiency Disorders

An **immunodeficiency disorder** (**im**-you-noh-deh-**FISH**-en-see) is a condition that occurs when one or more parts of the immune system are missing or not working properly.

- When the immune system is weakened in this manner, it is also described as being **compromised**.

- Some immunodeficiency disorders, such as **congenital immunodeficiency**, are hereditary. Other forms are caused by pathogens.

The Human Immunodeficiency Virus

The **human immunodeficiency virus**, also known as **HIV** (pronounced **H-I-V**), is a bloodborne pathogen that progressively damages or kills cells of the immune system.

- **Acquired immunodeficiency syndrome**, also known as **AIDS**, is the advanced stage of an HIV infection. At this stage, as shown in Figure 6.8, many pathologies are present throughout the body.

- **ELISA**, which is the acronym for **enzyme-linked immunosorbent assay**, is the blood test that is used to screen for the presence of HIV antibodies. However, this test may produce a false-positive

Table 6.2

EXAMPLES OF AUTOIMMUNE DISORDERS AND THE AFFECTED BODY SYSTEMS

Body System	Disorder
Skeletal System	**Rheumatoid arthritis** affects joints and connective tissue.
Muscular System	**Myasthenia gravis** affects nerve and muscle synapses.
Cardiovascular System	**Pernicious anemia** affects the red blood cells.
Digestive System	**Crohn's disease** affects the intestines, the ileum, or the colon.
Nervous System	**Multiple sclerosis** affects the brain and spinal cord.
Integumentary System	**Alopecia areata** affects the hair follicles.
	Lupus erythematosus affects the skin, connective tissue, and joints.
	Scleroderma affects the skin and connective tissues.
	Vitiligo affects melanin within the skin.
Endocrine System	**Type 1 diabetes mellitus**, affects the insulin-producing pancreatic cells.
	Graves' disease affects the thyroid gland.
	Hashimoto's thyroiditis affects the thyroid gland.

result. A *false positive* is an inaccurate test result that indicates the presence of HIV when HIV is not present.

- When the results of the ELISA test are positive, a **Western blot test** is performed to confirm the diagnosis. The Western blot test, which detects the presence of specific viral proteins, produces more accurate results.

Treatment Procedures of the Immune System

Immunotherapy

- **Immunotherapy** (ih-**myou**-noh-**THER**-ah-pee) is a treatment of disease that involves either stimulating or repressing the immune response (**immune/o** means immune and **-therapy** means treatment).
- In the treatment of allergies, immunotherapy is used to repress the immune response. *Repress* means to slow down or control.
- In the treatment of cancers, immunotherapy is used to stimulate the immune response to fight the malignancy.

Antibody Therapy

- **Synthetic immunoglobulins**, also known as **immune serum**, are used as a postexposure preventive measure against certain viruses including rabies and some types of hepatitis.
- **Synthetic interferon** is used in the treatment of multiple sclerosis, hepatitis C, and some cancers.
- **Monoclonal antibodies**, which may enhance a patient's immune response to the cancer, are used in the treatment of some non-Hodgkin's lymphoma, melanoma, and breast and colon cancers.

Immunosuppression

- **Immunosuppression** (**im**-you-noh-sup-**PRESH**-un) is treatment used to interfere with the ability of the immune system to respond to stimulation by antigens.
- An **immunosuppressant** (**im**-you-noh-soo-**PRES**-ant), which is a substance that prevents or reduces the body's normal immune response, is administered to prevent the rejection of donor tissue and to depress autoimmune disorders.

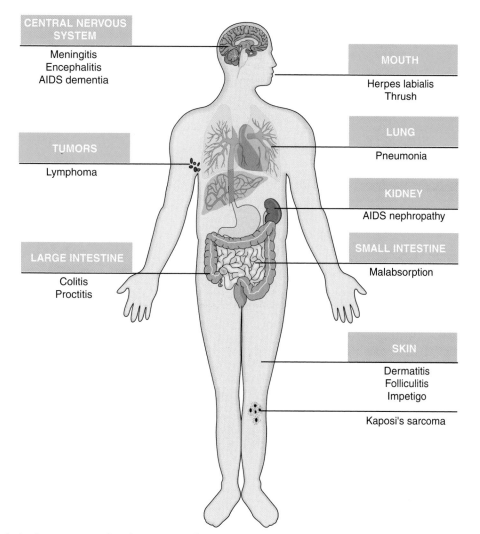

CENTRAL NERVOUS SYSTEM
Meningitis
Encephalitis
AIDS dementia

MOUTH
Herpes labialis
Thrush

LUNG
Pneumonia

TUMORS
Lymphoma

KIDNEY
AIDS nephropathy

SMALL INTESTINE
Malabsorption

LARGE INTESTINE
Colitis
Proctitis

SKIN
Dermatitis
Folliculitis
Impetigo

Kaposi's sarcoma

FIGURE 6.8   Pathologies associated with AIDS. (Each condition is discussed in the appropriate body system chapter.)

- A **corticosteroid drug** is a hormone-like preparation used primarily as an anti-inflammatory and as an immunosuppressant. The natural production of corticosteroids by the endocrine system is discussed in Chapter 13.

- A **cytotoxic drug** (**sigh**-toh-**TOK**-sick) kills or damages cells (**cyt/o** means cell, **tox** means poison and **-ic** means pertaining to). These drugs are used both as immunosuppressants and as antineoplastics. (See also the discussion of chemotherapy later in this chapter.)

PATHOGENIC ORGANISMS

A **pathogen** (**PATH**-oh-jen) is a microorganism that causes a disease (Figure 6.9). A *microorganism* is a living organism that is so small it can be seen only with the aid of a microscope.

Bacteria

Bacteria (back-**TEER**-ree-ah) are a group of one-celled microscopic organisms (singular, **bacterium**). The pathogenic types of bacteria include: bacilli, rickettsia, spirochetes, staphylococci, and streptococci.

- **Bacilli** (bah-**SILL**-eye) are rod-shaped spore-forming bacteria (singular, **bacillus**). **Tetanus** and **tuberculosis** are caused by bacilli (Figure 6.9).

- A **rickettsia** (rih-**KET**-see-ah) is a small bacterium that lives in lice, fleas, ticks, and mites (plural, **rickettsiae**). **Rocky Mountain spotted fever**, which is caused by *Rickettsia rickettsii*, is transmitted to humans by the bite of an infected tick.

- **Spirochetes** (**SPY**-roh-keets) are spiral-shaped bacteria that have flexible walls and are capable of movement (Figure 6.9). **Lyme disease**, which is caused by the spirochete *Borrelia burgdorferi*, is

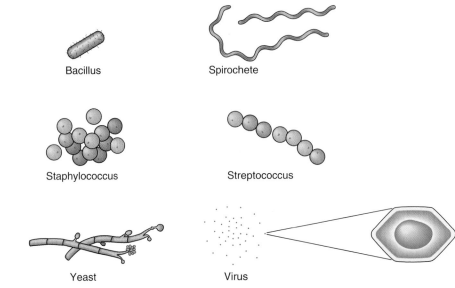

FIGURE 6.9 Types of pathogens. On the right, a single virus is magnified to illustrate its structure in detail.

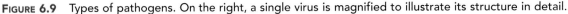

transmitted to humans by the bite of an infected deer tick.

- **Staphylococci** (**staf**-ih-loh-**KOCK**-sigh) are bacteria that form irregular groups or clusters (singular, **staphylococcus**) (Figure 6.9). *Staphylococcus aureus* causes a variety of pus-forming infections and superficial skin lesions such as boils and furuncles. (See Chapter 12.)

- **Streptococci** (**strep**-toh-**KOCK**-sigh) are bacteria that form a chain (singular, **streptococcus**) (Figure 6.9). **Severe pharyngitis**, commonly known as a **strep throat**, is caused by *Group A streptococci*.

Fungus, Yeast, and Parasites

- A **fungus** (**FUNG**-gus) is a simple parasitic plant. Some of these plants are harmless to humans and others are pathogenic (plural, **fungi**). **Aspergillosis** (**ass**-per-jil-**OH**-sis), which is an infection caused by a fungus of the genus *Aspergillus,* may cause inflammation and lesions on, or in, any organ. A *lesion* is a pathologic change of the tissues due to disease or injury.

- **Yeast** is a type of fungus (Figure 6.9). **Moniliasis** (mon-ih-**LYE**-ah-sis), which is caused by the pathogenic yeast *Candida albicans,* is an infection of the skin or mucous membranes. These infections are usually localized in the mouth or the vagina.

- A **parasite** (**PAR**-ah-sight) is a plant or animal that lives on or within another living organism at the expense of that organism. **Malaria** (mah-**LAY**-ree-ah), which is caused by a parasite that lives within

certain mosquitoes, is transferred to humans by the bite of an infected mosquito.

Viruses

- **Viruses** (**VYE**-rus-ez) are very small infectious agents that live only by invading cells (singular, **virus**) (Figure 6.9). Within the cell, the virus reproduces and then breaks the cell wall. The newly formed viruses are released so they can spread to other cells.

Viral Infections

- **Cytomegalovirus** (**sigh**-toh-**meg**-ah-loh-**VYE**-rus) is a group of large herpes-type viruses that cause a variety of diseases (**cyt/o** means cell, **megal/o** means large, **vir** means virus, and **-us** is a singular noun ending).

- **Infectious mononucleosis** (**mon**-oh-**new**-klee-**OH**-sis), which is caused by the **Epstein-Barr virus**, is characterized by fever, a sore throat, and enlarged lymph nodes.

- **Measles** is an acute, highly contagious infection caused by the rubeola virus and transmitted by respiratory droplets. Symptoms include fever, malaise, nasal congestion, a cough, photophobia, and a rash over the entire body. *Photophobia* means sensitivity to light. Complications of measles can be serious. Compare measles with *rubella*.

- **Mumps** is an acute viral disease characterized by the swelling of the parotid glands. The parotid glands are salivary glands located on the face just in front of the ears.

- **Rabies** (**RAY**-beez) is an acute viral infection that may be transmitted to humans by the blood, tissue, or saliva of an infected animal.

- **Rubella** (roo-**BELL**-ah), also known as **German measles** or **3-day measles**, is a viral infection characterized by fever and a diffuse, fine, red rash. If the mother has rubella during the early stages of pregnancy, the disease may cause congenital abnormalities in the developing child. Compare rubella with *measles*.

- **Varicella** (var-ih-**SEL**-ah) (**VZV**), also known as **chickenpox**, is caused by the herpes virus *Varicella zoster* and is highly contagious. VZV is characterized by fever and an itchy rash that eventually forms crusted scabs.

- **Herpes zoster** (**HER**-peez **ZOS**-ter), also known as **shingles**, is an acute viral infection characterized by painful skin eruptions that follow the underlying route of the inflamed nerve. This inflammation occurs when the dormant chickenpox virus is reactivated later in life. The duration of an outbreak is shortened by prompt treatment with antiviral drugs.

- The **West Nile virus**, which causes flulike symptoms, is carried by birds and transmitted to humans by mosquito or tick bites. If untreated, the inflammation can spread to the spinal cord and brain.

Medications to Control Infections

- **Antibiotics** are chemical substances capable of inhibiting growth or killing pathogenic microorganisms (**anti-** means against, **bio** means life, and **-tic** means pertaining to). *Inhibit* means to slow the growth or development. Antibiotics are used to combat bacterial infections; however, they are not effective against viruses.

- A **bactericide** (back-**TEER**-ih-sighd) is a substance that causes the death of bacteria (**bacteri** means bacteria and **-cide** means causing death). Bactericides include the antibiotic groups of penicillins and cephalosporins.

- A **bacteriostatic** (bac-**tee**-ree-oh-**STAT**-ick) is an agent that slows or stops the growth of bacteria (**bacteri** means bacteria and **-static** means causing control). Bacteriostatics include tetracycline, sulfonamide, and erythromycin.

- An **antifungal** (an-tih-**FUNG**-gul) is an agent that destroys or inhibits the growth of fungi (**anti-** means against, **fung** means fungus, and **-al** means pertain-

ing to). Lotrimin is an example of a topical antifungal that is applied to treat or prevent athlete's foot. This type of medication is also known as an **antimycotic** (an-tih-my-**KOT**-ick) (**anti-** means against, **myc/o** means fungus, and **-tic** means pertaining to).

- An **antiviral drug** (an-tih-**VYE**-ral), such as acyclovir, is used to treat viral infections or to provide temporary immunity (**anti-** means against, **vir** means virus, and **-al** means pertaining to).

ONCOLOGY

Oncology (ong-**KOL**-oh-jee) is the study of the prevention, causes, and treatment of tumors and cancer (**onc** means tumor and **-ology** means study of). The term **cancer** describes over 200 different kinds of malignancies. Cancer attacks all body systems and is the second leading cause of death in the United States. Most cancers are named for the part of the body where the cancer first starts. (Brain tumors are discussed in Chapter 10.)

Terms Related to Tumors

A **neoplasm** (**NEE**-oh-plazm), also known as a **tumor**, is a new and abnormal tissue formation in which the multiplication of cells is uncontrolled, abnormally rapid, and progressive (**neo-** means new or strange and **-plasm** means formation).

- **Angiogenesis** (an-jee-oh-**JEN**-eh-sis) is the process through which the tumor supports its growth by creating its own blood supply (**angi/o** means vessel and **-genesis** means reproduction). Compare with *antiangiogenesis*.

- **Antiangiogenesis** is a form of cancer treatment that disrupts this blood supply to the tumor (**anti-** means against, **angi/o** means vessel, and **-genesis** means reproduction). Compare with *angiogenesis*.

Benign Tumors

A **benign** tumor is not life-threatening and does not recur. *Memory aid:* Benign sounds like *be nice!* Although not life-threatening, these tumors can cause problems by placing pressure on adjacent structures. For example, a **myoma** (my-**OH**-mah) is a benign tumor made up of muscle tissue (**my** means muscle and **-oma** means tumor). Compare with *myosarcoma*.

Malignant Tumors

The term **malignant** means harmful, tending to spread, becoming progressively worse, and life-threatening. *Memory aid:* Malignant sounds like *malicious* or *mean*! Malignant tumors tend to spread to distant body sites.

- The term **carcinoma in situ** describes a malignant tumor in its original position that has not yet disturbed or invaded the surrounding tissues.

- An **invasive malignancy** grows and spreads into adjacent tissues. Figure 6.10 shows the progression as colorectal cancer invades the surrounding tissues.

Metastasis Compared with Metastasize

- **Metastasize** (meh-**TAS**-tah-sighz) is the verb that describes the process by which cancer spreads from one place to another. The cancer starts at the primary site and metastasizes (spreads) to a secondary site.

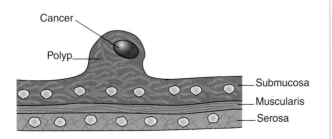

Class A colorectal cancer

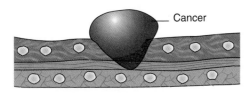

Class B colorectal cancer

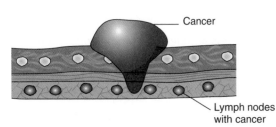

Class C colorectal cancer

FIGURE 6.10 Stages of colorectal cancer. *Class A:* The polyp has formed but has not yet invaded the surrounding tissue. *Class B:* The cancer has invaded the underlying tissue. *Class C:* The cancer has spread to surrounding lymph nodes.

- **Metastasis** (meh-**TAS**-tah-sis) is the noun that describes the new cancer site that results from the spreading process (**meta-** means beyond and **-stasis** means stopping). The metastasis may be within the same body system or in another body system at a distance from the primary site (plural, **metastases**).

Staging

Staging is the process of classifying tumors with respect to how far the disease has progressed, the potential for its responding to therapy, and the patient's prognosis. Specific staging systems are used for different types of cancer (Figure 6.10 and Table 6.3).

Carcinomas

A **carcinoma** (**kar**-sih-**NOH**-mah) is a malignant tumor that occurs in epithelial tissue (**carcin** means cancer and **-oma** means tumor). Epithelial tissue forms the protective covering for all of the internal and external surfaces of the body (Figure 6.11).

- Carcinomas tend to infiltrate and produce metastases that may affect any organ or part of the body.

- For example, an **adenocarcinoma** (**ad**-eh-noh-**kar**-sih-**NOH**-mah) is any one of a large group of carcinomas derived from glandular tissue (**aden/o** means gland, **carcin** means cancer, and **-oma** means tumor).

Sarcomas

A **sarcoma** (sar-**KOH**-mah) is a malignant tumor that arises from connective tissue (**sarc** means flesh and **-oma** means tumor) (plural, **sarcomas** or **sarcomata**).

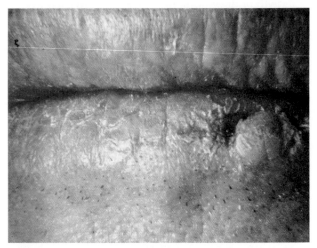

FIGURE 6.11 Carcinoma of the lip. (Courtesy of Dr. Joseph Konzelman, School of Dentistry, Medical College of Georgia.)

- Connective tissues include: hard tissues (bones and cartilage), soft tissues (fat, tissues surrounding and supporting organs), and liquid tissues (blood and lymph).

- Hard tissue sarcomas arise from bone or cartilage. (See also Chapter 3.) For example, an **osteosarcoma** (**oss**-tee-oh-sar-**KOH**-mah) is a malignant tumor usually involving the upper shaft of long bones, the pelvis, or knee (**oste/o** means bone, **sarc** means flesh, and **-oma** means tumor).

- Soft tissue sarcomas arise from tissues such as fat, muscle, and nerves. For example, a **myosarcoma** (**my**-oh-sahr-**KOH**-mah) is a malignant tumor derived from muscle tissue (**myo** means muscle, **sarc** means flesh, and **oma** means tumor). Compare with *myoma*.

- **Kaposi's sarcoma** (**KAP**-oh-seez sar-**KOH**-mah) may affect the skin, mucous membranes, lymph nodes, and internal organs. This form of cancer is frequently associated with HIV.

Lymphomas

Lymphoma (lim-**FOH**-mah) is a general term applied to malignancies that develop in the lymphatic system (**lymph** means lymph and **-oma** means tumor). The involved tissues include lymph nodes, spleen, liver, and bone marrow. The two most common types of lymphomas are Hodgkin's lymphoma and non-Hodgkin's lymphoma.

Hodgkin's Lymphoma

Hodgkin's lymphoma (**HODJ**-kinz lim-**FOH**-mah) (**HL**), also known as **Hodgkin's disease**, is distinguished by the presence of Reed-Sternberg cells, which are large cancerous lymphocytes. HL is staged using Roman numerals from I to IV.

Non-Hodgkin's Lymphoma

The term **non-Hodgkin's lymphoma** (non-**HODJ**-kinz lim-**FOH**-mah) (**NHL**) is used to describe all lymphomas *other than* Hodgkin's lymphoma.

- In NHL, the cells of the lymphatic system divide and grow without any order or control. This causes tumors to develop in different locations on the body and these cancer cells can also spread to other organs.

- This disease is described as three types: low-grade (growing slowly), intermediate-grade (growing moderately), and high-grade (growing rapidly).

Breast Cancer

Breast cancer is a malignant tumor that develops from the cells of the breast and may spread to adjacent lymph nodes and other body sites (Figure 6.12).

Types of Breast Cancer

- **Invasive ductal carcinoma**, also known as **infiltrating ductal carcinoma**, starts in the milk duct, breaks through the wall of that duct, and invades fatty breast tissue. This form of cancer accounts for the majority of all breast cancers.

- **Ductal carcinoma in situ** is breast cancer at its earliest stage (stage 0) before the cancer has broken through the wall of the milk duct. At this stage, the cure rate is nearly 100 percent.

- **Invasive lobular carcinoma**, also known as **infiltrating lobular carcinoma**, is cancer that starts in the milk glands (lobules), breaks through the wall of the gland, and invades the fatty tissue of the breast. Once the cancer reaches the lymph nodes, it can rapidly spread to distant parts of the body.

- **Male breast cancer** can occur in the small amount of breast tissue that is normally present in men. The types of cancers are similar to those occurring in women.

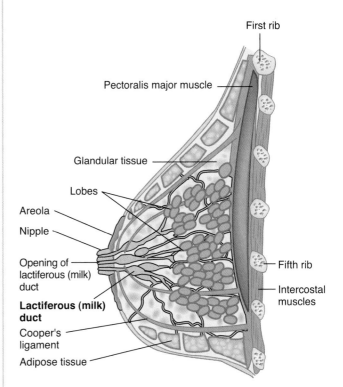

FIGURE 6.12   Invasive ductal carcinoma, which is the most common form of all breast cancers, begins in the lactiferons (milk) ducts.

Table 6.3

STAGING BREAST CANCER

Stage	Explanation
I	The cancer is no larger than two centimeters (about one inch) and has not spread outside the breast.
II	Any of the following may be true: The cancer is no larger than two centimeters but has spread to the axillary lymph nodes. The cancer is between two and five centimeters (from one to two inches) and may or may not have spread to the axillary lymph nodes. The cancer is larger than five centimeters (greater than two inches) but has not spread to the axillary lymph nodes.
IIIA	Either of the following is true: The cancer is smaller than five centimeters and has spread to the axillary lymph nodes and the lymph nodes are attached to each other or to other structures. The cancer is larger than five centimeters and has spread to the axillary lymph nodes.
IIIB	Either of the following is true: The cancer has spread to tissues near the breast (skin or chest wall, including the ribs and muscles of the chest). The cancer has spread to lymph nodes inside the chest wall along the breastbone.
IV	The cancer has spread to other organs of the body, most often the bones, lungs, liver, or brain. Or, the cancer has spread locally to the skin and lymph nodes inside the neck, near the collarbone.

Detection of Breast Cancer

Early detection is possible through **breast self-examination mammograms**, and professional palpation. These procedures are discussed in Chapter 14. A preliminary diagnosis is confirmed by biopsy.

- A **biopsy** (**BYE**-op-see) is the removal of a small piece of living tissue for examination to confirm or establish a diagnosis (**bi**- means pertaining to life and -**opsy** means view of). After a diagnosis has been established, treatment is then based on the stage of the cancer (Table 6.3).

- A **needle breast biopsy** is a technique in which an x-ray guided needle is used to remove small samples of tissue from the breast. It is less painful, less disfiguring (no scarring), and requires a shorter recovery time than surgical biopsy.

- **Lymph node dissection** is a diagnostic procedure in which all of the lymph nodes in a major group are removed to determine the spread of cancer. For example, an *axillary lymph node dissection* (ALND) is performed to diagnose the spread of breast cancer.

- A *sentinel node* is the first lymph node to come into contact with cancer cells as they leave the organ of origination and start spreading into the rest of the body. In a **sentinel-node biopsy (SNB)**, the sentinal node is identified and is the only node removed for biopsy. If the cancer has not spread, this spares the remaining nodes in that group.

Treatment of Breast Cancer

- A **lumpectomy** is the surgical removal of only the cancerous tissue and a margin of surrounding normal tissue (Figure 6.13).

- A **mastectomy** (mas-**TECK**-toh-mee) is the surgical removal of an entire breast (**mast** means breast and -**ectomy** means surgical removal).

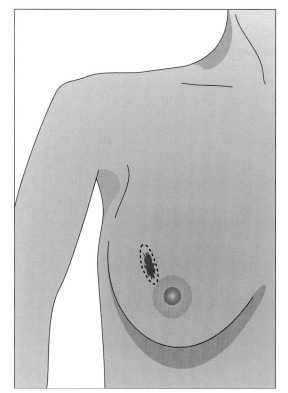

FIGURE 6.13 A lumpectomy is the removal of the cancerous tissue plus a margin of healthy tissue.

- A **modified radical mastectomy** is the surgical removal of the entire breast and axillary lymph nodes under the adjacent arm (Figure 6.14).

Cancer Treatments

The three most common forms of cancer treatments are surgery, chemotherapy, and radiation therapy.

Surgery

When possible, cancer surgery involves removing the malignancy plus a margin of normal surrounding tissue.

Chemotherapy

Chemotherapy is the use of chemical agents and drugs in combinations selected to destroy malignant cells and tissues.

- An **antineoplastic** (**an**-tih-nee-oh-**PLAS**-tick) is medication that blocks the development, growth, or proliferation of malignant cells (**anti-** means against, **ne/o** means new, **plast** means growth or formation, and **-tic** means pertaining to). *Proliferation* means to increase rapidly.

- Cytotoxic drugs, which are also used in chemotherapy, were discussed earlier in this chapter under immunosuppression.

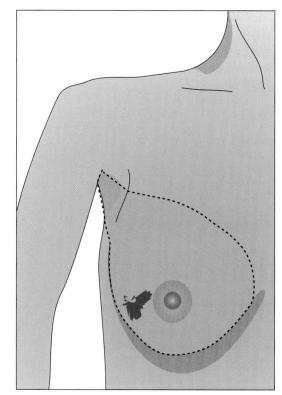

FIGURE 6.14 A modified radical mastectomy is the removal of the entire breast and the adjacent lymph nodes.

Radiation Therapies

Radiation therapy is the treatment of cancers through the use of x-rays. The goal of these therapies is to destroy the cancer while sparing healthy tissues.

- **Brachytherapy** (**brack**-ee-**THER**-ah-pee) is the use of radioactive materials in contact with, or implanted into, the tissues to be treated (**brachy-** means short and **-therapy** means treatment).

- **Teletherapy** (**tel**-eh-**THER**-ah-pee) is radiation therapy administered at a distance from the body (**tele-** means distant and **-therapy** means treatment). With three-dimensional computer imaging, it is possible to aim doses more precisely.

ABBREVIATIONS RELATED TO THE LYMPHATIC AND IMMUNE SYSTEMS

Table 6.4 presents an overview of the abbreviations related to the terms introduced in this chapter. *Note:* To avoid errors or confusion, always be cautious when using abbreviations.

Table 6.4

ABBREVIATIONS RELATED TO THE LYMPHATIC AND IMMUNE SYSTEMS

acquired immunodeficiency syndrome = AIDS	**AIDS** = acquired immunodeficiency syndrome
anaphylaxis = A	**A** = anaphylaxis
antibody = A, Ab	**A, Ab** = antibody
antigen = AG, Ag	**AG, Ag** = antigen
bacteria = BACT, Bact, bact	**BACT, Bact, bact** = bacteria
breast self-examination = BSE	**BSE** = breast self-examination
carcinoma = CA, Ca	**CA, Ca** = carcinoma
carcinoma in situ = CIS	**CIS** = carcinoma in situ
cytomegalovirus = CMV	**CMV** = cytomegalovirus
ductal carcinoma in situ = DCIS	**DCIS** = ductal carcinoma in situ
enzyme-linked immunosorbent assay = ELISA	**ELISA** = enzyme-linked immunosorbent assay
Epstein-Barr virus = EBV	**EBV** = Epstein-Barr virus
herpes zoster = HZ	**HZ** = herpes zoster
Hodgkin's lymphoma = HL	**HL** = Hodgkin's lymphoma
human immunodeficiency virus = HIV	**HIV** = human immunodeficiency virus
immunotherapy = IT	**IT** = immunotherapy
infectious mononucleosis = IM	**IM** = infectious mononucleosis
infiltrating ductal carcinoma, invasive ductal carcinoma = IDC	**IDC** = infiltrating ductal carcinoma, invasive ductal carcinoma
infiltrating lobular carcinoma, invasive lobular carcinoma = ILC	**ILC** = infiltrating lobular carcinoma, invasive lobular carcinoma
interferon, interstitial fluid = IF	**IF** = interferon, interstitial fluid
Kaposi's sarcoma = KS	**KS** = Kaposi's sarcoma
lymphedema = LE	**LE** = lymphedema
metastasis = MET	**MET** = metastasis
metastasize = met	**met** = metastasize
monoclonal antibodies = MABS	**MABS** = monoclonal antibodies
non-Hodgkin's lymphoma = NHL	**NHL** = non-Hodgkin's lymphoma
persistent generalized lymphadenopathy = PGL	**PGL** = persistent generalized lymphadenopathy
rickettsia = Rick	**Rick** = rickettsia
tuberculosis = TB	**TB** = tuberculosis

Learning Exercises

Matching Word Parts 1

Write the correct answer in the middle column.

Definition	Correct Answer	Possible Answers
6.1. lymph node	_____	carcin/o
6.2. lymph vessel	_____	lymphaden/o
6.3. eat, swallow	_____	lymphangi/o
6.4. cancer	_____	phag/o
6.5. poison	_____	tox/o

Matching Word Parts 2

Write the correct answer in the middle column.

Definition	Correct Answer	Possible Answers
6.6. formation	_____	immun/o
6.7. flesh	_____	onc/o
6.8. protected, safe	_____	-plasm
6.9. spleen	_____	sarc/o
6.10. tumor	_____	splen/o

● **Matching Types of Pathogens**

Write the correct answer in the middle column.

Definition	Correct Answer	Possible Answers
6.11. bacteria capable of movement	_____	parasite
6.12. chain-forming bacteria	_____	spirochete
6.13. cluster-forming bacteria	_____	staphylococci
6.14. live only by invading cells	_____	streptococci
6.15. lives within another organism	_____	viruses

● **Definitions**

Select the correct answer and write it on the line provided.

6.16. The _____ has/have a hemolytic function.

      adenoids   lymph nodes   spleen   tonsils

6.17. The term meaning inflammation of the lymph nodes is _____ .

      adenoiditis   lymphadenitis   lymphedema   lymphoma

6.18. Herpes zoster is commonly known as _____ .

      3-day measles   chickenpox   German measles   shingles

6.19. _____ is a family of proteins whose specialty is fighting viruses by slowing or stopping their multiplication.

      Complement   Immunoglobulin   Interferon   Synthetic immunoglobulin

6.20. The structure composed largely of lymphatic tissue that plays important roles in the immune and endocrine systems is the _____ .

      bone marrow   liver   spleen   thymus

6.21. The structures that form a protective ring of lymphatic tissue surrounding the internal openings of the nose and mouth are the _____ .

      adenoids   lacteals   lymph nodes   tonsils

6.22. Secondary _____ (SLE) may be due to cancer treatments, burns, or trauma.

       lymphadenitis   lymphangioma   lymphadenopathy   lymphedema

6.23. Fats and fat-soluble vitamins are absorbed by the _____ and carried into the

      bloodstream.

       lacteals   lymph nodes   Peyer's patches   spleen

6.24. _____ is carried by birds and transmitted to humans by mosquito or tick bites.

       Lyme disease   Malaria   Moniliasis   West Nile virus

6.25. A/An _____ protects the body by eating invading cells and by interacting with the

      other cells of the immune system.

       B lymphocyte   lymphokine   macrophage   T lymphocyte

● Matching Structures

Write the correct answer in the middle column.

Definition	Correct Answer	Possible Answers
6.26. acts as a physical barrier	_____	lymph nodes
6.27. filter harmful substances from lymph	_____	skin
6.28. has roles in lymphatic and endocrine systems	_____	spleen
6.29. lymphatic tissue hanging from the lower portion of the cecum	_____	thymus
6.30. stores extra erythrocytes	_____	vermiform appendix

● Which Word?

Select the correct answer and write it on the line provided.

6.31. The _____ direct the immune response by signaling between the cells of the immune system.

       lymphokines   macrophages

6.32. A _____ is used as an immunosuppressant and as an antineoplastic.

      corticosteroid   cytotoxic

6.33. Plasma cells develop from transformed _____ .

        B cells   T cells

6.34. Hepatitis B and C may be treated using _____ that was created in the laboratory.

      immunoglobulin   interferon

6.35. Infectious mononucleosis is a _____ infection.

        bacterial   viral

● Spelling Counts

Find the misspelled word in each sentence. Then write that word, spelled correctly, on the line provided.

6.36. A sarkoma is a malignant tumor that arises from connective tissue. _____

6.37. The nasopharyngeal tonsils are also known as the adenods. _____

6.38. Reubella is also known as 3-day measles. _____

6.39. Antiobiotics are used to combat bacterial infections. _____

6.40. The condition commonly known as chickenpox is caused by the herpes virus *Varicella soster*.

      _____

● Abbreviation Identification

In the space provided, write the words that each abbreviation stands for.

6.41. **AIDS**   _____

6.42. **Ca CA**   _____

6.43. **CMV**   _____

6.44. **ELISA**   _____

6.45. **HIV**   _____

● Term Selection

Select the correct answer and write it on the line provided.

6.46.   A/An _____ tumor is not life-threatening and not recurring.

    benign   in situ   malignant   neoplasm

6.47.   The condition that is frequently associated with an HIV infection is _____ .

    lymphoma   Hodgkin's disease   Kaposi's sarcoma   myoma

6.48.   Malaria is caused by a _____ and is transferred to humans by the bite of an infected mosquito.

    parasite   rickettsiae   spirochete   virus

6.49.   Bacilli, which are rod-shaped spore-forming bacteria, cause _____ .

    aspergillosis   Lyme disease   rubella   tuberculosis

6.50.   Photophobia is one of the symptoms of _____ .

    measles   mumps   shingles   rubella

● Sentence Completion

Write the correct term on the line provided.

6.51.   A systemic reaction, also described as _____, is a severe response to a foreign

    substance such as a drug, food, insect venom, or chemical.

6.52.   In _____, radioactive materials are implanted into the tissues to be treated.

6.53.   The _____ blot test is used to confirm a seropositive ELISA test for HIV.

6.54.   A/An _____ is a benign abnormal collection of lymphatic vessels forming a mass.

6.55.   Persistent generalized _____ is the continued presence of diffuse enlarged lymph nodes.

● Word Surgery

Divide each term into its component word parts. Write these word parts, in sequence, on the lines provided.

When necessary use a back slash (/) to indicate a combining vowel. (You may not need all of the lines provided.)

6.56.   An **antineoplastic** is a medication that blocks the development, growth, or proliferation of malignant cells.

    _____   _____   _____   _____

6.57. **Lymphangiography** is the radiographic examination of the lymphatic vessels after the injection of a contrast medium.

_____   _____   _____   _____

6.58. **Osteosarcoma** is a malignant tumor usually involving the upper shaft of long bones, the pelvis, or knee.

_____   _____   _____   _____

6.59. **Cytomegalovirus** is a group of large herpes-type viruses that cause a variety of diseases.

_____   _____   _____   _____

6.60. **Antiangiogenesis** is a form of cancer treatment that cuts off the blood supply to the tumor.

_____   _____   _____   _____

● True/False

If the statement is true, write **T** on the line. If the statement is false, write **F** on the line.

6.61. _____ Ductal carcinoma in situ has a very low cure rate.

6.62. _____ Lymph fluid always flows toward the thoracic cavity.

6.63. _____ Reed-Sternberg cells are present in non-Hodgkin's lymphoma.

6.64. _____ Invasive ductal carcinoma starts in fatty tissue and then invades the ducts of the breast.

6.65. _____ Breast cancer does not occur in males because they do not have breast tissue.

● Clinical Conditions

Write the correct answer on the line provided.

6.66. Dr. Wei diagnosed her patient as having an enlarged spleen. The medical term for this condition is

_____ .

6.67. The surgery to treat Juanita's breast cancer included a/an _____ node biopsy.

6.68. Mr. Grossman was treated with a _____ drug. This is a hormone-like preparation used primarily as an anti-inflammatory and as an immunosuppressant.

6.69. Soon after her breast cancer was diagnosed, Dorothy Pererson's doctor performed a/an

_____ . In this procedure, the tumor and a margin of healthy tissue are removed.

6.70. Since his kidney transplant, Mr. Lanning must take a/an _____ to prevent rejection of the donor organ.

6.71. José Sanchez received a poliomyelitis _____ to ensure his immunity to this disease.

6.72. Tarana Inglis complained that the glands in her neck were swollen. Dr. Neilson explained that these are the _____ lymph nodes.

6.73. Because he had chickenpox as a child, Rob Harris now has natural _____ immunity to this disease.

6.74. As a child, John Fogelman had a viral disease in which the parotid glands were swollen. John's doctor said he had the _____ .

6.75. Jane Doe is infected with HIV. One of her medications is acyclovir, which is a/an _____ drug.

● Which Is the Correct Medical Term?

Select the correct answer and write it on the line provided.

6.76. The yeast *Candida albicans* causes _____ .

    aspergillus   chickenpox   moniliasis   rubella

6.77. Of the diseases listed here, _____ is the only one that is *not* an autoimmune disorder.

    Crohn's disease   Graves' disease   lymphedema   psoriasis

6.78. Severe pharyngitis is a bacterial infection caused by *Group A* _____ .

    bacilli   spirochetes   staphylococci   streptococci

6.79. An example of a soft tissue sarcoma is _____ .

    adenocarcinoma   myosarcoma   neurosarcoma   osteosarcoma

6.80. A/an _____ is used either as an immunosuppressant or as an antineoplastic.

    corticosteroid   cytotoxic drug   monoclonal antibody   synthetic immunoglobulin

● Challenge Word Building

These terms are *not* found in this chapter; however, they are made up of the following familiar word parts. You may want to look in the textbook glossary or use a medical dictionary to check your answers.

adenoid/o	-ectomy
lymphaden/o	-itis
lymphang/o	-ology
immun/o	-oma
splen/o	-rrhaphy
tonsill/o	
thym/o	

6.81.   The study of the immune system is known as _____ .

6.82.   The term meaning surgical removal of the spleen is a/an _____ .

6.83.   The term meaning an inflammation of the thymus is _____ .

6.84.   The term meaning an inflammation of the lymph vessels is _____ .

6.85.   The term meaning to suture the spleen is _____ .

6.86.   The term meaning the surgical removal of the adenoids is a/an _____ .

6.87.   The term meaning the surgical removal of a lymph node is a/an _____ .

6.88.   The term meaning a tumor originating in the thymus is _____ .

6.89.   The term meaning an inflammation of the tonsils is _____ .

6.90.   The term meaning an inflammation of the spleen is _____ .

● Labeling Exercises

Identify the numbered items on the accompanying figures.

6.91. tonsils and _____

6.92. bone _____

6.93. appendix and _____ _____

6.94. _____

6.95. _____

6.96. _____ lymphatic duct

6.97. _____ lymph nodes

6.98. _____ duct

6.99. _____ lymph nodes

6.100. _____ lymph nodes

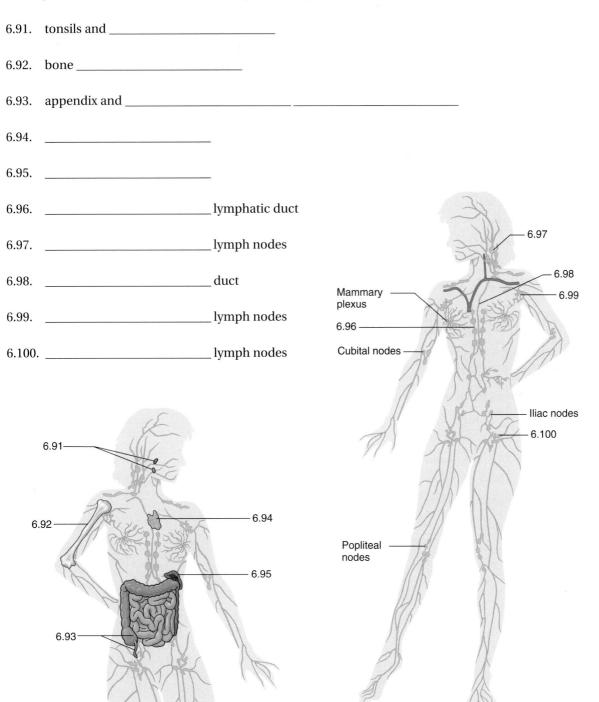

6.97

6.98

6.99

Mammary plexus

6.96

Cubital nodes

Iliac nodes

6.100

Popliteal nodes

6.91

6.92

6.94

6.95

6.93

THE HUMAN TOUCH: CRITICAL THINKING EXERCISE

The following story and questions are designed to stimulate critical thinking through class discussion or as a brief essay response. There are no right or wrong answers to these questions.

Hernani Fermin, a 35-year-old married father, was diagnosed HIV positive two years ago. He is a sales representative for a nationally recognized pharmaceutical company, and his hectic travel schedule was beginning to take a toll on his health. A few weeks ago, his doctor suggested he rethink his career goals. "You know, stress and this disease don't mix," Dr. Wettstein reminded him. "Why don't you look for something closer to home?"

That evening over lasagna his wife, Emily, suggested teaching. Hernani had enjoyed sharing the challenging concepts of math and science with seventh graders during the six years he had taught in a rural school upstate. It was only the financial demands of Kim and Kili's birth seven years ago that had tempted him into the better paying field of pharmaceuticals.

He sent out resumes for the next five weeks. Finally one was well received by South Hills Middle School. They had an opening in their math department, plus a need for someone to coach after-school athletics, and they wanted to meet with him. He hadn't interviewed since the twins were born. He thought about the questions normally asked—would there be some questions about his health? Being HIV positive shouldn't have any bearing on his ability to teach, but parents might be concerned. And it might disqualify him for the school's health insurance policy. Hernani believed in honesty, but what would happen to his family if he revealed his HIV status?

Suggested Discussion Topics:

1. Do you think Hernani should reveal his HIV status to South Hills Middle School? If so, why? If not, why not?

2. Do you think South Hills Middle School would hire Hernani if they knew he was HIV positive? Why or why not?

3. How would you feel if your child were on one of the teams Hernani would be coaching? Why?

4. Discuss the insurance problems Hernani might encounter by changing jobs.

5. Confidentiality is an important physician-patient issue. Discuss whether it would be Dr. Wettstein's duty to reveal Hernani's HIV status if asked about it.

The Respiratory System

Overview of Structures, Combining Forms, and Functions of the Respiratory System

MAJOR STRUCTURES	RELATED COMBINING FORMS	PRIMARY FUNCTIONS
Nose	nas/o	Exchanges air during inhaling and exhaling; warms, moisturizes, and filters inhaled air.
Sinuses	sinus/o	Provide mucus, make bones of the skull lighter, aids in sound production.
Pharynx	pharyng/o	Transports air back and forth between the nose and the trachea.
Larynx	laryng/o	Makes speech possible.
Epiglottis	epiglott/o	Closes off the trachea during swallowing.
Trachea	trache/o	Transports air back and forth between the pharynx and the bronchi.
Bronchi	bronch/o, bronchi/o	Transports air from the trachea into the lungs.
Alveoli	alveol/o	Air sacs that exchange gases with the pulmonary capillary blood.
Lungs	pneum/o, pneumon/o, pulmon/o	Bring oxygen into the body and remove carbon dioxide and some water waste from the body.

VOCABULARY RELATED TO THE RESPIRATORY SYSTEM

The items on this list have been identified as key word parts and terms for this chapter. However, all words in boldface in the text are important and may be included in the learning exercises and tests.

Word Parts

- [ ] atel/o
- [ ] bronch/o, bronchi/o
- [ ] cyan/o
- [ ] -ectasis
- [ ] laryng/o
- [ ] ox/i, ox/o, ox/y
- [ ] pharyng/o
- [ ] phon/o
- [ ] pleur/o
- [ ] -pnea
- [ ] pneum/o, pneumon/o, pneu-
- [ ] pulm/o, pulmon/o
- [ ] tachy-
- [ ] thorac/o, -thorax
- [ ] trache/o

Medical Terms

- [ ] **anoxia** (ah-**NOCK**-see-ah)
- [ ] **anthracosis** (**an**-thrah-**KOH**-sis)
- [ ] **antitussive** (**an**-tih-**TUSS**-iv)
- [ ] **aphonia** (ah-**FOH**-nee-ah)
- [ ] **apnea** (**AP**-nee-ah *or* ap-**NEE**-ah)
- [ ] **asbestosis** (**ass**-beh-**STOH**-sis)
- [ ] **asphyxia** (ass-**FICK**-see-ah)
- [ ] **asphyxiation** (ass-**fick**-see-**AY**-shun)
- [ ] **asthma** (**AZ**-mah)
- [ ] **atelectasis** (at-ee-**LEK**-tah-sis)
- [ ] **bradypnea** (**brad**-ihp-**NEE**-ah *or* **brad**-ee-**NEE**-ah)
- [ ] **bronchiectasis** (**brong**-kee-**ECK**-tah-sis)
- [ ] **bronchodilator** (**brong**-koh-dye-**LAY**-tor)
- [ ] **bronchorrhea** (**brong**-koh-**REE**-ah)
- [ ] **bronchoscopy** (brong-**KOS**-koh-pee)
- [ ] **Cheyne-Stokes respiration** (**CHAYN**-**STOHKS**)
- [ ] **croup** (**KROOP**)
- [ ] **cystic fibrosis** (**SIS**-tick figh-**BROH**-sis)

- [ ] **diphtheria** (dif-**THEE**-ree-ah)
- [ ] **dysphonia** (dis-**FOH**-nee-ah)
- [ ] **dyspnea** (**DISP**-nee-ah)
- [ ] **emphysema** (**em**-fih-**SEE**-mah)
- [ ] **empyema** (**em**-pye-**EE**-mah)
- [ ] **endotracheal intubation** (**en**-doh-**TRAY**-kee-al **in**-too-**BAY**-shun)
- [ ] **epistaxis** (**ep**-ih-**STACK**-sis)
- [ ] **hemoptysis** (hee-**MOP**-tih-sis)
- [ ] **hemothorax** (**hee**-moh-**THOH**-racks)
- [ ] **hypercapnia** (**high**-per-**KAP**-nee-ah)
- [ ] **hyperpnea** (**high**-perp-**NEE**-ah)
- [ ] **hypopnea** (**high**-poh-**NEE**-ah)
- [ ] **hypoxemia** (**high**-pock-**SEE**-mee-ah)
- [ ] **hypoxia** (high-**POCK**-see-ah)
- [ ] **laryngectomy** (**lar**-in-**JECK**-toh-mee)
- [ ] **laryngitis** (**lar**-in-**JIGH**-tis)
- [ ] **laryngoplegia** (**lar**-ing-goh-**PLEE**-jee-ah)
- [ ] **laryngoscopy** (**lar**-ing-**GOS**-koh-pee)
- [ ] **mediastinum** (**mee**-dee-as-**TYE**-num)
- [ ] **nebulizer** (**NEB**-you-lye-zer)
- [ ] **otolaryngologist** (**oh**-toh-**lar**-in-**GOL**-oh-jist)
- [ ] **pertussis** (per-**TUS**-is)
- [ ] **pharyngitis** (**far**-in-**JIGH**-tis)
- [ ] **pharyngoplasty** (fah-**RING**-goh-**plas**-tee)
- [ ] **pleurectomy** (ploor-**ECK**-toh-mee)
- [ ] **pleurisy** (**PLOOR**-ih-see)
- [ ] **pleurodynia** (**ploor**-oh-**DIN**-ee-ah)
- [ ] **pneumoconiosis** (**new**-moh-**koh**-nee-**OH**-sis)
- [ ] **pneumonectomy** (**new**-moh-**NECK**-toh-mee)
- [ ] **pneumothorax** (**new**-moh-**THOR**-racks)
- [ ] **polysomnography** (**pol**-ee-som-**NOG**-rah-fee)
- [ ] **pulmonologist** (**pull**-mah-**NOL**-oh-jist)
- [ ] **pulse oximeter** (ock-**SIM**-eh-ter)
- [ ] **pyothorax** (**pye**-oh-**THOH**-racks)
- [ ] **sinusitis** (**sigh**-nuh-**SIGH**-tis)
- [ ] **spirometry** (spy-**ROM**-eh-tree)
- [ ] **tachypnea** (**tack**-ihp-**NEE**-ah)
- [ ] **thoracentesis** (**thoh**-rah-sen-**TEE**-sis)
- [ ] **thoracostomy** (**thoh**-rah-**KOS**-toh-mee)
- [ ] **tracheostomy** (**tray**-kee-**OS**-toh-mee)
- [ ] **tracheotomy** (**tray**-kee-**OT**-oh-mee)
- [ ] **tuberculosis** (too-**ber**-kew-**LOH**-sis)

● OBJECTIVES

On completion of this chapter, you should be able to:

1. Identify and describe the major structures and functions of the respiratory system.

2. Recognize, define, spell, and pronounce terms related to the pathology and the diagnostic and treatment procedures of the respiratory system.

FUNCTIONS OF THE RESPIRATORY SYSTEM

The functions of the respiratory system are to:

● Bring oxygen-rich air into the body for delivery to the blood cells. The blood then delivers oxygen to body tissues.

● Expel waste products (carbon dioxide and some water waste) returned to the lungs by the blood.

● Produce the airflow through the larynx that makes speech possible.

STRUCTURES OF THE RESPIRATORY SYSTEM

For descriptive purposes, the respiratory system is divided into upper and lower respiratory tracts (Figure 7.1).

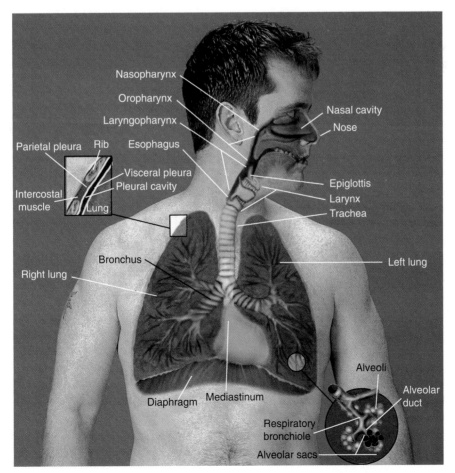

FIGURE 7.1   Structures of the respiratory system.

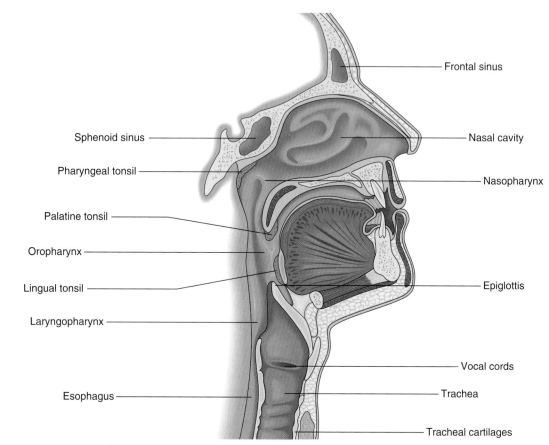

Frontal sinus

Sphenoid sinus

Nasal cavity

Pharyngeal tonsil

Nasopharynx

Palatine tonsil

Oropharynx

Lingual tonsil

Epiglottis

Laryngopharynx

Vocal cords

Esophagus

Trachea

Tracheal cartilages

FIGURE 7.2   Structures of the upper respiratory tract.

- The **upper respiratory tract** consists of the nose, mouth, pharynx, epiglottis, larynx, and trachea (Figure 7.2).

- The **lower respiratory tract** consists of the bronchial tree and lungs. These structures are protected within thoracic cavity.

The Nose

Air enters the body through the nose and passes through the **nasal cavity**, which is the interior portion of the nose.

- The **nasal septum** (**NAY**-zal **SEP**-tum) is a wall of cartilage that divides the nose into two equal sections. A *septum* is a wall that separates two chambers.

- **Cilia** (**SIL**-ee-ah), the thin hairs located just inside the nostrils, filter incoming air to remove debris.

- **Mucous membranes** (**MYOU**-kus) are the specialized tissues that line the respiratory, digestive, reproductive, and urinary systems.

- **Mucus** (**MYOU**-kus), which is secreted by the mucous membranes, protects and lubricates these tissues. In the nose mucus helps to moisten, warm,

and filter the air as it enters. *Notice the different spellings.* Mucous is the name of the tissue; mucus is the secretion that flows from the tissue.

- The **olfactory receptors** (ol-**FACK**-toh-ree) are nerve endings that act as the receptors for the sense of smell; they are also important to the sense of taste. These receptors are located in the mucous membrane in the upper part of the nasal cavity.

The Tonsils

The **tonsils,** which form a protective circle around the entrance to the respiratory system, are discussed in Chapter 6.

The Paranasal Sinuses

The **paranasal sinuses**, which are located in the bones of the skull, are connected to the nasal cavity via short ducts (**para-** means near, **nas** means nose, and **-al** means pertaining to).

A *sinus* is an air-filled cavity within a bone that is lined with mucous membrane. The functions of these sinuses are (1) to make the bones of the skull lighter, (2) to help produce sound by giving resonance to the voice, and (3) to produce mucus to provide additional lubrication for the tissues of the nasal cavity. The four paired sinuses are located on either side of the nose and are named for the bones in which they are located.

- The **frontal sinuses** are located in the frontal bone just above the eyebrows. An infection here can cause severe pain in this area (Figure 7.2).

- The **sphenoid sinuses**, which are located in the sphenoid bone, are close to the optic nerves, and an infection here can damage vision (Figures 3.9 and 3.10).

- The **maxillary sinuses**, which are the largest of the paranasal sinuses, are located in the maxillary bones. An infection here can cause pain in these teeth (Figures 3.9 and 3.10).

- The **ethmoid sinuses** (**ETH**-moid), which are located in the ethmoid bones, are irregularly shaped air cells that are separated from the orbital (eye) cavity by only a thin layer of bone (Figures 3.9 and 3.10).

The Pharynx

After passing through the nasal cavity, the air reaches the **pharynx** (**FAR**-inks), which is commonly known as the **throat** (Figure 7.2). The pharynx is made up of three divisions.

- The **nasopharynx** (**nay**-zoh-**FAR**-inks), the first division, is posterior to the nasal cavity and continues downward to behind the mouth (**nas/o** means nose and **-pharynx** means throat). This portion of the pharynx allows only the passage of air.

- The **oropharynx** (oh-roh-**FAR**-inks), the second division, is the portion that is visible when looking into the mouth (**or/o** means mouth and **-pharynx** means throat). The oropharynx, which is shared by the respiratory and digestive systems, transports air, food, and fluids downward to the laryngopharynx (Figure 8.2).

- The **laryngopharynx** (lah-**ring**-goh-**FAR**-inks), the third division, is also shared by both the respiratory and digestive systems (**laryng/o** means larynx and **-pharynx** means throat). Air, food, and fluids continue downward to the openings of the esophagus and trachea, where air enters the trachea and food and fluids flow into the esophagus. See the "Protective Swallowing Mechanisms" section.

The Larynx

The **larynx** (**LAR**-inks), also known as the **voice box,** is a triangular chamber located between the pharynx and the trachea (Figure 7.3).

- The larynx is protected and held open by a series of nine separate cartilages. The **thyroid cartilage** is the largest and when enlarged it is commonly known as the **Adam's apple**.

- The larynx contains the **vocal cords**. During breathing, the cords are separated to let air pass. During speech, they close together, and sound is produced as air expelled from the lungs causing the cords to vibrate against each other.

Protective Swallowing Mechanisms

The respiratory and digestive systems share part of the pharynx. During swallowing, there is the risk of a blocked airway or pneumonia caused by food or water entering the lungs instead of traveling into the esophagus. Two protective mechanisms act automatically during swallowing to ensure that *only* air goes into the lungs.

- During swallowing, the soft palate, which is the muscular posterior portion of the roof of the mouth, moves up and backward to close off the nasopharynx. This movement prevents food or liquid from going up into the nose. Structures of the mouth are discussed further in Chapter 8.

- At the same time, the **epiglottis** (ep-ih-**GLOT**-is), which is a lidlike structure located at the base of the tongue, swings downward and closes off the laryngopharynx so food does not enter the trachea and the lungs.

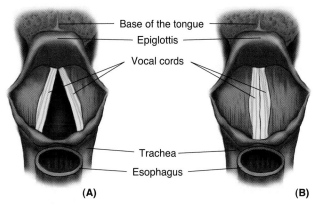

Base of the tongue
Epiglottis
Vocal cords
Trachea
Esophagus
(A)   (B)

FIGURE 7.3 View of the larynx and vocal cords from above. (A) The vocal cords are open during breathing. (B) The vocal cords vibrate together during speech.

The Trachea

Air passes from the larynx into the **trachea** (**TRAY**-kee-ah), the airway into the lungs commonly known as the **windpipe** (Figure 7.4).

- The trachea extends from the neck into the chest, directly in front of the esophagus, and is held open by a series of C-shaped cartilage rings. The wall between these rings is flexible and this makes it possible for the trachea to adjust to different body positions.

The Bronchial Tree

The trachea divides into two branches called **bronchi** (**BRONG**-kye). One branch goes into each lung (singular, **bronchus**).

- Within the lung, the bronchus divides and subdivides into increasingly smaller bronchi. **Bronchioles** (**BRONG**-kee-ohlz) are the smallest branches of the bronchi.
- Because of the similarity of these branching structures to an inverted tree, this is referred to as the **bronchial tree** (Figure 7.4).

The Alveoli

Alveoli (al-**VEE**-oh-lye), also known as **air sacs,** are the very small grape-like clusters found at the end of each bronchiole (singular, **alveolus**). Each lung contains millions of alveoli, which are filled with air from the bronchioles (Figures 7.1 and 7.4).

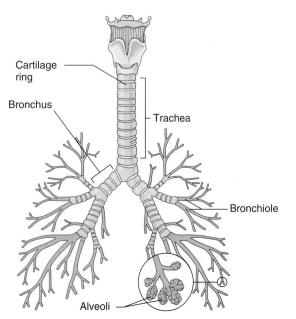

Cartilage ring

Bronchus

Trachea

Bronchiole

Alveoli

FIGURE 7.4   The trachea, bronchial tree, and alveoli.

- A network of microscopic pulmonary capillaries surrounds the thin, elastic walls of the alveoli.
- During respiration, the oxygen and carbon dioxide exchange between the alveolar air and the pulmonary capillary blood occurs through the walls of the alveoli.

The Lungs

The **lungs**, which are the organs of respiration, are divided into **lobes** (Figure 7.5).

- The **right lung** has three lobes: the superior, middle, and inferior.
- The **left lung** has only two lobes: the superior and inferior. It is slightly smaller than the right lung because of the space taken up by the heart.

The Mediastinum

The **mediastinum** (**mee**-dee-as-**TYE**-num), which is the cavity located between the lungs, contains connective tissue and organs including the heart and its veins and arteries, the esophagus, trachea, bronchi, the thymus gland and lymph nodes (Figure 7.1).

The Pleura

The **pleura** (**PLOOR**-ah) is the thin, moist, and slippery membrane that covers the outer surface of the lungs and lines the inner surface of the rib cage (plural, **pleurae**). A thin film of fluid separates the two layers of the pleura.

- The **parietal pleura** (pah-**RYE**-eh-tal **PLOOR**-ah) is the outer layer of the pleura that lines the walls of the thoracic cavity, covers the diaphragm, and forms the sac containing each lung. *Parietal* means relating to the walls of a cavity.
- The **visceral pleura** (**VIS**-er-al **PLOOR**-ah) is the inner layer of pleura that surrounds each lung. *Visceral* means pertaining to the internal organs.
- The **pleural space**, also known as the **pleural cavity**, is the airtight area between the layers of the pleural membranes containing a thin layer of fluid. This fluid allows the membranes to slide easily during breathing. *Pleural* means pertaining to the pleura.

The Diaphragm

The **diaphragm** (**DYE**-ah-fram) is the muscle that separates the thoracic cavity from the abdomen. It is the

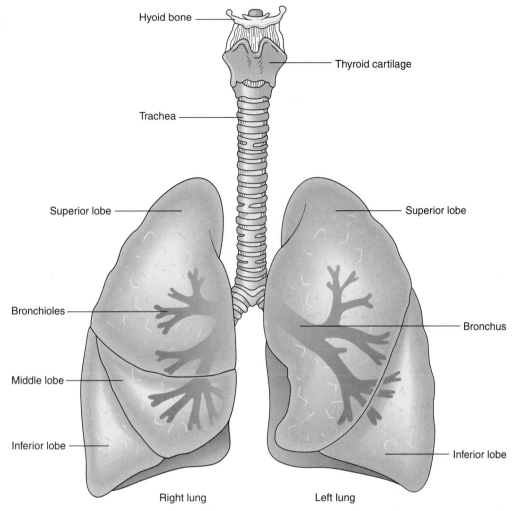

Hyoid bone

Thyroid cartilage

Trachea

Superior lobe

Superior lobe

Bronchioles

Bronchus

Middle lobe

Inferior lobe

Inferior lobe

Right lung

Left lung

FIGURE 7.5   External view of the lungs. Note the three lobes of the right lung and the two lobes of the left lung.

contraction and relaxation of this muscle that makes breathing possible (Figures 7.1 and 7.6).

- The **phrenic nerve** (**FREN**-ick) stimulates the diaphragm and causes it to contract (**phren** means diaphragm or mind, and -**ic** means pertaining to).

RESPIRATION

Respiration is the exchange of the gases oxygen and carbon dioxide that is essential to life. This occurs in the lungs as external respiration and on a cellular level as internal respiration.

External Respiration

External respiration, commonly known as **breathing**, is the act of bringing air into and out of the lungs. A single *respiration* consists of one inhalation and one

exhalation (Figure 7.6). The **intercostal muscles** (**in**-ter-**KOSS**-tul) move the rib cage during breathing (**inter**- means between, **cost** means ribs, and -**al** means pertaining to). See Figure 7.1.

Inhalation

Inhalation (**in**-hah-**LAY**-shun), which is also known as **inhaling,** is the act of taking in air as the diaphragm contracts and pulls downward. This action causes the thoracic cavity to expand. This expansion produces a vacuum within the thoracic cavity that draws air into the lungs (Figure 7.6, left).

Exhalation

Exhalation (**ecks**-hah-**LAY**-shun), also known as **exhaling**, is the act of breathing out. As the diaphragm relaxes, it moves upward causing the thoracic cavity to become narrower. This action forces air out of the lungs (Figure 7.6, right).

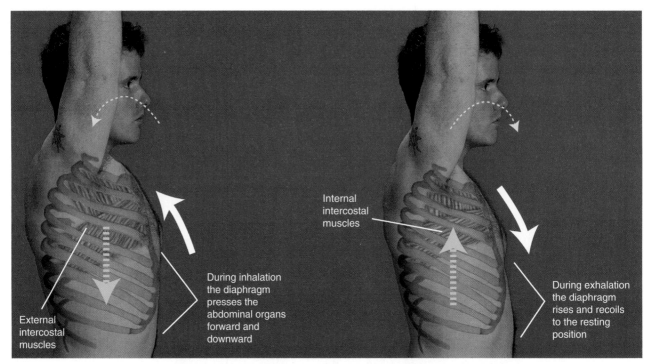

External intercostal muscles

During inhalation the diaphragm presses the abdominal organs forward and downward

Internal intercostal muscles

During exhalation the diaphragm rises and recoils to the resting position

FIGURE 7.6   Movements of the diaphragm and thoracic cavity during inhalation (left) and exhalation (right).

The Exchange of Gases Within the Lungs

As air moves in and out, there is an **exchange of gases** within the lungs (Figure 7.7A).

- As air is **inhaled** into the alveoli, oxygen (O_2) immediately passes into the surrounding capillaries and is carried by the erythrocytes (red blood cells) to all body cells.

- At the same time, the waste product carbon dioxide (CO_2) passes from the capillaries into the airspaces of the lungs to be **exhaled**.

Internal Respiration

Internal respiration is the exchange of gases within the cells of all the body organs and tissues. In this process, oxygen passes from the bloodstream into the tissue cells. At the same time, carbon dioxide passes from the tissue cells into the bloodstream (Figure 7.7B).

MEDICAL SPECIALTIES RELATED TO THE RESPIRATORY SYSTEM

- An **otolaryngologist** (**oh**-toh-**lar**-in-**GOL**-oh-jist), also known as an **otorhinolaryngologist** (**oh**-toh-**rye**-noh-**lar**-in-**GOL**-oh-jist), specializes in diagnosing and treating diseases and disorders of the ears, nose, and throat.

- A **pulmonologist** (**pull**-mah-**NOL**-oh-jist) is a physician who specializes in diagnosing and treating diseases and disorders of the lungs and associated tissues (**pulmon** means lung and **-ologist** means specialist).

PATHOLOGY OF THE RESPIRATORY SYSTEM

Chronic Obstructive Pulmonary Diseases

Chronic obstructive pulmonary disease is a general term used to describe a group of irreversible respiratory conditions, mainly emphysema and chronic bronchitis, which are characterized by chronic airflow limitations. These conditions are usually caused by smoking and are a common cause of death in the United States.

Emphysema

Emphysema (**em**-fih-**SEE**-mah) is the progressive loss of lung function that is commonly attributed to long-term smoking (Figure 7.8).

- This condition is characterized by (1) a decrease in the total number of alveoli, (2) the enlargement of the remaining alveoli, and (3) the progressive destruction of the walls of the remaining alveoli (Figure 7.8A).

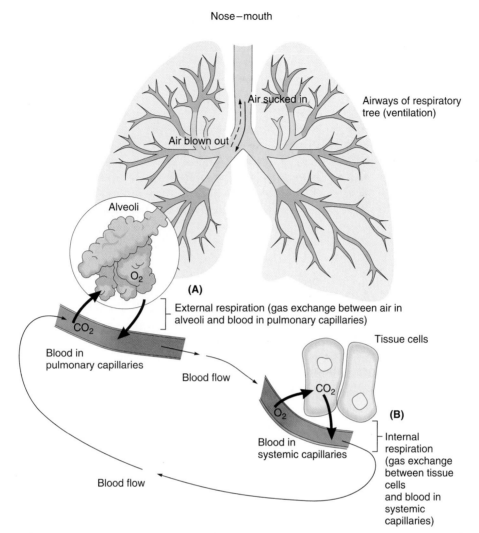

Nose—mouth

Air sucked in

Air blown out

Airways of respiratory tree (ventilation)

Alveoli

O_2

CO_2

(A)

External respiration (gas exchange between air in alveoli and blood in pulmonary capillaries)

Blood in pulmonary capillaries

Blood flow

Tissue cells

CO_2

O_2

(B)

Blood in systemic capillaries

Internal respiration (gas exchange between tissue cells and blood in systemic capillaries)

Blood flow

FIGURE 7.7   External and internal respiration compared. (A) External respiration, with the exchange of gases between the lungs and capillaries. (B) Internal respiration, with the exchange between the blood and tissues.

- As the alveoli are destroyed, breathing becomes increasingly rapid, shallow, and difficult. In an effort to compensate for the loss of capacity, the lungs expand and the chest sometimes assumes an enlarged barrel shape (Figure 7.8B).

Asthma

Asthma (**AZ**-mah) is a chronic allergic disorder characterized by episodes of severe breathing difficulty, coughing, and wheezing (Figure 7.9). An individual with asthma is referred to as an *asthmatic*. The incidence of asthma, and deaths from the condition, has been on the rise over the past decades for unknown reasons.

Breathing difficulty during an asthma attack is caused by several factors: (1) swelling and inflammation of the lining of the airways, (2) the production of thick mucus, and (3) tightening of the muscles that surround the airways. For treatment, see the bronchodilator description on page 203.

Upper Respiratory Diseases

- **Upper respiratory infection** and **acute nasopharyngitis** (**nay**-zoh-**far**-in-**JIGH**-tis) are among the terms used to describe the **common cold** (**nas/o** means nose, **pharyng** means pharynx, and **-itis** means inflammation). An upper respiratory infection can be caused by any one of 200 different viruses.

- **Allergic rhinitis** (rye-**NIGH**-tis), commonly referred to as an **allergy**, is an allergic reaction to airborne allergens that causes an increased flow of mucus (**rhin** means nose and **-itis** means inflammation).

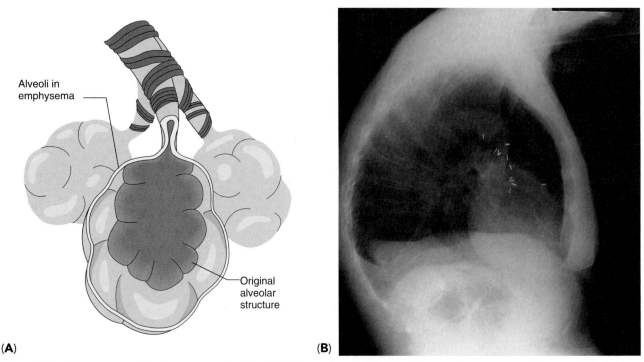

FIGURE 7.8   Emphysema. (A) Changes in the alveoli. (B) Lateral x-ray showing lung enlargement and abnormal barrel chest in emphysema.

- **Croup** (**KROOP**) is an acute respiratory syndrome in children and infants characterized by obstruction of the larynx, hoarseness, and a barking cough.
- **Diphtheria** (dif-**THEE**-ree-ah), now largely prevented through immunization, is an acute bacterial infection of the throat and upper respiratory tract. The diphtheria bacteria produce toxins that can damage the heart muscle and peripheral nerves.
- **Epistaxis** (ep-ih-**STACK**-sis), also known as a **nosebleed**, is bleeding from the nose that is usually caused by an injury, excessive use of blood thinners, or bleeding disorders.

- **Influenza** (**in**-flew-**EN**-zah), also known as **flu**, is an acute, highly contagious viral respiratory infection that is spread by respiratory droplets and occurs most commonly in epidemics during the colder months. There are many strains of the influenza virus, some strains can be prevented by annual immunization.
- **Pertussis** (per-**TUS**-is), also known as **whooping cough**, is a contagious bacterial infection of the upper respiratory tract that is characterized by recurrent bouts of a paroxysmal cough, followed by breathlessness, and a noisy inspiration. Pertussis

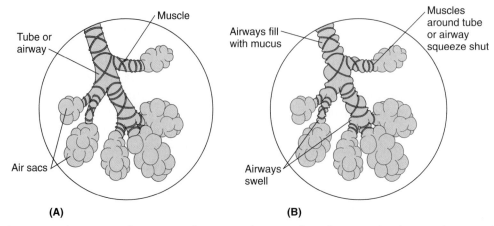

FIGURE 7.9   Changes in the airways during an asthma episode. (A) Before the episode, the muscles are relaxed and the airways are open. (B) During the episode, the muscles tighten and the airways fill with mucus.

can be prevented through immunization. *Paroxysmal* means sudden or spasm-like.

- **Rhinorrhea** (**rye**-noh-**REE**-ah), also known as a **runny nose,** is the watery flow of mucus from the nose (**rhin/o** means nose and **-rrhea** means abnormal discharge).

- **Sinusitis** (**sigh**-nuh-**SIGH**-tis) is an inflammation of the sinuses (**sinus** means sinus and **-itis** means inflammation).

Pharynx and Larynx

- **Pharyngitis** (**far**-in-**JIGH**-tis), also known as a **sore throat**, is an inflammation of the pharynx (**pharyng** means pharynx and **-itis** means inflammation).

- **Laryngoplegia** (**lar**-ing-goh-**PLEE**-jee-ah) is paralysis of the larynx (**laryng/o** means larynx and **-plegia** means paralysis).

- A **laryngospasm** (lah-**RING**-goh-spazm) is the sudden spasmodic closure of the larynx (**laryng/o** means larynx and **-spasm** means a sudden involuntary contraction).

Voice Disorders

- **Aphonia** (ah-**FOH**-nee-ah) is the loss of the ability of the larynx to produce normal speech sounds (**a-** means without, **phon** means voice or sound, and **-ia** means abnormal condition).

- **Dysphonia** (dis-**FOH**-nee-ah) is any change in vocal quality including hoarseness, weakness, or the cracking of a boy's voice in puberty (**dys-** means bad, **phon** means voice or sound, and **-ia** means abnormal condition).

- **Laryngitis** (**lar**-in-**JIGH**-tis) is an inflammation of the larynx (**laryng** means larynx and **-itis** means inflammation). This term is also commonly used to describe voice loss that is caused by this inflammation.

Trachea and Bronchi

- **Tracheorrhagia** (**tray**-kee-oh-**RAY**-jee-ah) is bleeding from the mucous membranes of the trachea (**trache/o** means trachea and **-rrhagia** means bleeding).

- **Bronchiectasis** (**brong**-kee-**ECK**-tah-sis) is the chronic, irreversible enlargement of bronchi or bronchioles (**bronchi** means bronchi and **-ectasis** means enlargement). This condition is often the result of a lung infection (Figure 7.10).

- **Bronchitis** (brong-**KYE**-tis) is an inflammation of the bronchial walls (**bronch** means bronchus and **-itis** means inflammation). Bronchitis is usually caused by an infection; however, it also can be caused by irritants such as smoking.

- **Bronchorrhea** (**brong**-koh-**REE**-ah) is an excessive discharge of mucus from the bronchi (**bronch/o** means bronchus and **-rrhea** means abnormal flow).

Pleural Cavity

- **Pleurisy** (**PLOOR**-ih-see), also known as **pleuritis**, is an inflammation of the pleura that produces sharp chest pain with each breath. Pleurisy can be caused by influenza or by damage to the lung beneath the pleura (**pleur** means pleura and **-isy** is a noun ending).

- **Pleurodynia** (**ploor**-oh-**DIN**-ee-ah) is pain in the pleura that occurs in relation to breathing movements (**pleur/o** means pleura and **-dynia** means pain).

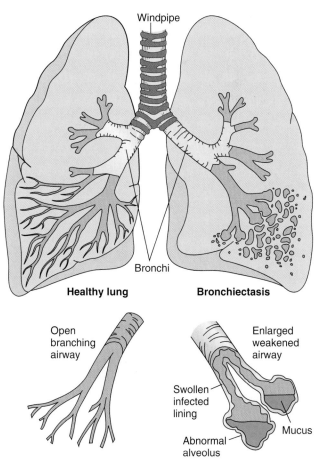

FIGURE 7.10   Bronchiectasis is the irreversible enlargement of bronchi or bronchioles that is commonly accompanied by chronic infection.

- A **pneumothorax** (**new**-moh-**THOR**-racks) is the accumulation of air in the pleural space causing a pressure imbalance that can make the lung collapse (**pneum/o** means lung or air and **-thorax** means chest). This may have an external cause, such as a stab wound, that perforates the chest wall. It also can be caused internally by a rupture in the pleura that allows air to leak into the pleural space (Figure 7.11).

- **Pleural effusion** (eh-**FEW**-zhun), which is the abnormal accumulation of fluid in the pleural space, produces a feeling of breathlessness because it prevents the lung from fully expanding. *Effusion* is the escape of fluid from blood or lymphatic vessels into the tissues or a cavity (Figure 7.12).

- **Empyema** (**em**-pye-**EE**-mah), also known as **pyothorax** (**pye**-oh-**THOH**-racks), is an accumulation of pus, or infected fluid, in the pleural cavity. This is usually the result of a primary infection of the lungs. The term *empyema* is also used to describe the presence of pus in other body cavities.

- **Hemothorax** (**hee**-moh-**THOH**-racks) is a collection of blood in the pleural cavity (**hem/o** means blood and **-thorax** means chest). This condition often results from chest trauma, such as a stab wound, but can also be caused by disease or surgery.

- **Hemoptysis** (hee-**MOP**-tih-sis) is coughing up of blood or bloodstained sputum derived from the lungs or bronchial tubes as the result of a pulmonary or bronchial hemorrhage (**hem/o** means blood and **-ptysis** means spitting).

Lungs

- **Severe acute respiratory syndrome (SARS),** which first appeared in China in 2003, is a sometimes fatal viral respiratory disorder that begins with a fever and progresses to a dry nonproductive cough and severe breathing difficulty.

- **Acute respiratory distress syndrome (ARDS)** is not a specific disease. Instead it is a form of sudden onset severe lung dysfunction affecting both lungs that makes breathing extremely difficult. ARDS is caused by trauma (injury), sepsis (systemic infection), diffuse pneumonia, or shock.

- **Pulmonary edema** (eh-**DEE**-mah) is an accumulation of fluid in lung tissues. *Edema* means swelling.

- **Pneumorrhagia** (**new**-moh-**RAY**-jee-ah) is bleeding from the lungs (**pneum/o** means lungs and **-rrhagia** means bleeding).

- **Atelectasis** (**at**-ee-**LEK**-tah-sis) is a condition in which the lung fails to expand completely because of shallow breathing or because the air passages are blocked (**atel** means incomplete and **-ectasis** means stretching). This term is also used to describe a condition in which the lungs of a fetus are not fully expanded at birth. Atelectasis can result in a partially or totally **collapsed lung.**

Tuberculosis

Tuberculosis (too-**ber**-kew-**LOH**-sis), which is an infectious disease caused by *Mycobacterium tuberculosis,* usually attacks the lungs; however, it can also affect other parts of the body. A healthy individual can carry TB without getting the disease. TB occurs most

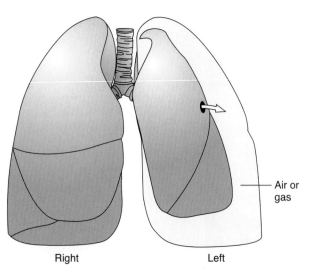

Right   Left

FIGURE 7.11 Pneumothorax is an accumulation of air or gas in the pleural space that causes the lung to collapse. In the left lung, a perforation in the pleura allowed air to escape into the pleural space.

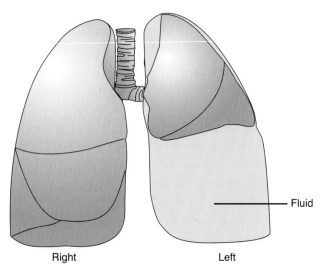

Right   Left

FIGURE 7.12 In pleural effusion, fluid in the pleural cavity prevents the lung from fully expanding.

commonly in individuals whose immune systems are weakened by another condition.

- **Multidrug-resistant tuberculosis** is a dangerous form of tuberculosis because the germs have become resistant to the effect of the primary TB drugs.

Pneumonia

Pneumonia (new-**MOH**-nee-ah) is a serious infection or inflammation of the lungs in which the smallest bronchioles and alveoli fill with pus and other liquid (**pneumon** means lung and **-ia** means abnormal condition). There are two types of pneumonia that are named for the parts of the lungs affected:

- **Bronchopneumonia** (**brong**-koh-new-**MOH**-nee-ah) is the form of pneumonia that affects patches of the bronchioles throughout both lungs (**bronch/o** means bronchial tubes, **pneumon** means lung, and **-ia** means abnormal condition). This form of pneumonia is a danger to the elderly, the very young, and the chronically ill.

- **Lobar pneumonia** affects one or more sections, or lobes, of a lung. **Double pneumonia** is lobar pneumonia involving both lungs, and is usually a form of bacterial pneumonia.

More than 30 different causes of pneumonia have been identified. These are primarily bacteria, viruses, infectious agents such as fungi, and various chemicals (Figure 7.13).

- **Bacterial pneumonia**, which is often caused by *Streptococcus pneumoniae,* is the only form of pneumonia that can be prevented through vaccination.

- **Viral pneumonia**, which is caused by several different types of viruses, accounts for approximately half of all pneumonias.

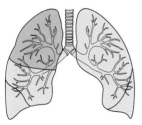 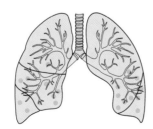

(A) Lobar pneumonia   **(B)** Bronchopneumonia

▨ Affected areas

Figure 7.13   Types of pneumonia are usually named for the causative agent or for the area of the lung that is involved.

- **Aspiration pneumonia** (**ass**-pih-**RAY**-shun) can occur when a foreign substance, such as vomit, is inhaled into the lungs. As used here, a*spiration* means inhaling or drawing a foreign substance into the upper respiratory tract. This term also means withdrawal by suction of fluids or gases from a body cavity.

- **Mycoplasma pneumonia** (**my**-koh-**PLAZ**-mah new-**MOH**-nee-ah), also known as **atypical** or **walking pneumonia**, is a milder but longer lasting form of the disease caused by the bacteria *Mycoplasma pneumoniae.*

- **Pneumocystis carinii pneumonia** (**new**-moh-**SIS**-tis kah-**RYE**-nee-eye new-**MOH**-nee-ah) is caused by an infection with the fungus *Pneumocystis carinii*. PCP is an opportunistic infection that frequently occurs when the immune system is weakened by an HIV infection.

Interstitial Lung Diseases

Interstitial lung diseases (**in**-ter-**STISH**-al), or ILDs, are a group of almost 200 diseases that cause inflammation and scarring of the alveoli and their supporting structures, the interstitium. *Interstitial* means pertaining to between, but not within, the parts of a tissue. As used here it refers to the supporting structures of the alveoli. ILD leads to a reduction of oxygen being transferred to the blood.

- **Interstitial fibrosis** is another name for the inflammation and thickening of the walls of the alveoli. *Fibrosis* is a condition in which normal tissue is replaced by fibrotic (hardened) tissue.

- Many connective tissue diseases, such as rheumatoid arthritis, scleroderma, and lupus can cause interstitial lung disease. Environmental and occupational toxins may cause ILD. Even activities such as keeping pet birds or bathing in hot tubs may result in the inhalation of some substance that causes an allergic reaction in certain individuals, leading to a form of ILD.

Environmental and Occupational Lung Diseases

- **Pneumoconiosis** (**new**-moh-**koh**-nee-**OH**-sis) is an abnormal condition caused by dust in the lungs that usually develops after years of environmental or occupational contact (**pneum/o** means lung, **coni** means dust, and **-osis** means abnormal condition). This causes fibrosis of the lung tissues. These disorders are named for the causative agents.

- **Anthracosis** (**an**-thrah-**KOH**-sis), also known as **coal worker's pneumoconiosis** or **black lung disease**, is caused by coal dust in the lungs (**anthrac** means coal dust and **-osis** means abnormal condition).

- **Asbestosis** (**ass**-beh-**STOH**-sis) is caused by asbestos particles in the lungs (**asbest** means asbestos and **-osis** means abnormal condition).

- **Byssinosis** (**biss**-ih-**NOH**-sis), also known as **brown lung disease**, is caused by inhaling cotton dust into the lungs and usually occurs in a textile factory environment (**byssin** means cotton dust and **-osis** means abnormal condition).

- **Silicosis** (**sill**-ih-**KOH**-sis) is a progressive lung disease caused by inhaling silica dust in the lungs (**silic** means glass and **-osis** means abnormal condition). Exposure can occur in many occupations including foundry work, quarrying, ceramics, glass work, and sandblasting.

Pulmonary Fibrosis

Pulmonary fibrosis (figh-**BROH**-sis) is the formation of scar tissue in the lung, resulting in decreased lung capacity and increased difficulty in breathing. This condition can be caused by autoimmune disorders, infections, dust, gases, toxins, and some drugs.

- *Idiopathic pulmonary fibrosis (IPF)* is a type of pulmonary fibrosis for which a cause cannot be identified. *Idiopathic* means without known cause.

Cystic Fibrosis

Cystic fibrosis (**SIS**-tick figh-**BROH**-sis), or CF, is a genetic disorder in which the lungs and pancreas are clogged with large quantities of abnormally thick mucus.

- Antibiotics are administered to control lung infections and daily physical therapies, known as *postural drainage* and *chest percussion*, are performed to remove excess mucus from the lungs.

- In CF, the digestive system is also impaired by mucus that interferes with digestive juices in the pancreas. Digestive enzymes are administered to aid the digestive system.

Breathing Disorders

- **Eupnea** (youp-**NEE**-ah) is easy or normal breathing (**eu-** means good and **-pnea** means breathing). This is the baseline for judging some breathing disorders (Figure 7.14A). Compare with *apnea*.

- **Tachypnea** (**tack**-ihp-**NEE**-ah) is an abnormally rapid rate of respiration usually of more than 20 breaths per minute (**tachy-** means rapid and **-pnea** means breathing) (Figure 7.14B). Compare with *bradypnea*.

- **Hyperventilation** (**high**-per-**ven**-tih-**LAY**-shun) occurs when an abnormally rapid rate of deep respiration results in a change in blood gas levels due to a decrease in carbon dioxide at the cellular level (**hyper-** means excessive and **-ventilation** means breathing). Compare with *hypernea*.

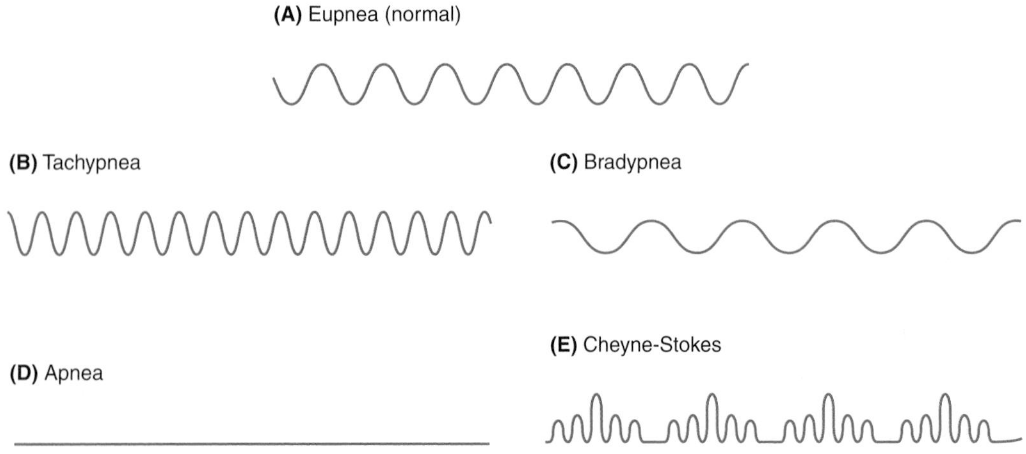

Figure 7.14 Respiratory patterns. (A) Eupnea is also known as normal breathing. (B) Tachypnea is also known as abnormally rapid breathing. (C) Bradypnea is also known as abnormally slow breathing. (D) Apnea is the absence of breathing. (E) Cheyne-Stokes is an alternating series of abnormal patterns.

- *Hyperventilation syndrome* is characterized by repeated episodes of the sensation of not being able to get enough air, and is usually caused by anxiety.

- **Bradypnea** (**brad**-ihp-**NEE**-ah *or* **brad**-ee-**NEE**-ah) is an abnormally slow rate of respiration, usually of less than 10 breaths per minute (**brady**- means slow and -**pnea** means breathing) (Figure 7.14C). Compare with *tachypnea*.

- **Apnea** (**AP**-nee-ah *or* ap-**NEE**-ah) is the absence of spontaneous respiration (**a**- means without and -**pnea** means breathing) (Figure 7.14D). Compare with *eupnea*.

- **Sleep apnea syndromes** are a group of potentially fatal disorders in which breathing repeatedly stops during sleep for long enough periods to cause a measurable decrease in blood oxygen levels. **Snoring**, which is noisy breathing caused by vibration of the soft palate during sleep, may be a symptom of sleep apnea.

- **Cheyne-Stokes respiration** (**CHAYN-STOHKS**) is a pattern of alternating periods of hypopnea (slow breathing) or apnea (the absence of breathing), followed by hyperpnea (rapid breathing) (Figure 7.14E).

- **Dyspnea** (**DISP**-nee-ah), also known as **shortness of breath**, is difficult or labored breathing (**dys**- means painful and -**pnea** means breathing). Shortness of breath is frequently one of the first symptoms of heart failure. It can also be caused by strenuous physical exertion or can be due to lung damage that produces dyspnea even at rest.

- **Hyperpnea** (**high**-perp-**NEE**-ah) is an increase in the depth and rate of the respiratory movements (**hyper**- means excessive and -**pnea** means breathing). Exercise commonly causes hyperpnea. Compare with *hyperventilation* and *hypopnea*.

- **Hypopnea** (**high**-poh-**NEE**-ah) is shallow or slow respiration (**hypo**- means decreased and -**pnea** means breathing). Compare with *hyperpnea*.

Lack of Oxygen

- In an **airway obstruction**, food or a foreign object blocks the airway and prevents air from entering or leaving the lungs. This is a life-threatening emergency requiring immediate action, usually by the abdominal (Heimlich) maneuver.

- **Smoke inhalation** is damage to the lungs in which particles from a fire coat the alveoli and prevent the normal exchange of gases.

- **Respiratory failure**, also known as **respiratory acidosis,** is a condition in which the level of oxygen in the blood becomes dangerously low or the level of carbon dioxide becomes dangerously high.

- **Anoxia** (ah-**NOCK**-see-ah) is the absence of oxygen from the body's gases, blood, or tissues (**an**- means without, **ox** means oxygen, and -**ia** means abnormal condition). If anoxia continues for more than four to six minutes, irreversible brain damage may occur.

- *Altitude anoxia,* also known as *altitude sickness*, is a condition that can be brought on by the decreased oxygen in the air at higher altitudes, usually above 8,000 feet.

- **Hypoxemia** (**high**-pock-**SEE**-mee-ah) is a condition of having below normal oxygen level in the blood (**hyp**- means deficient, **ox** means oxygen, and -**emia** means blood). This condition is less severe than anoxia. Compare with *hypoxia*.

- **Hypoxia** (high-**POCK**-see-ah), which is less severe than anoxia, is the condition of having below normal oxygen levels in the body tissues and cells (**hyp**- means deficient, **ox** means oxygen, and -**ia** means abnormal condition). Compare with *hypoxemia*.

- **Hypercapnia** (**high**-per-**KAP**-nee-ah) is the abnormal buildup of carbon dioxide in the blood (**hyper**- means excessive, **capn** means carbon dioxide, and -**ia** abnormal condition).

- **Asphyxia** (ass-**FICK**-see-ah) is the condition that occurs when the body cannot get the air it needs to function. In this life-threatening condition oxygen levels in the blood drop quickly, carbon dioxide levels rise, and unless the patient's breathing is restored within a few minutes, death or serious brain damage follows.

- **Asphyxiation** (ass-**fick**-see-**AY**-shun), also known as **suffocation,** is any interruption of breathing resulting in asphyxia. Asphyxiation can be caused by an airway obstruction, drowning, smothering, choking, or inhaling gases such as carbon monoxide.

- **Cyanosis** (**sigh**-ah-**NOH**-sis) is a bluish discoloration of the skin caused by a lack of adequate oxygen (**cyan** means blue and -**osis** means abnormal condition).

Sudden Infant Death Syndrome

Sudden infant death syndrome, also known as **SIDS** and **crib death**, is the sudden and unexplainable death of an apparently healthy infant between the ages of two weeks and one year that typically occurs while the infant is sleeping. This happens more often among babies who sleep on their stomach. For this reason, it is recommended that infants be put down to sleep on the back or side.

DIAGNOSTIC PROCEDURES OF THE RESPIRATORY SYSTEM

- **Respiration**, also known as **respiratory rate**, is an important vital sign and is discussed in Chapter 15.

- A **pulse oximeter** (ock-**SIM**-eh-ter) is an external monitor placed on the patient's finger or earlobe. The sensor measures the oxygen saturation level in the blood (**ox/i** means oxygen and **-meter** means to measure). In a normal reading, 95 to 100 percent of the blood is saturated by oxygen (Figure 7.15).

- **Spirometry** (spy-**ROM**-eh-tree) is a noninvasive test in which a patient breathes into a device that measures airflow, the length of time of each breath, and air volume (**spir/o** means to breathe and **-metry** means to measure).

- A **peak flow meter** is a handheld device often used to test those with asthma to measure how quickly they can expel air.

- **Pulmonary function tests** are a group of tests used to measure the capacity of the lungs to hold air as well as their ability to move air in and out and to exchange oxygen and carbon dioxide.

- **Phlegm** (**FLEM**) is thick mucus secreted by the tissues lining the respiratory passages. When phlegm is ejected through the mouth, it is called *sputum*.

Sputum (**SPYOU**-tum) may be examined for diagnostic purposes.

- **Polysomnography** (pol-ee-som-**NOG**-rah-fee), also known as a **sleep apnea study**, measures physiological activity during sleep and is most often performed to detect nocturnal defects in breathing associated with sleep apnea (**poly-** means many, **somn/o** means sleep, and **-graphy** means the process of recording).

- **Bronchoscopy** (brong-**KOS**-koh-pee) is the visual examination of the bronchi using a **bronchoscope** (**bronch/o** means bronchus and **-scopy** means direct visual examination). A bronchoscope is a flexible, fiber-optic device that is passed through the nose and down the airways. It may also be used for operative procedures such as tissue repair or the removal of a foreign object (Figure 7.16).

- **Laryngoscopy** (lar-ing-**GOS**-koh-pee) is the visual examination of the larynx using a laryngoscope inserted through the mouth and placed into the pharynx to examine the larynx (**laryng/o** means larynx and **-scopy** means a direct visual examination).

- *Mirror laryngoscopy* is a simpler version of this test in which the larynx is viewed by shining a light on an angled mirror held at the back of the soft palate.

- **Tuberculin skin testing** is a screening test for tuberculosis in which the skin of the arm is injected with a harmless antigen extracted from TB bacteria.

- One type of tuberculin testing is the *tuberculin tine test*, which is performed using an instrument with several small prongs called tines. A positive result

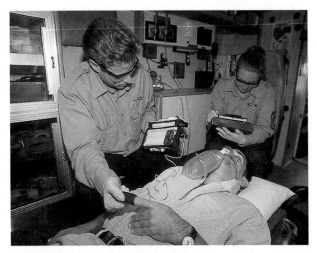

FIGURE 7.15   A pulse oximeter provides continuous reassessment of the levels of oxygenation.

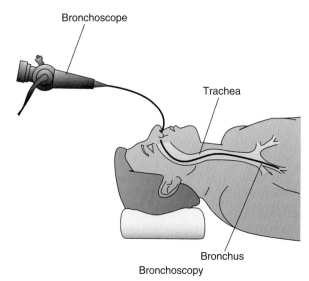

FIGURE 7.16   Bronchoscopy is the visual examination of the bronchi with the use of a bronchoscope.

indicates the possibility of exposure to the disease; this response warrants further testing.

- The **Mantoux PPD skin test** is considered more accurate for diagnosing tuberculosis. A very small amount of PPD tuberculin (a purified protein derivative) is injected just under the top layer of the skin on the forearm. The site is checked for a reaction 48 to 72 hours later.

- **Chest imaging**, also known as **chest x-rays**, is a valuable tool to show pneumonia, lung tumors, pneumothorax, pleural effusion, tuberculosis, and emphysema (Figure 7.8B).

TREATMENT PROCEDURES OF THE RESPIRATORY SYSTEM

Medications

- A **bronchodilator** (**brong**-koh-dye-**LAY**-tor) is an agent that expands the opening of the passages into the lungs. At the first sign of an asthma attack, the patient uses a metered dose inhaler to self-administer the bronchodilator.

- A **metered dose inhaler (MDI)** mixes a single dose of the medication with a puff of air and pushes it into the mouth via a chemical propellant (Figure 7.17). Compare with *nebulizer*.

- A **nebulizer** (**NEB**-you-lye-zer) dispenses larger doses of medication in the form of a mist that is

inhaled via a face mask or mouthpiece. Compare with *metered dose inhaler*.

- An **antitussive** (**an**-tih-**TUSS**-iv) is administered to prevent or relieve coughing (**anti-** means against, **tuss** means cough, and **-ive** means performs).

Nose and Throat

- **Septoplasty** (**SEP**-toh-**plas**-tee) is the surgical repair or alteration of parts of the nasal septum (**sept/o** means septum and **-plasty** means surgical repair).

- **Functional endoscopic sinus surgery** is a surgical procedure, performed using an endoscope, in which chronic sinusitis is treated by enlarging the opening between the nose and sinus.

- **Pharyngoplasty** (fah-**RING**-goh-**plas**-tee) is the surgical repair of the pharynx (**pharyng/o** means pharynx and **-plasty** means surgical repair).

- A **pharyngotomy** (**far**-ing-**GOT**-oh-mee) is a surgical incision of the pharynx (**pharyng** means pharynx and **-otomy** means a surgical incision).

- A **laryngectomy** (**lar**-in-**JECK**-toh-mee) is the surgical removal of the larynx (**laryng** means larynx and **-ectomy** means surgical removal).

- **Endotracheal intubation** (**en**-doh-**TRAY**-kee-al **in**-too-**BAY**-shun) is the passage of a tube through the nose or mouth into the trachea to establish or maintain an open airway (**endo-** means within, **trache** means trachea, and **-al** means pertaining to). *Intubation* is the insertion of a tube, usually for the passage of air or fluids.

Trachea

- **Tracheoplasty** (**TRAY**-kee-oh-**plas**-tee) is the surgical repair of the trachea (**trache/o** means trachea and **-plasty** means surgical repair).

- A **tracheotomy** (**tray**-kee-**OT**-oh-mee) is usually an emergency procedure in which an incision is made into the trachea to gain access to the airway below a blockage (**trache** means trachea and **-otomy** means surgical incision). This opening is usually temporary.

- A **tracheostomy** (**tray**-kee-**OS**-toh-mee) is the creation an opening into the trachea and inserting a tube to facilitate the passage of air or the removal of secretions (**trache** means trachea and **-ostomy** means surgically creating an opening). Placement of this tube may be temporary or permanent. The resulting opening is called a *stoma*.

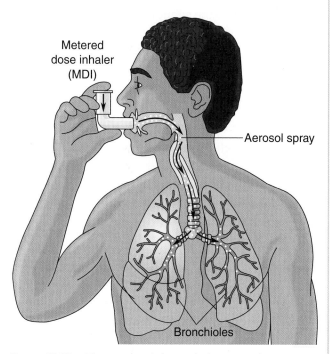

Metered dose inhaler (MDI)

Aerosol spray

Bronchioles

FIGURE 7.17   The metered dose inhaler aerosolizes medication for inhalation directly into the airways.

- A **stoma** (**STOH**-mah) is an opening on a body surface. A stoma can occur naturally (for example, a pore in the skin) or may be created surgically.

Lungs, Pleura, and Thorax

- A **pneumonectomy** (**new**-moh-**NECK**-toh-mee) is the surgical removal of all or part of a lung (**pneumon** means lung and -**ectomy** means surgical removal).

- A **lobectomy** (loh-**BECK**-toh-mee) is the surgical removal of a lobe of the lung (**lob** means lobe and -**ectomy** means surgical removal). This term also is used to describe the removal of a lobe of the liver, brain, or thyroid gland.

- A **pleurectomy** (ploor-**ECK**-toh-mee) is the surgical removal of part of the pleura (**pleur** means pleura and -**ectomy** means surgical removal).

- **Thoracentesis** (**thoh**-rah-sen-**TEE**-sis) is the surgical puncture of the chest wall with a needle to obtain fluid from the pleural cavity (**thora** means chest and -**centesis** means surgical puncture to remove fluid). This procedure is performed for diagnostic purposes or to drain excess fluid from severe pleural effusion (Figure 7.18). *Notice the spelling of this term.* It is *not* a simple combination of familiar word parts.

- A **thoracotomy** (thoh-rah-**KOT**-toh-mee) is a surgical incision through the chest wall (**thorac** means thorax or chest and -**otomy** means surgical incision). This incision is made into the pleural space for the visual examination of internal organs and the procurement of tissue specimens.

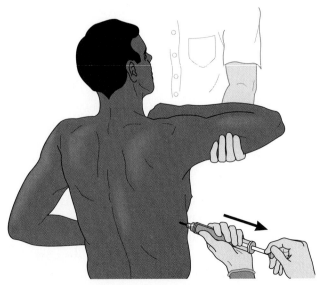

FIGURE 7.18 Fluid being removed from the pleural cavity by means of thoracentesis.

- A **thoracostomy** (**thoh**-rah-**KOS**-toh-mee) is the surgical creation of an opening into the chest cavity (**thorac** means thorax or chest and -**ostomy** means the surgical creation of an opening). This procedure is performed to establish drainage of empyema, which is pus in the pleural space.

Respiratory Therapy

- **Supplemental oxygen** can be administered through a nasal cannula, using either a rebreather or non-rebreather mask. A *nasal cannula* is a small tube that divides into two nasal prongs. In a *rebreather mask*, the exhaled breath is partially reused. A *non-rebreather mask* allows higher levels of oxygen to be added to the air taken in by the patient.

- **Postural drainage** is a procedure in which the patient is tilted head or chest downward to allow gravity to help drain secretions from the lungs. It is used with cystic fibrosis patients as well as those who have trouble coughing up sputum, such as postsurgical patients.

- A **ventilator** is a mechanical device for artificial ventilation of the lungs that is used to replace or supplement the patient's natural breathing function. The ventilator forces air into the lungs; exhalation takes place passively as the lungs contract.

- A **respirator** is a machine used for prolonged artificial respiration. For example, when a spinal cord injury destroys the natural breathing mechanism, the patient can continue to breathe through the use of a respirator. Note that the term *respirator* refers to any device controlling the quality of the air a person inhales, and therefore it can also mean a disposable dust mask or a piece of scuba diving equipment.

- **Positive pressure ventilation** is used to treat sleep apnea by pumping a steady supply of air into the nose all night through a tube and mask.

- **Diaphragmatic breathing,** also known as *abdominal breathing,* is a relaxation technique used to relieve anxiety.

ABBREVIATIONS RELATED TO THE RESPIRATORY SYSTEM

Table 7.1 presents an overview of the abbreviations related to the terms introduced in this chapter. *Note:* To avoid errors or confusion, always be cautious when using abbreviations.

Table 7.1

ABBREVIATIONS RELATED TO THE RESPIRATORY SYSTEM

acute respiratory distress syndrome = ARDS	**ARDS** = acute respiratory distress syndrome
asthma, asthmatic = AA	**AA** = asthma, asthmatic
bronchitis = BR, Br	**BR, Br** = bronchitis
bronchodilator = BD	**BD** = bronchodilator
bronchoscopy = BRO, bronch	**BRO, bronch** = bronchoscopy
Cheyne-Stokes breathing = CSB	**CSB** = Cheyne-Stokes breathing
chronic obstructive pulmonary disease = COPD	**COPD** = chronic obstructive pulmonary disease
coal worker's pneumoconiosis = CWP	**CWP** = coal worker's pneumoconiosis
cystic fibrosis = CF	**CF** = cystic fibrosis
diphtheria = diph	**diph** = diphtheria
emphysema = EMP	**EMP** = emphysema
endotracheal intubation = ETI	**ETI** = endotracheal intubation
functional endoscopic sinus surgery = FESS	**FESS** = functional endoscopic sinus surgery
hyperventilation = HVT	**HVT** = hyperventilation
interstitial lung diseases = ILD	**ILD** = interstitial lung diseases
larynx = lar, lx	**lar, lx** = larynx
laryngitis, laryngoscopy = laryn	**laryn** = laryngitis, laryngoscopy
lower respiratory tract = LRT	**LRT** = lower respiratory tract
multidrug-resistant tuberculosis = MDR-TB	**MDR-TB** = multidrug-resistant tuberculosis
nasopharynx = NP	**NP** = nasopharynx
oropharynx = OP	**OP** = oropharynx
Pneumocystis carinii pneumonia = PCP	**PCP** = Pneumocystis carinii pneumonia
pneumonia = PN, Pn, PNA, pneu, pneum	**PN, Pn, PNA, pneu, pneum** = pneumonia
pneumothorax = Pno	**Pno** = pneumothorax
positive pressure ventilation = PPV	**PPV** = positive pressure ventilation
postural drainage = PD	**PD** = postural drainage
pulmonary function test = PFT	**PFT** = pulmonary function test

(continues)

Table 7.1 (continued)

ABBREVIATIONS RELATED TO THE RESPIRATORY SYSTEM	
purified protein derivative = PPD	PPD = purified protein derivative
respiration = R, Resp	R, Resp = respiration
respiratory failure = RF	RF = respiratory failure
respiratory rate = RR	RR = respiratory rate
severe acute respiratory syndrome = SARS	SARS = severe acute respiratory syndrome
sleep apnea syndromes = SAS	SAS = sleep apnea syndromes
sudden infant death syndrome = SIDS	SIDS = sudden infant death syndrome
trachea = trach	trach = trachea
tuberculosis = TB	TB = tuberculosis
tuberculin skin testing = TST	TST = tuberculin skin testing
upper respiratory infection = URI	URI = upper respiratory infection
upper respiratory tract = URT	URT = upper respiratory tract

Learning Exercises

● Matching Word Parts 1

Write the correct answer in the middle column.

Definition	Correct Answer	Possible Answers
7.1. enlargement	_____	atel/o
7.2. voice box	_____	bronch/o
7.3. carries air into lungs	_____	cyan/o
7.4. blue	_____	-ectasis
7.5. incomplete	_____	laryng/o

● Matching Word Parts 2

Write the correct answer in the middle column.

Definition	Correct Answer	Possible Answers
7.6. lung	_____	ox/o
7.7. oxygen	_____	pharyng/o
7.8. multilayered membrane	_____	phon/o
7.9. throat	_____	pleur/o
7.10. voice or sound	_____	pneum/o

● Matching Word Parts 3

Write the correct answer in the middle column.

Definition	Correct Answer	Possible Answers
7.11. windpipe	_____	-pnea
7.12. rapid	_____	pulmon/o
7.13. lung	_____	tachy-
7.14. chest	_____	-thorax
7.15. breathing	_____	trache/o

● Definitions

Select the correct answer and write it on the line provided.

7.16.   The heart, aorta, esophagus, and trachea are located in the _____.

   dorsal cavity   manubrium   mediastinum   pleura

7.17.   The _____ acts as a lid over the entrance to the esophagus.

   Adam's apple   epiglottis   larynx   thyroid cartilage

7.18.   The innermost layer of the pleura is known as the _____.

   parietal pleura   pleural space   plural cavity   visceral pleura

7.19.   The _____ sinuses are located just above the eyes.

   ethmoid   frontal   maxillary   sphenoid

7.20.   The smallest divisions of the bronchial tree are the _____ .

   alveoli   alveolus   bronchioles   bronchi

7.21.   During respiration, the exchange of gases takes place through the walls of the _____ .

   alveoli   arteries   capillaries   veins

7.22.   The term meaning spitting blood or blood-stained sputum is _____ .

   effusion   epistaxis   hemoptysis   hemothorax

7.23.   Black lung disease is the lay term for _____ .

   anthracosis   byssinosis   pneumoconiosis   silicosis

7.24. The term _____ means an abnormally rapid rate of respiration.

      apnea   bradypnea   dyspnea   tachypnea

7.25. The term meaning any voice impairment is _____ .

      aphonia   dysphonia   laryngitis   laryngoplegia

● Matching Structures

Write the correct answer in the middle column.

Definition	Correct Answer	Possible Answers
7.26. first division of the pharynx	_____	laryngopharynx
7.27. second division of the pharynx	_____	larynx
7.28. third division of the pharynx	_____	nasopharynx
7.29. voice box	_____	oropharynx
7.30. windpipe	_____	trachea

● Which Word?

Select the correct answer and write it on the line provided.

7.31. The exchange of gases within the cells of the body is known as _____ respiration.

      external   internal

7.32. The term that describes the lung disease caused by cotton dust is _____ .

      anthracosis   byssinosis

7.33. The form of pneumonia that can be prevented through vaccination is _____

pneumonia.

      bacterial   viral

7.34. The term commonly known as shortness of breath is _____ .

      dyspnea   eupnea

7.35. The emergency procedure to gain access below a blocked airway is called a _____ .

      tracheostomy   tracheotomy

● Spelling Counts

Find the misspelled word in each sentence. Then write the word, spelled correctly, on the line provided.

7.36. The thick mucus secreted by the tissues that line the respiratory passages is called phlem.

_____

7.37. The medical term meaning an accumulation of pus in the pleural cavity is emphyema.

_____

7.38. The medical name for the disease commonly known as whooping cough is pertussosis.

_____

7.39. The medical term for the condition commonly known as TB is tuberculiosis. _____

7.40. An antitussiph is administered to prevent or relieve coughing. _____

● Abbreviation Identification

In the space provided, write the words that each abbreviation stands for.

7.41. **ARDS** _____

7.42. **COPD** _____

7.43. **SARS** _____

7.44. **SIDS** _____

7.45. **URI** _____

● Term Selection

Select the correct answer and write it on the line provided.

7.46. The term meaning the act of drawing a foreign substance into the upper respiratory tract is

_____ .

     aspiration   inhalation   inspiration   respiration

7.47. The term meaning abnormally rapid deep breathing is _____ .

     dyspnea   hyperpnea   hypopnea   hyperventilation

7.48.   The term meaning the surgical repair of the trachea is _____ .

pharyngoplasty   tracheoplasty   tracheostomy   tracheotomy

7.49.   The diaphragm is relaxed during _____ .

exhalation   inhalation   internal respiration   singultus

7.50.   During a/an _____ attack, the muscles of the airways contract.

allergic rhinitis   asthma   bronchiectasis   laryngospasm

● Sentence Completion

Write the correct term on the line provided.

7.51.   The term meaning an absence of spontaneous respiration is _____ .

7.52.   The sudden spasmodic closure of the larynx is a/an _____ .

7.53.   The acute infectious disease caused by the spore-forming bacterium *Bacillus anthracis* is known as

_____ .

7.54.   The term meaning pain in the pleura or in the side is _____ .

7.55.   The term meaning bleeding from the lungs is _____ .

● Word Surgery

Divide each term into its component word parts. Write these word parts, in sequence, on the lines provided.

When necessary use a back slash (/) to indicate a combining vowel. (You may not need all of the lines provided.)

7.56.   **Bronchorrhea** means an excessive discharge of mucus from the bronchi.

_____   _____   _____   _____

7.57.   Acute **nasopharyngitis** is among the terms used to describe the common cold.

_____   _____   _____   _____

7.58.   **Polysomnography** measures physiological activity during sleep and is most often performed to detect

nocturnal defects in breathing associated with sleep apnea.

_____   _____   _____   _____

7.59.   **Pneumorrhagia** is bleeding from the lungs.

_____   _____   _____   _____

7.60.   **Rhinorrhea**, also known as a runny nose, is an excessive flow of mucus from the nose.

_____   _____   _____   _____

● True/False

If the statement is true, write **T** on the line. If the statement is false, write **F** on the line.

7.61.   ____ A pulse oximeter is an internal monitor that measures the amount of oxygenated blood in the circulatory system.

7.62.   ____ In atelectasis the lung fails to expand because air cannot pass beyond the bronchioles that are blocked by secretions.

7.63.   ____ Croup is an allergic reaction to airborne allergens.

7.64.   ____ Hypoxemia is the condition of below normal oxygenation of arterial blood.

7.65.   ____ Emphysema is a chronic obstructive pulmonary disease.

● Clinical Conditions

Write the correct answer on the line provided.

7.66.   Baby Jamison was born with _____ _____ (CF). This is a genetic disorder in which the lungs are clogged with large quantities of abnormally thick mucus.

7.67.   Dr. Timkins surgically removed a portion of the pleura. This procedure is known as a/an

_____ .

7.68.   Wendy Barlow required the surgical repair of her larynx. This procedure is known as a/an

_____ .

7.69.   During his asthma attacks, Jamaal uses a metered dose inhaler containing a _____ .

This medication expands the opening of the passages into Jamaal's lungs.

7.70.   Mr. Partin received an immunization commonly known as a flu shot, to prevent

_____ .

7.71.   When hit during a fight, Marvin Roper's nose started to bleed. The medical term for this condition is

_____ .

7.72.   The doctor's examination revealed that Jean Marshall has an accumulation of blood in the pleural cavity. This diagnosis is recorded on her chart as a/an _____ .

7.73.   Duncan McClanahan had a/an _____ performed to correct damage to the septum of his nose.

7.74.   Suzanne Holderman is suffering from an inflammation of the bronchial walls. Suzanne's condition is _____ .

7.75.   Ted Coleman required the permanent placement of a breathing tube. The procedure for the placement of this tube is called a/an _____ .

Which Is the Correct Medical Term?

Select the correct answer and write it on the line provided.

7.76.   The irreversible enlargement of bronchi or bronchioles that is commonly accompanied by chronic infection is known as _____ .

| atelectasis | bronchiectasis | emphysema | pleurisy |

7.77.   The substance that is ejected through the mouth and used for diagnostic purposes in respiratory disorders is _____ .

| phlegm | pleural effusion | saliva | sputum |

7.78.   The term meaning a bluish discoloration of the skin caused by a lack of adequate oxygen is _____ .

| asphyxia | cyanosis | epistaxis | hypoxia |

7.79.   The term meaning paralysis of the vocal bands is _____ .

| aphonia | dysphonia | laryngitis | laryngoplegia |

7.80.   The pattern of alternating periods of rapid breathing, slow breathing, and the absence of breathing is known as _____ .

| anoxia | Cheyne-Stokes respiration | eupnea | tachypnea |

● **Challenge Word Building**

These terms are *not* found in this chapter; however, they are made up of the following familiar word parts. You may want to look in the textbook glossary or use a medical dictionary to check your answers.

bronch/o	-itis
epiglott/o	-ologist
laryng/o	-plasty
pharyng/o	-plegia
pneumon/o	-rrhagia
trache/o	-rrhea
	-scopy
	-stenosis

7.81. The term meaning an abnormal discharge from the pharynx is _____ .

7.82. The term meaning inflammation of the lungs is _____.

7.83. The term meaning a specialist in the study of the larynx is a/an _____ .

7.84. The term meaning bleeding from the larynx is _____ .

7.85. The term meaning inflammation of both the pharynx and the larynx is _____ .

7.86. The term meaning the abnormal narrowing of the lumen of the trachea is _____ .

7.87. The term meaning the surgical repair of a bronchial defect is _____ .

7.88. The term meaning an inflammation of the epiglottis is _____ .

7.89. The term meaning the inspection of both the trachea and bronchi through a bronchoscope is

_____ .

7.90. The term meaning paralysis of the walls of the bronchi is_____ .

● Labeling Exercises

Identify the parts of numbered items on accompanying figure.

7.91. _____

7.92. _____

7.93. _____

7.94. _____ muscle

7.95. _____

7.96. _____ cavity

7.97. _____

7.98. _____

7.99. _____ lung

7.100. _____ sacs

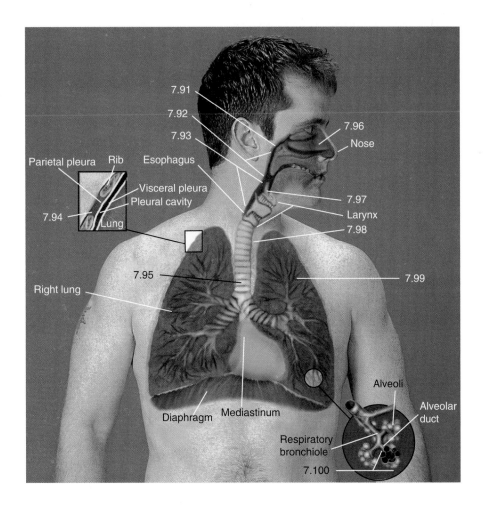

THE HUMAN TOUCH: CRITICAL THINKING EXERCISE

The following story and questions are designed to stimulate critical thinking through class discussion or as a brief essay response. There are no right or wrong answers to these questions.

Sylvia Gaylord works as a legal aide on the twelfth floor of an 18-story glass-and-steel monument to modern architectural technology in the center of the city. On clear days, the views are spectacular. From her cubicle, Sylvia's eye catches the edge of a beautiful blue and white skyscape as she reaches for her medi-haler. This is the third attack since she returned from lunch four hours ago—her asthma is really bad today. But if she leaves work early again, her boss will write her up. Sylvia concentrates on breathing normally.

Her roommate, Kelly, is a respiratory therapist at the county hospital. Kelly says Sylvia's asthma attacks are probably triggered by the city's high level of air pollution. That can't be true. They both run in the park every morning before work, and Sylvia rarely needs to use her inhaler. The problems start when she gets to work. The wheezing and coughing were so bad today that by the time she got up the elevator and into her cubicle she could hardly breathe.

Last night, the cable news ran a story on the unhealthy air found in some buildings. They called it "sick building syndrome" and reported that certain employees developed allergic reactions just by breathing the air. "Hmmm," she thought. "It seems like more and more people are getting sick in our office. John has had the flu twice. Sid's bronchitis turned into bronchopneumonia, and Nging complains of sinusitis. Could this building have an air quality problem?"

Suggested Discussion Topics:

1. Discuss which environmental factors might cause an asthma attack.
2. Discuss what Sylvia might do to find out if her building has an air quality problem.
3. Use proper medical terminology to describe what happens to Sylvia's airways during an asthma attack and how medications affect the symptoms.
4. Asthmatic medications, similar to Sylvia's inhaler, are easily available in drugstores without a prescription. Discuss the pros and cons of this practice.
5. If Sylvia's inhaler does not control her attack and her condition worsens, what steps should be taken promptly? Why?

The Digestive System

● Structures, Combining Forms, and Functions of the Digestive System

MAJOR STRUCTURES	RELATED COMBINING FORMS	PRIMARY FUNCTIONS
Mouth	or/o, stomat/o	Begins preparation of food for digestion.
Pharynx	pharyng/o	Transports food from the mouth to the esophagus.
Esophagus	esophag/o	Transports food from the pharynx to the stomach.
Stomach	gastr/o	Breaks down food and mixes it with digestive juices.
Small Intestine	enter/o	Completes digestion and absorption of most nutrients.
Large Intestine	col/o, colon/o	Absorbs excess water and prepares solid waste for elimination.
Rectum and Anus	an/o, proct/o, rect/o	Control the excretion of solid waste.
Liver	hepat/o	Secretes bile and enzymes to aid in the digestion of fats.
Gallbladder	cholecyst/o	Stores bile and releases it to the small intestine as needed.
Pancreas	pancreat/o	Secretes digestive juices and enzymes into small intestine as needed.

● VOCABULARY   RELATED TO THE DIGESTIVE SYSTEM

The items on this list have been identified as key word parts and terms for this chapter. However, all words in boldface in the text are important and may be included in the learning exercises and tests.

Word Parts

- [ ] an/o
- [ ] cec/o
- [ ] chol/e
- [ ] cholecyst/o
- [ ] col/o, colon/o
- [ ] enter/o
- [ ] esophag/o
- [ ] gastr/o
- [ ] hepat/o
- [ ] -lithiasis
- [ ] -pepsia
- [ ] pancreat/o
- [ ] proct/o
- [ ] rect/o
- [ ] sigmoid/o

Medical Terms

- [ ] amebic dysentery (ah-**MEE**-bik **DIS**-en-ter-ee)
- [ ] anastomosis (ah-**nas**-toh-**MOH**-sis)
- [ ] anorexia nervosa (**an**-oh-**RECK**-see-ah)
- [ ] anoscopy (ah-**NOS**-koh-pee)
- [ ] aphthous ulcers (**AF**-thus **UL**-serz)
- [ ] ascites (ah-**SIGH**-teez)
- [ ] bilirubin (bill-ih-**ROO**-bin)
- [ ] bolus (**BOH**-lus)
- [ ] borborygmus (**bor**-boh-**RIG**-mus)
- [ ] botulism (**BOT**-you-lizm)
- [ ] bruxism (**BRUCK**-sizm)
- [ ] bulimia nervosa (byou-**LIM**-ee-ah *or* boo-**LEE**-mee-ah)
- [ ] cholecystalgia (**koh**-lee-sis-**TAL**-jee-ah)
- [ ] cholecystectomy (**koh**-lee-sis-**TECK**-toh-mee)
- [ ] cholecystitis (**koh**-lee-sis-**TYE**-tis)
- [ ] choledocholithotomy (koh-**led**-oh-koh-lih-**THOT**-oh-mee)
- [ ] cholelithiasis (**koh**-lee-lih-**THIGH**-ah-sis)
- [ ] cholera (**KOL**-er-ah)
- [ ] cirrhosis (sih-**ROH**-sis)
- [ ] colonoscopy (**koh**-lun-**OSS**-koh-pee)

- [ ] colostomy (koh-**LAHS**-toh-mee)
- [ ] dental prophylaxis (**proh**-fih-**LACK**-sis)
- [ ] diverticulitis (**dye**-ver-tick-you-**LYE**-tis)
- [ ] diverticulosis (**dye**-ver-**tick**-you-**LOH**-sis)
- [ ] dyspepsia (dis-**PEP**-see-ah)
- [ ] dysphagia (dis-**FAY**-jee-ah)
- [ ] emesis (**EM**-eh-sis)
- [ ] emetic (eh-**MET**-ick)
- [ ] enteritis (**en**-ter-**EYE**-tis)
- [ ] eructation (eh-ruk-**TAY**-shun)
- [ ] esophageal reflux (eh-**sof**-ah-**JEE**-al **REE**-flucks)
- [ ] esophageal varices (eh-**sof**-ah-**JEE**-al **VAYR**-ih-seez)
- [ ] esophagogastroduodenoscopy (eh-**sof**-ah-goh-**gas**-troh-**dew**-oh-deh-**NOS**-koh-pee)
- [ ] gastroduodenostomy (**gas**-troh-**dew**-oh-deh-**NOS**-toh-mee)
- [ ] gastroenteritis (**gas**-troh-en-ter-**EYE**-tis)
- [ ] gingivitis (**jin**-jih-**VYE**-tis)
- [ ] hematemesis (**hee**-mah-**TEM**-eh-sis *or* **hem**-ah-**TEM**-eh-sis)
- [ ] hemoccult (**HEE**-moh-kult)
- [ ] hemorrhoidectomy (**hem**-oh-roid-**ECK**-toh-mee)
- [ ] hepatitis (**hep**-ah-**TYE**-tis)
- [ ] herpes labialis (**HER**-peez lay-bee-**AL**-iss)
- [ ] hiatal hernia (high-**AY**-tal **HER**-nee-ah)
- [ ] hyperemesis (**high**-per-**EM**-eh-sis)
- [ ] ileitis (**ill**-ee-**EYE**-tis)
- [ ] ileus (**ILL**-ee-us)
- [ ] intussusception (**in**-tus-sus-**SEP**-shun)
- [ ] jaundice (**JAWN**-dis)
- [ ] maxillofacial surgery (mack-**sill**-oh-**FAY**-shul)
- [ ] melena (meh-**LEE**-nah *or* **MEL**-eh-nah)
- [ ] morbid obesity (**MOR**-bid oh-**BEE**-sih-tee)
- [ ] nasogastric intubation (nay-zoh-**GAS**-trick in-too-**BAY**-shun)
- [ ] peristalsis (**pehr**-ih-**STAL**-sis)
- [ ] proctoplasty (**PROCK**-toh-**plas**-tee)
- [ ] pyrosis (pye-**ROH**-sis)
- [ ] regurgitation (ree-**gur**-jih-**TAY**-shun)
- [ ] salmonella (**sal**-moh-**NEL**-ah)
- [ ] sigmoidoscopy (**sig**-moi-**DOS**-koh-pee)
- [ ] ulcerative colitis (koh-**LYE**-tis)
- [ ] volvulus (**VOL**-view-lus)
- [ ] xerostomia (**zeer**-oh-**STOH**-mee-ah)

FUNCTIONS OF THE DIGESTIVE SYSTEM

The digestive system is also known as the **alimentary canal** (**al**-ih-**MEN**-tar-ee) (**aliment** means to nourish and **-ary** means pertaining to). The digestive system is responsible for:

- The intake and digestion of food
- The absorption of nutrients from digested food
- The elimination of solid waste products

STRUCTURES OF THE DIGESTIVE SYSTEM

The major structures of the digestive system include the **oral cavity** (mouth), **pharynx** (throat), **esophagus**, **stomach**, **small intestine**, **large intestine**, **rectum**, and **anus**.

Accessory organs related to the digestive system include the **liver**, **gallbladder**, and **pancreas** (Figure 8.1).

The Gastrointestinal Tract

The structures of the digestive system are also described as the **gastrointestinal** (**gas**-troh-in-**TESS**-tih-nal) or **GI tract** (**gastr/o** means stomach, **intestin** means intestine, and **-al** means pertaining to).

- The **upper GI tract** consists of the mouth, esophagus, and stomach.
- The **lower GI tract** is made up of the small intestine, large intestines, rectum, and anus. The intestines are sometimes referred to as the **bowels**.
- When these terms are used to describe diagnostic procedures, the small intestine is usually included with the upper GI tract.

The Oral Cavity

The major structures of the oral cavity, also known as the **mouth,** are the lips, hard and soft palates, salivary glands, tongue, teeth, and the periodontium (Figure 8.2).

The Lips

The **lips**, also known as **labia** (**LAY**-bee-ah), form the opening to the oral cavity (singular, **labium**). (The term *labia* is also applied to part of the female genitalia.) Another word part relating to the lips of the mouth is **cheil/o**. During eating, the lips hold food in the mouth and aid the tongue and cheeks in guiding

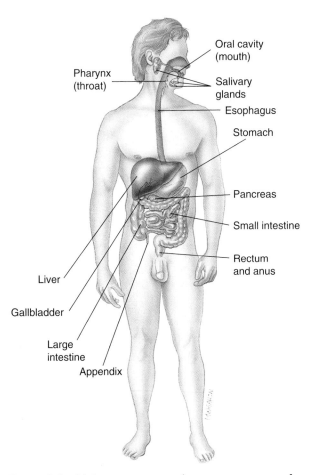

Pharynx (throat)

Oral cavity (mouth)

Salivary glands

Esophagus

Stomach

Pancreas

Small intestine

Rectum and anus

Liver

Gallbladder

Large intestine

Appendix

FIGURE 8.1   Major structures and accessory organs of the digestive system.

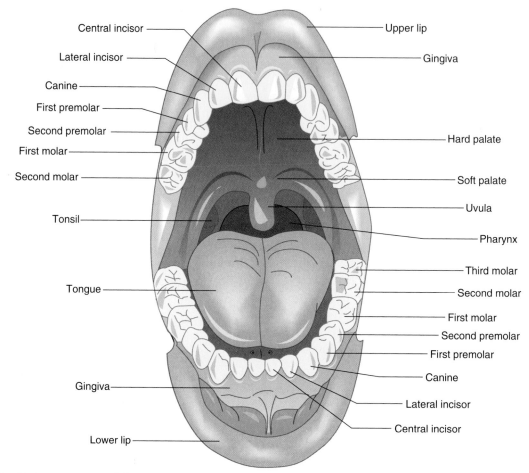

Figure 8.2   Major structures of the oral cavity. (The maxillary third molars are missing in this adult dentition.)

food between the teeth for chewing. The lips also have important roles in breathing, speaking, and the expression of emotions.

The Palate

The **palate** (**PAL**-at), which forms the roof of the mouth, consists of two parts: the hard and soft palates.

- The **hard palate** forms the bony anterior portion of the palate that is covered with specialized mucous membrane.

- **Rugae** (**ROO**-gay), which are irregular ridges or folds in the mucous membrane, cover the anterior portion of the hard palate. Rugae are also found in the stomach (singular, **ruga**).

- The **soft palate** forms the flexible posterior portion of the palate. It has the important role of closing off the nasal passage during swallowing so food and liquid do not move upward into the nasal cavity.

- The **uvula** (**YOU**-view-lah), which hangs from the free edge of the soft palate, moves upward with the soft palate during swallowing. Enlargement of the uvula is often associated with snoring problems**.**

The Tongue

The **tongue,** which is very strong and flexible, aids in speech and moves food during chewing and swallowing.

- The upper surface of the tongue has a tough protective covering and contains the papillae and the **taste buds,** which are the sensory receptors for the sense of taste.

- The underside of the tongue is highly vascular and covered with delicate tissue. *Highly vascular* means containing many blood vessels. It is this structure that makes it possible for medications placed under the tongue to be quickly absorbed into the bloodstream.

Terms Related to the Teeth

- The term **dentition** (den-**TISH**-un) refers to the natural teeth arranged in the **maxillary** (upper) and **mandibular** (lower) arches.

- **Edentulous** (ee-**DEN**-too-lus) means without teeth. This term is used after the natural teeth have been lost.

- Human dentition includes four types of teeth: **incisors** and **canines** (also known as **cuspids**) that are used for biting and tearing, plus **premolars** (also known as **bicuspids**) and **molars** that are used for chewing and grinding.

- The **primary dentition**, also known as the **deciduous dentition** (dee-**SID**-you-us) or **baby teeth**, consists of 20 teeth (eight incisors, four canines, eight molars, and no premolars). The primary teeth are lost normally and replaced by the permanent teeth.

- The **permanent dentition** consists of 32 teeth (eight incisors, four canines, eight premolars, and twelve molars). These teeth are designed to last a lifetime.

- As used in dentistry, **occlusion** (ah-**KLOO**-zhun) is any contact between the chewing surfaces of the maxillary (upper) and mandibular (lower) teeth. **Malocclusion** (**mal**-oh-**KLOO**-zhun) is any deviation from the normal positioning of the upper teeth against the lower teeth.

Structures and Tissues of the Teeth

- The **crown** of the tooth is the portion that is visible in the mouth. It is covered with **enamel,** the hardest substance in the body (Figure 8.3).

- The **root** holds the tooth securely in place within the dental arch. It is protected by **cementum,** which is not as hard as enamel.

- The crown and root meet at the **cervix**, or **neck**, of the tooth.

- **Dentin** makes up the bulk of the tooth and is protected by the enamel and cementum.

- The **pulp chamber** is the inner area of the crown of the tooth that runs downward to form the **root canals**. The **pulp** is made up of a rich supply of blood vessels and nerves.

The Periodontium

The **periodontium** (**pehr**-ee-oh-**DON**-shee-um) consists of the bone and soft tissues that surround and support the teeth (**peri-** means surrounding, **odonti** means the teeth, and **-um** is the noun ending).

- The **gingiva** (**JIN**-jih-vah), also known as the **gums**, is the specialized mucous membrane that surrounds the teeth, covers the bone of the dental arches, and continues to form the lining of the cheeks.

The Salivary Glands

The **salivary glands** (**SAL**-ih-ver-ee) secrete **saliva** that moistens food, begins the digestive process, and cleanses the mouth (Figure 8.1). There are three pairs of salivary glands.

- The **parotid glands** (pah-**ROT**-id) are located on the face in front of and slightly lower than each ear.

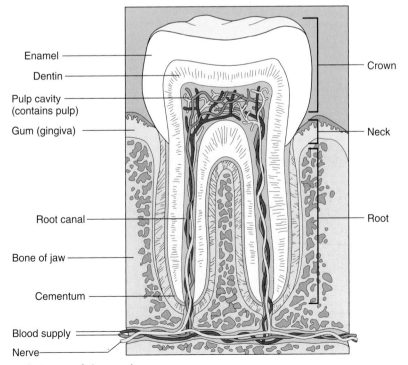

Enamel

Dentin

Pulp cavity (contains pulp)

Gum (gingiva)

Root canal

Bone of jaw

Cementum

Blood supply

Nerve

Crown

Neck

Root

FIGURE 8.3   Structures and tissues of the tooth.

- The **sublingual glands** are located on the underside of the tongue.
- The **submandibular glands** are located on the floor of the mouth.

The Pharynx

The **pharynx** (**FAR**-inks), also known as the **throat,** is the common passageway for both respiration and digestion (Chapter 7).

- During swallowing, food is prevented from moving from the pharynx into the lungs by the **epiglottis** (**ep**-ih-**GLOT**-is), which closes off the entrance to the trachea (windpipe). This closing allows food to move safely into the esophagus.

The Esophagus

The **esophagus** (eh-**SOF**-ah-gus), also known as the **gullet,** is a collapsible tube that leads from the pharynx to the stomach (Figure 8.1).

- The **lower esophageal sphincter** (**SFINK**-ter), also known as the **cardiac sphincter,** is a ringlike muscle that controls the flow between the esophagus and the stomach. A *sphincter* is a ringlike muscle that tightly constricts the opening of a passageway. When this muscle functions normally, stomach contents do not flow back into the esophagus.

- *Note:* The term *cardiac* means pertaining both to the heart and to the *cardia,* which is the area where the esophagus connects with the stomach.

The Stomach

The stomach is a saclike organ composed of the **fundus** (upper, rounded part), **body** (main portion), and **antrum** (lower part) (Figure 8.4).

- **Rugae** are the folds in the mucosa lining the stomach. Glands located within the folds produce the gastric juices that aid in digestion and mucus that forms the protective coating of the lining of the stomach.
- The **pylorus** (pye-**LOR**-us) is the narrow passage connecting the stomach with the small intestine.
- The **pyloric sphincter** (pye-**LOR**-ick) is the ring-like muscle that controls the flow from the stomach to the duodenum of the small intestine.

The Small Intestine

The **small intestine** extends from the pyloric sphincter to the first part of the large intestine. It is here that the nutrients from food are absorbed into the bloodstream. The small intestine is a coiled organ up to 20 feet in length; however, it is known as the small intestine because it is smaller in diameter than the large intestine (Figure 8.1).

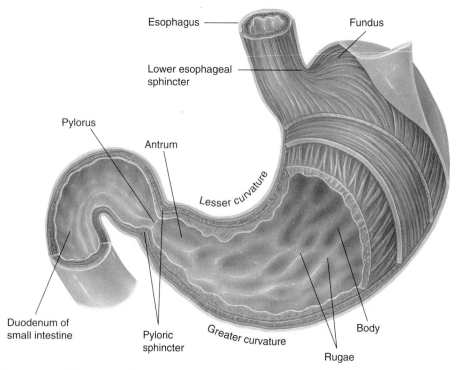

FIGURE 8.4   Structures of the stomach.

Parts of the Small Intestine

The small intestine consists of these three parts: the duodenum, jejunum, and ileum.

- The **duodenum** (**dew**-oh-**DEE**-num), the first portion of the small intestine, extends from the pylorus to the jejunum. The duodenum is where digestive fluids from the pancreas and liver are received.

- The **jejunum** (jeh-**JOO**-num), the middle portion of the small intestine, extends from the duodenum to the ileum. The jejunum secretes large amounts of digestive enzymes.

- The **ileum** (**ILL**-ee-um), the last and longest portion of the small intestine, extends from the jejunum to the cecum of the large intestine. The primary function of the ileum is in the absorption of nutrients. The **ileocecal sphincter** (**ill**-ee-oh-**SEE**-kull) is the ringlike muscle that controls the flow from the ileum of the small intestine into the cecum of the large intestine (Figure 8.5).

The Large Intestine

The large intestine extends from the end of the small intestine to the anus. It is about twice as wide as the small intestine, but only about one-fourth as long. It is here that the waste products of digestion are processed in preparation for excretion through the anus. The major parts of the large intestine are the cecum, colon, rectum, and anus (Figure 8.5).

The Cecum

The **cecum** (**SEE**-kum) is a pouch that lies on the right side of the abdomen. It extends from the end of the ileum to the beginning of the colon.

- The **vermiform appendix**, commonly called the **appendix**, hangs from the lower portion of the cecum. The term *vermiform* refers to its wormlike shape. The appendix, which consists of lymphatic tissue, is discussed in Chapter 6.

The Colon

The colon consists of the following four parts:

- The **ascending colon** travels upward from the cecum to the undersurface of the liver. *Ascending* means moving upward.

- The **transverse colon** passes horizontally from right to left toward the spleen. *Transverse* means moving across.

- The **descending colon** travels down the left side of the abdominal cavity to the sigmoid colon. *Descending* means moving downward.

- The **sigmoid colon** (**SIG**-moid) is an S-shaped structure that continues from the descending colon above and joins with the rectum below.

The Rectum and Anus

- The **rectum**, which is the last division of the large intestine, ends at the anus.

- The **anus** is the lower opening of the digestive tract. The flow of waste through the anus is controlled by the two **anal sphincter muscles**.

- The term **anorectal** (**ah**-noh-**RECK**-tal) refers to the anus and rectum as a single unit (**an/o** means anus, **rect** means rectum, and **-al** means pertaining to).

Accessory Digestive Organs

The following organs are referred to as accessory organs because they play a key role in the digestive process but are not part of the gastrointestinal tract (Figure 8.6).

The Liver

The liver is a large organ located in the right upper quadrant of the abdomen. It has several important functions related to removing toxins from the blood and turning food into the fuel and nutrients the body needs. The term **hepatic** (heh-**PAT**-ick) means

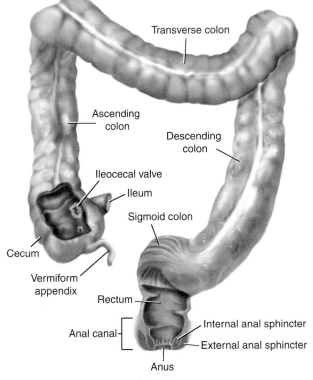

Transverse colon

Ascending colon

Descending colon

Ileocecal valve

Ileum

Sigmoid colon

Cecum

Vermiform appendix

Rectum

Anal canal

Internal anal sphincter

External anal sphincter

Anus

FIGURE 8.5 Structures of the large intestine.

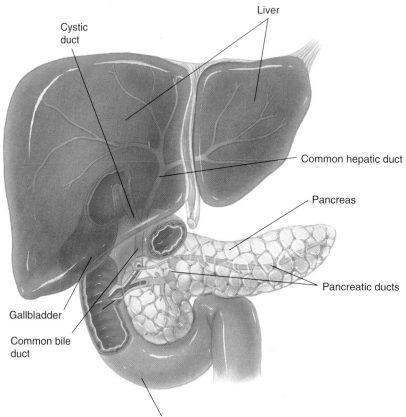

FIGURE 8.6 Accessory digestive organs: the liver, gallbladder, and pancreas.

pertaining to the liver (**hepat** means liver and **-ic** means pertaining to).

- The liver removes excess **glucose** (**GLOO**-kohs), also known as **blood sugar**, from the bloodstream and stores it as **glycogen** (**GLYE**-koh-jen), which is a form of starch. When the blood sugar level is low, the liver converts glycogen back into glucose and releases it for use by the body.

- The liver destroys old erythrocytes (red blood cells), removes toxins from the blood, and manufactures some blood proteins.

- **Bilirubin** (bill-ih-**ROO**-bin), a pigment produced from the destruction of hemoglobin, is released by the liver in bile. Excess bilirubin in the blood is associated with jaundice.

- The liver secretes **bile**, which is a yellowish-green fluid containing enzymes that break down fat. Bile travels from the liver to the gallbladder, where it is concentrated and stored.

The Biliary Tree

The **biliary tree** (**BILL**-ee-air-ee), also known as the **biliary system**, provides the channels through which bile is transported from the liver to the small intestine. *Biliary* means pertaining to bile.

- Small ducts in the liver join together like branches to form the biliary tree, with the trunk just outside the liver called the **common hepatic duct**.

- The bile travels from the liver through the common hepatic duct to the gallbladder where it enters and exits through a narrow tube called the **cystic duct**.

- The cystic duct leaving the gallbladder rejoins the common hepatic duct to form the **common bile duct.** The common bile duct joins the **pancreatic duct** and together they enter the duodenum of the small intestine.

The Gallbladder

The **gallbladder** is a pear-shaped organ about the size of an egg located under the liver. It stores and concentrates the bile for later use.

- The term **cholecystic** (**koh**-lee-**SIS**-tick) means pertaining to the gallbladder (**cholecyst** means gallbladder and **-ic** means pertaining to).

- When bile is needed, the gallbladder contracts, forcing the bile out through the biliary tree.

The Pancreas

The **pancreas** (**PAN**-kree-as) is a large feather-shaped organ located posterior to (behind) the stomach. It has important roles in both the digestive and endocrine systems. The endocrine functions, plus the pathology and procedures related to the pancreas, are discussed further in Chapter 13.

- The pancreas synthesizes and secretes **pancreatic juices.** These juices are made up of sodium bicarbonate (to help neutralize stomach acids) and digestive enzymes (to process the protein, carbohydrates, and fats in food).
- The pancreatic juices leave the pancreas through the **pancreatic duct** that joins the **common bile duct** just before the entrance into the duodenum.

DIGESTION

Digestion is the process by which complex foods are broken down into nutrients in a form the body can use. The flow of food through the digestive system is shown in Figure 8.7.

- **Enzymes** (**EN**-zimes) are responsible for the chemical changes that break foods down into simpler forms of nutrients for use by the body.

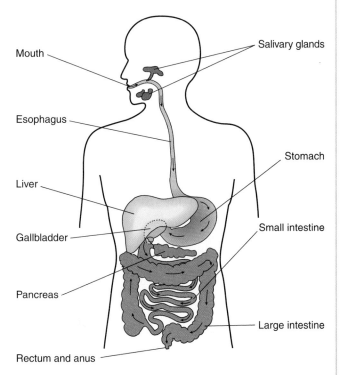

Mouth
Salivary glands
Esophagus
Stomach
Liver
Small intestine
Gallbladder
Pancreas
Large intestine
Rectum and anus

Figure 8.7   A schematic diagram showing the pathway of food through the digestive system.

- A **nutrient** is a substance, usually from food, that is necessary for normal functioning of the body. The primary nutrients are **carbohydrates**, **fats**, and **proteins**. **Vitamins** and **minerals** are essential nutrients, which are required only in small amounts.

Metabolism

Metabolism (meh-**TAB**-oh-lizm) is the sum of anabolism and catabolism. That is, metabolism includes *all* of the processes involved in the body's use of nutrients (**metabol** means change and **-ism** means condition).

- **Anabolism** (an-**NAB**-oh-lizm) is the building up of body cells and substances from nutrients.
- **Catabolism** (kah-**TAB**-oh-lizm), which is the opposite of anabolism, is the breaking down of body cells or substances, releasing energy and carbon dioxide.

Absorption

Absorption (ab-**SORP**-shun) is the process by which completely digested nutrients are taken into the circulatory system by passing through the capillaries located in the walls of the small intestine.

- Fats and fat-soluble vitamins are absorbed into the lymphatic system through **villi** (**VILL**-eye), the tiny hairlike projections that line the walls of the small intestine (singular, **villus**).

The Role of the Mouth, Salivary Glands, and Esophagus

- **Mastication** (**mass**-tih-**KAY**-shun), also known as **chewing**, breaks food down into smaller pieces and mixes it with saliva. Saliva contains an enzyme that begins the chemical breakdown to convert starches into sugar.
- A **bolus** (**BOH**-lus) is a mass of food that has been chewed and is ready to be swallowed. (The use of the term *bolus* in relation to the administration of medication is discussed in Chapter 15.)
- During swallowing, food travels from the mouth into the pharynx and on into the **esophagus**.
- In the esophagus food moves downward through the action of gravity and peristalsis. **Peristalsis** (**pehr**-ih-**STAL**-sis) is a series of wavelike contractions of the smooth muscles in a single direction.

The Role of the Stomach

- The **gastric juices** of the stomach contain **hydrochloric acid (HCl)** and digestive enzymes.

- Few nutrients enter the bloodstream through the walls of the stomach. Instead, the churning action of the stomach works with the gastric juices to convert the food to chyme.

- **Chyme** (**KYM**) is the semifluid mass of partly digested food that passes from the stomach, through the pyloric sphincter, and into the small intestine.

The Role of the Small Intestine

The conversion of food into usable nutrients is completed as the chyme is moved through the small intestine by peristaltic action.

- In the **duodenum**, chyme is mixed with pancreatic juice and bile. The bile breaks apart large fat globules so enzymes in the pancreatic juices can digest the fats. This action is called *emulsification* and must be completed before the nutrients can be absorbed into the body.

- In the **jejunum** additional digestive enzymes are added and the process of digestion continues.

- In the **ileum** the body absorbs the nutrients from the digested food.

The Role of the Large Intestine

The role of the entire large intestine is to receive the waste products of digestion and store them until they are eliminated from the body.

- Food waste enters the large intestine in liquid form. Excess water is reabsorbed into the body through the walls of the large intestine, helping to maintain the body's fluid balance, and the remaining waste forms into feces. **Feces** (**FEE**-seez), also known as **stools**, are solid body wastes expelled through the rectum and anus.

- **Defecation** (def-eh-**KAY**-shun), also known as a **bowel movement**, is the evacuation or emptying of the large intestine.

- The large intestine contains billions of bacteria, most of them harmless, which help break down organic waste material. This process produces gas. **Borborygmus** (bor-boh-**RIG**-mus) is the rumbling noise caused by the movement of gas in the intestine.

- **Flatulence** (**FLAT**-you-lens), also known as **flatus**, is the passage of gas out of the body through the rectum.

MEDICAL SPECIALTIES RELATED TO THE DIGESTIVE SYSTEM

- A **dentist** holds a Doctor of Dental Surgery (**DDS**) or Doctor of Medical Dentistry (**DMD**) degree and specializes in diagnosing and treating diseases and disorders of teeth and tissues of the oral cavity.

- A **gastroenterologist** (gas-troh-**en**-ter-**OL**-oh-jist) specializes in diagnosing and treating diseases and disorders of the stomach and intestines (**gastr/o** means stomach, **enter** means small intestine, and **-ologist** means specialist).

- An **internist** specializes in diagnosing and treating diseases and disorders of the internal organs and related body systems.

- An **orthodontist** (or-thoh-**DON**-tist) is a dental specialist who prevents or corrects malocclusion of the teeth and related facial structures (**orth** means straight or normal, **odont** means the teeth, and **-ist** means specialist).

- A **periodontist** (pehr-ee-oh-**DON**-tist) is a dental specialist who prevents or treats disorders of the tissues surrounding the teeth (**peri-** means surrounding, **odont** means the teeth, and **-ist** means specialist).

- A **proctologist** (prock-**TOL**-oh-jist) specializes in disorders of the colon, rectum, and anus (**proct** means anus and rectum and **-ologist** means specialist).

PATHOLOGY OF THE DIGESTIVE SYSTEM

Tissues of the Oral Cavity

- **Aphthous ulcers** (**AF**-thus **UL**-serz), also known as **canker sores** or **mouth ulcers**, are grey-white pits with a red border in the soft tissues lining the mouth. Although the exact cause is unknown, the appearance of these very common sores is associated with stress, certain foods, or fever.

- **Herpes labialis** (**HER**-peez lay-bee-**AL**-iss), also known as **cold sores** or **fever blisters** are blister-like sores on the lips and adjacent facial tissue that are caused by the **oral herpes simplex virus type 1** (**HSV-1**). Most adults have been infected by this extremely common virus, and in some it becomes re-activated periodically, causing cold sores.

- **Xerostomia** (**zeer**-oh-**STOH**-mee-ah), also known as **dry mouth**, is the lack of adequate saliva due to the absence or diminished secretions by the salivary glands (**xer/o** means dry and **-stoma** means mouth). This condition may be due to medications or radiation of the salivary glands, and can cause discomfort, difficulty in swallowing, changes in the taste of food, and dental decay.

- **Oral thrush** is an infection in infants characterized by white spots inside the mouth. It is caused by the fungus *Candida albicans*.

Cleft Lip and Cleft Palate

- A **cleft lip**, also known as a **harelip**, is a developmental defect resulting in a deep fissure of the lip running upward to the nose. As used here, a *fissure* is a deep groove or opening. As shown in Figure 8.8, a cleft lip usually can be surgically corrected.

- A **cleft palate** is the failure of the palate to close during the early development of the fetus. It can involve the upper lip, hard palate, and/or soft palate. If not corrected, this opening between the nose and mouth makes it difficult for the child to eat and speak. Cleft lip and cleft palate can occur singly or together (Figure 8.8).

Dental Diseases

- **Bruxism** (**BRUCK**-sizm) is involuntary grinding or clenching of the teeth that usually occurs during sleep and is associated with tension or stress. Bruxism wears away tooth structure, damages periodontal tissues, and injures the temporomandibular joint.

- **Dental caries** (**KAYR**-eez), also known as **tooth decay** or a **cavity,** is an infectious disease that destroys the enamel and dentin of the tooth. If the decay process is not arrested, the pulp can be exposed and become infected.

- **Dental plaque** (**PLACK**) is a soft deposit consisting of bacteria and bacterial by-products that builds up on the teeth and is a major cause of dental caries and periodontal disease. *Plaque* also means a patch or small differentiated area on a body surface or the buildup of deposits of cholesterol in blood vessels.

- **Dental calculus** (**KAL**-kyou-luhs), also known as tartar, is hardened dental plaque on the teeth that irritates the surrounding tissues. The term *calculus* also describes hard deposits, commonly known as **stones**, formed in any part of the body.

- **Periodontitis** (**pehr**-ee-oh-don-**TYE**-tis), also known **periodontal disease,** as is an inflammation of the tissues that surround and support the teeth (**peri-** means surrounding, **odont** means tooth or teeth, and **-itis** means inflammation). This progressive disease is classified according to the degree of tissue involvement.

- **Gingivitis** (**jin**-jih-**VYE**-tis), which is an inflammation of the gums, is the earliest stage of periodontal disease (**gingiv** means gums and **-itis** means inflammation).

- **Acute necrotizing ulcerative gingivitis**, also known as **trench mouth**, is caused by abnormal growth of bacteria in the mouth, and usually occurs in teens or young adults.

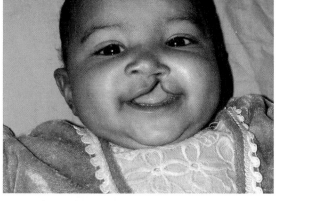
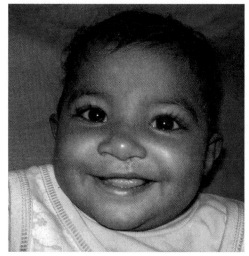

FIGURE 8.8 A child with a cleft palate before and after treatment. (Photos courtesy of The Smile Train: www.smiletrain.org.)

- **Halitosis** (hal-ih-**TOH**-sis), also known as **bad breath**, is an unpleasant odor coming from the mouth that may be caused by dental diseases or respiratory or gastric disorders (**halit** means breath and **-osis** means condition of).

- **Temporomandibular disorders** (**tem**-poh-roh-man-**DIB**-you-lar) **(TMD)** are a group of complex symptoms including pain, headache, or difficulty in chewing that are related to the functioning of the temporomandibular joint.

The Esophagus

- **Dysphagia** (dis-**FAY**-jee-ah) is difficulty in swallowing (**dys-** means difficult and **-phagia** means swallowing).

- **Gastroesophageal reflux disease**, also known as **esophageal reflux** (eh-**sof**-ah-**JEE**-al **REE**-flucks), is the upward flow of stomach acid into the esophagus and is a very common cause of indigestion (**gastr/o** means stomach, **esophag** means esophagus, and **-eal** means pertaining to). *Reflux* means a backward or return flow.

- **Pyrosis** (pye-**ROH**-sis), also known as **heartburn**, is the burning sensation caused by the return of acidic stomach contents into the esophagus (**pyr** means fever or fire and **-osis** means abnormal condition).

- **Esophageal varices** (eh-**sof**-ah-**JEE**-al **VAYR**-ih-seez) are enlarged and swollen veins at the lower end of the esophagus (singular, **varix**). Severe bleeding occurs if one of these veins ruptures.

- A **hiatal hernia** (high-**AY**-tal **HER**-nee-ah) is a protrusion of part of the stomach through the esophageal sphincter in the diaphragm (**hiat** means opening and **-al** means pertaining to). A *hernia* is the protrusion of a part or structure through the tissues that normally contain it. This condition can cause esophageal reflux and pyrosis (Figure 8.9).

The Stomach

- **Gastritis** (gas-**TRY**-tis) is a common inflammation of the stomach lining often caused by the bacterium *Helicobacter pylori* (**gastr** means stomach and **-itis** means inflammation).

- **Gastroenteritis** (gas-troh-en-ter-**EYE**-tis) is an inflammation of the mucous membrane lining the stomach and intestines (**gastr/o** means stomach, **enter** means small intestine, and **-itis** means inflammation).

- **Gastrorrhea** (**gas**-troh-**REE**-ah) is the excessive secretion of gastric juice or mucus in the stomach (**gastr/o** is stomach and **-rrhea** means flow or discharge).

Peptic Ulcers

Peptic ulcers (**UL**-serz) affect the mucous membranes of the digestive system (**pept** means digestion and **-ic** means pertaining to). Peptic ulcers can occur in the lower end of the esophagus, the stomach, or in the duodenum. An *ulcer* is an erosion of the skin or mucous membrane that is frequently caused by the bacterium *Helicobacter pylori*.

- A *perforating ulcer* involves erosion through the entire thickness of the organ wall.

- *Gastric ulcers* are peptic ulcers that occur in the stomach.

- *Duodenal ulcers* occur in the upper part of the small intestine, and are the most common form of peptic ulcer.

Eating Disorders

- **Anorexia** (an-oh-**RECK**-see-ah) is the loss of appetite for food, especially when caused by disease.

- **Anorexia nervosa** (an-oh-**RECK**-see-ah) is an eating disorder characterized by a false perception of body appearance. This leads to an intense fear of gaining

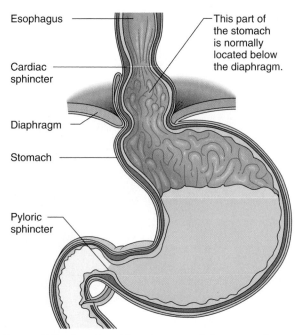

Esophagus

This part of the stomach is normally located below the diaphragm.

Cardiac sphincter

Diaphragm

Stomach

Pyloric sphincter

Figure 8.9   In a hiatal hernia, part of the stomach protrudes through the esophageal opening in the diaphragm.

weight and refusal to maintain a normal body weight. Compulsive dieting and excessive exercising often cause the patient to become emaciated.

- **Emaciated** (ee-**MAY**-shee-ayt-ed) means abnormally thin.
- **Bulimia nervosa** (byou-**LIM**-ee-ah *or* boo-**LEE**-mee-ah), also known as **bulimia**, is an eating disorder characterized by a false perception of body appearance leading to frequent episodes of binge eating followed by compensatory behaviors such as self-induced vomiting or the misuse of laxatives, diuretics, or other medications. *Bulimia* means continuous, excessive hunger.
- **Pica** (**PYE**-kah) is an eating disorder in which there is persistent eating of nonfood substances such as soil, chalk, starch, or clay. These abnormal cravings are sometimes associated with pregnancy.

Nutritional Conditions

- **Dehydration** is a condition in which fluid loss exceeds fluid intake and disrupts the body's normal electrolyte balance.
- **Malnutrition** is a lack of proper food or nutrients in the body, either due to a shortage of food or the improper absorption or distribution of nutrients.
- **Malabsorption** (**mal**-ab-**SORP**-shun) is a condition in which the small intestine cannot absorb nutrients from food that passes through it.

Obesity

Obesity (oh-**BEE**-sih-tee) is an excessive accumulation of fat in the body. The term *obese* is usually used to refer to individuals who are more than 20 percent to 30 percent over the established weight standards for their height, age, and sex.

- **Morbid obesity** (**MOR**-bid oh-**BEE**-sih-tee), also known as **clinically severe obesity,** is the condition of weighing two or three times, or more, than the ideal weight. As used here, *morbid* means pertaining to disease. Alternatively, a body mass index value greater than 39 may be used to diagnose morbid obesity.
- The *body mass index (BMI)*, a number that shows body weight adjusted for height, is one of many factors related to developing a chronic disease, such as heart disease, cancer, or diabetes. For adults aged 20 years or older, BMI falls into one of these categories: underweight, normal, overweight, or obese.

- *Bariatrics* is the branch of medicine concerned with the prevention and control of obesity and allied diseases.

Indigestion and Vomiting

- **Aerophagia** (**ay**-er-oh-**FAY**-jee-ah) is the excessive swallowing of air while eating or drinking, and is a common cause of gas in the stomach (**aer/o** means air and -**phagia** means swallowing).
- **Eructation** (eh-ruk-**TAY**-shun) is the act of belching or raising gas orally from the stomach.
- **Dyspepsia** (dis-**PEP**-see-ah), also known as **indigestion**, is pain or discomfort in digestion (**dys-** means painful and -**pepsia** means digestion).
- **Emesis** (**EM**-eh-sis), also known as **vomiting**, means to expel the contents of the stomach through the esophagus and out of the mouth.
- **Hematemesis** (**hee**-mah-**TEM**-eh-sis *or* **hem**-ah-**TEM**-eh-sis) is the vomiting of blood (**hemat** means blood and -**emesis** means vomiting).
- **Hyperemesis** (**high**-per-**EM**-eh-sis) is extreme, persistent vomiting (**hyper-** means excessive and -**emesis** means vomiting). This condition may lead to dehydration.
- **Nausea** (**NAW**-see-ah) is the sensation that leads to the urge to vomit.
- **Regurgitation** (ree-**gur**-jih-**TAY**-shun) is the return of swallowed food into the mouth.

Intestinal Disorders

- **Colorectal carcinoma** is a common form of cancer that often first manifests itself in polyps in the colon.
- A **diverticulum** (**dye**-ver-**TICK**-you-lum) is a pouch or sac occurring in the lining or wall of a tubular organ such as the colon (plural, **diverticula**). The formation of diverticula in the colon is associated with chronic constipation and straining to defecate.
- **Diverticulitis** (**dye**-ver-tick-you-**LYE**-tis) is the inflammation of one or more diverticula in the colon (**diverticul** means diverticulum and -**itis** means inflammation). Compare with *diverticulosis*.
- **Diverticulosis** (**dye**-ver-tick-you-**LOH**-sis) is the presence of a number of diverticula in the colon (**diverticul** means diverticulum and -**osis** means abnormal condition). Compare with *diverticulitis*.

- **Enteritis** (**en**-ter-**EYE**-tis) is an inflammation of the small intestine caused by eating or drinking substances contaminated with viral or bacterial pathogens such as *E. coli* (**enter** means small intestine and **-itis** means inflammation).

- **Ileus** (**ILL**-ee-us) is the partial or complete blockage of the small and/or large intestine. It is not caused by an obstruction, but by the cessation of intestinal peristalsis. Symptoms of ileus may include severe pain, cramping, abdominal distention, vomiting, and the failure to pass gas or stools. Postoperative ileus is often present for 24 to 72 hours after abdominal surgery.

Irritable Bowel Syndrome

Irritable bowel syndrome, or IBS, also known as **spastic colon**, is a common condition of unknown cause with symptoms that may include intermittent cramping, abdominal pain, bloating, constipation, and/or diarrhea. IBS, which is usually aggravated by stress, is *not* caused by pathogens (bacteria or viruses) or by structural changes.

Inflammatory Bowel Diseases

Inflammatory bowel disease is the general name for diseases that cause inflammation in the intestines. The two most common inflammatory bowel diseases are ulcerative colitis and Crohn's disease.

- These conditions are grouped together because both are chronic, incurable, and may affect the large and small intestines. They also have similar symptoms, which include abdominal pain, weight loss, fatigue, fever, rectal bleeding, and diarrhea.

- These conditions tend to occur at intervals of active disease (flares) and periods of remission. These disorders are treated with medication and surgery to remove diseased portions of the intestine.

Ulcerative Colitis

Ulcerative colitis (koh-**LYE**-tis) is a chronic condition of unknown cause in which repeated episodes of inflammation in the rectum and large intestine cause ulcers and irritation (**col** means colon and **-itis** means inflammation).

- Ulcerative colitis usually starts in the rectum and progresses upward to the lower part of the colon; however, it may affect the entire large intestine.

- Ulcerative colitis affects only the innermost lining and not the deep tissues of the colon. Compare with the tissues and structures affected by *Crohn's disease*.

Crohn's Disease

Crohn's disease is a chronic autoimmune disorder that can occur anywhere in the digestive tract; however, it is most often found in the ileum and in the colon.

- Crohn's disease generally penetrates every layer of tissue in the affected area. This commonly results in scarring and thickening of the walls of the affected structures. Compare with the tissues and structures affected by *ulcerative colitis*.

- **Ileitis** (**ill**-ee-**EYE**-tis) is an inflammation of the ileum (**ile** means ileum and **-itis** means inflammation). The term *regional ileitis* is used to describe Crohn's disease that affects the ileum.

- The term *Crohn's colitis* (koh-**LYE**-tis) is used to describe Crohn's disease that affects the colon (**col** means colon and **-itis** means inflammation). *Notice that colitis, as used here, is not the same as the condition ulcerative colitis.*

Intestinal Obstructions

An **intestinal obstruction** is the partial or complete blockage of the small and/or large intestine caused by a physical obstruction. This blockage may result from many causes such as scar tissue or a tumor.

- *Intestinal adhesions* abnormally hold together parts of the intestine where they normally should be separate. This condition, which is caused by inflammation or trauma, can lead to intestinal obstruction.

- In a *strangulating obstruction*, the blood flow to a segment of the intestine is cut off. This may lead to gangrene and perforation. *Gangrene* is tissue death that is usually associated with a loss of circulation. As used here, a *perforation* is a hole through the wall of a structure.

- **Volvulus** (**VOL**-view-lus) is the twisting of the intestine on itself that causes an obstruction (Figure 8.10). Volvulus is a condition that usually occurs in infancy.

- **Intussusception** (**in**-tus-sus-**SEP**-shun) is the telescoping of one part of the small intestine into the opening of an immediately adjacent part. This is a rare condition sometimes found in infants and young children (Figure 8.11).

- An **inguinal hernia** (**ING**-gwih-nal **HER**-nee-ah) is the protrusion of a small loop of bowel through a weak place in the lower abdominal wall or groin.

- A **strangulated hernia** occurs when a portion of the intestine is constricted inside the hernia and its blood supply is cut off.

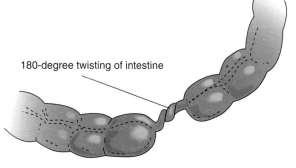

Volvulus

FIGURE 8.10   Volvulus is the twisting of the bowel on itself.

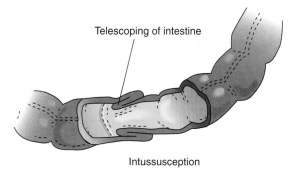

Intussusception

FIGURE 8.11   Intussusception is the telescoping of the bowel on itself.

Infectious Diseases of the Intestines

Infectious diseases of the intestines may be transmitted through contaminated food and water or through poor sanitation practices. The more common of these diseases are discussed in Table 8.1.

Anorectal Disorders

- An **anal fissure** is a small tear in the skin of the anus that can cause severe pain during a bowel movement. As used here, a *fissure* is a groove or crack-like sore of the skin.

Table 8.1

INFECTIOUS DISEASES OF THE INTESTINES

Disease and Mode of Transmission	Causative Agent and Symptoms
Amebic dysentery (ah-**MEE**-bik **DIS**-en-**ter**-ee), also known as *amebiasis*, is transmitted by food or water that is contaminated due to poor sanitary conditions.	*Caused by:* The one-celled parasite *E. histolytica*. *Symptoms:* Mild-form symptoms include loose stools, stomach pain, and stomach cramping. In the severe form, there are also bloody stools and fever.
Botulism (**BOT**-you-lizm), also known as food poisoning, is a rare condition transmitted through contaminated food or an infected wound.	*Caused by:* The bacterium *Clostridium botulinum*. *Symptoms:* Paralysis and sometimes death.
Cholera (**KOL**-er-ah) is transmitted through contact with contaminated food or water.	*Caused by:* The bacterium *Vibrio cholerae*. *Symptoms:* Starts with diarrhea and may progress to profuse diarrhea, vomiting, and rapid dehydration that can be fatal if not treated.
E. coli is transmitted through contaminated food that has not been properly cooked.	*Caused by:* The bacterium *Escherichia coli*. *Symptoms:* Bloody diarrhea and abdominal cramping that can be severe in the very young and the elderly.
Salmonella (**sal**-moh-**NEL**-ah) nontyphoidal, also known as salmonellosis, is transmitted by food contaminated by feces.	*Caused by:* The bacterium *Salmonella*. *Symptoms:* Severe diarrhea, nausea, and vomiting accompanied by a high fever.
Typhoid fever, also known as *enteric fever*, is caused by eating food that has been handled by a carrier. A *carrier* is someone who has the bacteria but is not sick.	*Caused by:* The bacterium *Salmonella typhi*. *Symptoms:* Headache, delirium, cough, watery diarrhea, rash, and a high fever.

- **Bowel incontinence** (in-**KON**-tih-nents) is the inability to control the excretion of feces. (Urinary incontinence refers to the inability to control urination and is discussed in Chapter 9.)

- **Constipation** is a decrease in frequency in the passage of stools, or difficulty in passing hard, dry stools.

- **Diarrhea** (dye-ah-**REE**-ah) is an abnormal frequency of loose or watery stools that may lead to dehydration (**dia** means through and **-rrhea** means flow or discharge).

- **Hemorrhoids** (**HEM**-oh-roids), also known as **piles,** occur when a cluster of veins, muscles, and tissues slip near or through the anal opening. The veins may become inflamed, resulting in pain, fecal leakage, and bleeding.

- **Melena** (meh-**LEE**-nah *or* **MEL**-eh-nah) is the passage of stools with a black and tarlike appearance that is caused by the presence of digested blood.

The Liver

Liver disorders are a major concern because the functioning of the liver is essential to the digestive process.

- **Hepatomegaly** (hep-ah-toh-**MEG**-ah-lee) is the abnormal enlargement of the liver (**hepat/o** means liver and **-megaly** means enlargement).

- **Jaundice** (**JAWN**-dis), also known as **icterus** (**ICK**-ter-us), is a yellow discoloration of the skin and eyes caused by greater-than-normal amounts of bilirubin in the blood.

Hepatitis

Hepatitis (hep-ah-**TYE**-tis) is an inflammation of the liver (**hepat** means liver and **-itis** means inflammation). This condition is usually caused by a virus, although *alcoholic hepatitis* may be caused by alcohol abuse. The five varieties of *viral hepatitis* are shown in Table 8.2.

Cirrhosis

Cirrhosis (sih-**ROH**-sis) is a progressive degenerative disease of the liver in which scar tissue replaces normal tissue (**cirrh** means yellow or orange and **-osis** means abnormal condition). Scar tissue blocks the flow of blood through the organ, which may result in jaundice (hence the name), ascites, and sometimes brain damage or kidney and liver failure (Figure 8.12).

- **Ascites** (ah-**SIGH**-teez) is an abnormal accumulation of serous fluid in the peritoneal cavity. As used here, the term *serous* means a substance having a watery consistency.

The Gallbladder

- **Cholecystalgia** (koh-lee-sis-**TAL**-jee-ah) is pain in the gallbladder (**cholecyst** means gallbladder and **-algia** means pain).

- **Cholecystitis** (koh-lee-sis-**TYE**-tis) is inflammation of the gallbladder, usually associated with gallstones blocking the flow of bile (**cholecyst** means gallbladder and **-itis** means inflammation).

Table 8.2

HEPATITIS FROM A TO E

A	**Hepatitis A virus (HAV)**, also known as **infectious hepatitis**, is transmitted by contaminated food and water, or close contact with an infected person. A vaccine is available.
B	**Hepatitis B virus (HBV)**, also known as **serum hepatitis**, is bloodborne and can be prevented through vaccination. HBV is frequently spread through sexual contact, IV drug abuse, and other sources of contact with contaminated blood.
C	**Hepatitis C virus (HCV)** is bloodborne, and there is no vaccine to prevent this disease. HCV is described as a silent epidemic because it can be present in the body for years and destroy the liver before any symptoms appear.
D	**Hepatitis D virus (HDV)** is bloodborne, and can only be acquired when the hepatitis B virus is already present in the individual.
E	**Hepatitis E virus (HEV)** is transmitted through contaminated food and water.

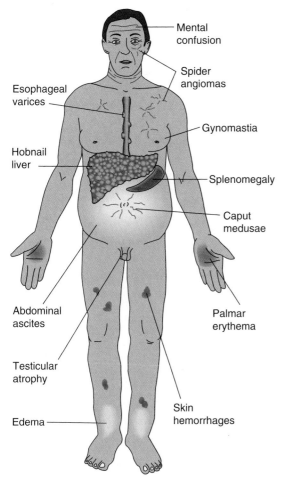

FIGURE 8.12   Clinical features of cirrhosis of the liver in the male.

Labels on figure: Mental confusion; Spider angiomas; Esophageal varices; Gynomastia; Hobnail liver; Splenomegaly; Caput medusae; Abdominal ascites; Palmar erythema; Testicular atrophy; Edema; Skin hemorrhages

- A **gallstone**, also known as **biliary calculus**, is a hard deposit that forms in the gallbladder and bile ducts (plural, **calculi**). The formation of stones is discussed further in Chapter 9.

- **Cholelithiasis** (**koh**-lee-lih-**THIGH**-ah-sis) is the presence of gallstones in the gallbladder or bile ducts (**chole** means bile or gall and -**lithiasis** means presence of stones).

The Pancreas

Disorders of the pancreas are discussed in Chapter 13.

DIAGNOSTIC PROCEDURES OF THE DIGESTIVE SYSTEM

- **Abdominal CT**, or **CT scan**, is a radiographic procedure that produces a detailed cross-section of the tissue structure within the abdomen, showing, for example, the presence of a tumor or obstruction. CT stands for **computerized tomography** (**tom/o**

means slice or cut and -**graphy** means the process of producing a picture or record).

- An **abdominal ultrasound** is a noninvasive test used to visualize internal organs by using very high frequency sound waves.

- The **Given Diagnostic Imaging System**, also known as known as a **capsule endoscopy**, is a tiny video camera in a capsule that the patient swallows. It records images of the walls of the small intestine, transmitting images to a data recorder worn on the patient's belt.

- An **esophagogastroduodenoscopy** (eh-**sof**-ah-goh-**gas**-troh-**dew**-oh-deh-**NOS**-koh-pee) is the examination of the esophagus, stomach, and upper duodenum through a specialized endoscope (**esophag/o** means esophagus, **gastr/o** means stomach, **duoden/o** means duodenum, and -**scopy** means visual examination).

- **Anoscopy** (ah-**NOS**-koh-pee) is the visual examination of the anal canal and lower rectum (**an/o** means anus and -**scopy** means visual examination). A short speculum called an **anoscope** (**AY**-no-skope) is used for this procedure. A *speculum* is an instrument used to enlarge the opening of any body cavity to facilitate inspection of its interior.

- An **upper GI series**, or **barium swallow**, and **lower GI series**, or **barium enema**, are radiographic studies to examine the digestive system. Barium, which is a contrast medium, is discussed further in Chapter 15.

- The term **enema** describes a solution placed into the rectum and colon to empty the lower intestine through bowel activity. One purpose of an enema is to clear the bowels in preparation for an endoscopic examination.

- **Hemoccult** (**HEE**-moh-kult), also known as the **fecal occult blood test**, is a laboratory test for hidden blood in the stools (**hem** means blood and -**occult** means hidden). A test kit may be used at home to obtain the specimens, which are then delivered to a laboratory or physician's office for evaluation.

- **Stool samples** are specimens of feces that are examined for content and characteristics. For example, fatty stools might indicate the presence of pancreatic problems. Cultures of the stool sample can be examined in the laboratory for the presence of bacteria or **O & P**, which are **ova** (parasite eggs) and **parasites**.

Endoscopic Procedures

An **endoscope** is an instrument used for visual examination of internal structures (**endo-** means within and **-scope** means an instrument for visual examination). Endoscopes are also used for obtaining biopsy samples, controlling bleeding, removing foreign objects, as well as for other surgical and treatment procedures. The endoscopes and procedures are named for the body parts being examined or treated.

- **Colonoscopy** (**koh**-lun-**OSS**-koh-pee) is the direct visual examination of the inner surface of the colon from the rectum to the cecum (**colon/o** means colon and **-scopy** means visual examination).

- **Sigmoidoscopy** (**sig**-moi-**DOS**-koh-pee) is the endoscopic examination of the interior of the rectum, sigmoid colon, and possibly a portion of the descending colon (**sigmoid/o** means sigmoid colon and **-scopy** is the visual examination).

TREATMENT PROCEDURES OF THE DIGESTIVE SYSTEM

Medications

- **Acid blockers,** which are taken before eating, block the effects of histamine that signals the stomach to produce acid.

- **Antacids** relieve indigestion or help peptic ulcers heal by neutralizing stomach acids.

- An **emetic** (eh-**MET**-ick), such as syrup of ipecac, is a medication that is administered to produce vomiting (**emet** means vomiting and **-ic** means pertaining to).

- An **antiemetic** (**an**-tih-ee-**MET**-ick) is administered to prevent or relieve nausea and vomiting (**anti-** means against, **emet** means vomiting, and **-ic** means pertaining to).

- **Laxatives** are medications, or foods, given to stimulate bowel movements. *Bulk-forming laxatives,* such as bran, treat constipation by helping fecal matter retain water and remain soft as it moves through the intestines.

- **Oral rehydration therapy** is a treatment in which a solution of electrolytes is administered in a liquid preparation to counteract the dehydration that may accompany severe diarrhea, especially in young children.

The Oral Cavity and Esophagus

- A **gingivectomy** (**jin**-jih-**VECK**-toh-mee) is the surgical removal of diseased gingival tissue (**gingiv** means gingival tissue and **-ectomy** means surgical removal).

- **Maxillofacial surgery** (mack-**sill**-oh-**FAY**-shul) is specialized surgery of the face and jaws to correct deformities, treat diseases, and repair injuries.

- **Palatoplasty** (**PAL**-ah-toh-**plas**-tee) is surgical repair of a cleft palate (**palat/o** means palate and **-plasty** means surgical repair).

- A **dental prophylaxis** (**proh**-fih-**LACK**-sis) is the professional cleaning of the teeth to remove plaque and calculus. The term *prophylaxis* also refers to a treatment, such as a vaccination or condom, intended to prevent a disease or stop it from spreading.

The Stomach

- A **gastrectomy** (gas-**TRECK**-toh-mee) is the surgical removal of all or a part of the stomach (**gastr** means stomach and **-ectomy** means surgical removal).

- A **gastric bypass**, which is used in the treatment of morbid obesity, is a surgical procedure in which the size of the stomach is drastically reduced. One technique for this is known as **stomach stapling**.

- **Nasogastric intubation** (**nay**-zoh-**GAS**-trick **in**-too-**BAY**-shun) is the placement of a tube through the nose and into the stomach.

The Intestines

- A **colectomy** (koh-**LECK**-toh-mee) is the surgical removal of all or part of the colon (**col** means colon and **-ectomy** means surgical removal).

- A **diverticulectomy** (**dye**-ver-**tick**-you-**LECK**-toh-mee) is the surgical removal of a diverticulum (**diverticul** means diverticulum and **-ectomy** means surgical removal).

- A **gastroduodenostomy** (**gas**-troh-**dew**-oh-deh-**NOS**-toh-mee) is the removal of the pylorus of the stomach and the establishment of an anastomosis between the upper portion of the stomach and the duodenum (**gastr/o** means stomach, **duoden** means first part of the small intestine, and **-ostomy** means surgically creating an opening). This procedure is performed to treat stomach cancer or to remove a malfunctioning pyloric valve (Figure 8.13). An **anastomosis** (ah-**nas**-toh-**MOH**-sis) is a surgical connection between two hollow or tubular structures (plural, **anastomoses**).

- A **hemorrhoidectomy** (**hem**-oh-roid-**ECK**-toh-mee) is the surgical removal of hemorrhoids (**hemorrhoid** means piles and **-ectomy** means surgical removal). *Rubber band ligation* is often used instead of surgery. Rubber bands cut off the circulation at the base of the hemorrhoid, causing it to eventually fall off. *Ligation* is the tying off of blood vessels or ducts.

- An **ileectomy** (**ill**-ee-**ECK**-toh-mee) is the surgical removal of the ileum (**ile** means the ileum and **-ectomy** means surgical removal. *Note:* This term is spelled with a double *e*.)

Ostomies

An **ostomy** (**OSS**-toh-mee) is a surgical procedure to create an artificial opening between an organ and the body surface. This opening is called a **stoma** (**STOH**-mah). *Ostomy* can be used alone as a noun to describe a procedure or as a suffix with the word part that describes the organ involved.

- A **gastrostomy** (gas-**TROS**-toh-mee) is the surgical creation of an artificial opening into the stomach (**gastr** means stomach and **-ostomy** means surgically creating an opening). This procedure is frequently performed for the placement of a permanent feeding tube.

- An **ileostomy** (**ill**-ee-**OS**-toh-mee) is the surgical creation of an artificial excretory opening between the ileum, at the end of the small intestine, and the outside of the abdominal wall (**ile** means small intestine and **-ostomy** means surgically creating an opening).

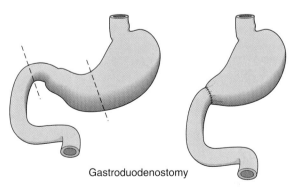

Gastroduodenostomy

FIGURE 8.13   In a gastroduodenostomy, an anastomosis is formed where the stomach and duodenum are surgically joined.

- A **colostomy** (koh-**LAHS**-toh-mee) is the surgical creation of an artificial excretory opening between the colon and the body surface (**col** means colon and **-ostomy** means surgically creating an opening). The entire segment of the intestine below the ostomy is usually removed and the fecal matter flows from the stoma into a disposable bag. A colostomy may be temporary, to divert feces from an area that needs to heal (Figure 8.14).

The Rectum and Anus

- A **proctectomy** (prock-**TECK**-toh-mee) is the surgical removal of the rectum (**proct** means rectum and **-ectomy** means surgical removal).

- **Proctopexy** (**PROCK**-toh-**peck**-see) is the surgical fixation of a prolapsed rectum to an adjacent tissue or organ (**proct/o** means rectum and **-pexy** means surgical fixation). *Prolapse* means the falling or dropping down of an organ or internal part.

- **Proctoplasty** (**PROCK**-toh-**plas**-tee) is the surgical repair of the rectum (**proct/o** means rectum and **-plasty** means surgical repair).

The Liver

- A **hepatectomy** (**hep**-ah-**TECK**-toh-mee) is the surgical removal of all or part of the liver (**hepat** means liver and **-ectomy** means surgical removal).

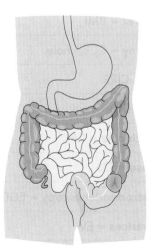

FIGURE 8.14   Colostomy sites are named for part of the bowel removed. Shown here is a sigmoid colostomy. The stoma is located at the end of the remaining intestine, which is shown in brown. The portion that has been removed is shown in blue.

Learning Exercises

● Matching Word Parts 1

Write the correct answer in the middle column.

Definition	Correct Answer	Possible Answers
8.1. anus	_____	enter/o
8.2. bile, gall	_____	an/o
8.3. large intestine	_____	cec/o
8.4. cecum	_____	chol/e
8.5. small intestine	_____	col/o

● Matching Word Parts 2

Write the correct answer in the middle column.

Definition	Correct Answer	Possible Answers
8.6. stomach	_____	-lithiasis
8.7. liver	_____	gastr/o
8.8. gallbladder	_____	esophag/o
8.9. esophagus	_____	hepat/o
8.10. presence of stones	_____	cholecyst/o

● Matching Word Parts 3

Write the correct answer in the middle column.

Definition	Correct Answer	Possible Answers
8.11. sigmoid colon	_____	-pepsia
8.12. anus and rectum	_____	pancreat/o
8.13. digestion	_____	proct/o
8.14. pancreas	_____	rect/o
8.15. rectum	_____	sigmoid/o

● Definitions

Select the correct answer and write it on the line provided.

8.16.   The visual examination of the anal canal and lower rectum is known as _____ .

   anoscopy   colonoscopy   proctoscopy   sigmoidoscopy

8.17.   The _____ glands are located on the face in front of each ear.

   maxillary   parotid   sublingual   submandibular

8.18.   The _____ are the posterior teeth used for grinding and chewing.

   canines   cuspids   incisors   molars

8.19.   The liver removes excess _____ from the bloodstream.

   bilirubin   glucose   glycogen   lipase

8.20.   The gallbladder stores _____ for later use.

   bile   glycogen   hydrochloric acid   pepsin

8.21.   The _____ colon travels upward from the cecum to the under surface of the liver.

   ascending   descending   sigmoid   transverse

8.22.   The process of breaking down substances is known as _____ .

   anabolism   catabolism   defecation   dentition

8.23.   The receptors of taste are located on the _____ .

   hard palate   rugae   tongue   uvula

8.24. Each tooth is surrounded by specialized mucous membrane known as the _____ .

cementum   dentin   gingiva   pulp

8.25. The condition characterized by the telescoping of one part of the intestine into another is called

_____ .

borborygmus   flatus   intussusception   volvulus

● Matching Structures

Write the correct answer in the middle column.

Definition	Correct Answer	Possible Answers
8.26. connects the small and large intestine	_____	cecum
8.27. major part of the large intestine leading into the rectum	_____	ileum
8.28. last division of the large intestine	_____	jejunum
8.29. middle portion of the small intestine	_____	rectum
8.30. last portion of the small intestine	_____	sigmoid colon

---

● Which Word?

Select the correct answer and write it on the line provided.

8.31. The word that means vomiting blood is _____ .

hematemesis   hyperemesis

8.32. The type of hepatitis that is transmitted by contaminated food and water is caused by the

_____ virus.

hepatitis A   hepatitis B

8.33. An often fatal form of food poisoning is _____ .

bulimia   botulism

8.34. The term meaning inflammation of the small intestine is _____ .

      colitis   enteritis

8.35. The _____ is the structure that hangs from the free edge of the soft palate.

      volvulus   uvula

● Spelling Counts

Find the misspelled word in each sentence. Then write that word, spelled correctly, on the line provided.

8.36. An ilectomy is the surgical removal of the last portion of the small intestine. _____

8.37. The cecum is connected to the ileum by the iliocecal sphincter. _____

8.38. The term hepatarrhaphy means surgical suturing of the liver. _____

8.39. A proctoplexy is the surgical fixation of the rectum to some adjacent tissue or organ.

      _____

8.40. Zerostomia is the lack of adequate saliva due to the absence of or diminished secretions by the salivary

      glands. _____

● Abbreviation Identification

In the space provided, write the words that each abbreviation stands for.

8.41. **BE**   _____

8.42. **CRC**   _____

8.43. **GERD**   _____

8.44. **IBS**   _____

8.45. **PU**   _____

● Term Selection

Select the correct answer and write it on the line provided.

8.46. Surgical removal of all or part of the stomach is known as a _____ .

      gastrectomy   gastritis   gastroenteritis   gastrotomy

8.47.   Difficulty in swallowing is known as _____ .

anorexia   dyspepsia   dysphagia   pyrosis

8.48.   The surgical removal of all or part of the colon is known as a _____ .

colectomy   colostomy   colotomy   proctectomy

8.49.   The progressive degeneration of the liver in which scar tissue replaces normal tissue is called

_____ .

cirrhosis   hepatomegaly   hepatitis   hepatorrhexis

8.50.   The pigment produced by the destruction of hemoglobin in the liver is called _____.

bile   bilirubin   hydrochloric acid   pancreatic juice

● Sentence Completion

Write the correct term on the line provided.

8.51.   The folds in the mucosa lining the mouth and of the stomach are known as _____.

8.52.   The return of swallowed food to the mouth is called _____ .

8.53.   A yellow discoloration of the skin caused by greater-than-normal amounts of bilirubin in the blood is

called _____.

8.54.   The flow from the stomach to the duodenum is controlled by the _____

_____.

8.55.   The medical term for the solid body wastes that are expelled through the rectum is/are

_____.

● Word Surgery

Divide each term into its component word parts. Write these word parts, in sequence, on the lines provided.

When necessary use a back slash (/) to indicate a combining vowel. (You may not need all of the lines provided.)

8.56.   An **esophagogastroduodenoscopy** is the examination of the esophagus, stomach, and upper duodenum

through a specialized endoscope.

_____   _____   _____   _____

8.57.   A **periodontist** is a dental specialist who prevents or treats disorders of the tissues surrounding the teeth.

_____   _____   _____   _____

8.58.   A **sigmoidoscopy** is the endoscopic examination of the interior of the rectum, sigmoid colon, and possibly a portion of the descending colon.

_____   _____   _____   _____

8.59.   An **antiemetic** is administered to prevent or relieve nausea and vomiting.

_____   _____   _____   _____

8.60.   A **gastroduodenostomy** is the establishment of an anastomosis between the upper portion of the stomach and the duodenum.

_____   _____   _____   _____

● True/False

If the statement is true, write **T** on the line. If the statement is false, write **F** on the line.

8.61.   _____ Hepatitis B can be prevented through immunization.

8.62.   _____ The Given Diagnostic Imaging System is also known as a capsule endoscopy.

8.63.   _____ Periodontitis is the progressive destruction of dental enamel.

8.64.   _____ Bruxism means to be without natural teeth.

8.65.   _____ A choledocholithotomy is an incision in the common bile duct for the removal of gallstones.

● Clinical Conditions

Write the correct answer on the line provided.

8.66.   James Ridgeview was treated for the temporary stoppage of intestinal peristalsis. The medical term for this condition is _____ .

8.67.   Chang Hoon suffers from _____. This condition is an abnormal accumulation of serous fluid in the peritoneal cavity.

8.68.   Dr. Martinson described the patient as being _____, which means he was without natural teeth.

8.69. Baby Kilgore was vomiting almost continuously. The medical term for this excessive vomiting is

_____.

8.70. A/An _____ was performed on Mr. Gonzalez to create an opening between his colon

and body surface.

8.71. After eating, Mr. Delahanty often suffers from heartburn. The medical term for this condition is

_____.

8.72. Catherine Baldwin's presenting symptom was the passage of black stools containing digested blood. The

medical term for this condition is _____ .

8.73. Alberta Roberts was diagnosed as having an inflammation of one or more diverticulum. The medical

term for this condition is _____ .

8.74. Jason Norton suffers from _____ labialis, which is also known as cold sores.

8.75. Lisa Wilson saw her dentist because she was concerned about bad breath. Her dentist refers to this con-

dition as _____ .

● Which Is the Correct Medical Term?

Select the correct answer and write it on the line provided.

8.76. The _____ test detects hidden blood in the stools.

anoscopy   colonoscopy   enema   hemoccult

8.77. In a patient with a colostomy, the effluent flows from the _____ .

colon   ileus   rectum   stoma

8.78. The term meaning the lack or loss of appetite is _____ .

anorexia   bulimia   nervosa   pica

8.79. The hardened deposit on the teeth that irritates the surrounding tissues is known as

_____ .

calculus   caries   gingiva   plaque

8.80. The surgical repair of the rectum is known as _____ .

anoplasty   palatoplasty   proctopexy   proctoplasty

● Challenge Word Building

These terms are *not* found in this chapter; however, they are made up of the following familiar word parts. You may want to look in the textbook glossary or use a medical dictionary to check your answers.

col/o	-algia
enter/o	-ectomy
esophag/o	-itis
gastr/o	-megaly
hepat/o	-ic
proct/o	-pexy
sigmoid/o	-rrhaphy

8.81.   The term meaning the surgical suturing of a stomach wound is _____ .

8.82.   The term meaning pain in the esophagus is _____.

8.83.   The term meaning the surgical removal of all or part of the sigmoid colon is _____.

8.84.   The term meaning pain in and around the anus and rectum is _____.

8.85.   The term meaning the surgical fixation of the stomach to correct displacement is

_____.

8.86.   The term meaning inflammation of the sigmoid colon is _____ .

8.87.   The term meaning the surgical removal of all or part of the esophagus and stomach is

_____.

8.88.   The term referring to the liver and intestines is _____.

8.89.   The term meaning abnormal enlargement of the liver is _____.

8.90.   The term meaning inflammation of the stomach, small intestine, and large intestine is

_____.

● Labeling Exercises

Identify the numbered items on the accompanying figure.

8.91. _____ glands

8.92. _____

8. 93. _____

8. 94. _____

8. 95. _____

8.96. _____

8.97. _____ intestine

8.98. vermiform _____

8.99. _____ intestine

8.100 _____ and anus

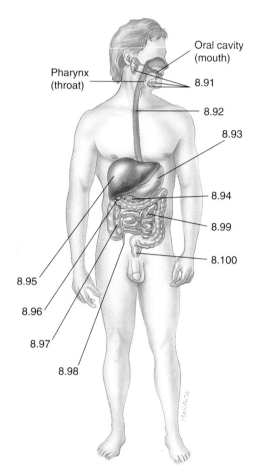

THE HUMAN TOUCH: CRITICAL THINKING EXERCISE

The following story and questions are designed to stimulate critical thinking through class discussion or as a brief essay response. There are no right or wrong answers to these questions.

"Stick the landing and our team walks away with the gold!" Coach Schaefer meant to be supportive as she squeezed Claire's shoulder. "What you mean is beat Leia's score for the Riverview team and we'll win," Claire thought sarcastically. She watched as Leia's numbers were shown from her last vault. A 6.8 out of a possible 7. "Great, just great! She chooses a less difficult vault, but with that toothpick body she gets more height than I ever will!" She wondered if Leia was naturally that thin, or did she use the secret method—you can't gain weight if the food doesn't stay in your stomach.

All season it had been that way. Everyone seemed to be watching the rivalry between West High's Claire and Riverview's "tiny-mighty" Leia. Claire was pretty sure that her 10-pound weight loss had improved both her floor routine and her tricky dismount off the beam. "I'm less than a half point behind, so coach should be happy," she thought. But just last week Coach Schaefer had a long talk with her when she got dizzy and fell off the balance beam. Coach had asked Claire the one question she swore she'd never answer: "Just what have you been doing to lose the weight?"

Claire felt her hands sweat. "Just stick the landing," she told herself, but her body had a different agenda. Starved for fuel, her muscles failed, and the gold slipped out of reach.

Suggested Discussion Topics:

1. Who do you think sets the standards for how a person thinks he or she should look?
2. List several eating disorders. What personality traits do you think cause a person to develop eating disorders?
3. Discuss why anorexia and bulimia usually occur in young women between the ages of 12 and 28.
4. Athletes sometimes abuse their bodies through dieting or drugs to achieve peak performances. What should the groups that oversee competitive athletics do about this practice?
5. Imagine you have a daughter. How would you know if she had an eating disorder? What kind of treatment might help her?

9 The Urinary System

● Overview of Structures, Combining Forms, and Functions of the Urinary System

MAJOR STRUCTURES	RELATED COMBINING FORMS	PRIMARY FUNCTIONS
Kidneys	nephr/o, ren/o	Filter the blood to remove waste products, maintain electrolyte concentrations, and remove excess water to maintain the fluid volume within the body.
Renal Pelvis	pyel/o	Collects urine produced by the kidney.
Urine	ur/o, urin/o	Liquid waste products to be excreted.
Ureters	ureter/o	Transport urine from the kidneys to the bladder.
Urinary Bladder	cyst/o	Stores urine until it is excreted.
Urethra	urethr/o	Transports urine from the bladder through the urethral meatus, where it is excreted from the body.

● VOCABULARY   RELATED TO THE URINARY SYSTEM

The items on this list have been identified as key word parts and terms for this chapter. However, all words in boldface in the text are important and may be included in the learning exercises and tests.

Word Parts

- ☐ dia-
- ☐ -cele
- ☐ cyst/o
- ☐ -ectasis
- ☐ glomerul/o
- ☐ lith/o
- ☐ -lysis
- ☐ nephr/o
- ☐ -pexy
- ☐ pyel/o
- ☐ -tripsy
- ☐ ur/o
- ☐ ureter/o
- ☐ urethr/o
- ☐ -uria

Medical Terms

- ☐ **anuria** (ah-**NEW**-ree-ah)
- ☐ **catheterization** (**kath**-eh-ter-eye-**ZAY**-shun)
- ☐ **cystitis** (sis-**TYE**-tis)
- ☐ **cystocele** (**SIS**-toh-seel)
- ☐ **cystolith** (**SIS**-toh-lith)
- ☐ **cystopexy** (**sis**-toh-**peck**-see)
- ☐ **cystoscopy** (sis-**TOS**-koh-pee)
- ☐ **diabetic nephropathy** (neh-**FROP**-ah-thee)
- ☐ **dialysis** (dye-**AL**-ih-sis)
- ☐ **diuretics** (**dye**-you-**RET**-icks)
- ☐ **dysuria** (dis-**YOU**-ree-ah)
- ☐ **enuresis** (**en**-you-**REE**-sis)
- ☐ **epispadias** (ep-ih-**SPAY**-dee-as)
- ☐ **glomerulonephritis** (gloh-**mer**-you-loh-neh-**FRY**-tis)
- ☐ **hemodialysis** (**hee**-moh-dye-**AL**-ih-sis)
- ☐ **hydronephrosis** (**high**-droh-neh-**FROH**-sis)
- ☐ **hydroureter** (**high**-droh-you-**REE**-ter)
- ☐ **hyperlipidemia** (**high**-per-**lip**-ih-**DEE**-mee-ah)
- ☐ **hyperproteinuria** (**high**-per-**proh**-tee-in-**YOU**-ree-ah)
- ☐ **hypoproteinemia** (**high**-poh-**proh**-tee-in-**EE**-mee-ah)

- ☐ **hypospadias** (**high**-poh-**SPAY**-dee-as)
- ☐ **incontinence** (in-**KON**-tih-nents)
- ☐ **interstitial cystitis** (**in**-ter-**STISH**-al sis-**TYE**-tis)
- ☐ **intravenous pyelogram** (**in**-trah-**VEE**-nus **PYE**-eh-loh-**gram**)
- ☐ **lithotomy** (lih-**THOT**-oh-mee)
- ☐ **lithotripsy** (**LITH**-oh-**trip**-see)
- ☐ **meatotomy** (**mee**-ah-**TOT**-oh-mee)
- ☐ **micturition** (**mick**-too-**RISH**-un)
- ☐ **nephrectasis** (neh-**FRECK**-tah-sis)
- ☐ **nephritis** (neh-**FRY**-tis)
- ☐ **nephrolith** (**NEF**-roh-lith)
- ☐ **nephrolithiasis** (**nef**-roh-lih-**THIGH**-ah-sis)
- ☐ **nephrolysis** (neh-**FROL**-ih-sis)
- ☐ **nephroptosis** (**nef**-rop-**TOH**-sis)
- ☐ **nephropyosis** (**nef**-roh-pye-**OH**-sis)
- ☐ **nephrostomy** (neh-**FROS**-toh-me)
- ☐ **nephrotic syndrome** (neh-**FROT**-ick)
- ☐ **nocturia** (nock-**TOO**-ree-ah)
- ☐ **oliguria** (**ol**-ih-**GOO**-ree-ah)
- ☐ **paraspadias** (**par**-ah-**SPAY**-dee-as)
- ☐ **percutaneous nephrolithotomy** (**per**-kyou-**TAY**-nee-us **nef**-roh-lih-**THOT**-oh-mee)
- ☐ **peritoneal dialysis** (**pehr**-ih-toh-**NEE**-al dye-**AL**-ih-sis)
- ☐ **polycystic kidney disease** (**pol**-ee-**SIS**-tick)
- ☐ **pyeloplasty** (**PYE**-eh-loh-**plas**-tee)
- ☐ **pyelotomy** (pye-eh-**LOT**-oh-mee)
- ☐ **suprapubic catheterization** (**soo**-prah-**PYOU**-bick **kath**-eh-ter-eye-**ZAY**-shun)
- ☐ **uremia** (you-**REE**-mee-ah)
- ☐ **ureterectasis** (you-**ree**-ter-**ECK**-tah-sis)
- ☐ **ureterolith** (you-**REE**-ter-oh-**lith**)
- ☐ **ureterorrhagia** (you-**ree**-ter-oh-**RAY**-jee-ah)
- ☐ **ureterorrhaphy** (**you**-ree-ter-**OR**-ah-fee)
- ☐ **ureterostenosis** (you-**ree**-ter-oh-steh-**NOH**-sis)
- ☐ **urethritis** (**you**-reh-**THRIGH**-tis)
- ☐ **urethropexy** (you-**REE**-throh-**peck**-see)
- ☐ **urethrorrhagia** (you-**ree**-throh-**RAY**-jee-ah)
- ☐ **urethrorrhea** (you-**ree**-throh-**REE**-ah)
- ☐ **urethrostenosis** (you-**ree**-throh-steh-**NOH**-sis)
- ☐ **urethrostomy** (**you**-reh-**THROS**-toh-mee)
- ☐ **vesicovaginal fistula** (**ves**-ih-koh-**VAG**-ih-nahl **FIS**-tyou-lah)
- ☐ **voiding cystourethrography** (**sis**-toh-you-ree-**THROG**-rah-fee)

On completion of this chapter, you should be able to:

1. Describe the major functions of the urinary system.

2. Name and describe the structures of the urinary system.

3. Recognize, define, spell, and pronounce terms related to the pathology and the diagnostic and treatment procedures of the urinary system.

FUNCTIONS OF THE URINARY SYSTEM

The urinary system performs many functions that are important in maintaining **homeostasis** (**hoh**-mee-oh-**STAY**-sis), which is a state of equilibrium that produces a constant internal environment throughout the body (**home/o** means sameness and **-stasis** means control). To achieve this, the urinary system:

- Maintains the proper balance of water, salts, and acids in the body fluids by removing excess fluids from the body or reabsorbing water as needed.

- Constantly filters the blood to remove urea and other waste materials from the bloodstream. **Urea** (you-**REE**-ah) is the major waste product of protein metabolism.

- Converts these waste products and excess fluids into **urine** in the kidneys and excretes them from the body via the urinary bladder.

STRUCTURES OF THE URINARY SYSTEM

The urinary system, also referred to as the **urinary tract**, consists of two kidneys, two ureters, one blad-

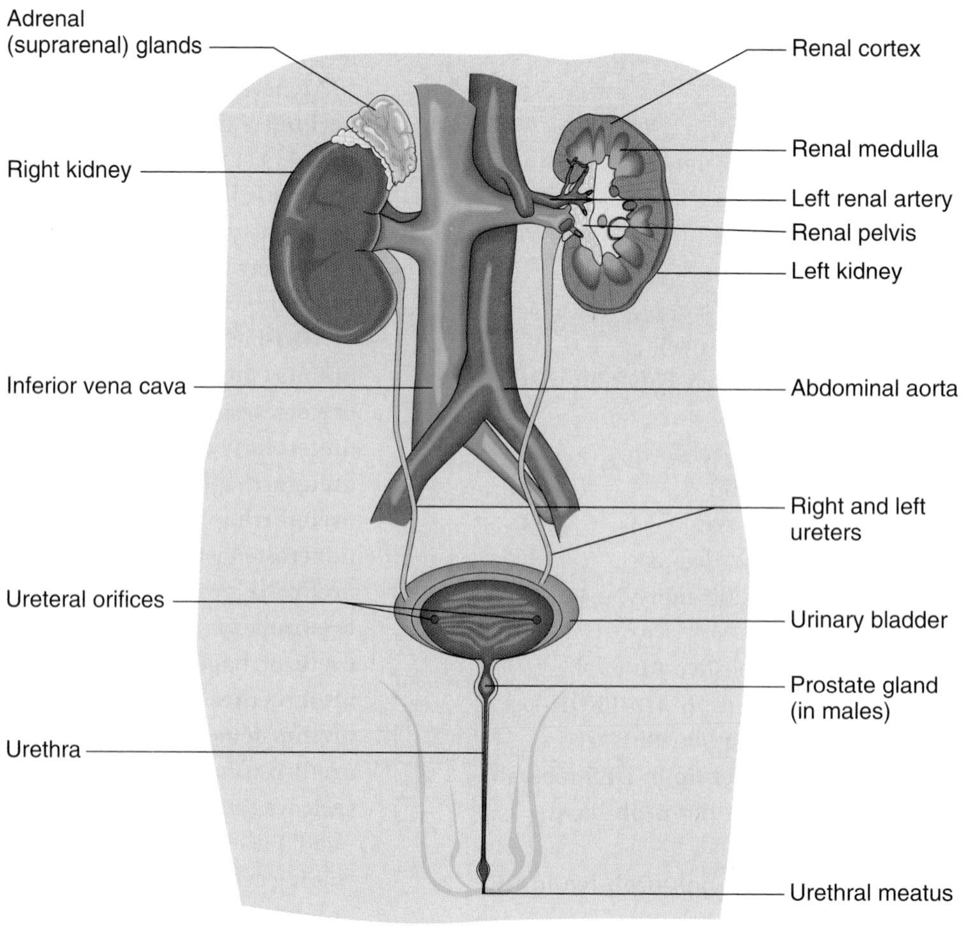

FIGURE **9.1**   The primary structures of the urinary system: the kidneys, ureters, urinary bladder, and urethra.

der, and a urethra (Figure 9.1). The adrenal glands, which are part of the endocrine system, are located on the top of the kidneys.

The Kidneys

The **kidneys** constantly filter the blood to remove waste products and excess water and salts. These are excreted as urine, which is 95 percent water and 5 percent other wastes (Figure 9.2A).

- The term **renal** (**REE**-nal) means pertaining to the kidneys.

- The two kidneys are located retroperitoneally with one on each side of the vertebral column below the diaphragm. *Retroperitoneally* means pertaining to being located behind the peritoneum. The *peritoneum* is the membrane that lines the abdominal cavity.

- The **renal cortex** (**REE**-nal **KOR**-tecks) is the outer rim of the kidney. It contains over one million microscopic units called **nephrons**.

- The **medulla** (meh-**DULL**-ah) is the inner region of the kidney; it contains most of the urine-collecting tubules. A *tubule* is a small tube.

- The **renal pelvis** is the funnel-shaped area within each kidney that is surrounded by these two layers.

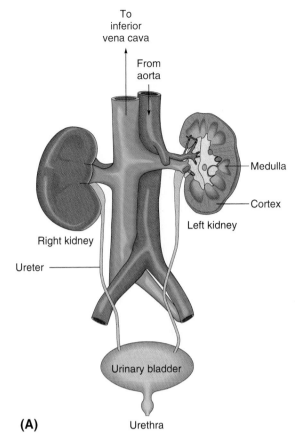

(A)

Figure 9.2A   Structures and blood flow of the kidneys, ureters, and bladder.

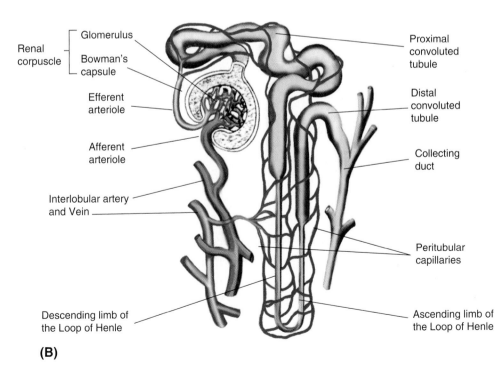

(B)

Figure 9.2B   A nephron unit and its associated structures.

The Nephrons

Nephrons (**NEF**-rons) are the functional units of the kidneys. They form urine by the processes of filtration, reabsorption, and secretion (Figure 9.2B).

- Each nephron contains a **glomerulus** (gloh-**MER**-you-lus), which is a cluster of capillaries surrounded by a cup-shaped membrane called the Bowman's capsule (plural, **glomeruli**).

- Blood enters the kidney through the renal artery and flows into the nephrons. It is filtered in the capillaries of the glomerulus and leaves the kidney through the renal vein.

- Waste products that have been filtered out of the blood remain behind, passing through a series of urine-collecting tubules before being transported to the **renal pelvis** and entering the ureters.

- **Urochrome** (**YOU**-roh-krome) is the pigment that gives urine its normal yellow-amber or straw color (**ur/o** means urine and **-chrome** means color). The color of urine can be influenced by normal factors such as the amount of liquid consumed, and can be changed by diseases and medications.

The Ureters

The **ureters** (you-**REE**-ters) are narrow tubes, each about 10 to 12 inches long. Each ureter carries urine

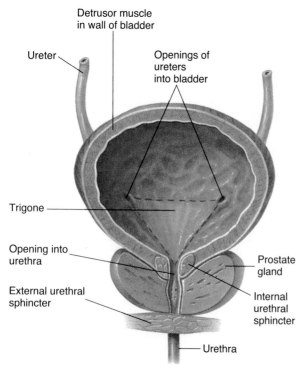

Detrusor muscle in wall of bladder
Ureter
Openings of ureters into bladder
Trigone
Opening into urethra
Prostate gland
External urethral sphincter
Internal urethral sphincter
Urethra

FIGURE 9.3 The anatomy of the urinary bladder in the male.

from a kidney to the urinary bladder. Peristalsis moves urine downward toward the bladder.

The Urinary Bladder

The **urinary bladder** (Figure 9.3) is a hollow muscular organ that is a reservoir for urine.

- The bladder is located in the anterior portion of the pelvic cavity behind the pubic symphysis. The bladder stores about one pint of urine.

- Like the stomach, the bladder is lined with rugae, which are folds that allow it to expand and contract.

The Urethra

The **urethra** (you-**REE**-thrah) is the tube extending from the bladder to the outside of the body. *Caution:* The spellings of *ureter* and *urethra* are very similar!

- Two **urinary sphincters,** one located at either end of the urethra, control the flow of urine from the bladder into the urethra and out of the urethra through the urethral meatus. A *sphincter* is a ring-like muscle that closes a passageway (Figure 9.3).

- The **urethral meatus** (you-**REE**-thrahl mee-**AY**-tus), also known as the **urinary meatus**, is the external opening of the urethra. A *meatus* is the external opening of a canal.

- The **female urethra** is approximately 1.5 inches long. The urethral meatus is located between the clitoris and the opening of the vagina. In the female, the urethra conveys only urine.

- The **male urethra** is approximately eight inches long, and the urethral meatus is located at the tip of the penis (Figure 9.3). In the male, the urethra conveys both urine and semen. The neck of the urethra is surrounded by the prostate gland, which is part of the reproductive system and is discussed further in Chapter 14.

THE EXCRETION OF URINE

As the bladder fills up, pressure is placed on the base of the urethra, resulting in the urge to **urinate** or **micturate.**

- **Urination**, also known as **micturition** (**mick**-too-**RISH**-un) or **voiding**, is the normal process of excreting urine.

- Urination requires the coordinated contraction of the bladder muscles and relaxation of the sphincters. This action forces the urine through the urethra and out through the urinary meatus.

MEDICAL SPECIALTIES RELATED TO THE URINARY SYSTEM

- A **nephrologist** (neh-**FROL**-oh-jist) specializes in diagnosing and treating diseases and disorders of the kidneys (**nephr** means kidney and **-ologist** means specialist).

- A **urologist** (you-**ROL**-oh-jist) specializes in diagnosing and treating diseases and disorders of the urinary system of females and the genitourinary system of males (**ur** means urine and **-ologist** means specialist). The term *genitourinary* refers to both the genital and urinary organs.

PATHOLOGY OF THE URINARY SYSTEM

Renal Failure

Renal failure, also known as **kidney failure**, is the inability of one or both of the kidneys to perform their functions. The body cannot replace damaged nephrons. When too many nephrons have been destroyed, the result is kidney failure.

- **Anuria** (ah-**NEW**-ree-ah) is the absence of urine formation by the kidneys (**an-** means without and **-uria** means urine).

- **Uremia** (you-**REE**-mee-ah), also known as **uremic poisoning**, is a toxic condition caused by excessive amount of urea and other waste products in the bloodstream (**ur** means urine and **-emia** means blood condition).

- **Acute renal failure** has sudden onset and is characterized by uremia. It can be fatal if not reversed promptly. This condition can be caused by many factors, including a drop in blood volume or blood pressure due to injury or surgery.

- **Chronic renal failure** is the progressive loss of renal function due to a variety of conditions, such as kidney disease, diabetes mellitus, or hypertension.

- **End-stage renal disease** refers to the late stages of chronic renal failure, in which there is irreversible loss of the function of both kidneys. Without dialysis or a kidney transplant, this condition is fatal.

Nephrotic Syndrome

Nephrotic syndrome (neh-**FROT**-ick) is a condition in which very high levels of protein are lost in the urine and low levels of protein are present in the blood (**nephr/o** means kidney and **-tic** means pertaining to).

This is the result of damage to the kidney's glomeruli. **Nephrosis** (neh-**FROH**-sis) is any degenerative kidney disease causing nephrotic syndrome *without* inflammation (**nephr** means kidney and **-osis** means abnormal condition). The following are characteristics of kidney malfunction diseases:

- **Edema** (eh-**DEE**-mah) is excessive fluid in the body tissues.

- **Hyperproteinuria** (**high**-per-**proh**-tee-in-**YOU**-ree-ah) is the presence of abnormally *high* concentrations of protein in the urine (**hyper-** means excessive, **protein** means protein, and **-uria** means urine).

- **Hypoproteinemia** (**high**-poh-**proh**-tee-in-**EE**-mee-ah) is the presence of abnormally *low* concentrations of protein in the blood (**hypo-** means deficient or decreased, **protein** means protein, and **-emie** means blood condition).

- **Hyperlipidemia** (**high**-per-**lip**-ih-**DEE**-mee-ah) is the presence of abnormally *large* amounts of lipids in the blood (**hyper-** means excessive, **lipid** means lipids [fat], and **-emia** means blood condition).

Nephropathy

The term **nephropathy** (neh-**FROP**-ah-thee) also means a disease of the kidney; however it includes both degenerative conditions and inflammatory diseases (**nephr** means kidney and **-pathy** means disease).

- **Diabetic nephropathy** is a kidney disease characterized by hyperproteinuria, which is the result of thickening and hardening of the glomeruli caused by long-term diabetes mellitus.

The Kidneys

- **Hydronephrosis** (**high**-droh-neh-**FROH**-sis) is the dilation (swelling) of one or both kidneys (**hydr/o** means water, **nephr** means kidney, and **-osis** means abnormal condition). This is the result of an obstruction in the flow of urine (Figure 9.4).

- **Nephrectasis** (neh-**FRECK**-tah-sis) is the distention of a kidney (**nephr** means kidney and **-ectasis** means enlargement or stretching). *Distention* means the state of being enlarged.

- **Nephritis** (neh-**FRY**-tis) is an inflammation of the kidney (**nephr** means kidney and **-itis** means inflammation).

- **Glomerulonephritis** (gloh-**mer**-you-loh-neh-**FRY**-tis) is a type of nephritis that involves primarily the

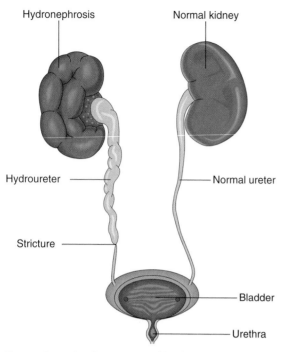

FIGURE 9.4 Hydroureter and hydronephrosis resulting from a urethral stricture.

glomeruli (**glomerul/o** means glomeruli, **nephr** means kidney, and **-itis** means inflammation).

- **Nephroptosis** (**nef**-rop-**TOH**-sis), also known as a **floating kidney**, is the prolapse, or downward displacement, of a kidney (**nephr/o** means kidney and **-ptosis** means dropping down). *Prolapse* means slipping or falling out of place.

- **Nephropyosis** (**nef**-roh-pye-**OH**-sis) is suppuration of the kidney (**nephr/o** means kidney, **py** means

pus, and **-osis** means condition). *Suppuration* means the formation or discharge of pus.

- **Polycystic kidney disease** (**pol**-ee-**SIS**-tick) is an inherited kidney disorder in which the kidneys become enlarged because of multiple cysts (**poly-** means many, **cyst** means cyst, and **-ic** means pertaining to) (Figure 9.5).

- **Pyelitis** (**pye**-eh-**LYE**-tis) is an inflammation of the renal pelvis (**pyel** means renal pelvis and **-itis** means inflammation).

- **Pyelonephritis** (**pye**-eh-loh-neh-**FRY**-tis) is an inflammation of the renal pelvis and of the kidney (**pyel/o** means renal pelvis, **nephr** means kidney, and **-itis** means inflammation).

- **Renal colic** (**REE**-nal **KOLL**-ick) is an acute pain in the kidney area that is caused by blockage during the passage of a kidney stone. *Colic* means spasmodic pains in the abdomen.

Stones

A **stone**, also known as **calculus** (**KAL**-kyou-luhs), is an abnormal mineral deposit (plural, **calculi**). These stones vary in size from small sandlike granules to the size of marbles and are named for the organ or tissue where they are located. Urinary stones are usually formed when waste products in the urine crystallize (Figure 9.6).

- **Nephrolithiasis** (**nef**-roh-lih-**THIGH**-ah-sis) is a disorder characterized by the presence of stones in the kidney (**nephr/o** means kidney and **-lithiasis** means the presence of stones). See Table 9.1.

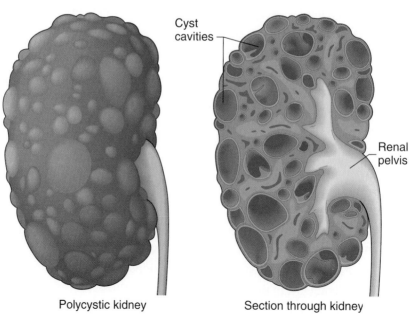

FIGURE 9.5 Polycystic kidney disease.

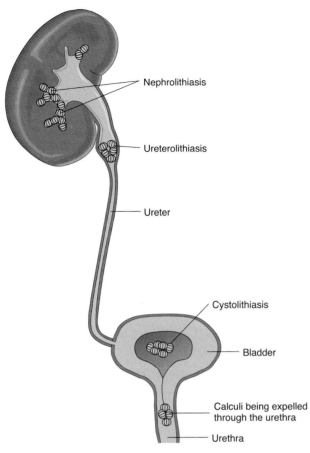

Nephrolithiasis

Ureterolithiasis

Ureter

Cystolithiasis

Bladder

Calculi being expelled
through the urethra

Urethra

FIGURE 9.6 Calculi of the urinary system.

The Ureters

- **Hydroureter** (**high**-droh-you-**REE**-ter) is the distention (stretching out) of the ureter with urine that cannot flow because the ureter is blocked (**hydr/o** means water and **-ureter** means ureter) (Figure 9.4).

- **Ureterectasis** (you-**ree**-ter-**ECK**-tah-sis) is the distention of a ureter (**ureter** means ureter and **-ectasis** means enlargement).

- **Ureterorrhagia** (you-**ree**-ter-oh-**RAY**-jee-ah) is the discharge of blood from the ureter (**ureter/o** means ureter and **-rrhagia** means bleeding).

- **Ureterostenosis** (you-**ree**-ter-oh-steh-**NOH**-sis) is a narrowing of the ureter due to a stricture caused by scar tissue (**ureter/o** means ureter and **-stenosis** means abnormal narrowing). This condition occurs almost exclusively in men. A *stricture* is an abnormal band of tissue narrowing a body passage.

The Urinary Bladder

- **Cystalgia** (sis-**TAL**-jee-ah) and **cystodynia** (**sis**-toh-**DIN**-ee-ah) both mean pain in the urinary bladder (**cyst** means bladder and **-algia** means pain).

- **Cystitis** (sis-**TYE**-tis) is an inflammation of the bladder (**cyst** mean bladder and **-itis** means inflammation).

- **Interstitial cystitis** (**in**-ter-**STISH**-al sis-**TYE**-tis) is a chronic inflammation within the wall of the bladder. The symptoms of this condition are similar to those of cystitis; however, they do not respond to traditional treatment. *Interstitial* means relating to spaces within a tissue or organ.

- A **cystocele** (**SIS**-toh-seel), also called a **fallen bladder**, is a hernia of the bladder through the vaginal wall (**cyst/o** means bladder and **-cele** means hernia).

- **Urinary tract infections (UTIs)** usually begin in the bladder. These infections occur more frequently in women because of the shortness of the urethra and the proximity of its opening to the vagina and rectum.

- A **vesicovaginal fistula** (**ves**-ih-koh-**VAG**-ih-nahl **FIS**-tyou-lah) is an abnormal opening between the bladder and vagina (**vesic/o** means bladder, **vagin** means vagina, and **-al** means pertaining to). A *fistula* is an abnormal passage between two internal organs.

Table 9.1

TYPES AND LOCATIONS OF URINARY STONES

Type of Stone	Word Parts	Location
Cystolith (**SIS**-toh-lith)	cyst/o means bladder and -lith means stone	Urinary bladder
Nephrolith (**NEF**-roh-lith), also known as **renal calculus** or a **kidney stone**	nephr/o means kidney and -lith means stone	Kidney
Ureterolith (you-**REE**-ter-oh-**lith**)	ureter/o means ureter and -lith means stone	Ureter

The Urethra

- **Urethritis** (**you**-reh-**THRIGH**-tis) is an inflammation of the urethra (**urethr** means urethra and **-itis** means inflammation).

- **Urethrorrhagia** (you-**ree**-throh-**RAY**-jee-ah) is bleeding from the urethra (**urethr/o** means urethra and **-rrhagia** means bleeding).

- **Urethrorrhea** (you-**ree**-throh-**REE**-ah) is an abnormal discharge from the urethra (**urethr/o** means urethra and **-rrhea** means flow or discharge).

- **Urethrostenosis** (you-**ree**-throh-steh-**NOH**-sis) is the stricture or narrowing of the urethra (**urethr/o** means urethra and **-stenosis** means tightening or narrowing).

Abnormal Urethral Openings

- **Epispadias** (**ep**-ih-**SPAY**-dee-as) is a congenital abnormality of the urethral opening. In the male with epispadias, the urethral opening is located on the upper surface of the penis. In the female with epispadias, the urethral opening is in the region of the clitoris.

- **Hypospadias** (**high**-poh-**SPAY**-dee-as) is a congenital abnormality of the urethral opening. In the male with hypospadias, the urethral opening is on the under surface of the penis. In the female with hypospadias the urethral opening is into the vagina.

- **Paraspadias** (**par**-ah-**SPAY**-dee-as) is a congenital abnormality in males in which the urethral opening is on the side of the penis.

Urination

- **Diuresis** (**dye**-you-**REE**-sis) is the increased excretion of urine (**diur** means increasing the output of urine and **-esis** means an abnormal condition).

- **Dysuria** (dis-**YOU**-ree-ah) is difficult or painful urination (**dys-** means painful and **-uria** means urination). This condition is frequently associated with UTIs.

- **Enuresis** (**en**-you-**REE**-sis) is the involuntary discharge of urine (**en-** means into and **-uresis** means urination). **Nocturnal enuresis**, which occurs during sleep, is also known as *bed-wetting*. *Nocturnal* means night.

- **Nocturia** (nock-**TOO**-ree-ah) is excessive urination during the night (**noct** means night and **-uria** means urination).

- **Oliguria** (**ol**-ih-**GOO**-ree-ah) means scanty urination (**olig** means scanty and **-uria** means urination). Compare with *polyuria*.

- **Polyuria** (**pol**-ee-**YOU**-ree-ah) means excessive urination (**poly-** means many and **-uria** means urination). Compare with *oliguria*.

- **Urinary hesitancy** is difficulty in starting a urinary stream. This condition is most common in older men with enlarged prostate glands. In younger people the inabililty to urinate when another person is present is known as *shy* or *bashful bladder syndrome*.

- **Urinary retention** is the inability to empty the bladder. This condition is also more common in men, and is frequently associated with an enlarged prostate gland.

Incontinence

Incontinence (in-**KON**-tih-nents) means the inability to control excretory functions.

- **Urinary incontinence** is the inability to control the voiding of urine.

- **Stress incontinence** is the inability to control the voiding of urine under physical stress such as running, sneezing, laughing, or coughing.

- **Overactive bladder**, also known as **urge incontinence**, occurs when the detrusor muscle in the wall of the bladder is too active (Figure 9.3). Symptoms may include urinary frequency, urgency, and accidental urination due to a sudden and unstoppable need to urinate.

DIAGNOSTIC PROCEDURES OF THE URINARY SYSTEM

- **Urinalysis** (**you**-rih-**NAL**-ih-sis) is the examination of urine to determine the presence of abnormal elements (**urin** means urine and **-analysis** means a study of the parts). These tests are discussed further in Chapter 15.

- **Catheterization** (**kath**-eh-ter-eye-**ZAY**-shun) is performed when a sterile specimen is required for diagnostic purposes.

- **Cystoscopy** (sis-**TOS**-koh-pee), also known as **cysto,** is the visual examination of the urinary bladder using a cystoscope (**cyst/o** means bladder and **-scopy** means visual examination). A **cystoscope** (**SIS**-toh-**skope**) is used for this examination and for treatment procedures such as the removal of tumors (Figure 9.7).

- An **intravenous pyelogram** (**in**-trah-**VEE**-nus **PYE**-eh-loh-**gram**) (**IVP**), is a radiographic study of the kidneys and ureters used to diagnose changes in the urinary tract resulting from kidney stones, enlarged prostate, internal injuries after an accident, or tumors (**pyel/o** means renal pelvis and **-gram** means a picture or record). Also known as **excretory urography** (you-**ROG**-rah-fee), an intravenously administered contrast medium is used to define these structures more clearly (Figure 9.8).

- **Computerized tomography (CT scan)** is frequently used instead of IVP as a primary tool for evaluation of the urinary system. A contrast medium is sometimes administered intravenously as part of this test, which uses an x-ray beam to produce cross-sections of the urinary system.

- A **KUB** (kidneys, ureters, bladder) is a radiographic study of these structures without the use of a contrast medium. This study is also referred to as a **flat-plate of the abdomen**.

- **Retrograde urography** is a radiograph of the urinary system taken after dye has been placed in the urethra through a sterile catheter and caused to flow upward (backward) through the urinary tract.

- **Cystography** (sis-**TOG**-rah-fee) is a radiographic examination of the bladder after instillation of a contrast medium via a urethral catheter. The resulting film is called a **cystogram** (**cyst/o** means bladder and **-gram** means a picture or record).

- **Voiding cystourethrography** (**sis**-toh-you-ree-**THROG**-rah-fee) (**VCUG**) is a diagnostic procedure in which a fluoroscope is used to examine the flow of urine from the bladder and through the urethra (**cyst/o** means bladder, **urethr/o** means urethra, and **-graphy** means the process of producing a picture or record). A VCUG is often performed after cystography.

TREATMENT PROCEDURES OF THE URINARY SYSTEM

Medications

- **Diuretics** (**dye**-you-**RET**-icks) are medications administered to increase urine secretion to rid the body of excess sodium and water.

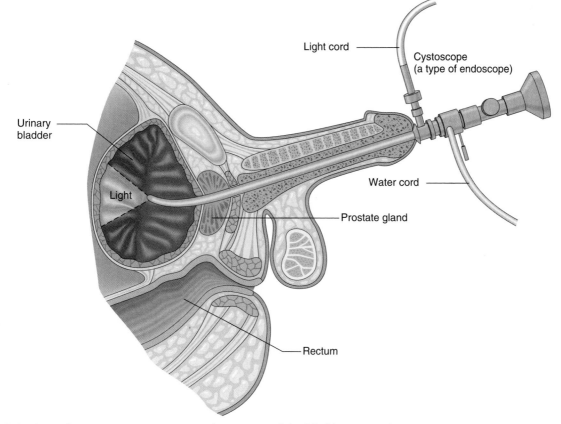

FIGURE 9.7   Use of a cystoscope to examine the interior of the bladder in a male.

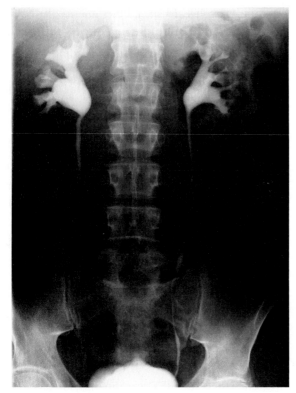

FIGURE 9.8   An IVP showing the internal structures of the kidneys and ureters.

Dialysis

Dialysis (dye-**AL**-ih-sis) is a procedure to remove waste products from the blood of patients whose kidneys no longer function (**dia-** means complete or through and **-lysis** means separation). The two types of dialysis in common use are hemodialysis and peritoneal dialysis.

Hemodialysis

Hemodialysis (**hee**-moh-dye-**AL**-ih-sis) **(HD)** filters waste products directly from the patient's blood (**hem/o** means blood, **dia** means complete or through, and **-lysis** means separation). This treatment takes several hours, and must be repeated about three times a week.

- A shunt implanted in the patient's arm is connected to the artifical kidney machine and arterial blood flows through the filters.
- The filters contain *dialysate*, a solution made up of water and electrolytes, which removes excess fluids and waste from the blood.
- After these are removed, the blood is returned to the body through a vein (Figure 9.9).

Peritoneal Dialysis

In **peritoneal dialysis** (**pehr**-ih-toh-**NEE**-al dye-**AL**-ih-sis), the lining of the peritoneal cavity acts as the filter

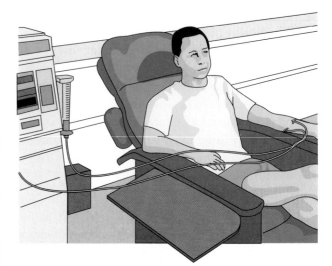

FIGURE 9.9   Hemodialysis filters waste from the patient's blood. A shunt implanted in the patient's arm allows blood to leave the body via an artery, be filtered by the dialysis machine, and returned via a vein.

to remove waste from the blood. Dialysate solution is run into the peritoneal cavity, and the fluid is exchanged through a catheter implanted in the abdominal wall. This type of dialysis is used for renal failure and certain types of poisoning (Figure 9.10).

- **Continuous ambulatory peritoneal dialysis (CAPD)** provides ongoing dialysis as the patient goes about his or her daily activities. In this procedure, a dialysate solution is instilled from a plastic container worn under the patient's clothing. About every four hours, the used solution is drained back into this bag and the bag is discarded. A new bag is then attached, the solution is instilled, and the process continues.
- **Continuous cycling peritoneal dialysis (CCPD)** uses a machine to cycle the dialysate fluid during the night while the patient sleeps.

The Kidneys

- A **renal transplantation**, also known as a **kidney transplant**, is the grafting of a donor kidney into the body to replace the recipient's failed kidneys (Figure 9.11). A single transplanted kidney, from either a living or nonliving donor, is capable of adequately performing all kidney functions.
- **Nephrolysis** (neh-**FROL**-ih-sis) is the freeing of a kidney from adhesions (**nephr/o** means kidney and **-lysis** means setting free). An *adhesion* is a band of fibers that holds structures together abnormally.

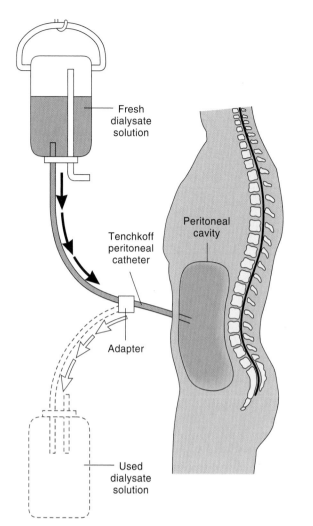

FIGURE 9.10 Peritoneal dialysis removes waste through a fluid exchange in the peritoneal cavity.

- *Note:* The suffix **-lysis** means setting free; however, it also means destruction. Therefore, the term *nephrolysis* can also describe a pathologic condition in which there is the destruction of kidney substance.

- **Nephropexy** (**NEF**-roh-**peck**-see) is the surgical fixation of a floating kidney (**nephr/o** means kidney and **-pexy** means surgical fixation).

- A **nephrostomy** (neh-**FROS**-toh-mee) is the establishment of an opening between the pelvis of the kidney to the exterior of the body (**nephr** means kidney and **-ostomy** means creating an opening). This allows a kidney suffering from hydronephrosis to be drained through the back, bypassing the ureter.

- **Pyeloplasty** (**PYE**-eh-loh-**plas**-tee) is the surgical repair of the renal pelvis (**pyel/o** means the renal pelvis and **-plasty** means surgical repair).

- A **pyelotomy** (pye-eh-**LOT**-oh-mee) is a surgical incision into the renal pelvis (**pyel** means the renal pelvis and **-otomy** means surgical incision).

Removal of Kidney Stones

- **Lithotripsy** (**LITH**-oh-**trip**-see), also known as **extracorporeal shockwave lithotripsy**, is the destruction of a kidney, urinary, or bladder stone with the use of high-energy ultrasonic waves traveling through water or gel (**lith/o** means stone and **-tripsy** means to crush). The fragments of the stone/s are then excreted in the urine. *Extracorporeal* means situated or occurring outside the body.

- A **nephrolithotomy** (**nef**-roh-lih-**THOT**-oh-mee) is the surgical removal of a kidney stone through an incision in the kidney (**nephr/o** means kidney, **lith** means stone, and **-otomy** means surgical incision).

- A **percutaneous nephrolithotomy** (**per**-kyou-**TAY**-nee-us **nef**-roh-lih-**THOT**-oh-mee) is performed by making a small incision in the back and inserting a nephroscope to crush and remove a kidney stone. *Percutaneous* means performed through the skin. A *nephroscope* is a specialized endoscope used in the treatment of the kidneys.

The Ureters

- A **ureterectomy** (**you**-ree-ter-**ECK**-toh-mee) is the surgical removal of a ureter (**ureter** means ureter and **-ectomy** means surgical removal).

- **Ureteroplasty** (you-**REE**-ter-oh-**plas**-tee) is the surgical repair of a ureter (**ureter/o** means ureter and **-plasty** means surgical repair).

- **Ureterorrhaphy** (**you**-ree-ter-**OR**-ah-fee) is the surgical suturing of a ureter (**ureter/o** means ureter and **-rrhaphy** means surgical suturing).

The Urinary Bladder

- A **cystectomy** (sis-**TECK**-toh-mee) is the surgical removal of all or part of the urinary bladder (**cyst** means bladder and **-ectomy** means surgical removal).

- **Cystopexy** (**sis**-toh-**peck**-see) is the surgical fixation of the bladder to the abdominal wall (**cyst/o** means bladder and **-pexy** means surgical fixation).

- **Cystorrhaphy** (sis-**TOR**-ah-fee) means the surgical suturing of the bladder (**cyst/o** means bladder and **-rrhaphy** means surgical suturing).

- A **lithotomy** (lih-**THOT**-oh-mee) is a surgical incision for the removal of a stone from the bladder (**lith** means stone and **-otomy** means surgical incision). This term also is used to describe a physical examination position. (See Chapter 15.)

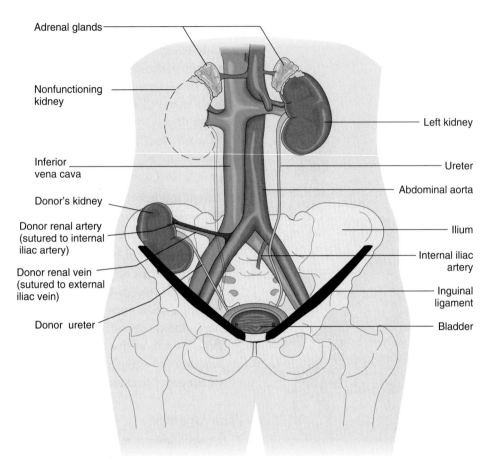

Adrenal glands

Nonfunctioning kidney

Inferior vena cava

Donor's kidney

Donor renal artery (sutured to internal iliac artery)

Donor renal vein (sutured to external iliac vein)

Donor ureter

Left kidney

Ureter

Abdominal aorta

Ilium

Internal iliac artery

Inguinal ligament

Bladder

Figure 9.11 In a kidney transplant, the donor kidney is sutured to the iliac vein and artery at a point lower than the nonfunctioning kidney, which is not removed.

Catheterization

Catheterization is performed to withdraw urine for diagnostic purposes, to control incontinence, or to place fluid, such as a chemotherapy solution, into the bladder (Figure 9.12).

- **Urethral catheterization** is performed by inserting a tube along the urethra and into the bladder.
- An **indwelling catheter** is one that remains inside the body for a prolonged time (Figure 9.12A).
- **Suprapubic catheterization** (**soo**-prah-**PYOU**-bick **kath**-eh-ter-eye-**ZAY**-shun) is the placement of a catheter into the bladder through a small incision made through the abdominal wall just above the pubic bone (Figure 9.12B).

The Urethra

- A **meatotomy** (**mee**-ah-**TOT**-oh-mee) is an incision of the urinary meatus to enlarge the opening (**meat** means meatus and **-otomy** means surgical incision).

- **Urethropexy** (you-**REE**-throh-**peck**-see), which is the surgical fixation of the urethra, is usually performed to correct urinary stress incontinence (**urethr/o** means urethra and **-pexy** means surgical fixation).

- A **urethrostomy** (**you**-reh-**THROS**-toh-mee) is the surgical creation of a permanent opening between the urethra and the skin (**urethr** means urethra and **-ostomy** means creating an opening).

- A **urethrotomy** (**you**-reh-**THROT**-oh-mee) is a surgical incision into the urethra for relief of a stricture (**urethr** means urethra and **-otomy** means surgical incision).

ABBREVIATIONS RELATED TO THE URINARY SYSTEM

Table 9.2 presents an overview of the abbreviations related to the terms introduced in this chapter. *Note:* To avoid errors or confusion, always be cautious when using abbreviations.

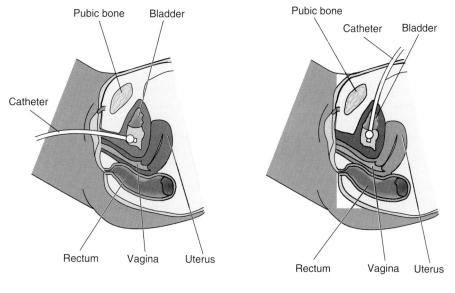

(A) Indwelling catheter   **(B) Suprapubic catheter**

FIGURE 9.12   Types of urinary catheterization. (A) An indwelling catheter. (B) A suprapubic catheter.

Table 9.2

ABBREVIATIONS RELATED TO THE URINARY SYSTEM

acute renal failure = ARF	**ARF** = acute renal failure
catheterization = cath	**cath** = catheterization
continuous ambulatory peritoneal dialysis = CAPD	**CAPD** = continuous ambulatory peritoneal dialysis
chronic renal failure = CRF	**CRF** = chronic renal failure
cystoscopy = cysto	**cysto** = cystoscopy
end-stage renal disease = ESRD	**ESRD** = end-stage renal disease
extracorporeal shock wave lithotripsy = ESWL	**ESWL** = extracorporeal shock wave lithotripsy
glomerulonephritis = GN	**GN** = glomerulonephritis
hemodialysis = HD, hemo	**HD, hemo** = hemodialysis
interstitial cystitis = IC	**IC** = interstitial cystitis
intravenous pyelogram = IVP	**IVP** = intravenous pyelogram
kidneys, ureters, bladder = KUB	**KUB** = kidneys, ureters, bladder
lithotripsy = litho	**litho** = lithotripsy
nephron = Neph	**Neph** = nephron
nephrotic syndrome = NS	**NS** = nephrotic syndrome

(continues)

Table 9.2 (continued)

ABBREVIATIONS RELATED TO THE URINARY SYSTEM

overactive bladder = OAB	**OAB** = overactive bladder
percutaneous nephrolithotomy = PCNL	**PCNL** = percutaneous nephrolithotomy
polycystic kidney disease = PCKD, PKD	**PCKD, PKD** = polycystic kidney disease
renal transplantation = RT	**RT** = renal transplantation
urinalysis = U/A, UA	**U/A, UA** = urinalysis
urinary bladder = UB	**UB** = urinary bladder
urinary tract infection = UTI	**UTI** = urinary tract infection
voiding cystourethrography = VCUG	**VCUG** = voiding cystourethrography
vesicovaginal fistula = VVF	**VVF** = vesicovaginal fistula

Learning Exercises

Matching Word Parts 1

Write the correct answer in the middle column.

Definition	Correct Answer	Possible Answers
9.1. bladder	_____	-cele
9.2. glomerulus	_____	cyst/o
9.3. hernia, tumor, cyst	_____	glomerul/o
9.4. kidney	_____	lith/o
9.5. stone, calculus	_____	nephr/o

Matching Word Parts 2

Write the correct answer in the middle column.

Definition	Correct Answer	Possible Answers
9.6. drooping down	_____	-lysis
9.7. setting free, separation	_____	-pexy
9.8. surgical fixation	_____	pyel/o
9.9. renal pelvis	_____	-ptosis
9.10. to crush	_____	-tripsy

● Matching Word Parts 3

Write the correct answer in the middle column.

Definition	Correct Answer	Possible Answers
9.11. urination, urine	_____	dia-
9.12. ureter	_____	ureter/o
9.13. urethra	_____	-ectasis
9.14. complete, through	_____	-uria
9.15. enlargement, stretching	_____	urethr/o

● Definitions

Select the correct answer and write it on the line provided.

9.16.   Urine is carried from the kidneys to the urinary bladder by the _____ .

glomeruli   nephrons   urethras   ureters

9.17.   A stone in the urinary bladder is known as a _____ .

cholecystolith   cystolith   nephrolith   ureterolith

9.18.   The increased excretion of urine is known as _____ .

anuria   diuresis   dysuria   oliguria

9.19.   Before entering the ureters, urine collects in the _____ .

glomeruli   renal cortex   renal pelvis   urinary bladder

9.20.   The flow of urine from the bladder is controlled by the _____ .

urethral meatus   urinary meatus   urinary sphincters   urinary strictures

9.21.   Urine gets its normal yellow-amber or straw color from the pigment known as _____ .

albumin   bilirubin   hemoglobin   urochrome

9.22.   In the male, the _____ carries both urine and semen.

nephron   renal pelvis   ureter   urethra

9.23.   A specialist who treats the genitourinary system of males is a/an _____ .

gynecologist   nephrologist   neurologist   urologist

9.24. In _____, the urethral opening is on one side of the penis.

     epispadias   hyperspadias   hypospadias   paraspadias

9.25. A/An _____ is a band of fibers that holds structures together abnormally.

     adhesion   distention   stricture   suppuration

● Matching Structures

Write the correct answer in the middle column.

Definition	Correct Answer	Possible Answers
9.26. the portion of a nephron active in filtering urine	_____	glomerulus
9.27. carries urine from a kidney to the urinary bladder	_____	meatus
9.28. external opening of the urethra	_____	renal cortex
9.29. outer layer of the kidney	_____	ureter
9.30. tube from the bladder to the outside of the body	_____	urethra

---

● Which Word?

Select the correct answer and write it on the line provided.

9.31. A surgical incision into the renal pelvis is _____ .

     pyelotomy   pyeloplasty

9.32. The discharge of blood from the ureter is _____ .

     ureterorrhagia   urethrorrhagia

9.33. The term meaning excessive urination is _____ .

     incontinence   polyuria

9.34. The term meaning an inflammation of the bladder is _____ .

     cystitis   pyelitis

9.35.   The major waste product of protein metabolism is _____ .

    urea   urine

● Spelling Counts

Find the misspelled word in each sentence. Then write that word, spelled correctly, on the line provided.

9.36.   Urinoalysis is the examination of the physical and chemical properties of urine to determine the

    presence of abnormal elements. _____

9.37.   Incontinance means being unable to control excretory functions. _____

9.38.   Catherozation is the process used to withdraw urine from the bladder. _____

9.39.   Urinary hesitency is difficulty in starting a urinary stream. _____

9.40.   Glomeronephritis is an inflammation of the kidney involving primarily the glomeruli.

    _____

● Abbreviation Identification

In the space provided, write the words that each abbreviation stands for.

9.41.   **ESWL**   _____

9.42.   **IVP**   _____

9.43.   **HD**   _____

9.44.   **NS**   _____

9.45.   **ESRD**   _____

● Term Selection

Select the correct answer and write it on the line provided.

9.46.   The term meaning the absence of urine formation by the kidneys is _____ .

    anuria   nocturia   oliguria   polyuria

9.47.   The term meaning the surgical suturing of the bladder is _____ .

    cystorrhaphy   cystorrhagia   cystorrhexis   nephrorrhaphy

9.48. The term meaning the freeing of a kidney from adhesions is _____ .

   nephrolithiasis   nephrolysis   nephropyosis   pyelitis

9.49. The term meaning scanty urination is _____ .

    diuresis   dysuria   enuresis   oliguria

9.50. The process of artificially filtering waste products from the patient's blood is known as

    _____ .

    diuresis   hemodialysis   homeostasis   hydroureter

● Sentence Completion

Write the correct term on the line provided.

9.51. An incision of the urinary meatus to enlarge the opening is a/an _____.

9.52. The condition of having a stone lodged in a ureter is known as _____.

9.53. The surgical creation of a permanent opening in the urethra is a/an _____.

9.54. The surgical fixation of the bladder to the abdominal wall is a/an _____.

9.55. Urination is also known as voiding or _____.

● Word Surgery

Divide each term into its component word parts. Write these word parts, in sequence, on the lines provided.

When necessary use a back slash (/) to indicate a combining vowel. (You may not need all of the lines provided.)

9.56. **Hyperproteinuria** is abnormally high concentrations of protein in the urine.

    _____   _____   _____   _____

9.57. **Hydronephrosis** is the dilation of the renal pelvis of one or both kidneys.

    _____   _____   _____   _____

9.58. Voiding **cystourethrography** uses a fluoroscope to examine the flow of urine from the bladder and

    through the urethra.

    _____   _____   _____   _____

9.59. A **nephrolithotomy** is the surgical removal of a kidney stone through an incision in the kidney.

    _____   _____   _____   _____

9.60. **Lithotripsy** is the destruction of a kidney stone with the use of ultrasonic waves traveling through water.

_____   _____   _____   _____

● True/False

If the statement is true, write **T** on the line. If the statement is false, write **F** on the line.

9.61. ____ Urge incontinence is difficulty in starting a urinary stream.

9.62. ____ A vesicovaginal fistula is an abnormal opening between the bladder and vagina.

9.63. ____ Urethrorrhea is bleeding from the urethra.

9.64. ____ A cystolith is a hernia of the urinary bladder.

9.65. ____ Acute renal failure has sudden onset and is characterized by uremia.

● Clinical Conditions

Write the correct answer on the line provided.

9.66. Mrs. Baldridge suffers from excessive urination during the night. The medical term for this is

_____ .

9.67. Rosita LaPinta inherited _____ kidney disease. Now her kidneys are enlarged

because of multiple cysts.

9.68. Doris Volk has a chronic bladder condition involving inflammation within the wall of the bladder. This is

known as _____ _____ .

9.69. John Danielson is being treated for abnormal narrowing of the ureter. This condition is known as

_____ .

9.70. Norman Smith was born with the opening of the urethra on the upper surface of the penis. This is known

as _____ .

9.71. Ralph Clark's kidneys failed. He is being treated with _____

_____ , which involves the removal of waste from his blood through a fluid

exchange in the abdominal cavity.

9.72. Roberta Gridley is scheduled for surgical repair of damage to the ureter. This procedure is a/an

_____ .

9.73. Letty Harding's physician ordered an indwelling _____ catheter. This is placed

into the bladder through a small incision made through the abdominal wall just above the pubic bone.

9.74. Mr. Morita was diagnosed as having an inflammation of the kidney. The medical term for this condition

is _____ .

9.75. Mrs. Franklin has _____ . This condition, which is downward displacement of the

kidney, is also known as a floating kidney.

● Which Is the Correct Medical Term?

Select the correct answer and write it on the line provided.

9.76.   The term that means a hernia of the bladder through the vaginal wall is _____.

        cystocele   cystolithiasis   cystopexy   vesicovaginal fistula

9.77.   The term meaning the inability to control the discharge of urine is _____ .

        incontinence   dysuria   enuresis   urinary retention

9.78.   The term meaning the distention of the ureter is _____ .

        ureteritis   ureterectasis   ureterolith   ureterostenosis

9.79.   The presence of abnormally *low* concentrations of protein in the blood is known as

        _____ .

        hypocalcemia   hyperproteinuria   hyperlipidemia   hypoproteinemia

9.80.   A specialist in diagnosing and treating diseases and disorders of the kidneys is a/an

        _____ .

        internist   nephrologist   proctologist   urologist

● Challenge Word Building

These terms are *not* found in this chapter; however, they are made up of the following familiar word parts. You may want to look in the textbook glossary or use a medical dictionary to check your answers.

cyst/o	-cele
nephr/o	-itis
pyel/o	-lysis
ureter/o	-malacia
urethr/o	-ostomy
	-otomy
	-plasty
	-ptosis
	-rrhexis
	-sclerosis

9.81. The creation of an artificial opening between the urinary bladder and the exterior of the body is a/an

_____ .

9.82. A surgical incision into the kidney is a/an _____ .

9.83. The term meaning abnormal hardening of the kidney is _____ .

9.84. The term meaning prolapse of the bladder into the urethra is _____ .

9.85. A hernia in the urethral wall is a/an _____ .

9.86. The procedure to separate adhesions around a ureter is _____ .

9.87. The term meaning abnormal softening of the kidney is _____ .

9.88. The term meaning an inflammation of the renal pelvis and kidney is _____ .

9.89. The term meaning rupture of the bladder is _____ .

9.90. The term meaning surgical repair of the bladder is _____ .

● **Labeling Exercises**

Identify the numbered items on the accompanying figure.

9.91. _____ gland

9.92. right _____

9.93. inferior _____

_____

9.94. _____

9.95. renal _____

9.96. renal _____

9.97. abdominal _____

9.98. right and left _____

9.99. urinary _____

9.100. urethral _____

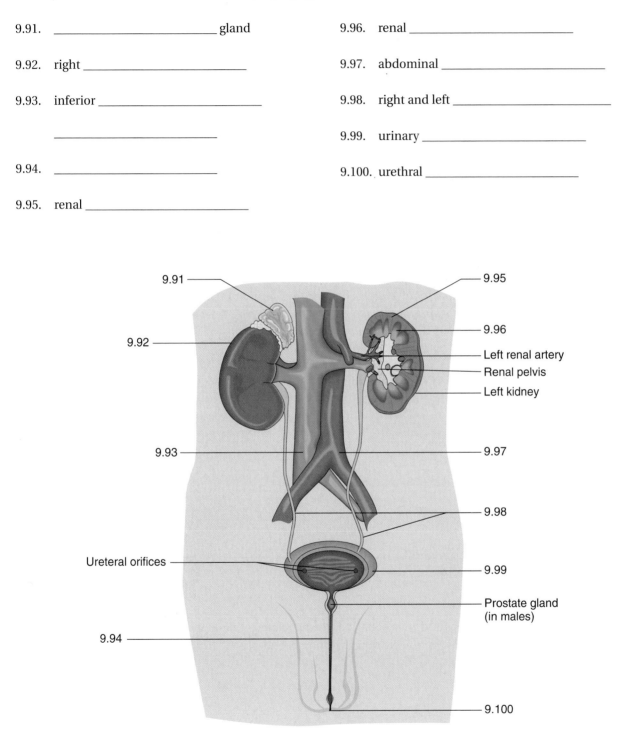

THE HUMAN TOUCH: CRITICAL THINKING EXERCISE

The following story and questions are designed to stimulate critical thinking through class discussion or as a brief essay response. There are no right or wrong answers to these questions.

"Mom, they want me to play for the National Women's Hockey League!" Josie yelled as she ran into the living room. She had just finished practice, and the scouts had told her afterwards how impressed they were with her moves. Finally, her life-long dream of winning an Olympic gold medal for Canada might actually come true! She'd had to make some sacrifices, like living at home after high school, but it looked like that would all pay off. As soon as she saw the looks on the faces of her parents, her smile disappeared.

"Honey, we just got back from the doctor. It turns out that your brother's recurrent bouts of pyelonephritis have led to irreversible renal damage. The nephrologist is recommending that Xavier have a kidney transplant," her mom explained with a pained look. "We know that he has a better chance if he has a related donor, but he could always go on hemodialysis and wait for a cadaver donor..."

Josie saw her dreams of a hockey career fade away. After Xavier's third bout with nephrotic syndrome, her whole family had been tested for compatibility in case he needed a transplant. Josie was the only one eligible, with a negative cross-match. The doctors had explained to her then what it would mean if she decided to donate one of her kidneys, but Josie had brushed it off, assuming that her brother would get better. Now the voices of the doctors came back to her. "No contact sports after a nephrectomy," she heard them say. "There's too big a risk of rupturing the remaining kidney."

Josie was faced with the toughest decision of all: she loved Xavier, but hockey was her life.

Suggested Discussion Topics:

1. Discuss the long-term repercussions of being a living organ donor.
2. There is an ongoing shortage of living and nonliving organ donors. What steps can be taken to remedy this?
3. Imagine that you are Josie's mom or dad and one of your children has the opportunity to save the life of another one of your children. Would you encourage him or her to donate an organ?
4. If Josie decides to donate her kidney and then later chooses to continue playing hockey, should her parents try to talk her out of it?
5. Discuss the pros and cons of having a living related organ donor, a living nonrelated organ donor, and a nonliving organ donor.

The Nervous System

Overview of Structures, Combining Forms, and Functions of the Nervous System

MAJOR STRUCTURES	RELATED COMBINING FORMS	PRIMARY FUNCTIONS
Brain	encephal/o	Coordinates all activities of the body by receiving and transmitting messages throughout the body.
Spinal Cord	myel/o	Transmits nerve impulses between the brain, limbs, and lower part of the body.
Nerves	neur/i, neur/o	Receive and transmit messages to and from all parts of the body.
Sensory Organs and Receptors		Receive external stimulation and transmit these stimuli to the sensory neurons.
• **Eyes (sight)**		See Chapter 11.
• **Ears (hearing)**		See Chapter 11.
• **Nose (smell)**		See Chapter 7.
• **Skin (touch)**		See Chapter 12.
• **Tongue (taste)**		See Chapter 8.

VOCABULARY   RELATED TO THE NERVOUS SYSTEM

The items on this list have been identified as key word parts and terms for this chapter. However, all words in boldface in the text are also important and may be included in learning exercises and tests.

Word Parts

- [ ] ambul/o
- [ ] cephal/o
- [ ] concuss/o
- [ ] contus/o
- [ ] ech/o
- [ ] encephal/o
- [ ] -esthesia
- [ ] klept/o
- [ ] mening/o
- [ ] myel/o
- [ ] narc/o
- [ ] neur/i, neur/o
- [ ] -phobia
- [ ] psych/o
- [ ] somn/o

Medical Terms

- [ ] **acrophobia** (**ack**-roh-**FOH**-bee-ah)
- [ ] **Alzheimer's disease** (**ALTZ**-high-merz)
- [ ] **amnesia** (am-**NEE**-zee-ah)
- [ ] **amobarbital** (**am**-oh-**BAR**-bih-tal)
- [ ] **amyotrophic lateral sclerosis** (ah-**my**-oh-**TROH**-fick)
- [ ] **analgesic** (an-al-**JEE**-zick)
- [ ] **anesthesia** (an-es-**THEE**-zee-ah)
- [ ] **anxiety disorders**
- [ ] **anxiolytic drugs** (ang-zee-oh-**LIT**-ick)
- [ ] **aphasia** (ah-**FAY**-zee-ah)
- [ ] **autistic disorders** (aw-**TISS**-tick)
- [ ] **Bell's palsy**
- [ ] **catatonic behavior** (kat-ah-**TON**-ick)
- [ ] **causalgia** (kaw-**ZAL**-jee-ah)
- [ ] **cerebral contusion** (**SER**-eh-bral *or* seh-**REE**-bral kon-**TOO**-zhun)
- [ ] **cerebral palsy** (**SER**-eh-bral *or* seh-**REE**-bral **PAWL**-zee)
- [ ] **cerebrovascular accident** (**ser**-eh-broh-**VAS**-kyou-lar)
- [ ] **claustrophobia** (**klaws**-troh-**FOH**-bee-ah)
- [ ] **cognition** (kog-**NISH**-un)
- [ ] **comatose** (**KOH**-mah-tohs)

- [ ] **concussion** (kon-**KUSH**-un)
- [ ] **cranial hematoma** (**hee**-mah-**TOH**-mah)
- [ ] **delirium** (dee-**LIR**-ee-um)
- [ ] **delirium tremens** (dee-**LIR**-ee-um **TREE**-mens)
- [ ] **delusion** (dee-**LOO**-zhun)
- [ ] **dementia** (dee-**MEN**-shee-ah)
- [ ] **dyslexia** (dis-**LECK**-see-ah)
- [ ] **dysthymia** (dis-**THIGH**-mee-ah)
- [ ] **echoencephalography** (**eck**-oh-en-**sef**-ah-**LOG**-rah-fee)
- [ ] **electroconvulsive therapy** (ee-**leck**-troh-kon-**VUL**-siv)
- [ ] **electroencephalography** (ee-**leck**-troh-en-**sef**-ah-**LOG**-rah-fee)
- [ ] **encephalitis** (**en**-sef-ah-**LYE**-tis)
- [ ] **epidural anesthesia** (**ep**-ih-**DOO**-ral **an**-es-**THEE**-zee-ah)
- [ ] **factitious disorder** (fack-**TISH**-us)
- [ ] **grand mal epilepsy** (**GRAN MAHL EP**-ih-**lep**-see)
- [ ] **Guillain-Barré syndrome** (gee-**YAHN**-bah-**RAY SIN**-drohm)
- [ ] **hallucination** (hah-**loo**-sih-**NAY**-shun)
- [ ] **hemorrhagic stroke** (**hem**-oh-**RAJ**-ick)
- [ ] **hydrocephalus** (high-droh-**SEF**-ah-lus)
- [ ] **hyperesthesia** (**high**-per-es-**THEE**-zee-ah)
- [ ] **hypochondriasis** (**high**-poh-kon-**DRY**-ah-sis)
- [ ] **lethargy** (**LETH**-ar-jee)
- [ ] **meningitis** (**men**-in-**JIGH**-tis)
- [ ] **meningocele** (meh-**NING**-goh-**seel**)
- [ ] **multiple sclerosis** (skleh-**ROH**-sis)
- [ ] **myelitis** (**my**-eh-**LYE**-tis)
- [ ] **myelography** (**my**-eh-**LOG**-rah-fee)
- [ ] **narcolepsy** (**NAR**-koh-**lep**-see)
- [ ] **paresthesia** (**par**-es-**THEE**-zee-ah)
- [ ] **Parkinson's disease**
- [ ] **peripheral neuropathy** (new-**ROP**-ah-thee)
- [ ] **petit mal epilepsy** (peh-**TEE MAHL EP**-ih-**lep**-see)
- [ ] **posttraumatic stress disorder**
- [ ] **Reye's syndrome**
- [ ] **schizophrenia** (**skit**-soh-**FREE**-nee-ah)
- [ ] **sciatica** (sigh-**AT**-ih-kah)
- [ ] **syncope** (**SIN**-koh-pee)
- [ ] **tetanus** (**TET**-ah-nus)
- [ ] **tic douloureux** (**TICK** doo-loo-**ROO**)
- [ ] **transient ischemic attack** (iss-**KEE**-mick)

FUNCTIONS OF THE NERVOUS SYSTEM

The nervous system, with the brain as its center, coordinates and controls all bodily activities. When the brain ceases functioning, the body dies.

STRUCTURES OF THE NERVOUS SYSTEM

The major structures of the nervous system are the nerves, brain, spinal cord, and sensory organs. The eyes and ears are discussed in Chapter 11.

Divisions of the Nervous System

For descriptive purposes, the nervous system is divided into two primary parts: the central and peripheral nervous systems (Figure 10.1).

- The **central nervous system**, which includes the brain and spinal cord, receives and processes information, and regulates all bodily activity.

- The **peripheral nervous system** includes the 12 pairs of cranial nerves extending from the brain and the 31 pairs of spinal nerves extending from the spinal cord.

The Nerves

A **nerve** is one or more bundles of **neurons** (impulse carrying fibers) that connect the brain and the spinal cord with other parts of the body.

- A **tract** is a bundle or group of nerve fibers located within the brain or spinal cord. **Ascending tracts** carry nerve impulses *toward* the brain. **Descending tracts** carry nerve impulses *away from* the brain.

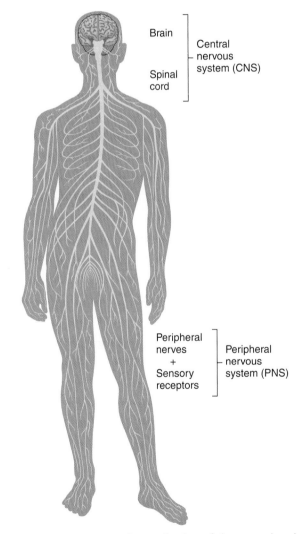

FIGURE 10.1 Structural organization of the central and peripheral nervous systems.

- A **ganglion** (**GANG**-glee-on) is a nerve center made up of a cluster of nerve cell bodies outside the central nervous system (plural, **ganglia** or **ganglions**). *Note:* This term may also mean a benign, tumor-like cyst.

- A **plexus** (**PLECK**-sus) is a network of intersecting nerves (plural, **plexuses**) (Figure 10.10). The term *plexus* also describes a network of intersecting blood or lymphatic vessels.

- **Innervation** (**in**-err-**VAY**-shun) is the supply of nerves to a body part. It also means the stimulation of a body part through the action of nerves.

- **Receptors** are sites in the sensory organs (eyes, ears, skin, nose, and taste buds) that receive external stimulation. The receptors send the stimulus through the sensory neurons to the brain for interpretation.

- A **stimulus** is anything that excites or activates a nerve and causes an impulse (plural, **stimuli**).

- An **impulse** is a wave of excitation transmitted through nerve fibers and neurons.

The Reflexes

A **reflex** (**REE**-flecks) is an automatic, involuntary response to some change, either inside or outside the body. Deep tendon reflexes are discussed in Chapter 4.

- Maintenance of the heart rate, breathing rate, and blood pressure are reflex actions.

- Coughing, sneezing, and reactions to painful stimuli are also reflex actions.

The Neurons

A **neuron** (**NEW**-ron) is the basic cell of the nervous system. The body has billions of neurons carrying neurological impulses throughout the body via an electrochemical process.

- This electrochemical process creates patterns of neuron electrical activity known as **brain waves**. Different types of brain waves are produced during periods of intense activity, rest, and sleep.

- There are three types of neurons and these are described according to their function. The system used for naming the neurons is summarized in Table 10.1. The memory aid **A-C-E** will help you remember their names, and **S-A-M** will help you remember their functions.

Neuron Parts

Each neuron consists of a cell body, several dendrites, a single axon, and terminal end fibers (Figure 10.2). The structures that extend out from the cell body, such as the dendrites and axon, are called **processes**.

- The **dendrites** (**DEN**-drytes) are the root-like processes that receive impulses and conduct them to the cell body.

- The **axon** (**ACK**-son) extends away from the cell body and conducts impulses away from the nerve cell. An axon can be more than three feet long. Many, but not all, axons are protected by a white fatty tissue covering called **myelin** (**MY**-eh-lin).

Table 10.1

TYPES OF NEURONS AND THEIR FUNCTIONS

Types of Neurons	Neuron Functions
"ACE"	"SAM"
Afferent neurons (**AF**-er-ent) *Afferent* means toward.	Also known as **sensory neurons**, they emerge from the skin or sense organs and carry impulses *toward* the brain and spinal cord.
Connecting neurons	Also known as **associative neurons**, they carry impulses from one neuron to another.
Efferent neurons (**EF**-er-ent) *Efferent* means away from.	Also known as **motor neurons**, they carry impulses *away from* the brain and spinal cord and toward the muscles and glands.

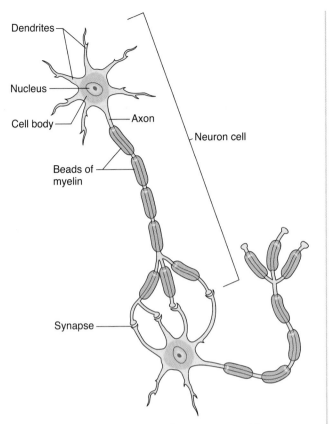

Dendrites

Nucleus

Cell body

Axon

Neuron cell

Beads of myelin

Synapse

FIGURE 10.2 The structures of two neurons. Messages are transmitted from one neuron to the other across the synapses.

- **Terminal end fibers** are the branching fibers at the end of the axon that lead the nervous impulse from the axon to the synapse.

Synapses

A **synapse** (**SIN**-apps) is the space between two neurons or between a neuron and a receptor organ. A neuron can have a few synapses, or several hundred.

Neurotransmitters

A **neurotransmitter** (**new**-roh-trans-**MIT**-er) is a chemical substance that makes it possible for messages to be transmitted by crossing the synapse from a neuron to the target receptor. There are between 200 and 300 known neurotransmitters. Each neurotransmitter is located within a specific group of neurons and has specific functions. Examples are shown in Table 10.2.

Glial Cells

Glial cells, also known as **neuroglia** (new-**ROG**-lee-ah), are the star-shaped supportive and connective cells of the nervous system. The brain contains 10 to 50 more glial cells than neurons. *Glial* means pertaining to glue and glial cells are sometimes referred to as *nerve glue.*

The Myelin Sheath

The term **myelinated** (**MY**-eh-lih-**nayt**-ed) means having a myelin sheath. A **myelin sheath** is the white protective covering that is made up of glial cells and covers some parts of the spinal cord, the white matter of the brain, and most peripheral nerves (Figure 10.3).

Table 10.2

EXAMPLES OF NEUROTRANSMITTERS AND THEIR FUNCTIONS

Acetylcholine (**ass**-eh-til-**KOH**-leen)	Released at some synapses in the spinal cord and at neuromuscular junctions; influences muscle action.
Dopamine (**DOH**-pah-meen)	Released within the brain; thought to be involved in mood and thought disorders and abnormal movement disorders such as Parkinson's disease.
Endorphins (en-**DOR**-fins)	Naturally occurring substances produced by the brain that are released to help relieve pain.
Norepinephrine (nor-ep-ih-**NEF**-rin)	Released at synaptic nerve endings; responds to hypotension and physical stress.
Serotonin (**sehr**-oh-**TOH**-nin *or* **seer**-oh-**TOH**-nin)	Released in the brain; has roles in sleep, hunger, pleasure recognition, and is sometimes linked to mood disorders.

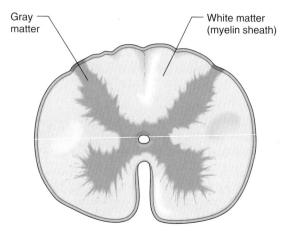

FIGURE 10.3   A cross section of the spinal cord showing the white matter (myelin sheath) that protects the gray matter (nerve tissue).

- **White matter** is the portion of the nerve fibers that *have* a myelin sheath. This covering gives these fibers their white color.

- **Gray matter** is the portion of the nerves that *does not* have a myelin sheath and is gray in color. These fibers make up the *gray matter* of the brain and spinal cord.

THE CENTRAL NERVOUS SYSTEM

The **central nervous system (CNS)** is made up of the brain and spinal cord. These structures are protected externally by the bones of the cranium and spinal column, which is discussed in Chapter 3. Within these bony structures, the brain and spinal cord are further protected by the meninges and cerebrospinal fluid (Figure 10.4).

The Meninges

The **meninges** (meh-**NIN**-jeez) are three layers of connective tissue membrane that enclose the brain and spinal cord. These are the dura mater, arachnoid membrane, and the pia mater (Figure 10.4).

The Dura Mater

The **dura mater** (**DOO**-rah **MAH**-ter *or* **DOO**-rah **MAY**-ter) is the thick, tough, outermost membrane of the meninges. *Dura* means hard and *mater* means mother.

- In the skull, the dura mater lines the inner surfaces of the cranium.

- In the vertebral column, the **epidural space** (**ep**-ih-**DOO**-ral) is located *above* the dura mater and within

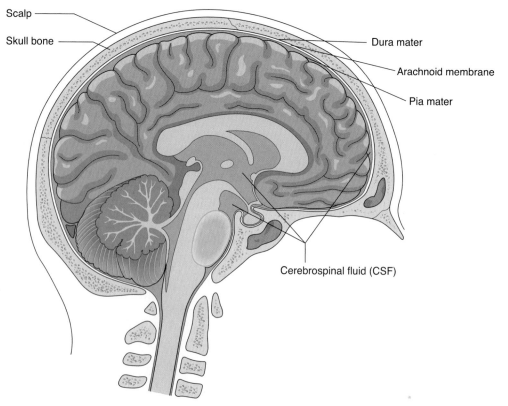

FIGURE 10.4   A cross section of the brain showing the protective coverings. The cerebrospinal fluid is shown in pink.

the surrounding walls of bone (**epi-** means above or upon and **-dural** means pertaining to dura mater). It contains fat and supportive connective tissues to cushion the dura mater.

- The **subdural space** (sub-**DOO**-ral) is located between the dura membrane and the arachnoid membrane (**sub-** means below and **-dural** means pertaining to dura mater).

The Arachnoid Membrane

The **arachnoid membrane** (ah-**RACK**-noid), which resembles a spider web, is the second layer of the meninges surrounding the brain and spinal cord. *Arachnoid* means having to do with spiders.

- The arachnoid membrane is loosely attached to the other meninges to allow space for fluid between the layers.
- The **subarachnoid space**, located below the arachnoid membrane and above the pia mater, contains cerebrospinal fluid.

The Pia Mater

The **pia mater** (**PEE**-ah **MAH**-ter *or* **PYE**-ah **MAY**-ter) the third layer of the meninges, is located nearest to the brain and spinal cord. It consists of delicate connective tissue with a rich supply of blood vessels. *Pia* means tender or delicate and *mater* means mother.

Cerebrospinal Fluid

Cerebrospinal fluid (CSF) (**ser**-eh-broh-**SPY**-nal *or* seh-**ree**-broh-**SPY**-nal), which is produced by special capillaries within the ventricles of the brain, is a clear, colorless, watery fluid that flows throughout the brain and around the spinal cord. The functions of CSF are to:

- Nourish, cool, and cushion these organs from shock or injury.
- Transports nutrients and chemical messengers throughout the brain and spinal cord.

Parts of the Brain

The brain parts are shown in Figures 10.5 and 10.8. The body functions controlled by these brain parts are summarized in Table 10.3. Notice that the functions vital to life support are located in the most protected portion of the brain.

Table 10.3

BRAIN PARTS AND THEIR FUNCTIONS	
Brain Part	**Functions**
Cerebrum—the largest and uppermost part of the brain, consisting of four lobes.	Controls the highest level of thought including judgment, memory, association, and critical thinking. It also processes sensations and controls all voluntary muscle activity.
Thalamus—located below the cerebrum	Relays sensory stimuli from the spinal cord and midbrain to the cerebral cortex, suppressing some and magnifying others.
Hypothalamus—located below the thalamus	Controls vital bodily functions (Table 10.4).
Cerebellum—located in the lower back of the cranium below the cerebrum	Coordinates muscular activity and balance for smooth and steady movements.
Brainstem, consisting of the midbrain, pons, and medulla—located in the base of the brain, forming the connection between the brain and spinal cord	The midbrain and the pons control reflexes for eye and head movements in response to visual and auditory stimuli, link some nerves to the cerebellum, and are involved in motor control and sensory analysis. The medulla, which is the most protected part of the brain, controls the basic vital functions of life, such as heart rate and breathing.

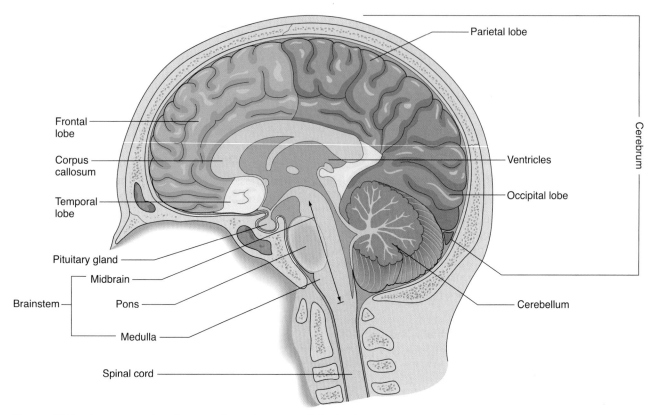

FIGURE **10.5** A cross section showing the major parts of the brain.

The Cerebrum

The **cerebrum** (seh-**REE**-brum) is the largest and uppermost portion of the brain. It is responsible for all thought, judgment, memory, and emotion, as well as for controlling and integrating motor and sensory functions. Note that *cerebrum* and *cerebellum* are similar words, but refer to different parts of the brain. *Memory aid:* The cere*bel*lum is *bel*ow the cerebrum.

- The term **cerebral** (**SER**-eh-bral *or* seh-**REE**-bral) means pertaining to the cerebrum or to the brain.

- The **cerebral cortex**, which is made up of gray matter, is the outer layer of the cerebrum and is arranged in deep folds known as fissures. As used here, a *fissure* is a normally occurring deep groove. Fissures are also crack-like sores in the skin; these are discussed in Chapter 12.

The Cerebral Hemispheres

- The cerebrum is divided into the **left** and **right** **hemispheres**, which are also referred to as the left brain and right brain (Figure 10.6).

- The two cerebral hemispheres are connected at the lower midpoint by the **corpus callosum** (**KOR**-pus kah-**LOH**-sum) (Figure 10.5).

The Lobes of the Cerebrum

Each hemisphere of the cerebrum is divided into four **lobes,** and each lobe is named for the bone of the cranium that covers it (Figure 10.7).

- The **frontal lobe** controls skilled motor functions, memory, and behavior.

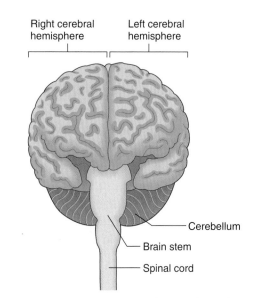

FIGURE **10.6** An anterior view showing how the brain is divided into right and left hemispheres.

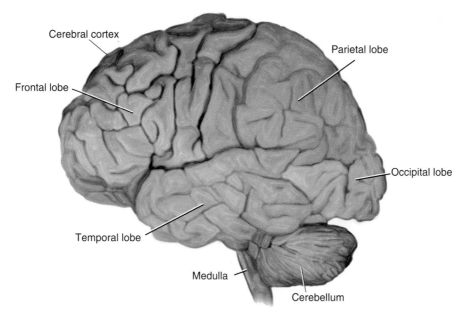

FIGURE 10.7   A left lateral view of the exterior of the brain with the lobes shown in color.

- The **parietal lobe** receives and interprets nerve impulses from sensory receptors in the tongue, skin, and muscles.
- The **occipital lobe** controls eyesight.
- The **temporal lobe** controls the senses of hearing and smell, and the ability to create, store, and access new information.

The Ventricles of the Cerebrum

The four **ventricles** located within the middle region of the cerebrum contain CSF (Figure 10.4). A *ventricle* is a small cavity, such as the ventricles of the brain and of the heart.

The Thalamus

The **thalamus** (**THAL**-ah-mus), which is located below the cerebrum, produces sensations by relaying impulses to and from the cerebrum and the sense organs of the body (Figure 10.8). *Note:* Be careful not confuse the *thalamus* with the *thymus,* which is part of the endocrine system and is discussed in Chapter 13.

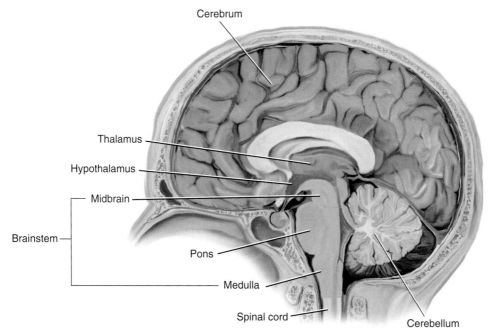

FIGURE 10.8   A schematic representation of the inner structures of the brain.

The Hypothalamus

The **hypothalamus** (**high**-poh-**THAL**-ah-mus), which is located below the thalamus, has seven major regulatory functions. These are summarized in Table 10.4.

The Cerebellum

The **cerebellum** (**ser**-eh-**BELL**-um) is the second-largest part of the brain. It is located at the back of the head below the posterior part of the cerebrum (Figures 10.7 and 10.8).

- The cerebellum receives incoming messages regarding movement within joints, muscle tone, and positions of the body. From here, messages are relayed to the different parts of the brain that control skeletal muscles.
- The general functions of the cerebellum are to produce smooth coordinated movements, to maintain equilibrium, and to sustain normal postures.

The Brainstem

The **brainstem** is the stalk-like portion of the brain that connects the cerebral hemispheres with the spinal cord. It is made up of three parts: the midbrain, pons, and medulla (Figure 10.8).

Table 10.4

REGULATORY FUNCTIONS OF THE HYPOTHALAMUS

1. Regulates and integrates the autonomic nervous system, thereby controlling heart rate, blood pressure, respiratory rate, and digestive tract activity

2. Regulates emotional responses, including fear and pleasure

3. Regulates body temperature

4. Regulates food intake by controlling hunger sensations

5. Regulates water balance and thirst

6. Regulates sleep-wakefulness cycles

7. Regulates the pituitary gland and endocrine system activity

The Midbrain and Pons

The **midbrain** and **pons** (**PONZ**) provide conduction pathways to and from higher and lower centers in the brain.

The Medulla

The **medulla** (meh-**DULL**-ah), also known as the **medulla oblongata** (meh-**DULL**-ah **ob**-long-**GAH**-tah), is located at the lowest part of the brainstem and is connected to the spinal cord. It controls basic life functions including the muscles of respiration, heart rate, and blood pressure, as well as reflexes for coughing, sneezing, swallowing, and vomiting.

The Spinal Cord

The **spinal cord** is the pathway for impulses going to and from the brain (Figure 10.1).

- The spinal cord contains all the nerves that affect the limbs and lower part of the body.
- The spinal cord is protected by CSF and is surrounded by the three meninges.
- The gray matter in the spinal cord, which is not protected by a myelin sheath, is located in the internal section. The myelinated white matter composes the outer portion of the spinal cord (Figure 10.3).

THE PERIPHERAL NERVOUS SYSTEM

The **peripheral nervous system (PNS)** consists of the 12 pairs of cranial nerves (extending from the brain) and the 31 pairs of spinal nerves (extending from the spinal cord). Three types of specialized peripheral nerves transmit signals to and from the central nervous system. See Table 10.5.

The Cranial Nerves

The 12 pairs of **cranial nerves** originate from the undersurface of the brain. Each nerve of a pair serves half of the body, and the two nerves of the pair are identical in function and structure.

- The cranial nerves are identified by Roman numerals and are named for the area or function they serve (Figure 10.9).

The Spinal Nerves

The 31 pairs of peripheral **spinal nerves** are usually grouped together based on the region of the body they innervate (Figure 10.10). The four regions are named

Table 10.5

TYPES OF PERIPHERAL NERVES	
Name	**Function**
Autonomic nerve fibers	Carry instructions to the organs and glands, and form the autonomic nerve system.
Sensory nerve fibers	Relay sensations from the outside world and also from inside the body.
Somatic nerve fibers (also known as **motor nerve fibers**)	Convey information that controls the body's voluntary muscular movements.

for the parts of the spine: the cervical (neck), the thoracic (the part of the back behind the chest), the lumbar (lower back), and sacral (the part connected to the pelvis).

- Within each region, the nerves are numbered. For example, the eight pairs of cervical nerves branching out from the part of the spinal column located in the neck are labeled C1 to C8.

- A spinal nerve sometimes joins with others to form a plexus to innervate a certain area. The lumbar plexus, as shown in Figure 10.10, is made up of the first four lumbar nerves (L1 to L4) and serves the lower back.

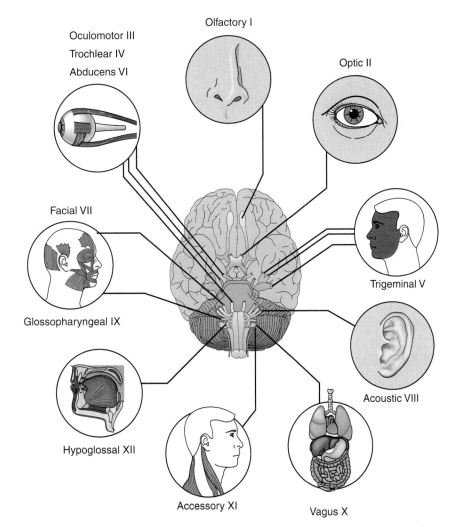

FIGURE 10.9 Cranial nerves are identified with Roman numerals and are named for the area or function they serve.

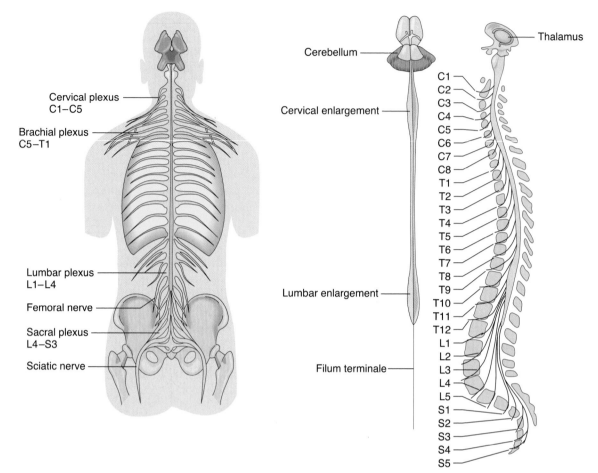

FIGURE 10.10   The spinal cord and nerves. Most spinal nerves are named for the corresponding vertebrae.

THE AUTONOMIC NERVOUS SYSTEM

The **autonomic nervous system** controls the involuntary actions of the body, such as the functioning of internal organs.

- The autonomic nervous system is organized into the **sympathetic** and **parasympathetic nervous systems**.
- One division balances the activity of the other to maintain homeostasis. **Homeostasis** (**hoh**-mee-oh-**STAY**-sis) is the process of maintaining the constant internal environment of the body.

The Sympathetic Nervous System

The **sympathetic nervous system (SNS)** prepares the body for emergencies and stress by increasing the breathing rate, heart rate, and blood flow to muscles.

The Parasympathetic Nervous System

The **parasympathetic nervous system (PNS)** returns the body to normal after a response to stress. It also maintains normal body functions during ordinary circumstances that are not emotionally or physically stressful.

MEDICAL SPECIALTIES RELATED TO THE NERVOUS SYSTEM

- An **anesthesiologist** (**an**-es-**thee**-zee-**OL**-oh-jist) is a physician who specializes in administering anesthetic agents before and during surgery (**an-** means without, **esthesi** means feeling, and **-ologist** means specialist).
- An **anesthetist** (ah-**NES**-theh-tist) is a person trained in administering anesthesia but who is not necessarily a physician, for example, a nurse anesthetist (**an-** means without, **esthet** means feeling, and **-ist** means specialist).
- A **neurologist** (new-**ROL**-oh-jist) specializes in diagnosing and treating diseases and disorders of the nervous system (**neur** means nerve and **-ologist** means specialist).
- A **neurosurgeon** is a physician who specializes in surgery of the nervous system.

- A **psychiatrist** (sigh-**KYE**-ah-trist) holds a Medical Doctor (MD) degree and specializes in diagnosing and treating chemical dependencies, emotional problems, and mental illness (**psych** means mind and **-iatrist** means specialist).

- A **psychologist** (sigh-**KOL**-oh-jist) holds an advanced degree other than a medical degree, and specializes in evaluating and treating emotional problems and mental illness (**psych** means mind and **-ologist** means specialist).

PATHOLOGY OF THE NERVOUS SYSTEM

The Head and Meninges

- **Cephalalgia** (**sef**-ah-**LAL**-jee-ah), also known as a **headache**, is pain in the head (**cephal** means head and **-algia** means pain).

- **Migraine headaches** (**MY**-grayn) are a headache syndrome characterized by sudden, throbbing, sharp pain that is usually more severe on one side of the head. This pain is often accompanied by nausea and sensitivity to light or sound. Compare with *cluster headaches.*

- **Cluster headaches** are characterized by concentrated pain on one side of the head. They are less common than migraines, but more painful, and often occur one or more times daily for weeks or months. Compare with *migraine headaches.*

- An **encephalocele** (en-**SEF**-ah-loh-**seel**), also known as a **craniocele** (**KRAY**-nee-oh-**seel**), is a congenital herniation of brain substance through a gap in the skull (**encephal/o** means brain and **-cele** means hernia). *Congenital* means present at birth and *herniation* means "protrusion." Compare this with a *meningocele.*

- A **meningocele** (meh-**NING**-goh-**seel**) is the congenital herniation of the meninges through a defect in the skull or spinal column (**mening/o** means meninges and **-cele** means hernia). Compare this with an *encephalocele.*

- **Hydrocephalus** (high-droh-**SEF**-ah-lus) is a condition in which there is an abnormally increased amount of CSF within the ventricles of the brain (**hydr/o** means water, **cephal** means head, and **-us** is a singular noun ending).

- **Meningitis** (men-in-**JIGH**-tis) is an inflammation of the meninges of the brain or spinal cord (**mening** means meninges and **-itis** means inflammation).

Meningitis is usually caused by a bacterial or viral infection. Compare with *encephalitis.*

Disorders of the Brain

- **Alzheimer's disease** (**ALTZ**-high-merz) is a group of disorders associated with degenerative changes in the brain structure that lead to symptoms including progressive memory loss, impaired cognition, and personality changes.

- **Cognition** (kog-**NISH**-un) is the mental activities associated with thinking, learning, and memory. *Mild cognitive impairment* is a memory disorder, usually associated with recently acquired information, that may be an early predictor of Alzheimer's disease.

- **Encephalitis** (**en**-sef-ah-**LYE**-tis) is an inflammation of the brain (**encephal** means brain and **-itis** means inflammation). Encephalitis can be caused by a viral infection such as rabies, or occur as a sequel to other diseases such as influenza and measles. Compare with *meningitis.*

- **Reye's syndrome** (RS), which is often fatal, affects all organs of the body but is most harmful to the brain and the liver. This syndrome commonly occurs during recovery from a viral infection with symptoms that include persistent vomiting, listlessness, and disorientation. The cause of RS is unknown; however, it has been linked to giving aspirin to children suffering from viral infections.

- **Parkinson's disease** is a chronic, degenerative CNS disorder in which there is a gradually progressive loss of control over movement resulting from inadequate levels of the chemical dopamine in the brain. The condition is characterized by fine muscle tremors, rigidity, and a slow or shuffling gait. *Gait* means manner of walking.

- **Tetanus** (**TET**-ah-nus), also known as **lockjaw,** is an acute and potentially fatal infection of the CNS caused by a toxin produced by the tetanus bacteria, typically acquired through a deep wound. Tetanus can be prevented through immunization.

Brain Injuries

- **Amnesia** (am-**NEE**-zee-ah) is a memory disturbance marked by a total or partial inability to recall past experiences that can be caused by a brain injury, illness, or psychological disturbance.

- A **concussion** (kon-**KUSH**-un) is a violent shaking up or jarring of the brain (**concuss** means shaken together and **-ion** means condition or state of) (Figure 10.11). A concussion may result in a temporary loss of awareness and function. Compare with *contusion*.

- A **cerebral contusion** (**SEB**-eh-bral *or* she-**REE**-bral kon-**TOO**-zhun), which is the bruising of brain tissue as a result of a head injury, sometimes causes swelling of the brain (**contus** means bruise and **-ion** means condition). Compare with *concussion*.

- A **cranial hematoma** (**hee**-mah-**TOH**-mah *or* **hem**-ah-**TOH**-mah) is a collection of blood trapped in the tissues of the brain (**hemat** means blood and **-oma** means tumor). Named for their location, the types of cranial hematomas include *epidural hematoma* and *subdural hematoma* (Figure 10.12).

Levels of Consciousness

Conscious, also known as **alert**, means being awake, aware, and responding appropriately. **Unconscious** is a state of being unaware, with the inability to respond to normal stimuli.

- **Syncope** (**SIN**-koh-pee), also known as **fainting**, is the brief loss of consciousness caused by the decreased flow of blood to the brain.

- **Lethargy** (**LETH**-ar-jee) is a lowered level of consciousness marked by listlessness, drowsiness, and apathy. As used here, *apathy* means indifference and a reduced level of activity. The term *lethargic* refers to a person who is at this level of consciousness.

- A **stupor** (**STOO**-per) is a state of impaired awareness in which the mind and senses are dulled to environmental stimuli.

- A **coma** (**KOH**-mah) is a profound (deep) state of unconsciousness marked by the absence of spontaneous eye movements, no response to painful stimuli, and no vocalization (speech). The term **comatose** (**KOH**-mah-tohs) refers to a person who is in a coma.

- A **persistent vegetative state** is a type of coma in which the patient exhibits a cyclic state of alternating sleep and wake cycles; however due to severe damage to certain areas of the brain, is unconscious even when appearing to be awake.

Delirium and Dementia

- **Delirium** (dee-**LIR**-ee-um) is a potentially reversible condition that comes on suddenly and is often associated with a high fever, intoxication, or shock. A *delirious* patient is confused, anxious, and unable to think clearly.

- **Dementia** (dee-**MEN**-shee-ah) is a slowly progressive decline in mental abilities including memory, thinking, and judgment, often accompanied by personality changes.

FIGURE 10.11   A concussion is the violent shaking up or jarring of the brain. The red lines in the anterior and posterior areas indicate injury and bleeding.

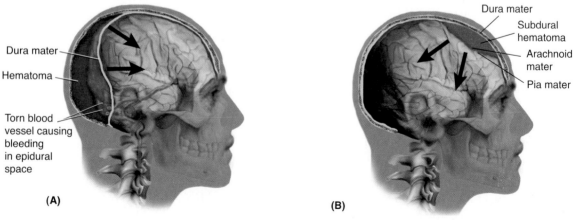

(A)   **(B)**

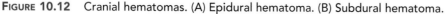

FIGURE 10.12   Cranial hematomas. (A) Epidural hematoma. (B) Subdural hematoma.

- **AIDS dementia complex** is a degenerative neurological condition that is the most common CNS complication of the HIV infection.

Brain Tumors

A **brain tumor** is an abnormal growth within the brain that may be either benign or malignant; however, both types can be life threatening.

- Any abnormal growth in the brain can cause damage in two ways. First, if the tumor is invasive, it destroys brain tissue. Second, because the skull is hard, the tumor can damage the brain tissue by causing pressure on it (Figure 10.13).

- A malignant brain tumor can originate in the brain as the primary site. When cancer metastasizes to the brain from another body system, this tumor is considered to be a secondary site.

- **Intracranial pressure** is the amount of pressure inside the skull (**intra-** means within, **crani** means cranium, and **-al** means pertaining to). Elevated intracranial pressure may be due to a tumor, an injury, or improper drainage of cerebrospinal fluid.

Cerebrovascular Accidents

A **cerebrovascular accident** (**ser**-eh-broh-**VAS**-kyou-lar), also known as a **stroke**, is damage to the brain that occurs when the blood flow to the brain is dis-

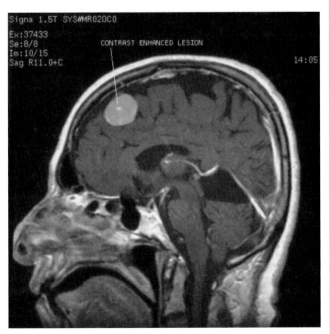

FIGURE 10.13   A brain tumor visualized by magnetic resonance imaging (MRI).

rupted because a blood vessel supplying it is either blocked or has ruptured (Figures 10.14 and 10.15). Note that *stroke* can also mean a sudden severe attack, such as the extreme reaction to heat exposure known as heat stroke.

Ischemic Attacks

Ischemic strokes, which are the most common type of stroke in older people, occur when the flow of blood to the brain is blocked (Figure 10.14A). This may be caused by narrowing of the carotid artery or by a cerebral thrombosis. A *cerebral thrombosis* occurs when a circulating blood clot blocks the artery. This disruption of blood flow usually affects the cerebrum and damages the controls of movement, senses, and speech.

- A **transient ischemic attack** (iss-**KEE**-mick), also known as a **T-I-A,** is the temporary interruption in the blood supply to the brain. *Transient* means passing quickly and *ischemic* means pertaining to the disruption of the blood supply. Symptoms of a TIA include numbness, blurred vision, dizziness, or loss of balance. A TIA passes in less than an hour; however, this incident is often a warning sign that the individual is at risk for a more serious and debilitating stroke.

- **Aphasia** (ah-**FAY**-zee-ah) is the loss of the ability to speak, write, and/or comprehend the written or spoken word (**a-** means without and **-phasia** means speech). Aphasia is often caused by brain damage associated with a stroke.

Hemorrhagic Stroke

A **hemorrhagic stroke** (**hem**-oh-**RAJ**-ick), also known as a **bleed,** occurs when a blood vessel in the brain leaks or ruptures. This type of stroke, which is sometimes due to an aneurysm, is less common than ischemic strokes, but is often fatal. A hemorrhagic stroke affects the area of the brain damaged by the leaking blood (Figures 10.14B and 10.15).

Sleep Disorders

- **Insomnia** is the prolonged or abnormal inability to sleep. This condition is usually a symptom of another problem such as depression, pain, or excessive caffeine (**in-** means without, **somn** means sleep, and **-ia** means abnormal condition).

- **Narcolepsy** (**NAR**-koh-**lep**-see) is a sleep disorder consisting of recurring episodes of falling asleep during the day (**narc/o** means stupor and **-lepsy**

as to cause marked impairment, psychosis, or hospitalization.

- **Dysthymia** (dis-**THIGH**-mee-ah), also known as **dysthymic disorder**, is a chronic depression present at least 50 percent of the time for more than two years (**dys-** means bad, **thym** means mind, and -**ia** means condition).

Anxiety Disorders

Anxiety disorders are characterized by anxiety or fear out of proportion to the real danger in a situation. Without treatment, anxiety disorders may become chronic.

- **Generalized anxiety disorder** is characterized by persistent, intrusive, excessive worry about multiple topics that is difficult to control, causes significant distress or impairment in functioning, and is associated with specific symptoms, such as muscle tension, sleep disturbance, and restlessness.

- An **obsessive-compulsive disorder** is characterized by obsessions and/or compulsions that are recurrent, persistent, and excessive. An *obsession* is a persistent idea, thought, or image that causes the individual anxiety or distress. A *compulsion* is a repetitive mental act or physical behavior that is performed to prevent, or reduce, anxiety or stress. Examples include patients whose obsessions about germs lead to compulsive handwashing or whose obsessions about harm to others lead to compulsive mental counting to certain numbers felt to be protective.

- **Posttraumatic stress disorder** is the development of characteristic symptoms after a traumatic event involving actual or threatened death or injury to the patient or someone else, during which the patient felt intense fear, helplessness, or horror. A shooting, natural disaster, or hostage situation can cause this reaction, with symptoms including numbed responsiveness to stimuli, anxiety, sleep disorders, persistent reliving of the event, and difficulty concentrating.

Panic Disorder

Panic disorder is characterized by having more than one panic attack, resulting in persistent fear of the attacks.

- A *panic attack* is an unanticipated recurrence of a group of symptoms characterized by intense feelings of apprehension, fearfulness, and terror.

Physical symptoms may include shortness of breath, feelings of unreality, sweating, heart palpitations, chest pain, and choking sensations. A panic attack is caused by sympathetic nervous system arousal, which is the body's fight or flight response to danger. Panic attacks can occur in any of the anxiety disorders.

Phobias

A **phobia** (**FOH**-bee-ah) is a persistent irrational fear of a specific thing or situation strong enough to cause significant distress and/or interfere with functioning. This fear causes predictable anxiety when facing the thing or situation, often leading to avoidance. There are countless types of phobias; they are named by adding -**phobia** to the name of the object, for example, a fear of spiders is *arachnophobia* (**arachn/o** means spider and -**phobia** means abnormal fear).

- **Acrophobia** (**ack**-roh-**FOH**-bee-ah) is an excessive fear of being in high places (**acr/o** means top and -**phobia** means abnormal fear).

- **Agoraphobia** (**ag**-oh-rah-**FOH**-bee-ah) is an excessive fear of situations in which having a panic attack seems likely and/or dangerous or embarrassing. An example is a person who fears leaving the familiar setting of home and going out in public because social situations may provoke anxiety (**agor/a** means market place and -**phobia** means abnormal fear).

- **Claustrophobia** (**klaws**-troh-**FOH**-bee-ah) is an abnormal fear of being in narrow or enclosed spaces (**claustr/o** means barrier and -**phobia** means abnormal fear).

- *Social phobia* is persistent, excessive anxiety in or avoidance of social or performance situations due to fear that one's actions will result in embarrassment or humiliation.

Somatoform Disorders

Somatoform disorders (soh-**MAT**-oh-**form**) are characterized by physical complaints or concerns about one's body which are out of proportion to any physical findings or disease. The person is not delusional, is truly distressed, and is not deliberately causing the symptoms. Compare with *factitious disorder*.

- **Somatization disorder** (soh-muh-ti-**ZAY**-shun) is characterized by years of physical complaints of many types (pain, gastrointestinal, sexual, and neurologic) that are not explained by a medical condition. In *undifferentiated somatoform disorder,* there are fewer types of complaints.

- A **conversion disorder** is characterized by a serious temporary or ongoing change in function, such as paralysis or blindness, triggered by psychological factors rather than any physical cause.

- Hypochondriasis (**high**-poh-kon-**DRY**-ah-sis) is characterized by misinterpretation of physical symptoms and fearing that one has a serious illness despite appropriate medical evaluation and reassurance. A person exhibiting this syndrome is called a *hypochondriac.*

Impulse-Control Disorders

The suffix -**mania**, meaning madness, is used in the names of many disorders in which a person repeatedly fails to resist an impulse despite potential negative consequences. For example:

- **Kleptomania** (**klep**-toh-**MAY**-nee-ah) is a disorder characterized by repeatedly stealing objects neither for personal use nor for their monetary value (**klept/o** means to steal and -**mania** means madness).

- **Pyromania** (**pye**-roh-**MAY**-nee-ah) is a disorder characterized by repeated, deliberate fire setting (**pyr/o** means fire and -**mania** means madness).

- **Trichotillomania** (**trick**-oh-**till**-oh-**MAY**-nee-ah) is a disorder characterized by the repeated pulling out of one's hair resulting in noticeable hair loss (**trichotill/o** means related to hair and -**mania** means madness).

Personality Disorders

A **personality disorder** is a chronic pattern of inner experience and behavior that causes serious problems with relationships and work. This pattern is pervasive and inflexible, has an onset in adolescence or early adulthood, is stable over time, and leads to distress or impairment.

- An *antisocial personality disorder* is a pattern of disregard for, and violation of, the rights of others. This pattern brings the individual into continuous conflict with society.

- A *borderline personality disorder* is characterized by impulsive actions, often with the potential for self-harm, as well as mood instability and chaotic relationships.

- A *narcissistic personality disorder* is a pattern of extreme preoccupation with the self and complete lack of empathy for others. *Empathy* is the ability to understand another person's mental and emotional state without becoming personally involved.

Factitious Disorders

A **factitious disorder** (fack-**TISH**-us) is a condition in which a person acts as if he or she has a physical or mental illness when he or she is not really sick. The term *factitious* means artificial, self-induced, or not naturally occurring. Compare with *somatoform disorder.*

- Most **factitious disorders**, previously known as *Munchausen syndrome,* are attempts by the patient to receive attention and sympathy.

- A **factitious disorder by proxy**, previously known as *Munchausen syndrome by proxy,* is a form of child abuse. Although seeming very concerned about the child's well-being, the abusive parent will falsify an illness in a child by making up or creating symptoms and then seeking medical treatment, even surgery, for the child.

- **Malingering** (mah-**LING**-ger-ing) is characterized by the intentional creation of false or grossly exaggerated physical or psychological symptoms, motivated by external incentives, such as avoiding work.

Medications to Treat Mental Disorders

Psychotropic drugs (**sigh**-koh-**TROP**-pick) are capable of affecting the mind, emotions, and behavior and are used in the treatment of mental illness.

- **Anxiolytic drugs** (**ang**-zee-oh-**LIT**-ick), also known as **antianxiety drugs** or **tranquilizers,** are administered to temporarily suppress anxiety (**anxi/o** means anxiety and -**lytic** means to destroy). Most of these medications also relax muscles and can be sedating. Nearly all are habit-forming and should not be suddenly stopped.

- **Stimulants** work by increasing activity in certain areas of the brain, thus increasing concentration and wakefulness. Drug therapies using stimulants have been effective in treating ADD and narcolepsy. The overuse of stimulants, including caffeine, can cause sleeplessness and palpitations.

- **Antipsychotic drugs** (**an**-tih-sigh-**KOT**-ick) are administered to treat symptoms of severe disorders of thinking and mood.

- **Mood stabilizing drugs** such as lithium and valproic acid (an anticonvulsant) are used to treat mood instability and bipolar disorders.

Antidepressant Drugs

Antidepressant drugs are administered to prevent or relieve depression. Some may also be used for obsessive-compulsive disorder, social anxiety disorder, and generalized anxiety disorders.

- **Selective serotonin reuptake inhibitor,** also known as **S-S-R-I,** is thought to work by reducing the re-entry of serotonin into nerve cells, thus allowing serotonin to build up in the nerve synapse.

- **Serotonin and norepinephrine reuptake inhibitor,** also known as **S-N-R-I,** is thought to work by inhibiting the reuptake of serotonin and norepinephrine.

- **Tricyclic antidepressants**, named for their chemical structure, are also used to treat depression.

Psychological Therapies to Treat Mental Disorders

In addition to drug treatments, mental disorders are often treated with individual or group therapy by a qualified psychotherapist.

- **Psychoanalysis** (**sigh**-koh-ah-**NAL**-ih-sis) is based on the idea that mental disorders have underlying causes stemming from childhood and can only be overcome by gaining insight into one's feelings and patterns of behavior.

- **Behavioral therapy** focuses on changing behavior by identifying problem behaviors, replacing them with appropriate behaviors, and using rewards or other consequences to make the changes.

- **Cognitive therapy** focuses on changing cognitions or thoughts that are affecting a person's emotions and actions. These are identified and then are challenged through logic, gathering evidence, and/or testing in action. The goal is to change problematic beliefs. *Cognitive-behavioral therapy* combines the techniques of cognitive and behavioral therapy.

- **Hypnotherapy** is the use of hypnosis to produce a relaxed state of focused attention in which the patient may be more willing to believe and act on suggestions.

ABBREVIATIONS RELATED TO THE NERVOUS SYSTEM

Table 10.6 presents an overview of the abbreviations related to the terms introduced in this chapter. *Note:* To avoid errors or confusion, always be cautious when using abbreviations.

Table 10.6

ABBREVIATIONS RELATED TO THE NERVOUS SYSTEM	
attention deficit disorder = ADD	**ADD** = attention deficit disorder
AIDS dementia complex = ADC	**ADC** = AIDS dementia complex
Alzheimer's disease = AD	**AD** = Alzheimer's disease
amyotrophic lateral sclerosis = AML	**AML** = amyotrophic lateral sclerosis
anesthesia = A	**A** = anesthesia
aphasia = Aph	**Aph** = aphasia
attention deficit disorder = ADD	**ADD** = attention deficit disorder
autonomic nerve system = ANS	**ANS** = autonomic nerve system
Bell's palsy = BP	**BP** = Bell's palsy
central nervous system = CNS	**CNS** = central nervous system
cerebral palsy = CP	**CP** = cerebral palsy
cerebrospinal fluid = CSF	**CSF** = cerebrospinal fluid
cerebrovascular accident = CVA	**CVA** = cerebrovascular accident

Table 10.6 (continued)

ABBREVIATIONS RELATED TO THE NERVOUS SYSTEM

complex regional pain syndrome = CRPS	**CRPS** = complex regional pain syndrome
computerized tomography = CT	**CT** = computerized tomography
delirium tremens = DT, DT's, DTs	**DT, DT's, DTs** = delirium tremens
developmental reading disorder = DRD	**DRD** = developmental reading disorder
electroconvulsive therapy = ECT	**ECT** = electroconvulsive therapy
electroencephalography = EECG	**EECG** = electroencephalography
encephalitis = E	**E** = encephalitis
epidural anesthesia = EDA	**EDA** = epidural anesthesia
epilepsy = epi, epil	**epi, epil** = epilepsy
generalized anxiety disorder = GAD	**GAD** = generalized anxiety disorder
Guillain-Barré syndrome = GBS	**GBS** = Guillain-Barré syndrome
hallucination = halluc	**halluc** = hallucination
intracranial pressure = ICP	**ICP** = intracranial pressure
level of consciousness = LOC	**LOC** = level of consciousness
meningitis = men, mgtis	**men, mgtis** = meningitis
mental retardation = MR	**MR** = mental retardation
multiple sclerosis = MS	**MS** = multiple sclerosis
obsessive-compulsive disorder = OCD	**OCD** = obsessive-compulsive disorder
Parkinson's disease = PD	**PD** = Parkinson's disease
peripheral neuropathy = PN, PNP	**PN, PNP** = peripheral neuropathy
parasympathetic nervous system, peripheral nervous system = PNS	**PNS** = parasympathetic nervous system, peripheral nervous system
persistent vegetative state = PVS	**PVS** = persistent vegetative state
posttraumatic stress disorder = PTSD	**PTSD** = posttraumatic stress disorder
reflex sympathetic dystrophy syndrome = RSDS	**RSDS** = reflex sympathetic dystrophy syndrome
seasonal affective disorder = SAD	**SAD** = seasonal affective disorder
serotonin and norepinephrine reuptake inhibitor = SNRI	**SNRI** = serotonin and norepinephrine reuptake inhibitor
selective serotonin reuptake inhibitor = SSRI	**SSRI** = selective serotonin reuptake inhibitor
tetanus = TE	**TE** = tetanus
transcutaneous electronic nerve stimulation = TENS	**TENS** = transcutaneous electronic nerve stimulation
transient ischemic attack = TIA	**TIA** = transient ischemic attack

Learning Exercises

● Matching Word Parts 1

Write the correct answer in the middle column.

Definition	Correct Answer	Possible Answers
10.1. brain	_____	ambul/o
10.2. bruise	_____	concuss/o
10.3. shaken together	_____	contus/o
10.4. sound	_____	ech/o
10.5. to walk	_____	encephal/o

● Matching Word Parts 2

Write the correct answer in the middle column.

Definition	Correct Answer	Possible Answers
10.6. brain covering	_____	-esthesia
10.7. sensation, feeling	_____	cephal/o
10.8. spinal cord	_____	klept/o
10.9. to steal	_____	mening/o
10.10. head	_____	myel/o

● Matching Word Parts 3

Write the correct answer in the middle column.

Definition	Correct Answer	Possible Answers
10.11. abnormal fear	_____	narc/o
10.12. mind	_____	neur/o
10.13. nerve	_____	-phobia
10.14. sleep	_____	psych/o
10.15. stupor	_____	somn/o

● Definitions

Select the correct answer and write it on the line provided.

10.16. The term that describes the space between two neurons or between a neuron and a receptor is

_____ .

dendrite	ganglion	plexus	synapse

10.17. The protective covering over some nerve cells is the _____ .

myelin sheath	neuroglia	neurotransmitter	pia mater

10.18. The rootlike structures of a nerve that receive impulses and conduct them to the cell body are the

_____ .

axons	dendrites	ganglions	terminal end fibers

10.19. The layer of the meninges that is located nearest the brain and spinal cord is the

_____ .

arachnoid membrane	dura mater	meninx	pia mater

10.20. Seven vital body functions are controlled by the _____ .

cerebral cortex	cerebellum	hypothalamus	thalamus

10.21. The division of the autonomic nervous system that is concerned with body functions under stress is the

_____ nervous system.

cranial	parasympathetic	peripheral	sympathetic

10.22. A network of intersecting nerves is a _____ .

     ganglion   plexus   synapse   tract

10.23. The cranial nerves are part of the _____ nervous system.

     autonomic   central   cranial   peripheral

10.24. Motor functions are controlled by the _____ lobe of the cerebrum.

     frontal   occipital   parietal   temporal

10.25. Impulses are carried away from the brain and spinal cord by the _____ neurons.

     afferent   associative   connecting   efferent

● Matching Structures

Write the correct answer in the middle column.

Definition	Correct Answer	Possible Answers
10.26. connects the brain and spinal cord	_____	cerebellum
10.27. uppermost layer of the brain	_____	cerebrum
10.28. most protected brain part	_____	hypothalamus
10.29. coordinates muscular activity	_____	medulla
10.30. controls vital body functions	_____	brainstem

● Which Word?

Select the correct answer and write it on the line provided.

10.31. A physician who specializes in administering anesthetic agents is an _____ .

     anesthetist   anesthesiologist

10.32. A lowered level of consciousness marked by listlessness and drowsiness is described as

     _____ .

     apathy   stupor

10.33. A disturbance in the memory marked by the inability to recall past experiences is known

     as_____ .

     amnesia   aphasia

10.34. A sense perception that has no basis in external stimulation is a/an _____ .

      delusion   hallucination

10.35. An excessive fear of heights is _____ .

      acrophobia   agoraphobia

● Spelling Counts

Find the misspelled word in each sentence. Then write that word, spelled correctly, on the line provided.

10.36. A miagraine headache is characterized by sudden, severe, sharp headache that is usually present only on one side. _____

10.37. Altzheimer's disease is a group of disorders associated with degenerative changes, including progressive memory loss, impaired thinking, and personality changes. _____

10.38. An anesthethic is the medication administered to block the normal sensation of pain.

_____

10.39. Epalepsy is a group of neurologic disorders characterized by recurrent episodes of convulsive seizure.

_____

10.40. Schiatica is a nerve inflammation that may result in pain through the thigh and leg.

_____

● Abbreviation Identification

In the space provided, write the words that each abbreviation stands for.

10.41. **CP** _____

10.42. **CVA** _____

10.43. **SNRI** _____

10.44. **OCD** _____

10.45. **PTSD** _____

● Term Selection

Select the correct answer and write it on the line provided.

10.46. A patient with a high fever who is confused, disoriented, and unable to think clearly is suffering from

_____ .

      delirium   dementia   lethargy   stupor

10.47. The term meaning inflammation of the spinal cord is _____ . This term also means inflammation of bone marrow.

      encephalitis   myelitis   myelosis   radiculitis

10.48. The medical term meaning an abnormal fear of being in narrow or enclosed spaces is

_____ .

      acrophobia   claustrophobia   kleptomania   pyromania

10.49. Trigeminal neuralgia is also known as _____ .

      Bell's palsy   Guillain-Barré syndrome   Lou Gehrig's disease   tic douloureux

10.50. The medical term for the condition commonly known as a reading disorder is _____ .

      attention deficit disorder   autism   dyslexia   mental retardation

● Sentence Completion

Write the correct term on the line provided.

10.51. The general term used to describe bruising of brain tissue as a result of a head injury is a cerebral

_____ .

10.52. A feeling of apprehension, tension, or uneasiness that stems from the anticipation of danger, the source of which is largely unknown or unrecognized, is a/an _____ state.

10.53. The term used to describe a disorder characterized by a recurrent failure to resist impulses to set fires is

_____ .

10.54. A/An _____ disorder by proxy is a form of child abuse.

10.55. Medication that is administered to prevent or relieve depression is known as a/an

_____ .

● Word Surgery

Divide each term into its component word parts. Write these word parts, in sequence, on the lines provided.

When necessary use a back slash (/) to indicate a combining vowel. (You may not need all of the lines provided.)

10.56. **Anesthesia** is the absence of normal sensation, especially sensitivity to pain.

_____   _____   _____   _____

10.57. **Somnambulism** is commonly known as sleepwalking.

_____   _____   _____   _____

10.58. **Electroencephalography (EEG)** is the process of recording the electrical activity of the brain through the use of electrodes attached to the scalp.

_____   _____   _____

10.59. **Echoencephalography** is the use of ultrasound imaging to diagnose a shift in the midline structures of the brain.

_____   _____   _____   _____

10.60. **Poliomyelitis** is a viral infection of the gray matter of the spinal cord that may result in paralysis.

_____   _____   _____   _____

● True/False

If the statement is true, write **T** on the line. If the statement is false, write **F** on the line.

10.61. _____ In a hemorrhagic stroke, a blood vessel in the brain leaks or ruptures.

10.62 _____ Selective serotonin reuptake inhibitors (SSRI) are a type of medication that is administered as an antidepressant.

10.63. _____ A sedative depresses the CNS and produces sleep.

10.64. _____ A pattern of repeated hand washing is a bipolar disorder.

10.65. _____ Anxiolytic drugs are administered to temporarily suppress anxiety.

● Clinical Conditions

Write the correct answer on the line provided.

10.66. Harvey Ikeman's chart listed him as being _____ . This means that he is in a coma.

10.67. After an auto accident, Anthony DeNicola required _____ to surgically suture the

severed nerve in his hand.

10.68. George Houghton suffered a transient _____ attack (TIA). Sometimes this is a

warning of an impending stroke.

10.69. Ted Duncan has Parkinson's disease. To control the tremors, his doctor performed a/an

_____ . This is a surgical incision into the thalamus.

10.70. Mary Beth Cawthorn was diagnosed as having _____ _____ , which

is also known as MS. This autoimmune disease is characterized by patches of demyelinated nerve fibers.

10.71. Joanne Ladner suffers from recurrent uncontrollable seizures of drowsiness and sleep. Her doctor diag-

nosed this condition as _____ .

10.72. After his stroke, Miguel Valladares was unable to understand written or spoken words. This condition is

called _____ .

10.73. Jill Beck said she fainted. The medical term for this brief loss of consciousness caused by a lack of oxygen

in the brain is _____ .

10.74. The Baily baby was born with _____ . This condition is an abnormally increased

amount of cerebrospinal fluid within the brain.

10.75. After the accident, the MRI indicated that Mrs. Hoshi had a collection of blood trapped in the tissues of

her brain. This condition is called a cranial _____ .

● Which Is the Correct Medical Term?

Select the correct answer and write it on the line provided.

10.76. The term that describes an intense, burning pain after an injury to a sensory nerve is

_____ .

    causalgia   hyperesthesia   hypoesthesia   paresthesia

10.77. Medication that usually produces sleep is known as a/an _____ .

analgesic   barbiturate   hypnotic   sedative

10.78. A/An _____ disorder is a mental condition characterized by a change in function

that suggests a physical disorder but has no physical cause.

anxiety   conversion   panic   posttraumatic stress

10.79. Only the surface of the tissues is affected when a/an _____ anesthetic is administered.

epidural   local   regional   topical

10.80. To control convulsions, _____ may be administered.

amobarbital   analgesics   phenobarbital   sedatives

● Challenge Word Building

These terms are *not* found in this chapter; however, they are made up of the following familiar word parts. You

may want to look in the textbook glossary or use a medical dictionary to check your answers.

poly-   encephal/o   -algia

mening/o   -itis

myel/o   -malacia

neur/o   -oma

-pathy

10.81. The term meaning pain in a nerve or nerves is _____ .

10.82. The term meaning abnormal softening of the meninges is _____ .

10.83. The term used to describe benign neoplasms made up of neurons and nerve fibers is a/an

_____ .

10.84. The term meaning any degenerative disease of the brain is _____ .

10.85. The term meaning an inflammation affecting many nerves is _____ .

10.86. The term meaning abnormal softening of nerve tissue is _____ .

10.87. The term meaning inflammation of the meninges and the brain is _____ .

10.88. The term meaning any pathological condition of the spinal cord is _____ .

10.89. The term meaning abnormal softening of the brain is _____.

10.90. The term meaning inflammation of the meninges, brain, and spinal cord is _____.

● **Labeling Exercises**

Identify the numbered items on the accompanying figures.

10.91. _____ cortex

10.92. _____ lobe

10.93. _____ lobe

10.94. _____ lobe

10.95. _____ lobe

10.96. _____

10.97. _____

10.98. _____

10.99. _____

10.100. _____

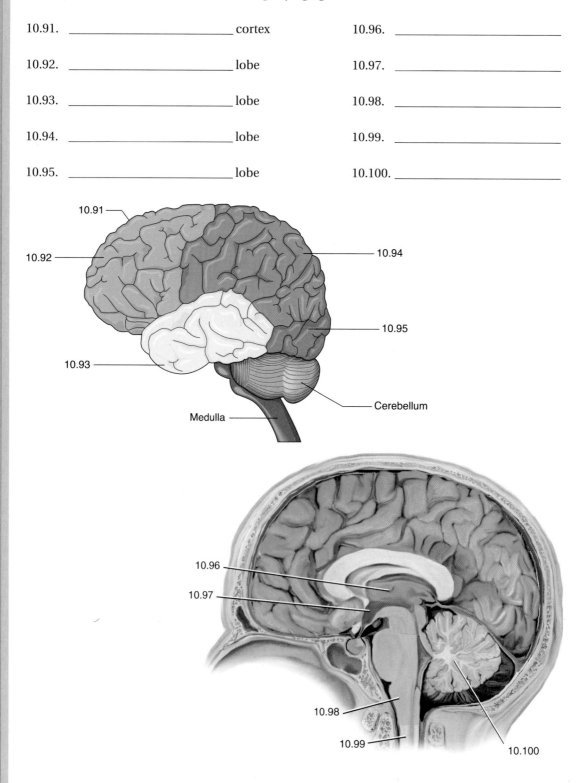

THE HUMAN TOUCH: CRITICAL THINKING EXERCISE

The following story and questions are designed to stimulate critical thinking through class discussion or as a brief essay response. There are no right or wrong answers to these questions.

Calle Washington read the information Dr. Thakker gave her with numb disbelief. "Multiple sclerosis is a neurological disorder characterized by demyelination of nerve fibers in the brain and spinal column. This disease may be progressively debilitating with symptoms that could include numbness, paralysis, ataxia, pain, and blindness. Some patients do experience life-threatening complications. This disease attacks young adults. It affects more women than men."

"Well, I sure fit the profile," thought Calle bitterly. She took a deep breath, trying to quiet the fluttering in her stomach. How could this happen now? Everything was so perfect. Her wedding gown was getting its last alterations, and the tickets for her honeymoon in Jamaica were in the desk drawer. Gabe was putting the final touches on the house where they planned on raising their family. Suddenly, her fairy tale life was turning into a nightmare.

She couldn't expect Gabe to waste his future caring for someone in a wheelchair, could she? And what would happen once her fellow teachers at the day care center noticed that her balance was sometimes off? She couldn't risk hurting one of the children, but if she lost her job she'd lose her health insurance. Dr. Thakker had said there were new drugs for MS, but he'd mentioned that they were very expensive. And what about the children that she and Gabe both wanted? Could she still have a baby and take care of it?

"Maybe I should take out an ad that says 'Twenty-five year old female seeks cure for deadly disease before marrying Prince Charming,'" she thought, trying to laugh through her tears . . .

Suggested Discussion Topics:

1. Discuss whether or not Calle and Gabe should go ahead with the wedding.

2. How might Calle's condition affect her job? Should she be asked to resign?

3. If Calle loses her job at the day care center and tries to find work elsewhere, should she disclose the fact that she has MS?

4. Insurance companies want the people they insure to have a physical and provide information about previous illnesses and diseases. Discuss whether you think this is an ethical practice. If you think it is not ethical, why do you think the insurance companies do it?

5. What federal legislation is designed to help individuals with disabilities? Do you think this law would apply to Calle's situation?

11 Special Senses: The Eyes and Ears

● Overview of Structures, Combining Forms, and Functions of the Eyes and Ears

MAJOR STRUCTURES	RELATED COMBINING FORMS	PRIMARY FUNCTIONS
Eyes (and Vision)	opt/i, opt/o, optic/o, ophthalm/o	Receptor organs for the sense of sight.
Adnexa of the Eye		Accessory structures that provide external protection and movement for the eyes.
Lacrimal Apparatus	dacryocyst/o, lacrim/o	Produces, stores, and removes tears.
Iris	ir/i, ir/o, irid/o, irit/o	Controls the amount of light entering the eye.
Lens	phac/o, phak/o	Focuses rays of light on the retina.
Retina	retin/o	Converts light images into electrical impulses and transmits them to the brain.
Ears (Hearing and Sound)	acous/o, acoust/o, audi/o, audit/o, ot/o	Receptor organs for the sense of hearing; also help to maintain balance.
Outer Ear	pinn/i	Transmits sound waves to the middle ear.
Middle Ear	myring/o, tympan/o	Transmits sound waves to the inner ear.
Inner Ear	labyrinth/o	Receives sound vibrations and transmits them to the brain.

● VOCABULARY RELATED TO THE SPECIAL SENSES

The items on this list have been identified as key word parts and terms for this chapter. However all words in boldface in the text are also important and may be included in learning exercises and tests.

Word Parts

- [ ] blephar/o
- [ ] -cusis
- [ ] irid/o
- [ ] kerat/o
- [ ] myring/o
- [ ] ophthalm/o
- [ ] -opia
- [ ] opt/o
- [ ] ot/o
- [ ] phak/o
- [ ] presby/o
- [ ] retin/o
- [ ] scler/o
- [ ] trop/o
- [ ] tympan/o

Medical Terms

- [ ] **adnexa** (ad-**NECK**-sah)
- [ ] **amblyopia** (**am**-blee-**OH**-pee-ah)
- [ ] **ametropia** (**am**-eh-**TROH**-pee-ah)
- [ ] **anisocoria** (**an**-ih-so-**KOH**-ree-ah)
- [ ] **astigmatism** (ah-**STIG**-mah-tizm)
- [ ] **barotrauma** (**bar**-oh-**TRAW**-mah)
- [ ] **blepharoptosis** (**blef**-ah-roh-**TOH**-sis *or* **blef**-ah-rop-**TOH**-sis)
- [ ] **cataract** (**KAT**-ah-rakt)
- [ ] **chalazion** (kah-**LAY**-zee-on)
- [ ] **conjunctivitis** (kon-**junk**-tih-**VYE**-tis)
- [ ] **convergence** (kon-**VER**-jens)
- [ ] **diplopia** (dih-**PLOH**-pee-ah)
- [ ] **ectropion** (eck-**TROH**-pee-on)
- [ ] **emmetropia** (em-eh-**TROH**-pee-ah)
- [ ] **entropion** (en-**TROH**-pee-on)
- [ ] **esotropia** (**es**-oh-**TROH**-pee-ah)
- [ ] **eustachitis** (**you**-stay-**KYE**-tis)
- [ ] **exotropia** (**eck**-soh-**TROH**-pee-ah)
- [ ] **fenestration** (fen-es-**TRAY**-shun)

- [ ] **fluorescein angiography** (**flew**-oh-**RES**-ee-in an-jee-**OG**-rah-fee)
- [ ] **glaucoma** (glaw-**KOH**-mah)
- [ ] **hemianopia** (**hem**-ee-ah-**NOH**-pee-ah)
- [ ] **hordeolum** (hor-**DEE**-oh-lum)
- [ ] **hyperopia** (**high**-per-**OH**-pee-ah)
- [ ] **iridectomy** (**ir**-ih-**DECK**-toh-mee)
- [ ] **iritis** (eye-**RYE**-tis)
- [ ] **keratitis** (**ker**-ah-**TYE**-tis)
- [ ] **labyrinthectomy** (**lab**-ih-rin-**THECK**-toh-mee)
- [ ] **laser trabeculoplasty** (trah-**BECK**-you-loh-**plas**-tee)
- [ ] **mastoidectomy** (**mas**-toy-**DECK**-toh-mee)
- [ ] **myopia** (my-**OH**-pee-ah)
- [ ] **myringitis** (**mir**-in-**JIGH**-tis)
- [ ] **myringotomy** (**mir**-in-**GOT**-oh-mee)
- [ ] **nyctalopia** (**nick**-tah-**LOH**-pee-ah)
- [ ] **nystagmus** (nis-**TAG**-mus)
- [ ] **ophthalmoscopy** (**ahf**-thal-**MOS**-koh-pee)
- [ ] **optometrist** (op-**TOM**-eh-trist)
- [ ] **otitis media** (oh-**TYE**-tis **MEE**-dee-ah)
- [ ] **otomycosis** (**oh**-toh-my-**KOH**-sis)
- [ ] **otopyorrhea** (**oh**-toh-**pye**-oh-**REE**-ah)
- [ ] **otorrhagia** (**oh**-toh-**RAY**-jee-ah)
- [ ] **otosclerosis** (**oh**-toh-skleh-**ROH**-sis)
- [ ] **papilledema** (**pap**-ill-eh-**DEE**-mah)
- [ ] **phacoemulsification** (**fay**-koh-ee-**mul**-sih-fih-**KAY**-shun *or* **fack**-koh-ee-**mul**-sih-fih-**KAY**-shun)
- [ ] **presbycusis** (**pres**-beh-**KOO**-sis)
- [ ] **presbyopia** (**pres**-bee-**OH**-pee-ah)
- [ ] **pterygium** (teh-**RIJ**-ee-um)
- [ ] **radial keratotomy** (**ker**-ah-**TOT**-oh-mee)
- [ ] **retinopexy** (**RET**-ih-noh-**peck**-see)
- [ ] **scleritis** (skleh-**RYE**-tis)
- [ ] **stapedectomy** (**stay**-peh-**DECK**-toh-mee)
- [ ] **strabismus** (strah-**BIZ**-mus)
- [ ] **tarsorrhaphy** (tahr-**SOR**-ah-fee)
- [ ] **tinnitus** (tih-**NIGH**-tus)
- [ ] **tonometry** (toh-**NOM**-eh-tree)
- [ ] **tympanometry** (**tim**-pah-**NOM**-eh-tree)
- [ ] **tympanostomy tubes** (**tim**-pan-**OSS**-toh-mee)
- [ ] **vertigo** (**VER**-tih-go)
- [ ] **vitrectomy** (vih-**TRECK**-toh-mee)
- [ ] **xerophthalmia** (**zeer**-ahf-**THAL**-mee-ah)

● OBJECTIVES

On completion of this chapter, you should be able to:

1. Describe the functions and structures of the eyes and their accessory structures.

2. Recognize, define, spell, and pronounce terms related to the pathology and the diagnostic and treatment procedures of the eyes and vision.

3. Describe the functions and structures of the ears.

4. Recognize, define, spell, and pronounce terms related to the pathology and the diagnostic and treatment procedures of the ears and hearing.

FUNCTIONS OF THE EYES

The two eyes are the receptor organs of sight; the abbreviations in Table 11.1 are used to describe them. The letter *O* stands for *oculus*, the Latin word for eye. The functions of the eyes are to receive images and transmit them to the brain.

- **Ocular** (**OCK**-you-lar) means pertaining to the eye (**ocul** means eye and **-ar** means pertaining to).

- **Extraocular** (**eck**-strah-**OCK**-you-lar) means outside the eyeball (**extra-** means on the outside, **ocul** means eye, and **-ar** means pertaining to).

- **Intraocular** (**in**-trah-**OCK**-you-lar) means within the eyeball (**intra-** means within, **ocul** means eye, and **-ar** means pertaining to).

- The term **optic** means pertaining to the eye or sight (**opt** means sight and **-ic** means pertaining to).

STRUCTURES OF THE EYES

Adnexa of the Eyes

The **adnexa** (ad-**NECK**-sah) of the eyes, also known as **adnexa oculi**, are the structures outside the eyeball: the orbit, eye muscles, eyelids, eyelashes, conjunctiva, and lacrimal apparatus (Figure 11.1). The term

adnexa, means the appendages or accessory structures of an organ.

The Orbit

The **orbit**, also known as the **eye socket**, is the bony cavity of the skull that contains and protects the eyeball and its associated muscles, blood vessels, and nerves.

The Eye Muscles

Six major muscles are attached to each eye and arranged into three pairs. These muscles make possible a wide range of very precise eye movements (Figure 11.2).

- The muscles of both eyes work together in coordinated movements that enable normal binocular vision. *Binocular* refers to the use of both eyes working together (**bin-** means two, **ocul** means eye, and **-ar** means pertaining to).

The Eyelids

The **upper** and **lower eyelids** of each eye protect the eyeball from foreign matter, excessive light, and impact (Figure 11.1).

- The **canthus** (**KAN**-thus) is the angle where the upper and lower eyelids meet (plural, **canthi**).

- The **inner canthus** is where the eyelids meet *nearest* the nose. The **epicanthus** (**ep**-ih-**KAN**-thus) is a vertical fold of skin on either side of the nose.

- The **outer canthus** is where the eyelids meet *farthest from* the nose.

- The **tarsus** (**TAHR**-suhs), also known as the **tarsal plate**, is the platelike framework within the upper and lower eyelids that provides stiffness and shape (plural, **tarsi**). *Caution: Tarsus* also refers to the seven tarsal bones of the instep.

Table 11.1

ABBREVIATIONS RELATING EYES	
OD	Right eye
OS	Left eye
OU	Each eye (or both eyes)

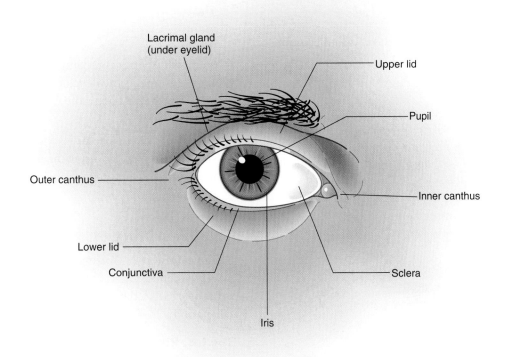

FIGURE 11.1   Major structures and adnexa of the right eye.

The Eyebrows and Eyelashes

The **eyebrows** and **eyelashes** prevent foreign matter from reaching the eyes.

- The edges of the eyelids contain small hairs called **cilia** (**SIL**-ee-ah), also known as **eyelashes**, and oil-producing sebaceous glands.

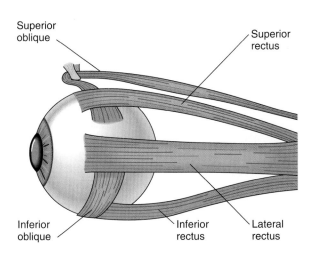

FIGURE 11.2   Six muscles, arranged in three pairs, make major eye movement possible. The medial rectus muscles are not visible here.

The Conjunctiva

The **conjunctiva** (**kon**-junk-**TYE**-vah) is the transparent mucous membrane that lines the underside of each eyelid and continues to form a protective covering over the exposed surface of the eyeball (plural, **conjunctivae**).

The Lacrimal Apparatus

The **lacrimal apparatus** (**LACK**-rih-mal), also known as the **tear apparatus**, consists of the structures that produce, store, and remove tears.

- The **lacrimal glands** are located above the outer corner of each eye. These glands secrete **lacrimal fluid**, which is also known as **tears**. The function of this fluid is to maintain moisture on the anterior surface of the eyeball. Blinking distributes the lacrimal fluid across the eye.

- The **lacrimal canal** (**LACK**-rih-mal) is made up of two ducts at the inner corner of each eye. These ducts collect tears and empty them into the lacrimal sacs. Crying is the overflowing of tears from the lacrimal canals.

- The **lacrimal sac**, also known the **tear sac**, is an enlargement of the upper portion of the lacrimal duct.

- The **lacrimal duct**, also known as the **nasolacrimal duct**, is the passageway that drains excess tears into the nose.
- **Lacrimation** (**lack**-rih-**MAY**-shun) is the secretion of tears, especially in excess.

The Eyeball

The eyeball, also known as the **globe**, is a one-inch sphere with only about one-sixth of its surface showing on the outside. The walls of the eyeball are made up of three layers: the sclera, choroid, and retina (Figure 11.3). The interior of the eye is divided into anterior and posterior segments.

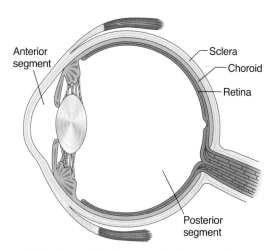

FIGURE 11.3 The walls of the eyeball are made up of the sclera, choroid, and retina.

The Sclera and Cornea

- The **sclera** (**SKLEHR**-ah), also known as the **white of the eye**, is the tough, fibrous tissue that forms the outer layer of the eye, except for the part covered by the cornea. It maintains the shape of the eye and protects the delicate inner layers of tissue. *Caution:* **scler/o** means the white of the eye; it also means hard.
- The **cornea** (**KOR**-nee-ah) is the transparent outer surface of the eye covering the iris and pupil. It is the primary structure focusing light rays entering the eye (Figure 11.4).

The Uveal Tract

The **uveal tract** (**YOU**-vee-ahl), also known as the **uvea** (**YOU**-vee-ah), is the vascular layer of the eye. The iris is in the front, and behind it are the choroid and the ciliary body (Figure 11.4).

The Iris, Pupil, and Lens

- The **iris** is the pigmented (colored) muscular layer that surrounds the pupil. The color of the iris is determined by the amount of melanin that is present. *Melanin* is the pigment that also determines the color of the skin. The skin is discussed in Chapter 12.
- The **pupil** is the black circular opening in the center of the iris that permits light to enter the eye.
- Muscles within the iris control the amount of light that is allowed to enter. To *decrease* the amount of light, these circular muscles contract and make the pupil smaller. To *increase* the amount of light, the muscles dilate (relax) and make the pupil larger.

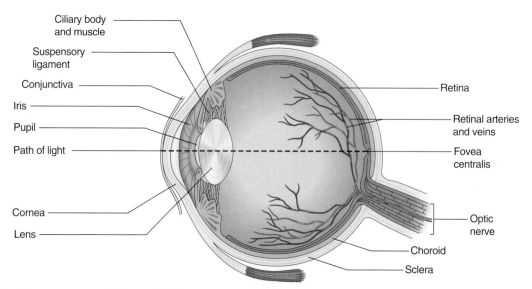

FIGURE 11.4 The structures of the eyeball shown in cross section.

- The **lens**, also known as the **crystalline lens**, is the clear, flexible, curved structure that focuses images on the retina. The lens is contained within a clear capsule located behind the iris and pupil.

The Choroid

The **choroid** (**KOH**-roid), also known as the **choroid coat**, is the opaque middle layer of the eyeball that contains many blood vessels and provides the blood supply for the entire eye. *Opaque* means that light cannot pass through this substance.

The Ciliary Body

The **ciliary body** (**SIL**-ee-ehr-ee), which is located within the choroid, is a set of muscles and suspensory ligaments that adjust the thickness of the lens to refine the focus of light rays on the retina (Figure 11.4).

- To focus on nearby objects, these muscles adjust the lens to make it *thicker.*

- To focus on distant objects, these muscles stretch the lens so it is *thinner.*

The Retina

- The **retina** (**RET**-ih-nah) is the sensitive innermost layer that lines the posterior segment of the eye (Figure 11.3).

- The retina contains specialized light-sensitive cells called **rods** (black and white receptors) and **cones** (color receptors).

- These rods and cones receive images and convert them into nerve impulses, which are sent to the brain via the optic nerve.

The Macula and Fovea Centralis

- The **macula** (**MACK**-you-lah), also known as the **macula lutea**, is a clearly defined yellow area in the center of the retina (**macula** means spot and **lutea** means yellow). This is the area of sharpest central vision (Figure 11.5B).

- The **fovea centralis** (**FOH**-vee-ah sen-**TRAH**-lis) is a pit in the middle of the macula. Color vision is best in this area because it contains a high concentration of cones and no rods (Figure 11.5B).

The Optic Disk and Nerve

- The **optic disk**, also known as the **blind spot**, is a small region in the eye where the nerve endings of the retina enter the optic nerve. It is called the blind spot because it does not contain any rods or cones to convert images into nerve impulses.

- The **second cranial nerve**, also known as the **optic nerve**, transmits the nerve impulses from the retina to the brain. Cranial nerves are discussed in Chapter 10.

Segments of the Eye

The interior of the eye is divided into the anterior and posterior segments. Both segments are filled with fluid that is produced by the ciliary body (Figure 11.5A).

Anterior Segment of the Eye

The front one-third of the eyeball, known as the **anterior segment**, is divided into anterior and posterior chambers.

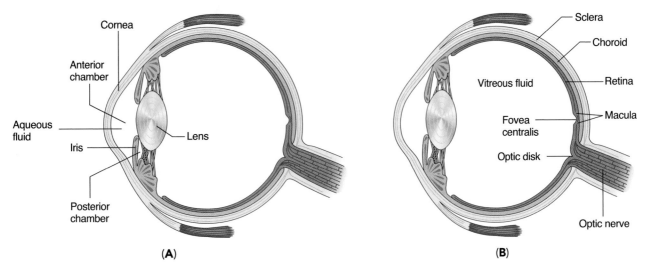

(A)   (B)

FIGURE 11.5 Segments of the eye. (A) The anterior segment of the eye is divided into anterior and posterior chambers. (B) The posterior segment.

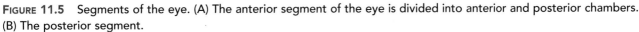

- The **anterior chamber** is located behind the cornea and in front of the iris. The **posterior chamber** is located behind the iris and in front of the ligaments holding the lens in place. *Note:* Don't confuse the posterior chamber with the posterior segment.

- These chambers are filled with **aqueous fluid**, also known as **aqueous humor**. As used here, a *humor* is any clear body liquid or semifluid substance.

- Aqueous fluid helps the eye maintain its shape and nourishes the intraocular structures. This fluid is constantly filtered and drained through the **trabecular meshwork** and the **canal of Schlemm** (Figure 11.6).

- This constant drainage regulates **intraocular pressure (IOP)**. See Diagnostic Procedures of the Eye and Vision, later in this chapter.

Posterior Segment of the Eye

The posterior two-thirds of the eyeball is known as the **posterior segment**. **Vitreous humor** (VIT-ree-us), also known as **vitreous gel**, is the soft, clear, jellylike mass that fills this segment to aid the eye in maintaining its shape. The posterior segment is lined with the retina and its related structures (Figure 11.5).

Normal Action of the Eyes

- **Accommodation** (ah-**kom**-oh-**DAY**-shun) is the process whereby the eyes make adjustments for seeing objects at various distances. These adjustments include constriction (narrowing) and dila-tion (widening) of the pupil, movement of the eyes, and changes in the shape of the lens.

- **Convergence** (kon-**VER**-jens) is the simultaneous inward movement of the eyes toward each other in an effort to maintain single binocular vision as an object comes nearer.

- **Emmetropia** (em-eh-**TROH**-pee-ah) **(EM)** is the normal relationship between the refractive power of the eye and the shape of the eye that enables light rays to focus correctly on the retina (**emmetr** means in proper measure and **-opia** means vision condition). Compare with *hyperopia* and *myopia*.

- **Refraction** is the ability of the lens to bend light rays to help them focus on the retina (Figure 11.11A).

Visual Acuity

Visual acuity is the ability to distinguish object details and shape at a distance. *Acuity* means sharpness.

- A **Snellen chart** is used to measure visual acuity. The results for each eye are recorded as two numbers in fraction form (Figure 11.7).

- The **first number** indicates the distance from the chart, which is always standardized at 20 feet. The **second number** indicates the deviation from the norm based on the ability to read progressively smaller lines of letters on the chart.

- For example, a person with 20/40 vision can read at 20 feet what someone with "normal" vision could read from a distance of 40 feet. Although normal vision has been standardized at 20/20, many people have vision of 20/15 or better.

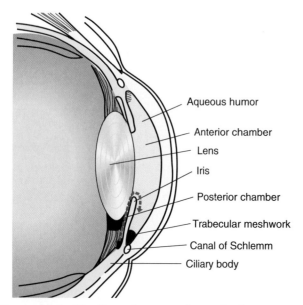

Aqueous humor
Anterior chamber
Lens
Iris
Posterior chamber
Trabecular meshwork
Canal of Schlemm
Ciliary body

Figure 11.6 The flow of aqueous humor in the anterior segment of the eye.

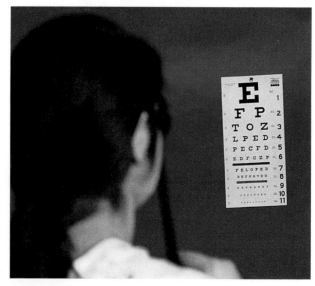

Figure 11.7 A Snellen chart is used to measure visual acuity.

MEDICAL SPECIALTIES RELATED TO THE EYES

- An **ophthalmologist** (ahf-thal-**MOL**-oh-jist) holds an MD degree and specializes in diagnosing and treating diseases and disorders of the eyes and vision (**ophthalm** means eye and **-ologist** means specialist).

- An **optometrist** (op-**TOM**-eh-trist) holds a Doctor of Optometry degree and specializes in measuring the accuracy of vision to determine whether corrective lenses are needed (**opt/o** means vision and **-metrist** means one who measures).

PATHOLOGY OF THE EYES AND VISION

The Eyelids

- **Blepharoptosis** (blef-ah-roh-**TOH**-sis *or* blef-ah-rop-**TOH**-sis) is drooping of the upper eyelid that is usually due to paralysis (**blephar/o** means eyelid and **-ptosis** means drooping or sagging).

- **Ectropion** (eck-**TROH**-pee-on) is the eversion (turning outward) of the edge of an eyelid (**ec-** mean out, **trop** means turn, and **-ion** means condition). This usually affects the lower lid, thereby exposing the inner surface to irritation and preventing tears from draining (Figure 11.8A). Compare with *entropion*.

- **Entropion** (en-**TROH**-pee-on) is the inversion (turning inward) of the edge of an eyelid (**en-** means in, **trop** means turn, and **-ion** means condition). This usually affects the lower lid, thereby

causing the eyelashes to rub against the cornea (Figure 11.8B). Compare with *ectropion*.

- A **hordeolum** (hor-**DEE**-oh-lum), also known as a **stye**, is a pus-filled lesion on the eyelid resulting from an infection in a sebaceous gland.

- A **chalazion** (kah-**LAY**-zee-on), also known as an **internal stye**, is a localized swelling inside the eyelid resulting from obstruction of one of the sebaceous glands.

Additional Adnexa Pathology

- **Conjunctivitis** (kon-**junk**-tih-**VYE**-tis), also known as **pinkeye**, is an inflammation of the conjunctiva, usually caused by an infection or allergy (**conjunctiv** means conjunctiva and **-itis** means inflammation).

- **Subconjunctival hemorrhage** is bleeding between the conjunctiva and the sclera. This common condition, usually caused by an injury, causes a red area over the white of the eye.

- **Xerophthalmia** (**zeer**-ahf-**THAL**-mee-ah), also known as **dry eye**, is drying of eye surfaces, including the conjunctiva, that may be due to disease or to a lack of vitamin A in the diet (**xer** means dry, **ophthalm** means eye, and **-ia** means abnormal condition).

Sclera, Cornea, and Iris

- **Scleritis** (skleh-**RYE**-tis) is an inflammation of the sclera (**scler** means white of eye and **-itis** means inflammation). *Note:* **scler/o** also means hard.

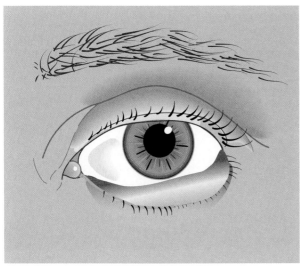

(A)   (B)

FIGURE 11.8   Disorders of the eyelid. (A) Ectropion. (B) Entropion.

- **Keratitis** (ker-ah-**TYE**-tis) is an inflammation of the cornea (**kerat** means cornea and **-itis** means inflammation). *Note:* **kerat/o** also means hard.

- A **corneal abrasion** is an injury, such as a scratch or irritation, to the outer layers of the cornea. Compare with *corneal ulcer*.

- A **corneal ulcer** is a pitting of the cornea caused by an infection or injury. Although these ulcers heal with treatment, they may leave a cloudy scar that impairs vision. Compare with *corneal abrasion*.

- A **pterygium** (teh-**RIJ**-ee-um) is a noncancerous growth that develops on the cornea and can grow large enough to distort vision.

- **Iritis** (eye-**RYE**-tis) is an inflammation of the iris (**ir** means iris and **-itis** means inflammation).

- **Synechia** (sigh-**NECK**-ee-ah) is an adhesion that binds the iris to an adjacent structure such as the lens or cornea (plural, **synechiae**). An *adhesion* holds structures together abnormally.

The Eye

- **Anisocoria** (**an**-ih-so-**KOH**-ree-ah) is a condition in which the pupils are unequal in size (**anis/o** means unequal, **cor** means pupil, and **-ia** means abnormal condition). This may be congenital (present at birth) or caused by a head injury, aneurysm, or pathology of the central nervous system.

- A **cataract** (**KAT**-ah-rakt) is the loss of transparency of the lens. This may be congenital or caused by trauma (injury) or disease; however, the formation of most cataracts is associated with aging (Figure 11.9B).

- **Floaters**, also known as **vitreous floaters**, are particles of cellular debris that float in the vitreous fluid and

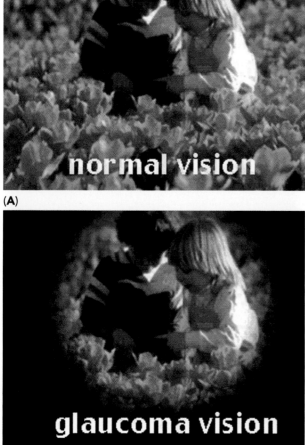

(A)

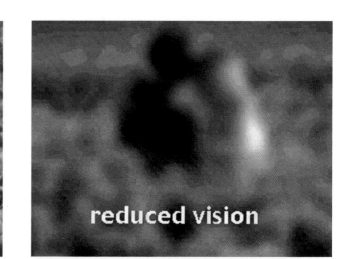

(B)

(C)

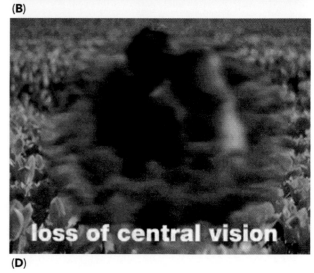

(D)

FIGURE 11.9   Normal vision and pathologic vision changes. (A) Normal vision. (B) Vision reduced by cataracts. (C) The loss of peripheral vision caused by untreated glaucoma. (D) The loss of central vision due to macular degeneration.

cast shadows on the retina. Floaters occur normally with aging or in association with vitreous detachments, retinal tears, or intraocular inflammations.

- **Nystagmus** (nis-**TAG**-mus) is an involuntary, constant, rhythmic movement of the eyeball. It may be congenital, or caused by neurological injury or drug use.

- **Papilledema** (**pap**-ill-eh-**DEE**-mah), also known as **choked disk**, is swelling and inflammation of the optic nerve at the point of entrance into the eye through the optic disk (**pappill** means nipple-like and -**edema** means swelling). This swelling is caused by increased intracranial pressure and may be due to a tumor pressing on the optic nerve.

- In a **detached retina**, also known as a **retinal detachment**, the retina is pulled away from its normal position of being attached to the choroid in the back of the eye. A *retinal tear* occurs when a hole develops in the retina as it is pulled away from its normal position.

- **Uveitis** (**you**-vee-**EYE**-tis) is an inflammation anywhere in the uveal tract (**uve** means uveal tract and -**itis** means inflammation). It may affect the choroid, iris, or ciliary body and has many possible causes, including diseases elsewhere in the body. Uveitis can rapidly damage the eye and produce complications including cataracts, swelling of the retina, and glaucoma.

Glaucoma

Glaucoma (glaw-**KOH**-mah) is a group of diseases characterized by increased intraocular pressure (IOP), resulting in damage to the retinal nerve fibers and the optic nerve. The increase in pressure is caused by a blockage in the flow of fluid out of the eye. If left untreated, this pressure can cause the loss of peripheral vision and eventually blindness (Figure 11.9C).

- *Open-angle glaucoma,* also known as *chronic glaucoma*, is the most common form of this condition. Here the trabecular meshwork gradually becomes blocked and this causes a buildup of pressure. Symptoms of this condition are not noticed by the patient until the optic nerve has been damaged; however, it can be detected earlier through regular eye examinations including tonometry and visual field testing. See Diagnostic Procedures of the Eyes, later in this chapter.

- In *closed-angle glaucoma*, also known as *acute glaucoma*, the opening between the cornea and iris narrows so that fluid cannot reach the trabecular meshwork. This narrowing may cause a sudden increase in the intraocular pressure that produces severe pain, nausea, redness of the eye, and blurred vision. Without immediate treatment, blindness may occur in as little as two days.

Macular Degeneration

Macular degeneration (**MACK**-you-lar) is a gradually progressive condition in which the macula at the center of the retina is damaged, resulting in the loss of central vision but not in total blindness (**macul** means spot and -**ar** mean pertaining to). This condition, also known as **age-related macular degeneration**, most frequently affects older people and is the leading cause of legal blindness in those over 60 (Figure 11.9D).

- *Dry type macular degeneration*, which accounts for 90 percent of cases, is caused by the deterioration of the cells of the macula.

- *Wet type macular degeneration* is caused by the formation of new blood vessels that produce small hemorrhages damaging the macula.

Functional Defects

- **Diplopia** (dih-**PLOH**-pee-ah), also known as **double vision**, is the perception of two images of a single object (**dipl** means double and -**opia** means vision condition). It is sometimes a symptom of a serious underlying disorder such as multiple sclerosis or a brain tumor.

- **Hemianopia** (**hem**-ee-ah-**NOH**-pee-ah) is blindness in one half of the visual field (**hemi-** mean half, **an-** means without, and -**opia** means vision). Sometimes spelled **hemianopsia**.

- **Monochromatism** (**mon**-oh-**KROH**-mah-tizm), also known as **color blindness**, is the inability to distinguish certain colors (**mon/o** means one, **chromat** means color, and -**ism** means condition). This condition, which is usually inherited, is caused by defects in the cones of the retina.

- **Nyctalopia** (**nick**-tah-**LOH**-pee-ah), also known as **night blindness**, is a condition in which an individual with normal daytime vision has difficulty seeing at night (**nyctal** means night and -**opia** means vision condition).

- The term **presbyopia** (**pres**-bee-**OH**-pee-ah) describes the common changes in the eyes that occur with aging (**presby** means old age and -**opia** means vision condition). After about age 40, near vision declines noticeably as the lens becomes less flexible and the muscles of the ciliary body become weaker. The result is that the eyes are no longer able to focus the image properly on the retina.

Strabismus

Strabismus (strah-**BIZ**-mus), also known as **squint**, is a disorder in which the eyes point in different directions or are not aligned correctly because the eye muscles are unable to focus together (Figure 11.10).

- **Esotropia** (**es**-oh-**TROH**-pee-ah), also known as **cross-eyes**, is strabismus characterized by an inward deviation of one eye or both eyes (**eso-** means inward, **trop** means turn, and **-ia** means abnormal condition). Compare with *exotropia*.

- **Exotropia** (**eck**-soh-**TROH**-pee-ah), also known as **walleye**, is strabismus characterized by the outward deviation of one eye relative to the other (**exo-** means outward, **trop** means turn, and **-ia** means abnormal condition). Compare with *esotropia*.

Refractive Disorders

A **refractive disorder** is a focusing problem that occurs when the lens and cornea do not bend light so that it focuses properly on the retina.

- **Ametropia** (**am**-eh-**TROH**-pee-ah) is any error of refraction in which images do not focus properly on the retina (**ametr** means out of proportion and **-opia** means vision condition). Astigmatism, hyperopia, and myopia are all forms of ametropia (Figure 11.11).

- **Astigmatism** (ah-**STIG**-mah-tizm) is a condition in which the eye does not focus properly because of uneven curvatures of the cornea.

- **Hyperopia** (**high**-per-**OH**-pee-ah), also known as **farsightedness**, is a defect in which light rays focus

beyond the retina (**hyper-** means excessive and **-opia** means vision condition). This condition may occur in childhood, but usually causes difficulty after age 40 (Figure 11.11B). Compare with *myopia*.

- **Myopia** (my-**OH**-pee-ah) **(MY)**, also known as **nearsightedness**, is a defect in which light rays focus in front of the retina. This condition occurs most commonly around puberty (Figure 11.11C). Compare with *hyperopia*.

Blindness

Blindness is the inability to see. Although some sight remains, **legal blindness** is the point at which, under law, an individual is considered to be blind. A commonly used standard is that a person is legally blind when his or her best-corrected vision is reduced to 20/200 or less. See Normal Action of the Eyes, earlier in this chapter.

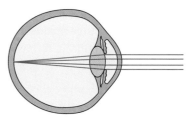

(A) Normal eye
Light rays focus on the retina.

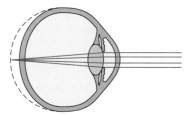

(B) Hyperopia (farsightedness)
Light rays focus beyond the retina.

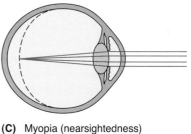

(C) Myopia (nearsightedness)
Light rays focus in front of the retina.

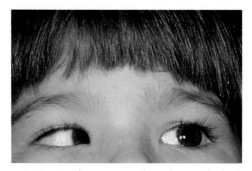

FIGURE 11.10 Strabismus is a disorder in which the eyes cannot be directed in a parallel manner toward the same object.

FIGURE 11.11 Refraction. (A) Normal eye. (B) Hyperopia (farsightedness). (C) Myopia (nearsightedness).

- **Amblyopia** (**am**-blee-**OH**-pee-ah) is a dimness of vision or the partial loss of sight, especially in one eye, without detectable disease of the eye (**ambly** means dim or dull and **-opia** means vision condition).

- **Scotoma** (skoh-**TOH**-mah), also known as **blind spot**, is an abnormal area of absent or depressed vision surrounded by an area of normal vision.

DIAGNOSTIC PROCEDURES OF THE EYES AND VISION

- **Visual acuity measurement** (ah-**KYOU**-ih-tee) is an evaluation of the eye's ability to distinguish object details and shape. See Normal Action of the Eyes.

- **Refraction** is an examination procedure to determine an eye's refractive error and the best corrective lenses to be prescribed.

- A **diopter** (dye-**AHP**-tur) is the unit of measurement of a lens's refractive power.

- **Tonometry** (toh-**NOM**-eh-tree) is the measurement of intraocular pressure (**ton/o** means tension and **-metry** means to measure). Abnormally high pressure may be an indication of glaucoma.

- **Ophthalmoscopy** (ahf-thal-**MOS**-koh-pee), also known as **funduscopy**, is the visual examination of the fundus of the eye with an ophthalmoscope (Figure 15.8). The *fundus* is that portion of a hollow organ that is opposite, or farthest from, it's opening.

- When ophthalmoscopy is performed as part of a routine eye examination, dilation is required. *Dilation* in preparation for an examination of the interior of the eye is the artificial enlargement of the pupil through the use of mydriatic drops.

- **Mydriatic drops** (**mid**-ree-**AT**-ick) are medication placed into the eyes in the form of eye drops that produce temporary paralysis. This paralysis forces the pupils to remain dilated (wide open) even in the presence of bright light.

- **Slit-lamp ophthalmoscopy** (ahf-thal-**MOS**-koh-pee) is a diagnostic procedure in which a narrow beam of light is focused onto parts of the eye to permit the ophthalmologist to examine the structures at the front of the eye, including the cornea, iris, and lens.

Specialized Diagnostic Procedures

- **Fluorescein staining** (**flew**-oh-**RES**-ee-in) is the application of fluorescent dye to the surface of the eye. This dye causes a corneal abrasion to appear bright green.

- **Fluorescein angiography** (**flew**-oh-**RES**-ee-in **an**-jee-**OG**-rah-fee) is a radiographic study of the blood vessels in the retina of the eye following the intravenous injection of a fluorescein dye as a contrast medium. The resulting **angiograms** are used to determine whether there is proper circulation in the retinal vessels.

- **Visual field testing**, also known as **perimetry**, is performed to determine losses in peripheral vision (Figure 11.9). *Peripheral* means occurring away from the center. Blank sections in the visual field may be symptomatic of glaucoma or an optic nerve disorder.

TREATMENT PROCEDURES OF THE EYES AND VISION

The Orbit and Eyelids

- An **orbitotomy** (or-bih-**TOT**-oh-mee) is a surgical incision into the orbit for biopsy, abscess drainage, or the removal of a tumor or foreign object (**orbit** means bony socket and **-otomy** means surgical incision).

- **Tarsorrhaphy** (tahr-**SOR**-ah-fee) is the partial, or complete, suturing together of the upper and lower eyelids (**tars/o** means eyelid and **-rrhaphy** means surgical suturing). This procedure is performed to protect the eye when the lids are paralyzed and unable to close normally.

- Cosmetic procedures relating to the eyelids are discussed in Chapter 12.

The Conjunctiva and Eyeball

- **Conjunctivoplasty** (**kon**-junk-**TYE**-voh-**plas**-tee) is the surgical repair of the conjunctiva (**conjunctiv** means conjunctiva and **-plasty** means surgical repair).

- A **corneal transplant**, also known as **keratoplasty** (**KER**-ah-toh-**plas**-tee), is the surgical replacement of a scarred or diseased cornea with clear corneal tissue from a donor (**kerat/o** means cornea and **-plasty** means surgical repair).

- An **ocular prosthesis** may be fitted to wear over a malformed eye or to replace an eyeball this is either congenitally missing or has been surgically removed. A *prosthesis* is a replacement part.

- An **iridectomy** (**ir**-ih-**DECK**-toh-mee) is the surgical removal of a portion of the tissue of the iris (**irid** means iris and -**ectomy** means surgical removal).

- **Radial keratotomy** (**ker**-ah-**TOT**-oh-mee) is a surgical procedure to correct myopia (**kerat** means cornea and -**otomy** means surgical incision). During the surgery, incisions are made partially through the cornea that cause it to flatten. Compare with *LASIK* later in this chapter.

- **Vitrectomy** (vih-**TRECK**-toh-mee) is the removal of the vitreous fluid and its replacement with a clear solution (**vitr** means vitreous fluid and -**ectomy** means removal). This procedure is sometimes performed to treat a retinal detachment or diabetic retinopathy. Diabetic retinopathy is discussed in Chapter 13.

Cataract Surgery

- **Lensectomy** (len-**SECK**-toh-mee) is the general term used to describe the surgical removal of a cataract-clouded lens (**lens** means lens and -**ectomy** means surgical removal).

- **Phacoemulsification** (**fack**-koh-ee-**mul**-sih-fih-**KAY**-shun) is the use of ultrasonic vibration to shatter and break up a cataract making removal easier.

- **Pseudophakia** (**soo**-doh-**FAY**-kee-ah) is an eye in which the natural lens has been replaced with an intraocular lens (**pseudo/o** means false, **phak** means lens, and -**ia** means abnormal condition). An **intraocular lens** is an artificial lens that is surgically implanted to replace the natural lens (**intra-** means within, **ocul** means eye, and -**ar** means pertaining to) (Figure 11.12).

Corrective Lenses

Refractive errors in the eye can often be corrected with lenses that alter the angle of light rays before they reach the cornea. *Concave lenses* (curved inward) are used for myopia, or nearsightedness, and *convex lenses* (curved outward) for hyperopia, or farsightedness.

- Corrective lenses can combine two or three different refractive powers, one above the other, to allow for better distance vision when looking up and near vision when looking down. *Bifocals* are lenses with two powers. *Trifocals* are lenses with three powers.

- Strabismus is sometimes treated with corrective lenses, or an eye patch, covering the stronger eye and thus strengthening the muscles in the weaker eye.

- *Contact lenses* are refractive lenses that float directly on the tear film in front of the eye. Rigid and gas-permeable lenses cover the central part of the cornea, and disposable soft lenses cover the entire cornea.

Laser Treatments of the Eyes

In the treatment of eye disorders, lasers are used for many reasons. For more details on how lasers work, see Chapter 12.

- **Laser iridotomy** (**ir**-ih-**DOT**-oh-mee) is used to treat acute, or closed-angle, glaucoma by creating an opening in the iris to allow drainage (**irid** means iris and -**otomy** means surgical incision).

- **Laser trabeculoplasty** (trah-**BECK**-you-loh-**plas**-tee) is used to treat chronic, or open-angle, glaucoma by creating an opening in the trabecular meshwork to allow fluid to drain properly.

- **LASIK** is an acronym for **L**aser-**A**ssisted in **Si**tu **K**eratomileusis (**kerat/o** means cornea, -**mileusis** means carving, and *in situ* means in its original place). LASIK is used to treat vision conditions, such as myopia, that are caused by the shape of the cornea. During this procedure, a flap is opened in the surface of the cornea and then a laser is used to change the shape of a deep corneal layer. Compare with *radial keratotomy*.

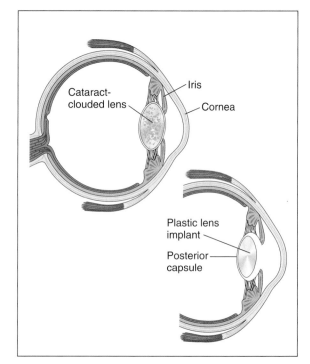

FIGURE 11.12   After the cataract-clouded lens has been removed, it is replaced with an intraocular lens (IOL).

- **Photo-refractive keratectomy** (**ker**-ah-**TECK**-toh-mee) is used to correct refractive errors by shaving away some of the top layer of the cornea.
- **Retinopexy** (**RET**-ih-noh-**peck**-see) is used to reattach the detached area in a retinal detachment.
- **Photocoagulation** is the use of lasers to treat some forms of macular degeneration by sealing leaking or damaged blood vessels.
- Lasers are used to treat retinal tears by sealing the torn portion.
- Lasers are used to remove clouded tissue that may have formed in the posterior portion of the lens capsule after cataract extraction.

FUNCTIONS OF THE EARS

The ears are the receptor organs of hearing; the abbreviations in Table 11.2 are used to describe them. The letter A stands for *auris*, the Latin word for ear.

Table 11.2

ABBREVIATIONS RELATING TO THE EARS	
AD	Right ear
AS	Left ear
AU	Each ear or both ears

The functions of the ears are to receive sound impulses and transmit them to the brain. The inner ear also helps to maintain balance.

- The term **auditory** (**AW**-dih-**tor**-ee) means pertaining to the sense of hearing (**audit** means hearing or sense of hearing and **-ory** means pertaining to).
- **Acoustic** (ah-**KOOS**-tick) means relating to sound or hearing (**acous** means hearing or sound and **-tic** means pertaining to).

STRUCTURES OF THE EARS

The ear is divided into three separate regions: the outer ear, the middle ear, and the inner ear (Figure 11.13).

The Outer Ear

- The **pinna** (**PIN**-nah), also known as the **auricle**, is the external portion of the ear. This structure catches sound waves and transmits them into the external auditory canal.
- The **external auditory canal** transmits sound waves from the pinna to the middle ear.
- **Cerumen** (seh-**ROO**-men), also known as **earwax**, is secreted by ceruminous glands that line the auditory canal. This sticky yellow-brown substance has protective functions as it traps small insects, dust, debris, and certain bacteria to prevent them from entering the middle ear.

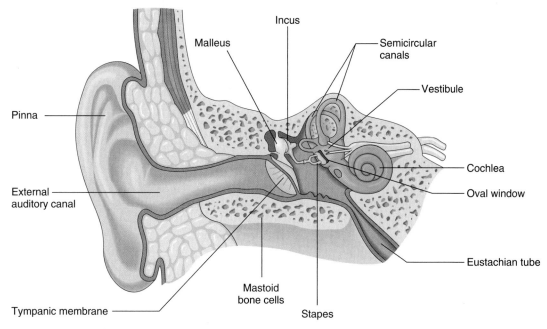

FIGURE 11.13   Structures of the ear shown in cross section.

The Middle Ear

- The **tympanic membrane** (tim-**PAN**-ick), also known as the **eardrum**, is located between the outer and middle ear (Figure 11.14). (**myring/o** and **tympan/o** both mean tympanic membrane.) The eardrum seals the inner end of the ear canal.

- When sound waves reach the eardrum, this membrane transmits the sound by vibrating.

- The middle ear is surrounded by the **mastoid bone cells**, which are hollow air spaces located in the mastoid process of the temporal bone. An infection in the middle ear can rapidly spread to these cells.

The Auditory Ossicles

The **auditory ossicles** (**OSS**-ih-kulz) are three small bones found in the middle ear (Figure 11.13). These bones transmit the sound waves from the eardrum to the inner ear by vibration. These bones, which are named for the Latin terms that describe their shapes, are the

- **Malleus** (**MAL**-ee-us), also known as the **hammer**

- **Incus** (**ING**-kus), also known as the **anvil**

- **Stapes** (**STAY**-peez), also known as the **stirrup**

The Eustachian Tubes

The **eustachian tubes** (you-**STAY**-shun), also known as the **auditory tubes**, are narrow tubes that lead from the middle ear to the nasal cavity and the throat. The

purpose of the tubes is to equalize the air pressure in the middle ear with that of the outside atmosphere.

The Inner Ear

The **inner ear**, also known as the **labyrinth** (**LAB**-ih-rinth), contains the sensory receptors for hearing and balance (Figure 11.13).

- The **oval window**, which is located under the base of the stapes, is the membrane that separates the middle ear from the inner ear. Vibrations enter the inner ear through this passage.

- The **cochlea** (**KOCK**-lee-ah) is the spiral passage that leads from the oval window.

- The **cochlear duct**, located within the cochlea, is filled with fluid that vibrates when the sound waves strike it.

- The **organ of Corti**, also located within the cochlea, is the receptor site that receives these vibrations and relays them to the **auditory nerve fibers**, which transmit them to the auditory center of the brain's cerebral cortex, where they are heard and interpreted.

- The three **semicircular canals**, also located within the inner ear, contain **endolymph** (a liquid) and sensitive hairlike cells. The bending of these hairlike cells in response to the movements of the head sets up impulses in nerve fibers to help maintain equilibrium. *Equilibrium* is the state of balance.

- The **acoustic nerves** (cranial nerve VIII) transmit this information to the brain, and the brain sends messages to muscles in all parts of the body to ensure that equilibrium is maintained.

Normal Action of the Ears

- **Air conduction** is the process by which sound waves enter the ear through the pinna. These waves then travel down the external auditory canal and strike the tympanic membrane between the outer and middle ear.

- **Bone conduction** occurs as the eardrum vibrates and moves the auditory ossicles. These bones then conduct the sound waves through the middle ear to the inner ear.

- **Sensorineural conduction** occurs when sound vibrations reach the inner ear via the oval window. From here the structures of the inner ear receive the sound waves and relay them to auditory nerve for transmission to the brain.

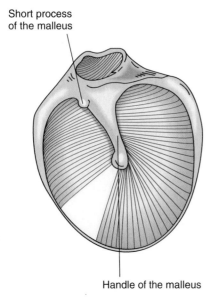

Short process
of the malleus

Handle of the malleus

FIGURE 11.14   Schematic of the normal tympanic membrane as viewed from the auditory canal.

MEDICAL SPECIALTIES RELATED TO THE EARS

- An **audiologist** (**aw**-dee-**OL**-oh-jist) specializes in the measurement of hearing function and in the rehabilitation of persons with hearing impairments (**audi** means hearing and **-ologist** means specialist).

PATHOLOGY OF THE EARS AND HEARING

The Outer Ear

- **Impacted cerumen** is an accumulation of cerumen, or earwax, that forms a solid mass adhering to the walls of the external auditory canal. *Impacted* means lodged or wedged firmly in place.
- **Otalgia** (oh-**TAL**-gee-ah), also known as an **earache**, is pain in the ear (**ot** means ear and **-algia** means pain).
- **Otitis** (oh-**TYE**-tis) means any inflammation of the ear (**ot** means ear and **-itis** means inflammation). The second part of the term (*externa, media,* and *interna*) gives the location of the inflammation.
- *Otitis externa* is an inflammation of the external auditory canal.
- **Otomycosis** (**oh**-toh-my-**KOH**-sis), also known as **swimmer's ear**, is a fungal infection of the external auditory canal (**ot/o** means ear, **myc** means fungus, and **-osis** means abnormal condition).
- **Otopyorrhea** (**oh**-toh-**pye**-oh-**REE**-ah) is the flow of pus from the ear (**ot/o** means ear, **py/o** means pus, and **-rrhea** means flow or discharge).
- **Otorrhagia** (**oh**-toh-**RAY**-jee-ah) is bleeding from the ear (**ot/o** means ear and **-rrhagia** means bleeding).

The Middle Ear

- **Barotrauma** (**bar**-oh-**TRAW**-mah) is pressure-related ear discomfort often caused by changes in pressure when flying, driving in the mountains, or scuba diving, when the eustachian tube is blocked (**bar/o** means pressure and **-trauma** means injury).
- **Eustachitis** (**you**-stay-**KYE**-tis) is inflammation of the eustachian tube (**eustach** means eustachian tube and **-itis** means inflammation).
- **Mastoiditis** (**mas**-toy-**DYE**-tis) is an inflammation of any part of the mastoid process (**mastoid** means mastoid process and **-itis** means inflammation).

- **Myringitis** (**mir**-in-**JIGH**-tis) is an inflammation of the tympanic membrane (**myring** means eardrum and **-itis** means inflammation).
- **Otosclerosis** (**oh**-toh-skleh-**ROH**-sis) is the ankylosis of the bones of the middle ear resulting in a conductive hearing loss (**ot/o** means ear and **-sclerosis** means abnormal hardening). *Ankylosis* means fused together. This condition is treated with a stapedectomy.
- **Patulous eustachian tube** (**PAT**-you-lus) is distention of the eustachian tube. *Patulous* means extended, spread wide open.

Otitis Media

Otitis media (oh-**TYE**-tis **MEE**-dee-ah) is an inflammation of the middle ear.

- **Acute otitis media** (oh-**TYE**-tis **MEE**-dee-ah) is usually associated with an upper respiratory infection and is most commonly seen in young children. This condition can lead to a *ruptured eardrum* due to the buildup of pus or fluid in the middle ear.
- **Serous otitis media** (**SEER**-us oh-**TYE**-tis **MEE**-dee-ah) is a fluid buildup in the middle ear that may follow acute otitis media or may be caused by obstruction of the eustachian tube (Figure 11.15A).
- **Acute purulent otitis media** is a buildup of pus within the middle ear (Figure 11.15B). *Purulent* means producing or containing pus.

The Inner Ear

- **Labyrinthitis** (**lab**-ih-rin-**THIGH**-tis) is an inflammation of the labyrinth that can result in vertigo and deafness (**labyrinth** means labyrinth and **-itis** means inflammation).
- **Vertigo** (**VER**-tih-goh) is a sense of whirling, dizziness, and the loss of balance, often combined with nausea and vomiting. Although it is a symptom of many disorders, recurrent vertigo is sometimes associated with inner ear problems such as Ménière's syndrome.
- **Ménière's syndrome** is a rare chronic disease in which the amount of fluid in the inner ear increases intermittently, producing attacks of vertigo, a fluctuating hearing loss (usually in one ear), and tinnitus.
- **Tinnitus** (tih-**NIGH**-tus) is a ringing, buzzing, or roaring sound in one or both ears. It is often associated with hearing loss, and is more likely to occur when there has been prolonged exposure to loud noises.

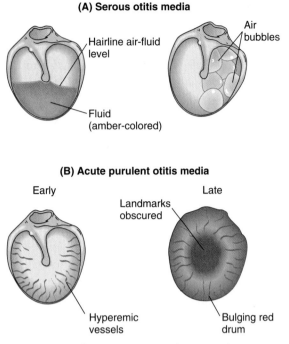

FIGURE 11.15 The tympanic membrane in the presence of otitis media. (A) Serous otitis media. (B) Acute purulent otitis media. *Hyperemic* means increased blood within these vessels.

Hearing Loss

- **Deafness** is the complete or partial loss of the ability to hear. It may range from the inability to hear sounds of a certain pitch or intensity to a complete loss of hearing.

- **Presbycusis** (pres-beh-**KOO**-sis) is a gradual loss of sensorineural hearing that occurs as the body ages (**presby** means old age and **-cusis** means hearing).

- A **conductive hearing loss** occurs when sound waves are prevented from passing from the air to the fluid-filled inner ear. Causes of this hearing loss include by a buildup of earwax, infection, fluid in the middle ear, a punctured eardrum, otosclerosis, and scarring.

- A **sensorineural hearing loss**, also known as **nerve deafness**, develops when the auditory nerve or hair cells in the inner ear are damaged. The source of this hearing loss may be located in the inner ear, in the nerve from the inner ear to the brain, or in the brain.

- A **noise-induced hearing loss** is a type of nerve deafness due to damage caused by repeated exposure to very intense noise such as aircraft engines, noisy equipment, or loud music.

DIAGNOSTIC PROCEDURES OF THE EARS AND HEARING

- **Audiometry** (aw-dee-**OM**-eh-tree) is the use of an audiometer to measure hearing acuity (**audi/o** means hearing and **-metry** means to measure).

- An **audiometer** (aw-dee-**OM**-eh-ter) is an electronic device that produces acoustic stimuli of a set frequency and intensity (**audi/o** means hearing and **-meter** means to measure).

- Sound is measured in two different ways. A **hertz** is a measure of sound frequency that determines how high or low a pitch is. Sound volume is measured in **decibels**, with normal conversation measuring about 60 dB. An *audiometry trace* plots the patient's ability to perceive both frequency and volume.

- **Speech audiometry** measures the threshold of speech reception (hearing speech sounds) and speech discrimination (understanding speech sounds).

- **Tympanometry** (tim-pah-**NOM**-eh-tree) is the measurement of acoustical energy absorbed or reflected by the middle ear through the use of a probe placed in the ear canal (**tympan/o** means eardrum and **-metry** means to measure). In a conductive hearing loss, the middle ear absorbs relatively less sound and reflects relatively more sound. This test is used to test for middle ear effusion (fluid buildup) or eustachian tube obstruction. The resulting record is a *tympanogram*.

- **Monaural testing** (mon-**AW**-rahl) involves one ear (**mon-** means one, **aur** means hearing, and **-al** means pertaining to). Compare with *binaural testing*.

- **Binaural testing** (bye-**NAW**-rul *or* bin-**AW**-rahl) involves both ears (**bi-** means two, **aur** means hearing, and **-al** means pertaining to). Compare with *monaural testing*.

TREATMENT PROCEDURES OF THE EARS AND HEARING

The Outer Ear

- **Otoplasty** (**OH**-toh-**plas**-tee) is the surgical repair of the pinna (**ot/o** means ear and **-plasty** means surgical repair).

The Middle Ear

- A **mastoidectomy** (mas-toy-**DECK**-toh-mee) is the surgical removal of mastoid cells (**mastoid** means mastoid process and **-ectomy** means surgical removal). This procedure is used to treat a mastoid infection that cannot be controlled with antibiotics.

- A **myringotomy** (**mir**-in-**GOT**-oh-mee) is the surgical incision of the eardrum to create an opening for the placement of tympanostomy tubes (**myring** means eardrum and **-otomy** means surgical incision).

- **Tympanostomy tubes** (**tim**-pan-**OSS**-toh-mee), also known as **pediatric ear tubes**, are tiny ventilating tubes placed through the eardrum to provide ongoing drainage for fluids and to relieve pressure that can build up after childhood ear infections.

- **Tympanoplasty** (**tim**-pah-noh-**PLAS**-tee) is the surgical correction of a damaged middle ear, either to cure chronic inflammation or to restore function (**tympan/o** means eardrum and **-plasty** means a surgical repair).

- A **stapedectomy** (**stay**-peh-**DECK**-toh-mee) is the surgical removal of the top portion of the stapes bone and the insertion of a small prosthetic device called a piston that conducts sound vibrations to the inner ear.

The Inner Ear

- **Fenestration** (**fen**-es-**TRAY**-shun) is a surgical procedure in which a new opening is created in the labyrinth to restore hearing (**fenestra** means window and **-tion** means process).

- A **hearing aid** is an external electronic device that amplifies sounds through a small speaker.

Sensorineural hearing loss can sometimes be corrected with a hearing aid.

- A **labyrinthectomy** (**lab**-ih-rin-**THECK**-toh-mee) is the surgical removal of all or a portion of the labyrinth (**labyrinth** means labyrinth and **-ectomy** means surgical removal). This procedure is performed to relieve uncontrolled vertigo; however, this causes a complete hearing loss in the affected ear.

- A **labyrinthotomy** (**lab**-ih-rin-**THOT**-oh-mee) is a surgical incision between two of the fluid chambers of the labyrinth to allow the pressure to equalize (**labyrinth** means labyrinth and **-otomy** means a surgical incision). This procedure is performed to relieve severe vertigo; however, about half of patients suffer some loss of high-tone hearing in the affected ear.

Cochlear Implant

A **cochlear implant** (**KOCK**-lee-ar) is an electronic device implanted behind the ear that receives sound signals and transmits these signals to electrodes implanted in the cochlea. This stimulation of the cochlea allows individuals with severe-to-profound hearing loss to perceive sound.

ABBREVIATIONS RELATED TO THE SPECIAL SENSES

Table 11.3 presents an overview of the abbreviations related to the terms introduced in this chapter. *Note:* To avoid errors or confusion, always be cautious when using abbreviations.

Table 11.3

ABBREVIATIONS RELATED TO THE SPECIAL SENSES	
age-related macular degeneration = AMD	**AMD** = age-related macular degeneration
astigmatism = AS	**AS** = astigmatism
cataract = CAT	**CAT** = cataract
conjunctivitis = CI	**CI** = conjunctivitis
convergence = C	**C** = convergence
decibel = dB	**dB** = decibel
diopter = D, diopt, Dptr	**D, diopt, Dptr** = diopter
esotropia, eustachian tube = ET	**ET** = esotropia, eustachian tube
fluorescein angiography = FA	**FA** = fluorescein angiography
glaucoma = G, glau, glc	**G, glau, glc** = glaucoma
hertz = Hz	**Hz** = hertz
hyperopia = H	**H** = hyperopia
intraocular lens = IOL	**IOL** = intraocular lens
myopia = M, MY, Myop	**M, MY, Myop** = myopia
nystagmus = ny, nst	**ny, nst** = nystagmus
otitis media = OM	**OM** = otitis media
photo-refractive keratectomy = PRK	**PRK** = photo-refractive keratectomy
presbyopia = P, Pb, Pr	**P, Pb, Pr** = presbyopia
retinal detachment = RD	**RD** = retinal detachment
radial keratotomy = RK	**RK** = radial keratotomy
serous otitis media = SOM	**SOM** = serous otitis media
Snellen chart = SC	**SC** = Snellen chart
strabismus = strab	**strab** = strabismus
tympanic membrane = TM	**TM** = tympanic membrane
visual acuity = V, VA	**V, VA** = visual acuity
xerophthalmia = X	**X** = xerophthalmia

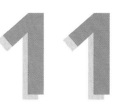
Learning Exercises

● Matching Word Parts 1

Write the correct answer in the middle column.

Definition	Correct Answer	Possible Answers
11.1. cornea, hard	_____	blephar/o
11.2. to measure	_____	-cusis
11.3. eyelid	_____	kerat/o
11.4. hearing	_____	opt/o
11.5. eyes, vision	_____	-metry

● Matching Word Parts 2

Write the correct answer in the middle column.

Definition	Correct Answer	Possible Answers
11.6. eye, vision	_____	myring/o
11.7. eardrum	_____	irid/o
11.8. iris of the eye	_____	-opia
11.9. old age	_____	ophthalm/o
11.10. vision condition	_____	presby/o

● Matching Word Parts 3

Write the correct answer in the middle column.

Definition	Correct Answer	Possible Answers
11.11. retina	_____	ot/o
11.12. hard, white of eye	_____	retin/o
11.13. turn	_____	scler/o
11.14. ear	_____	tympan/o
11.15. eardrum	_____	trop/o

● Definitions

Select the correct answer and write it on the line provided.

11.16. The structure that maintains the shape of the eye and protects the delicate inner tissues is the

_____ .

      choroid   conjunctiva   cornea   sclera

11.17. The structure that is a spiral-shaped passage leading from the oval window of the inner ear is the

_____ .

      cochlea   eustachian tube   organ of Corti   semicircular canal

11.18. The structure also known as the blind spot is the _____ .

      fovea centralis   macula   optic disk   optic nerve

11.19. The structure that lies between the outer ear and the middle ear is/are the _____ .

      mastoid cells   oval window   pinna   tympanic membrane

11.20. The structure that separates the middle ear from the inner ear is the _____ .

      eustachian tube   inner canthus   oval window   tympanic membrane

11.21. The auditory ossicle that is also known as the anvil is the _____ .

      incus   labyrinth   malleus   stapes

11.22. The term meaning lessening of the accommodation of the lens that occurs normally with aging is

_____ .

      ametropia   amblyopia   presbyopia   presbycusis

11.23. The term that describes reattachment of a detached retina by using a laser is _____ .

keratoplasty   laser trabeculoplasty   photo-refractive keratectomy   retinopexy

11.24. The term meaning turning inward of the edge of the eyelid is _____ .

ectropion   emmetropia   entropion   esotropia

11.25. The condition of _____ otitis media involves a buildup of pus in the middle ear.

acute   effusive   purulent   serous

● Matching Conditions

Write the correct answer in the middle column.

Definition	Correct Answer	Possible Answers
11.26. squint	_____	diplopia
11.27. nearsightedness	_____	esotropia
11.28. farsightedness	_____	hyperopia
11.29. double vision	_____	myopia
11.30. cross-eyes	_____	strabismus

● Which Word?

Select the correct answer and write it on the line provided.

11.31. The turning outward of an eyelid is called _____ .

ectropion   entropion

11.32. The term meaning bleeding from the ears is _____ .

otorrhagia   otorrhea

11.33. The surgical placement of a ventilating tube through the eardrum to drain fluid is a

_____ .

myringotomy   tympanostomy

11.34. A visual field test to determine losses in peripheral vision is used to diagnose _____ .

cataracts   glaucoma

11.35. A hearing test that involves both ears is _____ .

binaural   binocular

● Spelling Counts

Find the misspelled word in each sentence. Then write that word, spelled correctly, on the line provided.

11.36. The euctachian tubes lead from the middle ear to the pharynx. _____

11.37. Cerunem, which is also known as earwax, is secreted by glands that line the external auditory canal.

_____

11.38. Astegmatism is a condition in which the eye does not focus properly because of unequal curvatures of

the cornea. _____

11.39. The surgical procedure in which a new opening is made in the labyrinth of the inner ear is known as a

fenistration. _____

11.40. A Snellan chart is used to measure visual acuity. _____

● Abbreviation Identification

In the space provided, write the words that each abbreviation stands for.

11.41. **AMD**   _____

11.42. **AS**   _____

11.43. **IOL**   _____

11.44. **PRK**   _____

11.45. **OD**   _____

● Term Selection

Select the correct answer and write it on the line provided.

11.46. The condition known as _____ may be treated by radial keratotomy.

astigmatism   cataracts   hyperopia   myopia

11.47. The term that describes a condition in which the pupils are unequal in size is _____ .

    anisocoria   choked disk   macular degeneration   synechia

11.48. The term that describes the surgical repair of the pinna of the ear is _____ .

    keratoplasty   myringoplasty   otoplasty   tympanoplasty

11.49. The loss of central vision is frequently caused by _____ .

    glaucoma   macular degeneration   presbyopia   uveitis

11.50. The condition also known as a stye is _____ .

    blepharoptosis   chalazion   hordeolum   subconjunctival hemorrhage

---

● Sentence Completion

Write the correct term on the line provided.

11.51. The ability of the lens to bend light rays to help focus them on the retina is known as

_____ .

11.52. A sense of whirling, dizziness, and the loss of balance is called _____ .

11.53. A specialist in measuring the accuracy of vision is a/an _____ .

11.54. The medical term meaning an inflammation of the cornea is _____ .

11.55. The medical term for color blindness is _____ .

● Word Surgery

Divide each term into its component word parts. Write these word parts, in sequence, on the lines provided.

When necessary use a back slash (/) to indicate a combining vowel. (You may not need all of the lines provided.)

11.56. **Ophthalmoscopy** is the visual examination of the fundus of the eye.

_____   _____   _____   _____

11.57. **Emmetropia** is the normal relationship between the refractive power of the eye and the shape of the eye

that enables light rays to focus correctly on the retina.

_____   _____   _____   _____

11.58. **Otopyorrhea** is the flow of pus from the ear.

_____   _____   _____   _____

11.59. **Presbycusis** is a progressive hearing loss occurring in old age.

_____   _____   _____   _____

11.60. **Xerophthalmia** is drying of eye surfaces.

_____   _____   _____   _____

● True/False

If the statement is true, write **T** on the line. If the statement is false, write **F** on the line.

11.61. ____ Rods in the retina are the receptors for color.

11.62. ____ Aqueous fluid is drained through the canal of Schlemm.

11.63. ____ A cochlear implant is prescribed to treat presbycusis.

11.64. ____ LASIK is an acronym for Laser-Assisted in Situ Keratomileusis.

11.65. ____ Tarsorrhaphy is the suturing together of the upper and lower eyelids.

● Clinical Conditions

Write the correct answer on the line provided.

11.66. Following a boxing match, Jack Lawson required _____ to repair the pinna of his injured ear.

11.67. Sheila McClelland suffers from a/an _____ hearing loss because the middle ear does not conduct sound vibrations to the inner ear normally.

11.68. Edward Cooke was treated for an inflammation of mastoid cells. The medical term for this condition is

_____ .

11.69. Margo Wilkins was diagnosed as having blindness in one half of the visual field. The medical term for this condition is _____ .

11.70. Mr. Eisner required the diagnostic test in which a dye is injected into a vein in the arm and pictures are taken as the dye passes through the blood vessels in the retina. The medical term for this test is _____ angiography.

11.71. Juan Gutierrez has an earache caused by a buildup of fluid in the middle ear. His doctor referred to this condition as serous _____ _____.

11.72. Adrienne Jacobus says she suffers from night blindness. The medical term for this condition is _____.

11.73. Maude Colson is troubled by _____, which is a ringing sound in her ears.

11.74. Paul Ogelthorpe has closed-angle glaucoma. This was treated with laser _____.

11.75. Mrs. Liu's hearing loss was diagnosed as being caused by ankylosis of the bones of the middle ear. The medical term for this condition is _____ .

● Which Is the Correct Medical Term?

Select the correct answer and write it on the line provided.

11.76. The medical term for the condition that is also known as choked disk, is _____ .

    eustachitis   papilledema   tinnitus   xerophthalmia

11.77. The term describing an adhesion that binds the iris to an adjacent structure is _____ .

    blepharoptosis   convergence   scleritis   synechia

11.78. Astigmatism, hyperopia, and myopia are all forms of _____ .

    ametropia   diplopia   esotropia   hemianopia

11.79. The medical term that describes the condition commonly known as farsightedness is _____ .

    amblyopia   exotropia   hyperopia   myopia

11.80. The term that describes an accumulation of earwax in the auditory canal is _____ .

    conjunctivitis   impacted cerumen   otitis externa   pseudophakia

● **Challenge Word Building**

These terms are *not* found in this chapter; however, they are made up of the following familiar word parts. You may want to look in the textbook glossary or use a medical dictionary to check your answers.

blephar/o	-algia
irid/o	-ectomy
lacrim/o	-edema
ophthalm/o	-itis
labyrinth/o	-ology
retin/o	-otomy
	-pathy

11.81. The term meaning pain felt in the iris is _____ .

11.82. The term meaning inflammation of the eyelid is _____ .

11.83. The term meaning an incision into the iris is a/an _____ .

11.84. The term meaning any disease of the retina is _____ .

11.85. The term meaning the study of the eye is _____ .

11.86. The term meaning swelling of the eyelid is _____ .

11.87. The term meaning a surgical incision into the lacrimal duct is a/an _____ .

11.88. The term meaning the surgical removal of the labyrinth of the inner ear is a/an

_____ .

11.89. The term meaning any disease of the iris is _____ .

11.90. The term meaning inflammation of the retina is _____ .

● Labeling Exercises

Identify the numbered items on the accompanying figures.

11.91. _____

11.92. _____ chamber

11.93. crystalline _____

11.94. _____

11.95. _____ centralis

11.96. _____ or _____

11.97. external _____ canal

11.98. _____ membrane

11.99. _____ tube

11.100. _____

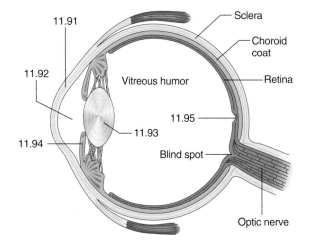

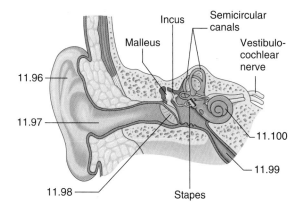

THE HUMAN TOUCH: CRITICAL THINKING EXERCISE

The following story and questions are designed to stimulate critical thinking through class discussion or as a brief essay response. There are no right or wrong answers to these questions.

William Davis is 62 years old. He was employed as a postal worker until his declining eyesight forced him into early retirement a few months ago. His wife, Mildred, died last year of complications from diabetes after a prolonged and expensive hospitalization. Mr. Davis does not trust the medical community and because of this distrust, he has not been to a doctor since his wife's death.

Mr. Davis is not considered legally blind, but his presbyopia and the advancing cataract in his right eye are starting to interfere with his ability to take care of himself. He still drives to the market once a week, but angry drivers honk and yell at him. He pays for his groceries with a credit card because he is afraid the checker will cheat him if he accidentally gives her the wrong bills from his wallet. He complains that the cleaning lady hides things from him and deliberately leaves the furniture out of place. When she leaves, he can't find his slippers or an ashtray. Yesterday, he put his lit pipe down in a wooden bowl by accident.

His son insists on taking him to see the ophthalmologist who treated his wife's diabetic retinopathy. Dr. Hsing believes Mr. Davis's sight can be improved in the right eye by performing cataract surgery. Mr. Davis listens in fear as the doctor explains. "Without this procedure your sight will only get worse."

Mr. Davis thinks about all the medical procedures that were tried on Mildred, and she died anyway. He doesn't want to go into the hospital, and he doesn't want any operations. But his son is talking about taking away his car if he doesn't do something about his failing sight. "What more can be taken away from me?" he thinks bitterly. "First my wife, then my job, and now my independence."

Suggested Discussion Topics:

1. Discuss how Mr. Davis's loss of sight is affecting the way he treats others and is treated by them.

2. Mr. Davis is a patient at the clinic where you work. Discuss the ways you would adjust your usual routine to accommodate his needs.

3. Close your eyes and keep them closed for 15 minutes while a classmate or friend leads you around. Discuss how you feel and what could have been done to make the experience less stressful.

4. Discuss why cataract surgery would be scary to Mr. Davis and what Dr. Hsing and his staff could do to ease his apprehension.

5. If Mr. Davis does not go ahead with the surgery, support groups might help him cope with his vision loss. What groups might be available to help him deal with his grief and depression?

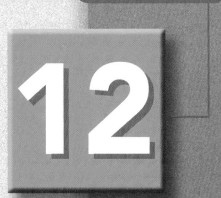

Skin: The Integumentary System

Overview of Structures, Combining Forms, and Functions of the Integumentary System

MAJOR STRUCTURES	RELATED COMBINING FORMS	PRIMARY FUNCTIONS
Skin	cutane/o, dermat/o, derm/o	Intact skin is the first line of defense for the immune system.
		Skin also waterproofs the body and is the major receptor for the sense of touch.
Sebaceous Glands	seb/o	Secrete sebum (oil) to lubricate the skin and discourage the growth of bacteria on the skin.
Sweat Glands	hidr/o	Secrete sweat to regulate body temperature and water content and excrete some metabolic waste.
Hair	pil/i, pil/o	Aids in controlling the loss of body heat.
Nails	onych/o, ungu/o	Protect the dorsal surface of the last bone of each finger and toe.

The items on this list have been identified as key word parts and terms for this chapter. However all words in boldface in the text are also important and may be included in learning exercises and tests.

Word Parts

- [ ] albin/o
- [ ] bi/o
- [ ] derm/o, dermat/o
- [ ] erythr/o
- [ ] hidr/o
- [ ] kerat/o
- [ ] lip/o
- [ ] melan/o
- [ ] myc/o
- [ ] onych/o
- [ ] pedicul/o
- [ ] pil/o
- [ ] rhytid/o
- [ ] seb/o
- [ ] xer/o

Medical Terms

- [ ] actinic keratosis (ack-**TIN**-ick **kerr**-ah-**TOH**-sis)
- [ ] albinism (**AL**-bih-niz-um)
- [ ] alopecia (**al**-oh-**PEE**-shee-ah)
- [ ] blepharoplasty (**BLEF**-ah-roh-**plas**-tee)
- [ ] bulla (**BULL**-ah)
- [ ] carbuncle (**KAR**-bung-kul)
- [ ] cellulitis (**sell**-you-**LYE**-tis)
- [ ] chloasma (kloh-**AZ**-mah)
- [ ] cicatrix (sick-**AY**-tricks)
- [ ] comedo (**KOM**-eh-doh)
- [ ] debridement (day-breed-**MON**)
- [ ] decubitus ulcer (dee-**KYOU**-bih-tus)
- [ ] dermatitis (**der**-mah-**TYE**-tis)
- [ ] diaphoresis (**dye**-ah-foh-**REE**-sis)
- [ ] dysplastic nevi (dis-**PLAS**-tick **NEE**-vye)
- [ ] ecchymosis (**eck**-ih-**MOH**-sis)
- [ ] eczema (**ECK**-zeh-mah)
- [ ] erythema (**er**-ih-**THEE**-mah)
- [ ] erythroderma (eh-**rith**-roh-**DER**-mah)

- [ ] exfoliative cytology (ecks-**FOH**-lee-**ay**-tiv sigh-**TOL**-oh-jee)
- [ ] folliculitis (foh-**lick**-you-**LYE**-tis)
- [ ] furuncles (**FYOU**-rung-kulz)
- [ ] granuloma (**gran**-you-**LOH**-mah)
- [ ] hematoma (**hee**-mah-**TOH**-mah)
- [ ] hirsutism (**HER**-soot-izm)
- [ ] ichthyosis (**ick**-thee-**OH**-sis)
- [ ] impetigo (**im**-peh-**TYE**-go)
- [ ] keloid (**KEE**-loid)
- [ ] keratosis (**kerr**-ah-**TOH**-sis)
- [ ] koilonychia (**koy**-loh-**NICK**-ee-ah)
- [ ] lipedema (lip-eh-**DEE**-mah)
- [ ] lipoma (lih-**POH**-mah)
- [ ] lupus erythematosus (**LOO**-pus er-ih-**thee**-mah-**TOH**-sus)
- [ ] macule (**MACK**-youl)
- [ ] malignant melanoma (mel-ah-**NOH**-mah)
- [ ] miliaria (**mill**-ee-**AYR**-ee-ah)
- [ ] necrotizing fasciitis (**fas**-ee-**EYE**-tis)
- [ ] onychocryptosis (**on**-ih-koh-krip-**TOH**-sis)
- [ ] onychomycosis (**on**-ih-koh-my-**KOH**-sis)
- [ ] papilloma (**pap**-ih-**LOH**-mah)
- [ ] papule (**PAP**-youl)
- [ ] paronychia (**par**-oh-**NICK**-ee-ah)
- [ ] pediculosis (pee-**dick**-you-**LOH**-sis)
- [ ] petechiae (pee-**TEE**-kee-ee)
- [ ] pruritus (proo-**RYE**-tus)
- [ ] psoriasis (soh-**RYE**-uh-sis)
- [ ] purpura (**PUR**-pew-rah)
- [ ] purulent (**PYOU**-roo-lent)
- [ ] rhytidectomy (**rit**-ih-**DECK**-toh-mee)
- [ ] rosacea (roh-**ZAY**-shee-ah)
- [ ] scabies (**SKAY**-beez)
- [ ] scleroderma (**sklehr**-oh-**DER**-mah *or* **skleer**-oh-**DER**-mah)
- [ ] seborrhea (seb-oh-**REE**-ah)
- [ ] strawberry hemangioma (hee-**man**-jee-**OH**-mah)
- [ ] tinea (**TIN**-ee-ah)
- [ ] urticaria (**ur**-tih-**KAR**-ree-ah)
- [ ] verrucae (veh-**ROO**-see)
- [ ] vitiligo (vit-ih-**LYE**-goh)
- [ ] wheal (**WHEEL**)
- [ ] xeroderma (zee-roh-**DER**-mah)

On completion of this chapter, you should be able to:

1. Identify and describe the functions and structures of the integumentary system.

2. Identify the medical specialists associated with the integumentary system.

3. Recognize, define, spell, and pronounce the terms used to describe the pathology and

the diagnostic and treatment procedures related to the skin.

4. Recognize, define, spell, and pronounce terms used to describe the pathology and the diagnostic and treatment procedures related to hair, nails, and sebaceous glands.

FUNCTIONS OF THE INTEGUMENTARY SYSTEM

The **integumentary system** (in-**teg**-you-**MEN**-tah-ree), which makes up the outer covering of the body and includes the related structures, serves many important functions beyond appearance.

Functions of the Skin

- The skin waterproofs the body and prevents fluid loss.
- Intact (unbroken) skin plays important roles in the immune system (see Chapter 6).
- Skin is the major receptor for the sense of touch.
- Skin helps the body synthesize (manufacture) vitamin D from the sun's ultraviolet light, while screening out some harmful ultraviolet radiation.

Functions of Related Structures

- **Sebaceous glands** (seh-**BAY**-shus), also known as **oil glands**, secrete **sebum**, a lipid (oil) that lubricates the skin and discourages the growth of bacteria on the skin.
- **Sweat glands** help regulate body temperature and water content by secreting sweat. Also, a small amount of metabolic waste is excreted through the sweat glands.
- **Hair** helps control the loss of body heat.
- **Nails** protect the dorsal surface of the last bone of each toe and finger.

STRUCTURES OF THE INTEGUMENTARY SYSTEM

The integumentary system consists of the skin and its related structures: sebaceous glands, sweat glands, hair, and nails (Figure 12.1).

THE SKIN

Skin covers the external surfaces of the body. The average adult has two square yards of skin, making it the largest bodily organ. The terms **derma** and **cutaneous** (kyou-**TAY**-nee-us) are both used to describe the skin (**cutane** means skin and **-ous** means pertaining to).

The skin is a complex system of specialized tissues and is made up of two basic layers, the epidermis and dermis, with an underlying, or subcutaneous, layer of fatty tissue (Figure 12.2).

The Epidermis

The **epidermis** (ep-ih-**DER**-mis), which is the outermost layer of the skin, is made up of several specialized epithelial tissues. **Epithelial tissues** (ep-ih-**THEE**-lee-al) form a protective covering for *all* of the internal and external surfaces of the body. *Epithelial* means relating to or consisting of epithelium.

- **Squamous epithelial tissue** (**SKWAY**-mus), which forms the upper layer of the epidermis, consists of flat, scaly cells. (*Squamous* means scale-like.) This layer is continuously shed by the sloughing off of cells.

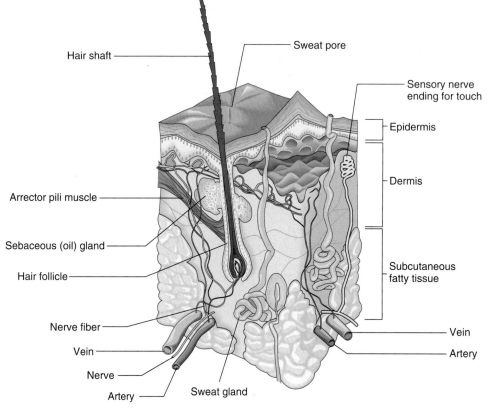

FIGURE 12.1 Structures of the skin.

- The epidermis does not contain any blood vessels or connective tissue and is dependent on lower layers for nourishment.
- Cells are produced in the lowest **basal layer** of the epidermis and pushed upward. When these cells

reach the surface, they die and become filled with keratin.
- **Keratin** (**KER**-ah-tin) is a fibrous, water-repellent protein. Soft keratin is a primary component of the epidermis. Hard keratin is found in the hair and nails.

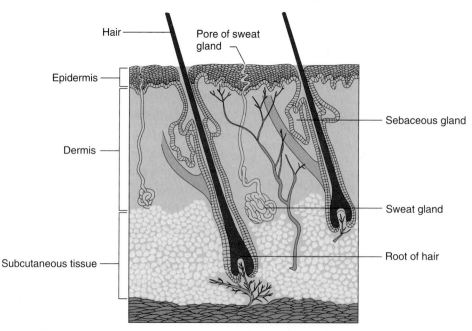

FIGURE 12.2 Layers of the skin.

- The basal cell layer also contains special cells called **melanocytes** (**MEL**-ah-noh-sights *or* meh-**LAN**-oh-sights). These cells produce and contain a dark brown to black pigment called **melanin** (**MEL**-ah-nin). The type and amount of melanin pigment determines the color of the skin. It also produces spots of color such as freckles.

- Melanin also protects the skin against some of the harmful ultraviolet rays of the sun. **Ultraviolet (UV)** refers to light that is beyond the visible spectrum at the violet end. Some UV rays help the skin produce vitamin D, but others can cause damage.

The Dermis

The **dermis** (**DER**-mis), also known as the **corium**, is the thick layer of living tissue directly below the epidermis. It contains connective tissue, blood and lymph vessels, and nerve fibers. It also contains the associated structures of the skin, which are the hair follicles and the sebaceous and sweat glands.

Sensitive nerve endings in the dermis receive impulses that enable the body to recognize sensory stimuli such as touch, temperature, pain, and pressure.

- **Tactile** (**TACK**-til) means pertaining to the sense of touch.

- **Perception** is the ability to recognize sensory stimuli. A *stimulus* causes a response in the affected tissues (plural *stimuli*).

Tissues Within the Dermis

- **Collagen** (**KOL**-ah-jen), which means glue, is a tough, yet flexible, fibrous protein material. In addition to being found in the skin, collagen is also found in bone, cartilage, tendons, and ligaments.

- **Mast cells**, which are found in the connective tissue of the dermis, respond to injury, infection, or allergy by producing and releasing substances including heparin and histamine.

- **Heparin** (**HEP**-ah-rin), which is released in response to injury, is an anticoagulant.

- **Histamine** (**HISS**-tah-meen), which is released in response to allergens, causes itching and increased mucus secretion.

The Subcutaneous Layer

The **subcutaneous layer**, located just below the skin, connects the skin to the surface muscles.

- This layer is made up of loose connective tissue and fatty **adipose tissue** (**AD**-ih-pohs). *Adipose* means fat.

- **Cellulite** is a term that was coined in European salons and spas to describe deposits of dimpled fat found on the thighs and buttocks of many women. This is not a medical term and medical authorities agree that cellulite is simply ordinary fatty tissue.

- **Lipocytes** (**LIP**-oh-sights), also known as **fat cells**, are predominant in the subcutaneous layer where they manufacture and store large quantities of fat (**lip/o** means fat and **-cytes** means cells).

ASSOCIATED STRUCTURES OF THE INTEGUMENTARY SYSTEM

The following structures are associated with the integumentary system (Figure 12.3):

- Sebaceous glands
- Sweat glands
- Hair
- Nails

The Sebaceous Glands

Sebaceous glands (seh-**BAY**-shus) are located in the dermis layer of the skin and are closely associated with hair follicles.

- These glands secrete **sebum** (**SEE**-bum), which is released through ducts opening into the hair follicles.

- From here, the sebum moves onto the surface and lubricates the skin.

- Because sebum is slightly acidic, it also discourages the growth of bacteria on the skin.

Mammary Glands

The milk-producing **mammary glands**, which are modified sebaceous glands, are often classified with the integumentary system. However, they also are part of the reproductive system and are discussed in Chapter 14.

The Sweat Glands

Sweat glands, also known as **sudoriferous glands**, are tiny, coiled glands found on almost all body surfaces. They are most numerous in the palms of the hands, the soles of the feet, the forehead, and the armpits.

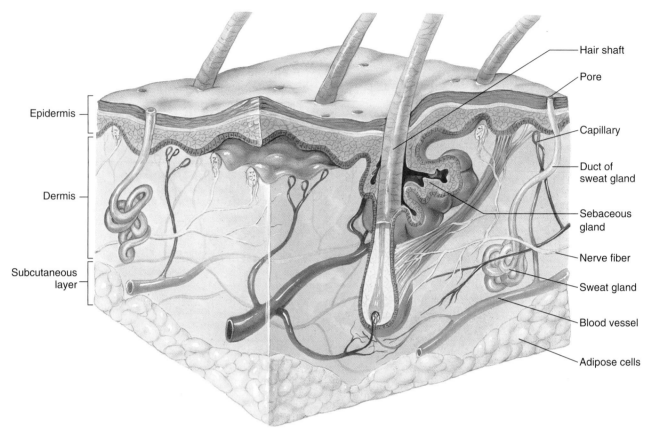

FIGURE 12.3   Glands and associated structures of the skin.

Ducts from sweat glands open on the surface of the skin through **pores**.

- **Sweat**, also known as **perspiration**, is secreted by sweat glands and is made up of 99 percent water plus some salt and metabolic waste products.

- **Perspiring**, or secreting sweat, is a means of excreting excess water. It also cools the body as the sweat evaporates into the air. Body odor associated with sweat comes from the interaction of the perspiration with bacteria on the skin's surface.

- **Hidrosis** (high-**DROH**-sis) means the production and excretion of sweat.

The Hair

Hair fibers are rodlike structures composed of tightly fused, dead protein cells filled with hard keratin. The darkness and color of the hair is determined by the amount and type of melanin produced by the melanocytes that surround the core of the hair shaft.

- **Hair follicles** are the sacs that hold the **root** of the hair fibers. The shape of the follicle determines whether the hair is straight or curly.

- Although hair is dead tissue, it appears to grow because the cells at the base of the follicle divide rapidly and push the old cells upward. As these cells are pushed upward, they harden and undergo pigmentation.

- The **arrector pili** (ah-**RECK**-tor **PYE**-lye), also known as the **erector muscles**, are tiny muscle fibers attached to the hair follicles that cause the hair to stand erect. In response to cold or fright, these muscles contract, causing raised areas of skin known as goose bumps. This action reduces heat loss through the skin.

The Nails

A nail, also known as an **unguis** (**UNG**-gwis), is the keratin plate protecting the dorsal surface of the last bone of each finger and toe (plural, **ungues**). Each nail consists of these parts (Figure 12.4).

- The **nail body**, which is translucent, is closely molded to the surface of the underlying tissues. It is made up of hard, keratinized plates of epidermal cells.

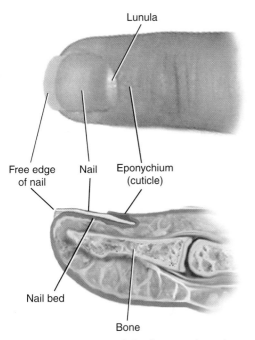

Lunula

**Free edge
of nail**   **Nail**   **Eponychium
(cuticle)**

Nail bed

Bone

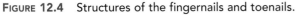

FIGURE 12.4   Structures of the fingernails and toenails.

- The **nail bed**, which joins the nail body to the underlying connective tissue, nourishes the nail. The blood vessels here give the nail its characteristic pink color.

- The **free edge**, which is the portion of the nail not attached to the nail bed, extends beyond the tip of the finger or toe.

- The **lunula** (**LOO**-new-lah) is a pale half-moon-shaped region at every nail root, generally easiest seen in the thumbnail (plural, **lunulae**). This is the active area of the nail, where new keratin cells form. *Lunula* means little moon.

- The **cuticle** is a narrow band of epidermis attached to the surface of the nail just in front of the root, protecting the new keratin cells as they form. *Cuticle* means little skin.

- The **root** fastens the nail to the finger or toe by fitting into a groove in the skin.

MEDICAL SPECIALTIES RELATED TO THE INTEGUMENTARY SYSTEM

- A **dermatologist** (**der**-mah-**TOL**-oh-jist) specializes in diagnosing and treating disorders of the skin (**dermat** means skin and **-ologist** means specialist).

- A **cosmetic surgeon**, also known as a **plastic surgeon**, specializes in the surgical restoration and reconstruction of body structures. As used here, *plastic* refers to the suffix **-plasty** meaning surgical repair.

PATHOLOGY OF THE INTEGUMENTARY SYSTEM

The Sebaceous Glands

- **Acne vulgaris** (**ACK**-nee vul-**GAY**-ris), the most common type of **acne**, is a chronic inflammatory disease that is characterized by pustular eruptions of the skin caused by an overproduction of sebum. Although often triggered by hormones in puberty and adolescence, it also occurs in adults. *Vulgaris* is a Latin term for common.

- A **comedo** (**KOM**-eh-doh) is a noninfected lesion formed by the buildup of sebum and keratin in a hair follicle (plural, **comedones**). Comedones are often associated with acne vulgaris. When the sebum plug is exposed to air, it oxidizes and becomes a **blackhead**.

- A **sebaceous cyst** (seh-**BAY**-shus **SIST**) is a sebaceous gland containing yellow, fatty material. These cysts may appear anywhere on the skin, including the scalp or the outer lips of the vagina.

- **Seborrhea** (seb-oh-**REE**-ah) is any of several common skin conditions in which there is an overproduction of sebum (**seb/o** means sebum and **-rrhea** means flow or discharge).

- **Seborrheic dermatitis** (seb-oh-**REE**-ick **der**-mah-**TYE**-tis) is an inflammation that causes scaling and itching of the upper layers of the skin or scalp. Extensive *dandruff* is a form of seborrheic dermatitis, as is the scalp rash in infants known as *cradle cap*. In contrast, mild dandruff is usually caused by a yeast-like fungus on the scalp.

- A **seborrheic keratosis** (seb-oh-**REE**-ick **kerr**-ah-**TOH**-sis) is a benign growth that has a waxy "pasted-on" look. These growths, which vary in color form light tan to black, occur most commonly in the elderly.

The Sweat Glands

- **Anhidrosis** (an-high-**DROH**-sis) is the abnormal condition of lacking sweat in response to heat (**an-** means without, **hidr** means sweat, and **-osis** means abnormal condition).

- **Hyperhidrosis** (high-per-high-**DROH**-sis) is a condition of excessive sweating in one area or over the whole body (**hyper-** means excessive, **hidr** means sweat, and **-osis** means abnormal condition).

- **Diaphoresis** (dye-ah-foh-**REE**-sis) is profuse sweating (**dia-** means through or complete, **phor** means movement, and **-esis** means abnormal condition). This is a normal condition when brought on by heat or exertion, but may also be the body's response to emotional or physical distress.

- **Miliaria** (**mill**-ee-**AYR**-ee-ah), also known as **heat rash** and **prickly heat**, is an intensely itchy rash caused by blockage of the sweat glands by bacteria and dead cells. *Caution:* Do not confuse this condition with the infectious disease *malaria*.

The Hair

Folliculitis (foh-**lick**-you-**LYE**-tis) is an inflammation of the hair follicles that is especially common on the limbs and in the beard area on men (**follicul** means the hair follicle and **-itis** means inflammation). This condition is frequently associated with AIDS, which is discussed in Chapter 6.

Excessive Hairiness

Hirsutism (**HER**-soot-izm) is the presence of excessive bodily and facial hair in women, usually occurring in a male pattern (**hirsut** means hairy and **-ism** means condition). This condition may be hereditary, or caused by a hormonal imbalance.

Abnormal Hair Loss

- **Alopecia** (al-oh-**PEE**-shee-ah), also known as **baldness**, is the partial or complete loss of hair, most commonly on the scalp (**alopec** means baldness and **-ia** means condition).
- *Alopecia areata* is an autoimmune disorder that attacks the hair follicles, causing well-defined bald areas on the scalp or elsewhere on the body. It often begins in childhood. *Areata* means occurring in patches.
- *Alopecia capitis totalis* is an uncommon condition characterized by the loss of all the hair on the scalp. *Capitis* means head.
- *Alopecia universalis* is the total loss of hair on all parts of the body. *Universalis* means total.
- *Female pattern baldness* is a condition in which the hair thins in the front and on the sides of the scalp and sometimes on the crown. It rarely leads to total hair loss.
- *Male pattern baldness* is a common hair loss pattern in men, with the hairline receding from the front to the back until only a horseshoe-shaped area of hair remains in the back and at the temples.

The Nails

- **Clubbing** is abnormal curving of the nails that is often accompanied by enlargement of the fingertips. This condition can be hereditary, but usually is caused by changes associated with oxygen deficiencies related to coronary or pulmonary disease.
- **Koilonychia** (**koy**-loh-**NICK**-ee-ah), also known as **spoon nail**, is a malformation of the nails in which the outer surface is concave or scooped out like the bowl of a spoon (**koil** means hollow or concave, **onych** means fingernail or toenail, and **-ia** means condition). Koilonychia is often an indication of iron-deficiency anemia.
- **Onychia** (oh-**NICK**-ee-ah), also known as **onychitis** (on-ih-**KYE**-tis), is an inflammation of the matrix of the nail (**onych** means fingernail or toenail and **-ia** means condition).
- **Onychocryptosis** (**on**-ih-koh-krip-**TOH**-sis) means ingrown toenail (**onych/o** means fingernail or toenail, **crypt** means hidden, and **-osis** means abnormal condition). The edges of a toenail, usually on the big toe, curve inward and cut into the skin. The affected area is prone to inflammation.
- **Onychomycosis** (**on**-ih-koh-my-**KOH**-sis) is a fungal infection of the nail (**onych/o** means fingernail or toenail, **myc** means fungus, and **-osis** means abnormal condition). Depending on what type of fungus is involved, this condition may cause the nails to turn white, yellow, green, or black and become thick or brittle.
- **Onychophagia** (**on**-ih-koh-**FAY**-jee-ah) means nail biting or nail eating (**onych/o** means fingernail or toenail and **-phagia** means eating or swallowing).
- **Paronychia** (par-oh-**NICK**-ee-ah) is an acute or chronic infection of the skin fold around a nail (**par-** means near, **onych** means fingernail or toenail, and **-ia** means condition).

Skin Pigmentation

- **Albinism** (**AL**-bih-niz-um) is an inherited deficiency or absence of pigment in the skin, hair, and irises due to a missing enzyme necessary for the production of melanin (**albin** means white and **-ism** means condition). A person with this condition is said to be an *albino*.
- **Chloasma** (kloh-**AZ**-mah), also known as **melasma** or the **mask of pregnancy**, is a pigmentation disorder characterized by brownish spots on the face.

This may occur during pregnancy, especially among women with dark hair and fair skin, and usually disappears after delivery.

- **Melanosis** (**mel**-ah-**NOH**-sis) is any condition of unusual deposits of black pigment in different parts of the body (**melan** means black and **-osis** means abnormal condition).

- **Vitiligo** (**vit**-ih-**LYE**-goh), believed to be an autoimmune disorder, is characterized by a loss of melanin resulting in whitish areas of skin, usually on the face and hands. This condition is more apparent in people with dark skin.

Bruises

- A **contusion** (kon-**TOO**-zhun), also known as a **bruise**, is an injury that does not break the skin and is characterized by discoloration and pain (**contus** means bruise and **-ion** means condition). The discoloration is caused by hemorrhaging (bleeding) within the skin.

- **Petechiae** (pee-**TEE**-kee-ee) are small pinpoint hemorrhages that are *less than* 2 mm in diameter (singular, **petechia**). These hemorrhages sometimes result from severe fevers.

- **Purpura** (**PUR**-pew-rah) is a condition that causes spontaneous bruises that are 2 mm to 10 mm in diameter, as well as hemorrhages in the internal organs and other tissues (**purpur** means purple and **-a** is a noun ending).

- An **ecchymosis** (**eck**-ih-**MOH**-sis) is an irregular area of purplish discoloration that is larger than 10 mm in diameter (**ecchym** means pouring out of juice and **-osis** means abnormal condition) (plural, **ecchymoses**). These bruises are sometimes the result of a blood disorder.

- A **hematoma** (hee-mah-**TOH**-mah) is a swelling of clotted blood trapped in the tissues that is usually caused by an injury (**hemat** means blood, and **-oma** means tumor). The body eventually resorbs this blood. A hematoma is often named for the area where it occurs. For example, a *subungual hematoma* (sub-**UNG**-gwal) is blood trapped under the nail. *Subungual* means under the nail.

Surface Lesions

A **lesion** (**LEE**-zhun) is a pathologic change of the tissues due to disease or injury. Skin lesions are described by their appearance, location, color, and size as measured in centimeters (cm) (Figure 12.5).

- A **crust**, also known as **scab**, is a collection of dried serum and cellular debris (Figure 12.6A).

- A **macule** (**MACK**-youl), or **macula**, is a discolored, flat spot that is less than 1 cm in diameter. Freckles, or flat moles, are examples of macules (Figure 12.6B).

- A **papule** (**PAP**-youl) is a small, raised red lesion that is *less than* 0.5 cm in diameter. Small pimples and insect bites are types of papules (Figure 12.6C). A papule does not contain pus. Compare with *pustule*.

- A **nodule** is a solid raised skin lesion that is larger than 0.5 cm in diameter and deeper than a papule. In acne vulgaris, nodules may cause scarring. The term *nodule* is also means a small node, or cluster of cells.

- A **plaque** (**PLACK**) is a scaly, solid raised area of closely spaced papules. For example, the lesions of psoriasis are plaques (Figure 12.11). *Note:* The term *plaque* also means a fatty buildup in the arteries and a soft substance that forms on the teeth.

- **Scales** are flakes or dry patches made up of excess dead epidermal cells. Some shedding of scales is normal; however, excessive shedding is associated with skin disorders such as psoriasis.

- **Verrucae** (veh-**ROO**-see), also known as **warts**, are small, hard skin lesions caused by the human papilloma virus (singular, **verruca**). *Plantar warts* develop on the sole of the foot.

- A **wheal** (**WHEEL**), also known as a **welt**, is a small bump that itches. Wheals can appear as a symptom of an allergic reaction (Figure 12.6D).

Fluid-Filled Lesions

- An **abscess** (**AB**-sess) is a closed pocket containing pus that is caused by a purulent bacterial infection. **Purulent** (**PYOU**-roo-lent) means producing or containing pus. An abscess can appear on the skin or elsewhere in the body.

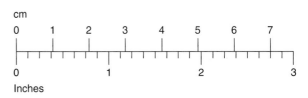

Figure 12.5   Lesions are described by length in centimeters. (*Note:* 2.5 centimeters equals one inch.)

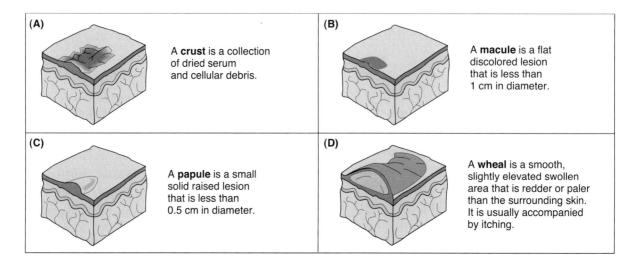

FIGURE 12.6   Surface lesions of the skin. (A) A crust. (B) A macule. (C) A papule. (D) A wheal.

- A **cyst** (**SIST**) is a deep closed sac just under the skin containing soft or semisolid material (Figure 12.7A). The term *cyst* can also refer to a sac or vesicle elsewhere in the body. The most common type of skin cyst is a sebaceous cyst.
- A **pustule** (**PUS**-tyoul), also known as a **pimple**, is a small, circumscribed lesion containing pus (Figure 12.7B). *Circumscribed* means contained within a limited area. Pustules can be caused by acne vulgaris or by impetigo, smallpox, and other infections.
- A **vesicle** (**VES**-ih-kul) is a small blister, less than 0.5 cm in diameter, containing watery fluid (Figure

12.7C). For example, the rash of poison oak consists of vesicles (Figure 12.10).
- A **bulla** (**BULL**-ah) is a large blister that is usually *more than* 0.5 cm in diameter (plural, **bullae**) (Figure 12.7D).

Lesions Through the Skin

- An **abrasion** (ah-**BRAY**-zhun) is an injury in which superficial layers of skin are scraped or rubbed away. The term *abrasion* also describes a treatment that involves scraping or rubbing away skin. See dermabrasion later in this chapter.

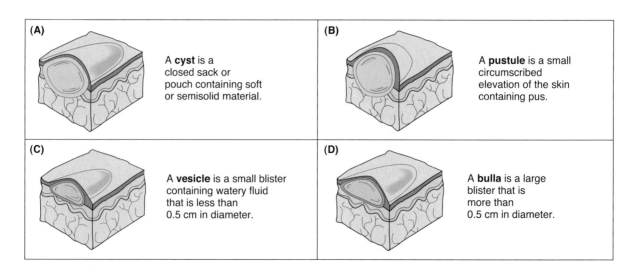

FIGURE 12.7   Fluid filled lesions. (A) A cyst. (B) A pustule. (C) A vesicle. (D) A bulla.

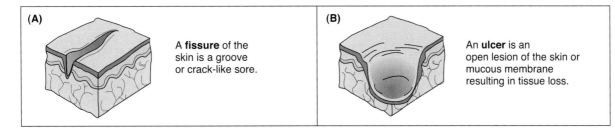

FIGURE 12.8 Lesions through the skin. (A) A fissure. (B) An ulcer.

- A **fissure** of the skin is a groove or crack-like sore (Figure 12.8A). The term *fissure* also describes normal folds in the contours of the brain.

- A **laceration** (**lass**-er-**AY**-shun) is a jagged wound or an accidental cut.

- A **puncture wound** is a deep hole made by a sharp object such as a nail. The risk for infection, especially tetanus, is greater with this type of wound. A *needlestick injury* is an accidental puncture with a hypodermic needle, and can transmit infection if the needle is not sterile.

- An **ulcer** (**UL**-ser) is an open lesion of the skin or mucous membrane resulting in tissue loss around the edges (Figure 12.8B). *Note:* Ulcers also occur inside the body. Those associated with the digestive system are discussed further in Chapter 8.

- A **decubitus ulcer** (dee-**KYOU**-bih-tus), also known as a **pressure ulcer** or **bedsore**, is an ulcerated area

in which prolonged pressure causes tissue death. Without proper care, open sores quickly become infected. *Decubitus* means lying down.

Birthmarks

- A **port-wine stain** is a large, reddish purple discoloration of the face or neck. This discoloration *will not* resolve without treatment (Figure 12.9A). See Laser Treatments of Skin Conditions later in this chapter.

- A **strawberry hemangioma** (hee-**man**-jee-**OH**-mah) is a soft raised dark, reddish purple birthmark. A *hemangioma* is a benign tumor made up of newly formed blood vessels (**hemangi/o** means blood vessels and **-oma** means tumor). These birthmarks usually resolve, without treatment, by about age five (Figure 12.9B).

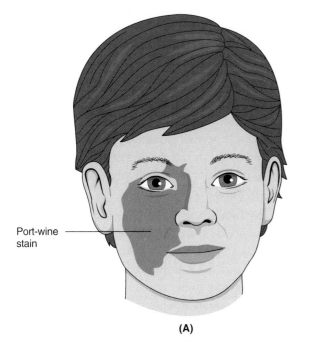

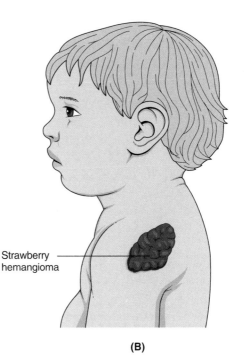

Port-wine stain

Strawberry hemangioma

(A) (B)

FIGURE 12.9 Types of birthmarks. (A) A port-wine stain is flat and is made up of pigmented cells. (B) A strawberry hemangioma is raised and is made up of blood vessels.

Dermatitis

The term **dermatitis** (der-mah-TYE-tis) means an inflammation of the skin (**dermat** means skin and **-itis** means inflammation). This condition, which takes many forms, usually includes redness, swelling, and itching. Compare with *dermatosis*.

- **Pruritus** (proo-RYE-tus), also known as **itching**, is associated with most forms of dermatitis (**prurit** means itching and **-us** is a singular noun ending).

- **Eczema** (ECK-zeh-mah) is a form of dermatitis that is usually associated with severe itching. In the early stages of eczema, the affected skin can be red, blistering, or oozing. In later stages, the affected skin can become scaly, brownish, or thickened.

- **Contact dermatitis** is a localized allergic response caused by contact with an irritant or allergen, such as an allergic reaction to latex gloves (Figure 12.10).

Erythema

Erythema (er-ih-THEE-mah) is any redness of the skin due to dilated capillaries, including a nervous blush, inflammation, or sunburn (**erythem** means flushed and **-a** is a noun ending).

- *Erythema multiforme* is damage to the blood vessels of the skin, with subsequent damage to the skin tissues, usually resulting from an allergic reaction to medication or infection. The mucous membranes are often also affected.

- *Fifth's disease*, also known as *erythema infectiosum*, is a mildly contagious viral infection common in childhood. It produces a red lacelike rash that may last as long as a month.

- *Chilblains*, also known as *erythema pernio*, are itchy, reddish-purple swellings on the fingers or toes caused by exposure to cold and moisture. The affected areas begin to itch when warmth restores full circulation.

- *Sunburn* is a form of erythema in which the cells of the skin are damaged by the ultraviolet rays in sunlight. This damage increases the chances of later developing skin cancer.

- **Erythroderma** (eh-**rith**-roh-**DER**-mah), also known as **exfoliative dermatitis (ED)**, is a condition in which there is widespread erythema accompanied by scaling of the skin (**erythr/o** means red and **-derma** means skin). This condition may result from skin diseases such as psoriasis, infections related to AIDS, or drug reactions.

General Skin Conditions

- **Pyoderma (pye**-oh-**DER**-mah) is any acute, inflammatory, pus-forming bacterial skin infection such as impetigo (**py/o** means pus and **-derma** means skin).

- **Dermatosis (der**-mah-**TOH**-sis) is a general term used to denote skin lesions or eruptions of any type that are *not* associated with inflammation (**dermat** means skin and **-osis** means abnormal condition). Compare with *dermatitis*.

- **Ichthyosis (ick**-thee-**OH**-sis) is a group of hereditary disorders that are characterized by dry, thickened, and scaly skin (**ichthy** means dry or scaly and **-osis** means abnormal condition). These conditions are caused either by the slowing of the skin's natural shedding process or by a rapid increase in the production of the skin's cells.

- **Lupus erythematosus (LOO**-pus er-ih-**thee**-mah-**TOH**-sus), also known as **systemic lupus erythematosus**, is an autoimmune disorder that is characterized by a red, scaly rash on the face and upper trunk. In addition to the skin, LE also attacks the connective tissue in other body systems, especially the joints.

- **Lipedema (lip**-eh-**DEE**-mah) is a chronic swelling caused by the collection of fat and fluid under the

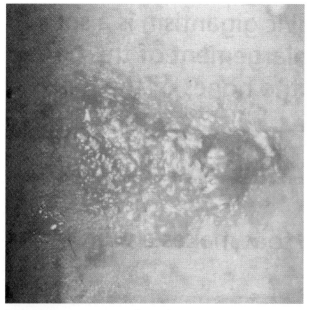

FIGURE **12.10** Contact dermatitis caused by poison oak. (*Courtesy of Timothy Berger, MD, Clinical Professor, Dept. of Dermatology, University of California, San Francisco.*)

skin (**lip** means fat and **-edema** means swelling). This swelling, which usually affects women in middle age, occurs commonly between the calf and ankle but does not involve the feet.

- **Psoriasis** (soh-**RYE**-uh-sis) is a common skin disorder characterized by flare-ups in which red papules covered with silvery scales occur on the elbows, knees, scalp, back, or buttocks (Figure 12.11).

- **Rosacea** (roh-**ZAY**-shee-ah) is a chronic condition of unknown cause that produces redness, tiny pimples, and broken blood vessels. It usually occurs on the central area of the face and appears most often in people over 30.

- **Rhinophyma** (rye-noh-**FIGH**-muh), also known as **bulbous nose**, is hyperplasia (overgrowth) of the tissues of the nose and is associated with advanced rosacea, but usually only in older men (**rhin/o** means nose and **-phyma** means growth) (Figure 12.16).

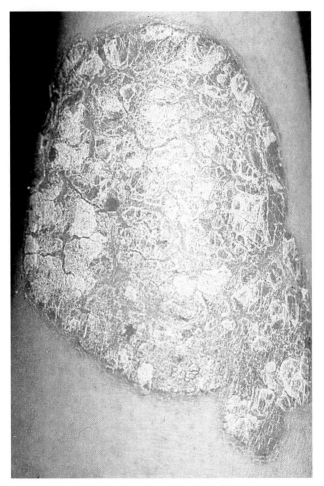

FIGURE 12.11 Psoriasis is characterized by silvery scales. (*Courtesy of Robert A. Silverman, MD, Pediatric Dermatology, Georgetown University.*)

- **Scleroderma** (sklehr-oh-**DER**-mah *or* skleer-oh-**DER**-mah) is an autoimmune disorder in which the connective tissues become thickened and hardened, causing the skin to become hard and swollen (**scler/o** means hard and **-derma** means skin). This condition may also affect the joints and internal organs.

- **Urticaria** (ur-tih-**KAR**-ree-ah), also known as **hives**, are wheals caused by an allergic reaction (**urtic** means rash and **-aria** means connected with).

- **Xeroderma** (zee-roh-**DER**-mah), also known as **xerosis**, is excessively dry skin (**xer/o** means dry and **-derma** means skin).

Bacterial Skin Infections

- **Furuncles** (**FYOU**-rung-kulz), also known as **boils**, are large tender, swollen, areas caused by a staphylococcal infection around hair follicles or sebaceous glands.

- A **carbuncle** (**KAR**-bung-kul) is a cluster of connected furuncles (boils).

- **Cellulitis** (**sell**-you-**LYE**-tis) is an acute, rapidly spreading infection within the connective tissue that is characterized by malaise, swelling, warmth, and red streaks. *Malaise* is a feeling of general discomfort or uneasiness that is often the first indication of an infection or other disease.

- **Gangrene** (**GANG**-green) is tissue necrosis (death) that is most commonly caused by a loss of circulation to the affected tissues. The tissue death is followed by bacterial invasion that causes putrefaction; if this infection enters the bloodstream it can be fatal. **Putrefaction** (**pyou**-treh-**FACK**-shun) is decay that produces foul-smelling odors.

- **Impetigo** (**im**-peh-**TYE**-goh) is a highly contagious bacterial skin infection characterized by isolated pustules that become crusted and rupture.

- **Necrotizing fasciitis** (**fas**-ee-**EYE**-tis) (**NF**), also known as **flesh-eating bacteria**, is caused by *Group A strep* (*necrotizing* means causing tissue death and *fasciitis* is inflammation of fascia). *Group A strep* normally live harmlessly on the skin; however if they enter the body through a skin wound, this serious infection may result. If untreated, the infected body tissue is destroyed and the illness can be fatal.

Fungal Skin Infections

Tinea (**TIN**-ee-ah) is a fungal infection that can grow on the skin, hair, or nails. This condition is also known as **ringworm** not because a worm is involved, but because as the fungus grows it spreads out in a circle, leaving normal-looking skin in the middle.

- *Tinea capitis* is found on the scalps of children. *Capitis* means head.
- *Tinea corporis* is a fungal infection of the skin on the body. *Corpus* means body.
- *Tinea cruris*, also known as *jock itch*, is found in the genital area.
- *Tinea pedis*, also known as *athlete's foot*, is found between the toes and on the feet. *Pedis* means foot.
- **Pityriasis versicolor** (pit-ih-**RYE**-ah-sis **VER**-sih-**kol**-or), also known as **tinea versicolor**, is a fungal infection that causes painless, discolored areas on the skin (**pity** means branlike, referring to bran-like scales, and **-iasis** means disease). The term *versicolor* means changing in color.

Parasitic Skin Infestations

An **infestation** is the dwelling of microscopic parasites on external surface tissue. Some parasites live temporarily on the skin. Others lay eggs and reproduce there.

- **Scabies** (**SKAY**-beez) is a skin infection caused by an infestation with the itch mite that produces distinctive brown lines and an itchy rash.
- **Pediculosis** (pee-**dick**-you-**LOH**-sis) is an infestation with **lice** (**pedicul** means lice and **-osis** means abnormal condition). The lice eggs, known as *nits*, must be destroyed in order to get rid of the infestation. There are three types of lice, each attracted to a specific part of the body.
- *Pediculosis capitis* is an infestation with head lice.
- *Pediculosis corporis* is an infestation with body lice.
- *Pediculosis pubis* is an infestation with lice in the pubic hair and pubic region.

Skin Growths

- A **callus** (**KAL**-us) is a thickening of part of the skin on the hands or feet caused by repeated rubbing. Compare with *callus* in Chapter 3. A *clavus*, or *corn*, is a callus in the keratin layer of the skin covering the joints of the toes, usually caused by ill-fitting shoes.
- A **cicatrix** (sick-**AY**-tricks) is a normal scar resulting from the healing of a wound (plural, **cicatrices**).

- **Granulation tissue** is the tissue that normally forms during the healing of a wound. It is this tissue that becomes the scar tissue.
- **Granuloma** (**gran**-you-**LOH**-mah) is a general term used to describe small knotlike swellings of granulation tissue in the epidermis (**granul** meaning granular and **-oma** means tumor). Granulomas may result from inflammation, injury, or infection.
- A **keloid** (**KEE**-loid) is an abnormally raised or thickened scar that expands beyond the boundaries of the incision (**kel** means growth or tumor and **-oid** means resembling). A tendency to form keloids is often inherited, and is more common among people with darkly pigmented skin.
- A **keratosis** (**kerr**-ah-**TOH**-sis) is any skin growth, such as a wart or a callus, in which there is overgrowth and thickening of the skin (**kerat** means hard or horny and **-osis** means abnormal condition). *Note:* **kerat/o** also refers to the cornea of the eye (plural, **keratoses**).
- A **lipoma** (lih-**POH**-mah) is a benign fatty deposit under the skin that causes a bump (**lip** means fatty and **-oma** means tumor).
- **Nevi** (**NEE**-vye), also known as **moles**, are small dark skin growths that develop from melanocytes in the skin (singular, **nevus**). Normally, these growths are benign.
- **Dysplastic nevi** (dis-**PLAS**-tick **NEE** vye) are atypical moles that may develop into skin cancer.
- A **papilloma** (**pap**-ih-**LOH**-mah) is a benign, superficial wartlike growth on the epithelial tissue or elsewhere in the body, such as in the bladder (**papill** means resembling a nipple and **-oma** means tumor).
- **Polyp** (**POL**-ip) is a general term used most commonly to describe a mushroom-like growth from the surface of a mucous membrane, such as a polyp in the nose. These growths have many causes and are not necessarily malignant.
- **Skin tags** are small flesh-colored or light brown polyps that hang from the body by fine stalks. Skin tags are benign and tend to enlarge with age.

Skin Cancer

Skin cancer is the most common form of cancer today, but fortunately most skin cancers are curable. Sun exposure is one of the main factors in predicting skin cancer. There are three main types of skin cancer: basal cell carcinoma, squamous cell carcinoma, and melanoma.

- **Basal cell carcinoma**, which is the most frequent and least harmful type of skin cancer, is a malignant tumor of the basal cell layer of the epidermis. It occurs mainly on the face or neck, is slow growing and rarely spreads to other parts of the body. The lesions are usually pink, smooth, raised, with a depression in the center, and they tend to bleed easily (Figure 12.12).

- **Squamous cell carcinoma** (**SKWAY**-mus) begins as a malignant tumor of the thin, scaly squamous cells of the epithelium; however, it can quickly spread to other body systems. These cancers begin as skin lesions that appear to be sores that will not heal or sores with a crusted, heaped-up look (Figure 12.13).

- **Malignant melanoma** (mel-ah-**NOH**-mah), also known as **melanoma**, is a type of skin cancer that occurs in the melanocytes (**melan** means black and **-oma** means tumor). The first sign of melanoma is often a change in the size, shape, or color of a mole. Melanoma may spread to other parts of the body through the lymphatic system, or the blood, and although the least common skin cancer, it is the most dangerous and is sometimes fatal (Figure 12.14).

- An **actinic keratosis** (ack-**TIN**-ick **kerr**-ah-**TOH**-sis) is a skin lesion caused by excessive exposure to the sun. Actinic keratoses (plural) are rough, red or brown scaly patches on the skin that may be precancerous.

Burns

A **burn** is an injury to body tissues caused by heat, flame, electricity, sun, chemicals, or radiation. The severity of a burn is described according to the percentage of the total body skin surface affected (more than 15 percent is considered serious). It is also described according to the depth or layers of skin involved (Table 12.1 and Figure 12.15).

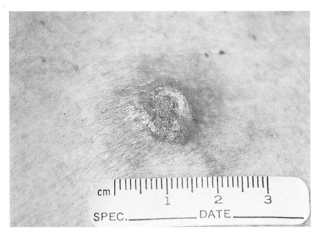

FIGURE 12.12   Basal cell carcinoma. (*Courtesy of Robert A. Silverman, MD, Pediatric Dermatology, Georgetown University.*)

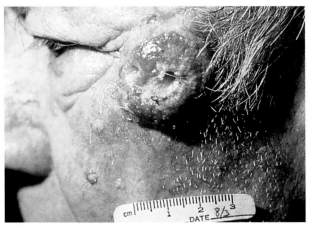

FIGURE 12.13   Squamous cell carcinoma. (*Courtesy of Robert A. Silverman, MD, Pediatric Dermatology, Georgetown University.*)

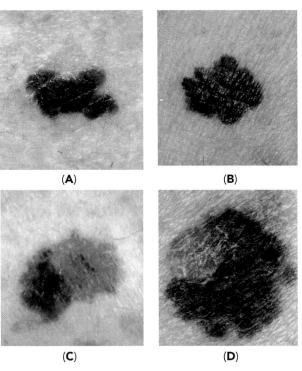

FIGURE 12.14   The signs of melanoma. (A) Asymmetry. (B) Border irregularity. (C) Color. (D) Diameter. (*Reprinted with permission from the American Academy of Dermatology. All rights reserved.*)

Table 12.1

CLASSIFICATION OF BURN SEVERITY

Type of Burn	Also Known As	Layers of Skin Involved
First-degree	Superficial burns, sunburn	No blisters, superficial damage to the epidermis
Second-degree	Partial thickness burns	Blisters, damage to the epidermis and the second layer (dermis)
Third-degree	Full thickness burns	Damage to the epidermis, dermis, and subcutaneous layers and possibly also the muscle below

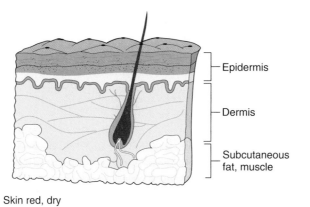

Skin red, dry

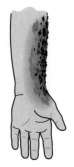

First-degree, superficial

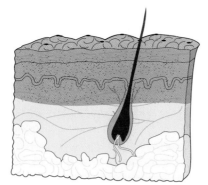

Blistered, skin moist, pink or red

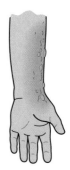

Second-degree, partial thickness

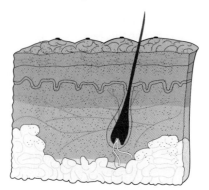

Charring, skin black, brown, red

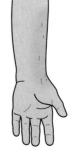

Third-degree, full thickness

FIGURE 12.15   The degree of a burn is determined by the layers of skin involved.

DIAGNOSTIC PROCEDURES OF THE INTEGUMENTARY SYSTEM

A **biopsy** (**BYE**-op-see) is the removal of a small piece of living tissue for examination to confirm or establish a diagnosis (**bi** means pertaining to life and **-opsy** means view of).

- In an *incisional biopsy* a piece, but not all, of the tumor or lesion is removed. *Incision* means to cut into.

- In an *excisional biopsy* the entire tumor or lesion and a margin of surrounding tissue are removed. *Excision* means the complete removal of a lesion or organ.

- In a *needle biopsy*, a hollow needle is used to remove a core of tissue for examination.

- **Exfoliative cytology** (ecks-**FOH**-lee-**ay**-tiv sigh-**TOL**-oh-jee) is a technique in which cells are scraped from the tissue and examined under a microscope.

TREATMENT PROCEDURES OF THE INTEGUMENTARY SYSTEM

Transdermal Medications

The skin is able to absorb certain drugs and other chemical substances used to treat problems ranging from acne to angina attacks.

- A **topical** application is one that pertains to a specific location. Topical medication is put on the skin to treat the area it is applied to.

  Cortisone ointment is applied topically to relieve itching and speed healing.

  Topical steroids, which are anti-inflammatory drugs, are used to treat many skin diseases by suppressing the inflammatory response in the area of application.

- **Transdermal** medication is applied to unbroken skin so that it is absorbed continuously to produce a systemic effect (**trans-** means through or across, **derm** means skin, and **-al** means pertaining to). A transdermal patch may be used to convey medications such as nitroglycerin for angina pectoris, hormones for hormone replacement therapy, or scopolamine for motion sickness.

Preventive Measures

Sunscreen that blocks out the harmful ultraviolet B (UVB) rays is sometimes measured in terms of the strength of the **sun protection factor**. Some sunscreens also give protection against ultraviolet A (UVA) rays.

Tissue Removal

- **Cauterization** (**kaw**-ter-eye-**ZAY**-zhun) is the destruction of tissue by burning.

- **Curettage** (**kyou**-reh-**TAHZH**) is the removal of material from the surface by scraping. This technique is used to remove and destroy basal cell tumors.

- **Chemical peel**, also known as **chemabrasion** (keem-ah-**BRAY**-shun), is the use of chemicals to remove the outer layers of skin to treat acne scaring, fine wrinkling, and general keratoses.

- **Cryosurgery** is the destruction or elimination of abnormal tissue cells, such as warts or tumors, through the application of extreme cold, often by using liquid nitrogen (**cry/o** means cold and **-surgery** means operative procedure).

- **Debridement** (day-breed-**MON**) is the removal of dirt, foreign objects, damaged tissue, and cellular debris from a wound to prevent infection and to promote healing.

- **Dermabrasion** (**der**-mah-**BRAY**-zhun) is a form of abrasion involving the use of a revolving wire brush or sandpaper. It is used to remove acne and chickenpox scars as well as for facial skin rejuvenation.

- **Incision and drainage** (I & D) involves incision (cutting open) of a lesion, such as an abscess, and draining the contents.

- **Mohs' surgery** is a technique of excising skin tumors by removing tumor tissue, layer-by-layer, examining the removed portion microscopically for malignant cells, and repeating the procedure until the entire tumor is removed.

Laser Treatment of Skin Conditions

Lasers are used to treat skin and many conditions affecting other body conditions. The term **laser** is an acronym. The letters stand for *light amplification by stimulated emission of radiation*. A laser tube can be filled with a solid, liquid, or gas substance that is stimulated to emit light to a specific wavelength. Some wavelengths are capable of destroying all skin tissue; others target tissue of a particular color.

- **Rhinophyma** is treated by using a laser to reshape the nose by vaporizing the excess tissue (Figure 12.16).

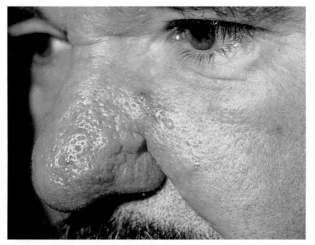

FIGURE 12.16 Rhinophyma before laser treatment. (*Courtesy of Robert A. Silverman, MD, Pediatric Dermatology, Georgetown University.*)

- **Port-wine stain** is treated using short pulses of laser light to remove the birthmark (Figure 12.9A). Treatment may require many sessions, because only a small section is treated at a time.
- Tattoos are removed by using lasers that target particular colors.
- Lasers are also used in the treatment of some skin cancers, precancer of the lip, and warts that recur around nails and on the soles of feet.

Cosmetic Procedures

- **Blepharoplasty** (**BLEF**-ah-roh-**plas**-tee), also known as a **lid lift**, is the surgical reduction of the upper and lower eyelids by removing excess fat, skin, and muscle (**blephar/o** means eyelid and **-plasty** means surgical repair).
- **Botox** is a formulation of botulinum toxin type A. This is the neurotoxin that is responsible for the form of food poisoning known as botulism. Botox injections, which temporarily block the nerve signals to the injected muscle, improve the appearance of moderate to severe frown lines for up to three to four months. *Frown lines* are located between the eyebrows.

- **Collagen replacement therapy** is a form of soft-tissue augmentation used to soften facial lines or scars or to make lips appear fuller. Tiny quantities of collagen are injected under a line or scar to boost the skin's natural supply of collagen. The effect usually lasts from three to 12 months.
- **Dermatoplasty** (**DER**-mah-toh-**plas**-tee), also known as a **skin graft**, is the replacement of damaged skin with healthy tissue taken from a donor site on the patient's body (**dermat/o** means skin and **-plasty** means surgical repair).
- **Electrolysis** is the use of an electric current to destroy hair follicles; it produces relatively permanent removal of undesired hair.
- **Lipectomy** (lih-**PECK**-toh-mee) is the surgical removal of fat beneath the skin (**lip** means fat and **-ectomy** means surgical removal).
- **Liposuction** (**LIP**-oh-**suck**-shun *or* **LYE**-poh-**suck**-shun), also known as **suction-assisted lipectomy**, is the surgical removal of fat beneath the skin with the aid of suction.
- **Rhytidectomy** (**rit**-ih-**DECK**-toh-mee), also known as a **facelift**, is the surgical removal of excess skin and fat for the elimination of wrinkles (**rhytid** means wrinkle and **-ectomy** means surgical removal).
- **Sclerotherapy** (**sklehr**-oh-**THER**-ah-pee) is used in the treatment of spider veins. *Spider veins* are small, nonessential veins that can be seen through the skin. This treatment involves injecting a sclerosing solution (saline solution) into the vein being treated. This solution irritates the tissue, causing the veins to collapse and disappear.

ABBREVIATIONS RELATED TO THE INTEGUMENTARY SYSTEM

Table 12.2 presents an overview of the abbreviations related to the terms introduced in this chapter. *Note:* To avoid errors or confusion, always be cautious when using abbreviations.

Table 12.2

ABBREVIATIONS RELATED TO THE INTEGUMENTARY SYSTEM

alopecia areata = AA	**AA** = alopecia areata
basal cell carcinoma = BCC	**BCC** = basal cell carcinoma
cauterization = caut	**caut** = cauterization
contact dermatitis = CD	**CD** = contact dermatitis
cryosurgery = CRYO	**CRYO** = cryosurgery
debridement = debr	**debr** = debridement
decubitus ulcer = du	**du** = decubitus ulcer
eczema = Ez	**Ez** = eczema
histamine = HA, Hi, hist	**HA, Hi, hist** = histamine
incision and drainage = I & D	**I & D** = incision and drainage
lupus erythematosus = LE	**LE** = lupus erythematosus
malignant melanoma = MM	**MM** = malignant melanoma
necrotizing fasciitis = NF	**NF** = necrotizing fasciitis
psoriasis = PS, Ps	**PS, Ps** = psoriasis
sclerotherapy = ST	**ST** = sclerotherapy
squamous cell carcinoma = SCC	**SCC** = squamous cell carcinoma
sun protection factor = SPF	**SPF** = sun protection factor
systemic lupus erythematosus = SLE	**SLE** = systemic lupus erythematosus

Learning Exercises

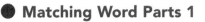

● Matching Word Parts 1

Write the correct answer in the middle column.

Definition	Correct Answer	Possible Answers
12.1. life	_____	albin/o
12.2. red	_____	rhytid/o
12.3. wrinkle	_____	erythr/o
12.4. sweat	_____	bi/o
12.5. white	_____	hidr/o

● Matching Word Parts 2

Write the correct answer in the middle column.

Definition	Correct Answer	Possible Answers
12.6. black, dark	_____	dermat/o
12.7. fat, lipid	_____	kerat/o
12.8. lice	_____	lip/o
12.9. horny, hard	_____	melan/o
12.10. skin	_____	pedicul/o

● Matching Word Parts 3

Write the correct answer in the middle column.

Definition	Correct Answer	Possible Answers
12.11. dry	_____	**onych/o**
12.12. fungus	_____	**pil/o**
12.13. hair	_____	**seb/o**
12.14. nail	_____	**xer/o**
12.15. sebum	_____	**myc/o**

● Definitions

Select the correct answer and write it on the line provided.

12.16. The term that describes a diffuse infection of connective tissue is _____.

      abscess   cellulitis   fissure   ulcer

12.17. The biopsy technique in which only part of the lesion is cut out is a/an _____

    biopsy.

      excisional   exfoliative   incisional   needle

12.18. The autoimmune disorder in which there are well-defined bald areas, is known as

    _____ _____ .

      alopecia areata   alopecia capitis   alopecia universalis   psoriasis

12.19. An ecchymosis is commonly known as a/an _____ .

      abscess   bruise   scar   ulcer

12.20. The term meaning profuse sweating is _____ .

      anhidrosis   diaphoresis   hidrosis   miliaria

12.21. The term that describes a normal scar left by a wound is a _____ .

      cicatrix   keloid   keratosis   papilloma

12.22. The type of treatment used to remove a port-wine stain is _____ .

    abrasion   cryosurgery   laser   Mohs' chemosurgery

12.23. The removal of dirt, foreign objects, damaged tissue, and cellular debris from a wound is called

    _____ .

    debridement   drainage   excision   incision

12.24. A burn that has no blisters, and only superficial damage to the epidermis, is described as a

    _____ burn.

    first-degree   fourth-degree   second-degree   third-degree

12.25. The lesions caused by the human papillomavirus, commonly known as warts, are

    _____ .

    nevi   petechiae   scabies   verrucae

● Matching Structures

Write the correct answer in the middle column.

Definition	Correct Answer	Possible Answers
12.26. secrete sebum	_____	dermis
12.27. finger and toenails	_____	keratin
12.28. fibrous protein found in hair, nails, and skin	_____	mammary glands
12.29. the layer of skin below the epidermis	_____	sebaceous glands
12.30. milk-producing sebaceous glands	_____	unguis

● Which Word?

Select the correct answer and write it on the line provided.

12.31. The medical term for the condition commonly known as an ingrown toenail is _____ .

    onychomycosis   onychocryptosis

12.32. A contagious, superficial skin infection usually seen in young children is _____ .

impetigo   xeroderma

12.33. A torn or jagged wound or an accidental cut wound is known as a _____ .

laceration   lesion

12.34. The lesions of _____ carcinoma tend to bleed easily.

basal cell   squamous cell

12.35. Group A strep, also known as flesh-eating bacteria, causes _____

_____ .

lupus erythematosus   necrotizing fasciitis

● **Spelling Counts**

Find the misspelled word in each sentence. Then write that word, spelled correctly, on the line provided.

12.36. Soriasis is a chronic disease of the skin characterized by itching and by red papules covered with silvery

scales. _____

12.37. Exema is an inflammatory skin disease with erythema, papules, and scabs. _____

12.38. An abcess is a localized collection of pus. _____

12.39. Onyochia is an inflammation of the nail bed, resulting in the loss of the nail. _____

12.40. Skleroderma is an autoimmune disorder in which the skin becomes taut, firm, and swollen.

_____

● **Abbreviation Identification**

In the space provided, write the words that each abbreviation stands for.

12.41. **BCC**   _____

12.42. **I & D**   _____

12.43. **NF**   _____

12.44. **MM**   _____

12.45. **SLE**   _____

● **Term Selection**

Select the correct answer and write it on the line provided.

12.46. A small, knotlike swelling of granulation tissue that may result from inflammation, injury, or infection is a

_____ .

        cicatrix   granuloma   keratosis   petechiae

12.47. The term meaning an infestation of body lice is _____ .

    pediculosis capitis   pediculosis corpus   pediculosis pubis   scabies

12.48. The term meaning any redness of the skin is _____ .

        dermatitis   ecchymosis   erythema   urticaria

12.49. A dry patch made up of excessive dead epidermal cells is a _____ .

        bulla   macule   plaque   scale

12.50. A cluster of boils is known as a/an _____ .

        acne vulgaris   carbuncle   comedo   furuncle

● **Sentence Completion**

Write the correct term on the line provided.

12.51. The term meaning producing or containing pus is _____ .

12.52. The term meaning a fungal infection of the nail is _____ .

12.53. Tissue death followed by bacterial invasion and putrefaction is known as _____ .

12.54. Any condition of unusual deposits of black pigment is known as _____ .

12.55. The medical term for the condition commonly known as hives is _____ .

● **Word Surgery**

Divide each term into its component word parts. Write these word parts, in sequence, on the lines provided.

When necessary use a back slash (/) to indicate a combining vowel. (You may not need all of the lines provided.)

12.56. A **rhytidectomy** is the surgical removal of excess skin for the elimination of wrinkles.

_____   _____   _____   _____

12.57. **Onychomycosis** is any fungal infection of the nail.

_____   _____   _____   _____

12.58. **Folliculitis** is an inflammation of the hair follicles that is especially common on the limbs and in the beard area on men.

_____   _____   _____   _____

12.59. **Pruritus** is also known as itching.

_____   _____   _____   _____

12.60. **Ichthyosis** is a group of hereditary disorders that are characterized by dry, thickened, and scaly skin.

_____   _____   _____   _____

● True/False

If the statement is true, write **T** on the line. If the statement is false, write **F** on the line.

12.61. ____ Putrefaction is decay that produces foul-smelling odors.

12.62. ____ A skin tag that enlarges in the elderly is malignant.

12.63. ____ The arrector pili are tiny muscles that cause the hair to stand erect.

12.64. ____ An abnormally raised scar is known as a keratosis.

12.65. ____ A lipoma is a benign tumor made up of mature fat cells.

● Clinical Conditions

Write the correct answer on the line provided.

12.66. Roberta Harris underwent _____ for the treatment of spider veins.

12.67. Jordan Caswell has an inherited deficiency or absence of pigment in the skin, hair, and eyes due to an abnormality in production of melanin. This disorder is called _____ .

12.68. Mike Young hit his thumb with a hammer and soon there was a collection of blood beneath the nail. This is called a/an _____ _____ .

12.69. When Trisha fell off her bicycle, she scraped off the superficial layers on skin on her knees. The type of injury is known as a/an _____ .

12.70. Rosita Chavez was diagnosed as suffering from a disorder with bleeding beneath the skin that causes

spontaneous bruising. The medical term for this condition is _____ .

12.71. Henry Walton was treated for a skin infection caused by the itch mite. This was entered on his chart as

treatment for _____ .

12.72. Dr. Liu found that Jeanette Isenberg had an abnormal skin lesion caused by excessive exposure to the

sun. The medical term for this is a/an _____ _____.

12.73. Mrs. Garrison had cosmetic surgery that is commonly known as a lid lift. The medical term for this treat-

ment is a/an _____ .

12.74. When Manuel fell he suffered a painful injury that caused swelling and discoloration but did not break

the skin. The medical term for this condition is a/an _____.

12.75. Agnes Farrington uses a patch to prevent motion sickness. This is known as _____

administration.

● Which Is the Correct Medical Term?

Select the correct answer and write it on the line provided.

12.76. The term that refers to an acute infection of the fold of skin at the margin of a nail is

_____ .

    onychia   onychocryptosis   paronychia   vitiligo

12.77. When the sebum plug of a _____ is exposed to air, it oxidizes and becomes a black-

head.

    comedo   macule   pustule   sebaceous cyst

12.78. In a/an _____ biopsy the entire lesion is removed.

    dermabrasion   excisional   incisional   needle

12.79. The medical term referring to a malformation of the nail is _____ . This condition

is also called spoon nail.

    clubbing   koilonychia   onychomycosis   paronychia

12.80. Also known as moles, _____ are small dark skin growths that develop from

melanocytes in the skin.

keloids   nevi   papilloma   verrucae

● **Challenge Word Building**

These terms are *not* found in this chapter; however, they are made up of the following familiar word parts. You

may want to look in the textbook glossary or use a medical dictionary to check your answers.

an-	dermat/o	-ia
hypo-	hidr/o	-ectomy
	melan/o	-itis
	myc/o	-malacia
	onych/o	-oma
	py/o	-derma
	rhin/o	-osis
		-pathy
		-plasty

12.81. The term meaning abnormal softening of the nails is _____ .

12.82. The term meaning an abnormal condition resulting in the diminished flow of perspiration is

_____ .

12.83. The term meaning plastic surgery to change the shape or size of the nose is _____ .

12.84. The term meaning a tumor arising from the nail bed is _____ .

12.85. The term meaning any pus-forming skin disease is _____ .

12.86. The term meaning the surgical removal of a finger or toenail is a/an _____ .

12.87. The term meaning pertaining to the absence of finger or toenails is _____ .

12.88. The term meaning any disease of the skin is _____ .

12.89. The term meaning any disease caused by a fungus is _____ .

12.90. The term meaning that an excess of melanin is present in an area of inflammation of the skin is

_____ .

● Labeling Exercises

Identify the numbered items on the accompanying figures.

12.91. _____

12.92. _____

12.93. _____

12.94. _____

12.95. _____

12.96. _____

12.97. _____

12.98. _____ tissue

12.99. _____ gland

12.100. _____ gland

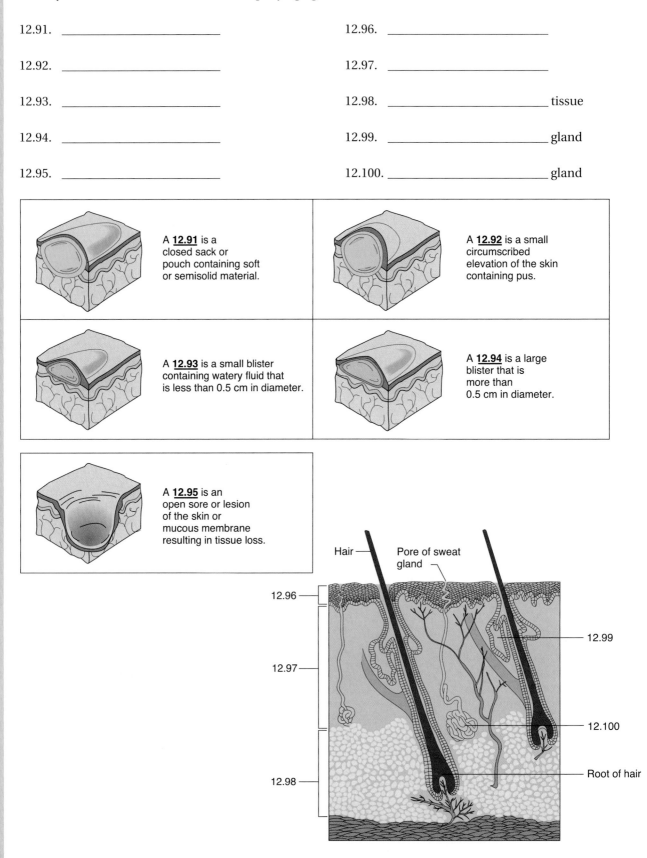

A **12.91** is a closed sack or pouch containing soft or semisolid material.

A **12.92** is a small circumscribed elevation of the skin containing pus.

A **12.93** is a small blister containing watery fluid that is less than 0.5 cm in diameter.

A **12.94** is a large blister that is more than 0.5 cm in diameter.

A **12.95** is an open sore or lesion of the skin or mucous membrane resulting in tissue loss.

Hair

Pore of sweat gland

12.96

12.97

12.98

12.99

12.100

Root of hair

THE HUMAN TOUCH: CRITICAL THINKING EXERCISE

The following story and questions are designed to stimulate critical thinking through class discussion or as a brief essay response. There are no right or wrong answers to these questions.

"OK, guys, we're late again." Shaylene Boulay calls out to her two oldest sons, Nathan Jr., 10, and Carl, 12. Grabbing the lunches Nate Sr. packed, she walks out the back door. "Come on Michel, school time!" Shaylene peers under the porch for her five-year-old. Their house is only a mile from the waterfront, and he loves to race cars between their dog Bubba's big paws in the cool sand underneath the porch. "Look at you!" As Shaylene dusts him off and heads to the truck, she notices that the rash of blisters on his leg is still bright red. "Must be ant bites, she thinks."

"Have a good day!" Shaylene hands Nathan and Carl their lunches as they hop out of the truck at the middle school. Next stop, Oak Creek Elementary. As Michel starts to get out, clutching his brown lunch bag tightly, his kindergarten teacher comes rushing over. "Michel, what are you doing here today? Didn't you give your mother the note from the nurse?"

"What note? Michel honey, did you forget to give Mama something from school?" Michel smiles sheepishly and reaches into his shorts pocket for a wadded up piece of paper. The note says: "We believe Michel has impetigo on his leg. This condition is very contagious. Please consult your doctor as soon as possible. We will need a note from him before we can allow Michel to reenter class."

"Oh no," Shaylene thinks. "I'm due for my shift at the diner in 15 minutes. Nobody's home to watch Michel. We don't have the money to see Dr. Gaines again already. And what if this rash on my arm is that thing Michel has?" She sits clutching the wheel of the old pickup, asking herself over and over, "What am I gonna do?"

Suggested Discussion Topics:

1. Look up *impetigo* in a medical dictionary and read its description. Discuss how Shaylene could mistake the symptoms for something else.

2. You work in Dr. Gaines's office and the Boulays have an appointment today. What precautions would you take while seeing this family?

3. Shaylene is having difficulty understanding Dr. Gaines. She asks you to explain. Using information from a medical dictionary and terminology she can understand, describe the symptoms and treatment of impetigo.

4. Discuss Shaylene's responsibility to her children, her job, and the school. Provide her with a solution to her question, "What am I gonna do?"

5. What should Shaylene do to prevent her other children from getting impetigo?

13 The Endocrine System

● Overview of Structures, Combining Forms, and Functions of the Endocrine System

MAJOR STRUCTURES	RELATED COMBINING FORMS	PRIMARY FUNCTIONS
Adrenal Glands (2)	adren/o	Regulate electrolyte levels, influence metabolism, and respond to stress.
Gonads • Male testicles (2) • Female ovaries (2)	gonad/o	Regulate development and maintenance of secondary sex characteristics.
Pancreatic Islets	pancreat/o	Control blood sugar levels and glucose metabolism.
Parathyroid Glands (4)	parathyroid/o	Regulate calcium levels throughout the body.
Pineal Gland (1)	pineal/o	Influences the sleep-wakefulness cycle.
Pituitary Gland (1)	pituit/o, pituitar/o	Secretes hormones that control the activity of the other endocrine glands.
Thymus (1)	thym/o	Plays a major role in the immune reaction.
Thyroid Gland (1)	thyr/o, thyroid/o	Stimulates metabolism, growth, and the activity of the nervous system.

● VOCABULARY   RELATED TO THE ENDOCRINE SYSTEM

The items on this list have been identified as key word parts and terms for this chapter. However, all words in boldface in the text are important and may be included in the learning exercises and tests.

Word Parts

- ☐ acr/o
- ☐ adren/o
- ☐ crin/o
- ☐ -dipsia
- ☐ gonad/o
- ☐ -ism
- ☐ pancreat/o
- ☐ parathyroid/o
- ☐ pineal/o
- ☐ pituitar/o
- ☐ poly-
- ☐ somat/o
- ☐ thym/o
- ☐ thyr/o, thyroid/o
- ☐ -tropin

Medical Terms

- ☐ **acromegaly** (**ack**-roh-**MEG**-ah-lee)
- ☐ **Addison's disease** (**AD**-ih-sonz)
- ☐ **adrenalitis** (ah-**dree**-nal-**EYE**-tis)
- ☐ **aldosteronism** (al-**DOSS**-teh-roh-**niz**-em *or* al-doh-**STER**-ohn-izm)
- ☐ **anabolic steroids** (**an**-ah-**BOL**-ick **STEHR**-oidz)
- ☐ **calcitonin** (**kal**-sih-**TOH**-nin)
- ☐ **chemical thyroidectomy** (**thigh**-roi-**DECK**-toh-mee)
- ☐ **cretinism** (**CREE**-tin-izm)
- ☐ **Cushing's syndrome** (**KUSH**-ingz **SIN**-drohm)
- ☐ **diabetes insipidus** (**dye**-ah-**BEE**-teez in-**SIP**-ih-dus)
- ☐ **diabetes mellitus** (**dye**-ah-**BEE**-teez mel-**EYE**-tus *or* **MEL**-ih-tus)
- ☐ **diabetic retinopathy** (**ret**-ih-**NOP**-ah-thee)
- ☐ **electrolytes** (ee-**LECK**-troh-lytes)
- ☐ **epinephrine** (**ep**-ih-**NEF**-rin)
- ☐ **estrogen** (**ES**-troh-jen)
- ☐ **exophthalmos** (**eck**-sof-**THAL**-mos)
- ☐ **fructosamine test** (fruck-**TOHS**-ah-meen)
- ☐ **gestational diabetes mellitus** (jes-**TAY**-shun-al **dye**-ah-**BEE**-teez mel-**EYE**-tus *or* **MEL**-ih-tus)

- ☐ **gigantism** (jigh-**GAN**-tiz-em)
- ☐ **glucagon** (**GLOO**-kah-gon)
- ☐ **Graves' disease** (**GRAYVZ** dih-**ZEEZ**)
- ☐ **gynecomastia** (**guy**-neh-koh-**MAS**-tee-ah)
- ☐ **Hashimoto's thyroiditis** (hah-shee-**MOH**-tohz **thigh**-roi-**DYE**-tis)
- ☐ **hypercalcemia** (**high**-per-kal-**SEE**-mee-ah)
- ☐ **hypercrinism** (**high**-per-**KRY**-nism)
- ☐ **hyperglycemia** (**high**-per-glye-**SEE**-mee-ah)
- ☐ **hypergonadism** (**high**-per-**GOH**-nad-izm)
- ☐ **hyperinsulinism** (**high**-per-**IN**-suh-lin-izm)
- ☐ **hyperpituitarism** (**high**-per-pih-**TOO**-ih-tah-rizm)
- ☐ **hyperthyroidism** (**high**-per-**THIGH**-roid-izm)
- ☐ **hypocalcemia** (**high**-poh-kal-**SEE**-mee-ah)
- ☐ **hypocrinism** (**high**-poh-**KRY**-nism)
- ☐ **hypoglycemia** (**high**-poh-gly-**SEE**-mee-ah)
- ☐ **hypogonadism** (**high**-poh-**GOH**-nad-izm)
- ☐ **hypopituitarism** (**high**-poh-pih-**TOO**-ih-tah-rizm)
- ☐ **hypothyroidism** (**high**-poh-**THIGH**-roid-izm)
- ☐ **insulinoma** (**in**-suh-lin-**OH**-mah)
- ☐ **laparoscopic adrenalectomy** (ah-**dree**-nal-**ECK**-toh-mee)
- ☐ **myxedema** (**mick**-seh-**DEE**-mah)
- ☐ **oxytocin** (**ock**-sih-**TOH**-sin)
- ☐ **pancreatalgia** (**pan**-kree-ah-**TAL**-jee-ah)
- ☐ **pancreatitis** (**pan**-kree-ah-**TYE**-tis)
- ☐ **pheochromocytoma** (fee-oh-**kroh**-moh-sigh-**TOH**-mah)
- ☐ **pinealectomy** (**pin**-ee-al-**ECK**-toh-mee)
- ☐ **pituitarism** (pih-**TOO**-ih-tar-izm)
- ☐ **pituitary adenoma** (pih-**TOO**-ih-**tair**-ee ad-eh-**NOH**-mah)
- ☐ **polydipsia** (**pol**-ee-**DIP**-see-ah)
- ☐ **polyphagia** (**pol**-ee-**FAY**-jee-ah)
- ☐ **polyuria** (**pol**-ee-**YOU**-ree-ah)
- ☐ **progesterone** (proh-**JES**-ter-ohn)
- ☐ **prolactinoma** (proh-**lack**-tih-**NOH**-mah)
- ☐ **testosterone** (tes-**TOS**-teh-rohn)
- ☐ **tetany** (**TET**-ah-nee)
- ☐ **thymectomy** (thigh-**MECK**-toh-mee)
- ☐ **thymitis** (thigh-**MY**-tis)
- ☐ **thymoma** (thigh-**MOH**-mah)
- ☐ **thymosin** (**THIGH**-moh-sin)
- ☐ **thyromegaly** (**thigh**-roh-**MEG**-ah-lee)
- ☐ **thyrotoxicosis** (**thy**-roh-**tock**-sih-**KOH**-sis)
- ☐ **thyroxine** (thigh-**ROCK**-sin)

● OBJECTIVES

● OBJECTIVES

On completion of this chapter, you should be able to:

1. Describe the role of the endocrine glands in maintaining homeostasis.

2. Name and describe the functions of the primary hormones secreted by each of the endocrine glands.

3. Recognize, define, spell, and pronounce terms relating to the pathology and the diagnostic and treatment procedures of the endocrine glands.

FUNCTIONS OF THE ENDOCRINE SYSTEM

The primary function of the endocrine system is to produce hormones. Because hormones are secreted directly into the bloodstream, they are able to reach cells and organs throughout the body.

A **hormone** is a chemical messenger with a specialized function. The major hormones, their sources, and functions are described in Table 13.1.

Steroid Hormones

Steroid hormones help control metabolism, inflammation, immune functions, salt and water balance, development of sexual characteristics, and the ability to withstand illness and injury.

- The term **steroid** (**STEHR**-oid) describes both hormones produced by the body and artificially produced medications that duplicate the action of the naturally occurring steroids.

Anabolic Steroids

Anabolic steroids (**an**-ah-**BOL**-ick **STEHR**-oidz), which are chemically related to the male sex hormone testosterone, have been used illegally by athletes to increase strength and muscle mass.

- Serious side effects of anabolic steroid use include liver damage, altered body chemistry, testicular shrinkage, and breast development in males, plus unpredictable mood swings and violence.

- Steroid use by teenagers also stops long bone development, resulting in shortened stature.

- The use of steroids usually can be detected through the testing of either blood or urine.

STRUCTURES OF THE ENDOCRINE SYSTEM

There are 13 major glands in the endocrine system (Figure 13.1).

- One **pituitary gland** (divided into two lobes)
- One **thyroid gland**
- Four **parathyroid glands**
- Two **adrenal glands**
- One **pancreas** (**pancreatic islets**)

Table 13.1

HORMONES FROM A TO T		
Hormone	**Source**	**Functions**
Aldosterone	Adrenal cortex	Aids in regulating the levels of salt and water in the body.
Androgens	Adrenal cortex and gonads	Influence sex-related characteristics.
Adrenocorticotropic hormone	Pituitary gland	Stimulates the growth and secretions of the adrenal cortex.
Antidiuretic hormone	Pituitary gland	Helps control blood pressure by reducing the amount of water that is excreted.

Table 13.1 (continued)

HORMONES FROM A TO T		
Hormone	**Source**	**Functions**
Calcitonin	Thyroid gland	Works with the parathyroid hormone to regulate calcium levels in the blood and tissues.
Cortisol	Adrenal cortex	Regulates the metabolism of carbohydrates, fats, and proteins in the body. Also has an anti-inflammatory action.
Epinephrine	Adrenal medulla	Stimulates the sympathetic nervous system.
Estrogen	Ovaries	Develops and maintains the female secondary sex characteristics and regulates the menstrual cycle.
Follicle-stimulating hormone	Pituitary gland	In the female, stimulates the secretion of estrogen and the growth of ova (eggs). In the male, stimulates the production of sperm.
Glucagon	Pancreatic islets	Increases the level of glucose in the bloodstream.
Growth hormone	Pituitary gland	Regulates the growth of bone, muscle, and other body tissues.
Human chorionic gonadotropin	Placenta	Stimulates the secretion of the hormones required to maintain pregnancy.
Insulin	Pancreatic islets	Regulates the transport of glucose to body cells and stimulates the conversion of excess glucose to glycogen for storage.
Lactogenic hormone	Pituitary gland	Stimulates and maintains the secretion of breast milk.
Luteinizing hormone	Pituitary gland	In the female, stimulates ovulation. In the male, stimulates testosterone secretion.
Melatonin	Pineal gland	Influences the sleep-wakefulness cycles.
Norepinephrine	Adrenal medulla	Stimulates the sympathetic nervous system.
Oxytocin	Pituitary gland	Stimulates uterine contractions during childbirth. Causes milk to flow from the mammary glands after childbirth.
Parathyroid hormone	Parathyroid glands	Works with calcitonin to regulate calcium levels in the blood and tissues.
Progesterone	Ovaries	Completes preparation of the uterus for possible pregnancy.
Testosterone	Testicles	Stimulates the development of male secondary sex characteristics.
Thymosin	Thymus	Plays an important role in the immune system.
Thyroid hormones	Thyroid gland	Regulate the rate of metabolism.
Thyroid-stimulating hormone	Pituitary gland	Stimulates the secretion of hormones by the thyroid gland.

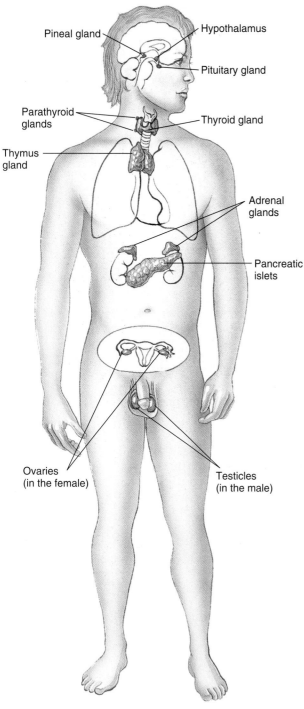

FIGURE 13.1   Structures of the endocrine system.

- One **thymus**
- One **pineal gland**
- Two **gonads** (ovaries in females, testes in males)

MEDICAL SPECIALTIES RELATED TO THE ENDOCRINE SYSTEM

- An **endocrinologist** (en-doh-krih-**NOL**-oh-jist) specializes in diagnosing and treating diseases and malfunctions of the glands of internal secretion (**endo-** means within, **crin** means to secrete, and **-ologist** means specialist).

PATHOLOGY OF THE ENDOCRINE SYSTEM

- **Endocrinopathy** (en-doh-krih-**NOP**-ah-thee) is any disease due to a disorder of the endocrine system (**endo-** means within, **crin/o** means to secrete, and **-pathy** means disease).
- **Hypercrinism** (**high**-per-**KRY**-nism) is a condition caused by excessive secretion of any gland, especially an endocrine gland (**hyper-** means excessive, **crin** means to secrete, and **-ism** means condition). Compare with *hypocrinism.*
- **Hypocrinism** (**high**-poh-**KRY**-nism) is a condition caused by deficient secretion of any gland, especially an endocrine gland (**hypo-** means deficient, **crin** means to secrete, and **-ism** means condition). Compare with *hypercrinism.*

DIAGNOSTIC PROCEDURES RELATED TO THE ENDOCRINE SYSTEM

- Nuclear medicine and imaging techniques are used to diagnose and treat disorders affecting the endocrine system.
- Hormone levels are measured by blood or urine tests. These laboratory tests and diagnostic techniques are described in Chapter 15.

THE PITUITARY GLAND

The pea-sized **pituitary gland** (pih-**TOO**-ih-**tair**-ee) is located at the base of the brain just below the hypothalamus and is composed of anterior and posterior lobes (Figure 13.1).

Functions of the Pituitary Gland

The primary function of the pituitary gland is to secrete hormones that control the activity of the other endocrine glands (Figure 13.2).

- The pituitary acts in response to stimuli from the hypothalamus. This creates a system of checks and balances that maintains an appropriate blood level of each hormone.

The Hypothalamus

The **hypothalamus** (**high**-poh-**THAL**-ah-mus), which is part of the brain, secretes neurohormones that

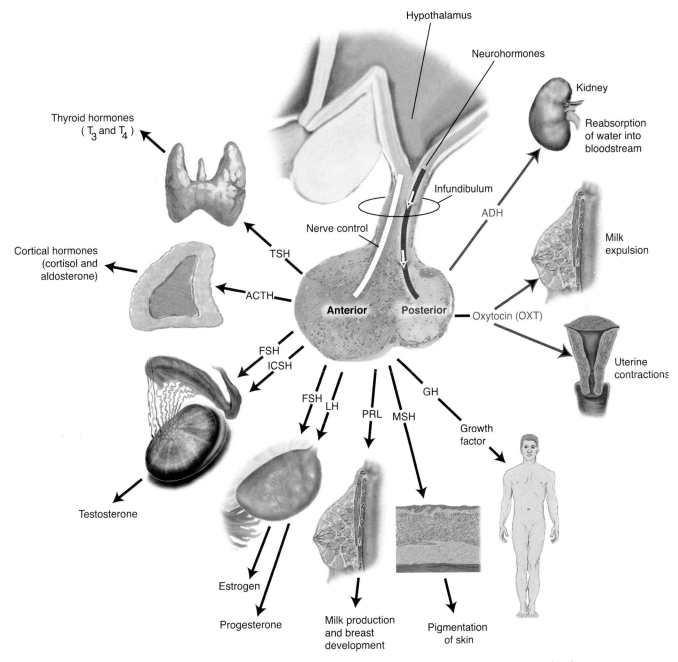

Figure 13.2   The pituitary gland secretes hormones that control the activities of other endocrine glands.

enable it to communicate with other parts of the body. A *neurohormone* is unlike a hormone secreted by the endocrine glands because the neurohormone is secreted by, or acts on, a part of the nervous system.

Secretions of the Pituitary Gland: Anterior Lobe

- The **adrenocorticotropic hormone**, also known as **adrenotropin**, stimulates the growth and secretions of the adrenal cortex (**adren/o** means adrenal glands and **-tropin** means to stimulate).

- The **follicle-stimulating hormone**, also known as **follitropin**, in the female stimulates the secretion of estrogen and the growth of ova (eggs) in the ovaries. In the male, it stimulates the production of sperm in the testicles.

- The **growth hormone**, also known as **somatotropin**, regulates the growth of bone, muscle, and other body tissues (**somat/o** means body and **-tropin** means to stimulate).

- The **lactogenic hormone**, also known as **prolactin**, stimulates and maintains the secretion of breast milk after childbirth (**lact/o** means milk, **gen** means production, and **-ic** means pertaining to).

- The **interstitial cell-stimulating hormone**, also known as **luteinizing hormone** or **luteotropin**, stimulates ovulation in the female. In the male, it stimulates the secretion of testosterone.

- The **melanocyte-stimulating hormone**, also known as **melanotropin**, increases pigmentation of the skin (**melan/o** means black and **-tropin** means to stimulate).

- The **thyroid-stimulating hormone**, also known as **thyrotropin**, stimulates the growth and secretions of the thyroid gland (**thyr/o** means thyroid and **-tropin** means to stimulate).

Secretions of the Pituitary Gland: Posterior Lobe

- The **antidiuretic hormone** maintains the water balance within the body by promoting the reabsorption of water through the kidneys, which are discussed in Chapter 9. When more antidiuretic hormone is secreted, less urine is produced. In contrast, a *diuretic* is a medication that is administered to increase urine secretion.

- **Oxytocin** (**ock**-sih-**TOH**-sin) stimulates uterine contractions during childbirth **oxy-** means swift and **-tocin** means labor). *Pitocin*, a synthetic form of oxytocin, is administered to induce or speed up labor. After childbirth, oxytocin stimulates the flow of milk from the mammary glands.

Pathology of the Pituitary Gland

- **Acromegaly** (**ack**-roh-**MEG**-ah-lee) is enlargement of the extremities (hands and feet) caused by excessive secretion of growth hormone *after* puberty (**acr/o** means extremities and **-megaly** means abnormal enlargement). Compare with *gigantism*.

- **Gigantism** (jigh-**GAN**-tiz-em), also known as **giantism** (**JIGH**-en-tiz-em), is abnormal overgrowth of the body caused by excessive secretion of the growth hormone *before* puberty. Compare with *acromegaly*.

- **Hyperpituitarism** (**high**-per-pih-**TOO**-ih-tah-rizm) is pathology that results in the excessive secretion by the anterior lobe of the pituitary gland (**hyper-** means excessive, **pituitar** means pituitary, and **-ism** means condition). Compare with *hypopituitarism*.

- **Hypopituitarism** (**high**-poh-pih-**TOO**-ih-tah-rizm) is a condition of reduced secretion due to the partial, or complete, loss of the function of the anterior lobe of the pituitary gland (**hypo-** means deficient, **pituitar** means pituitary, and **-ism** means condition). Compare with *hyperpituitarism*.

- **Pituitarism** (pih-**TOO**-ih-tar-izm) is any disorder of pituitary function (**pituitar** means pituitary and **-ism** means condition).

- A **pituitary adenoma** (ad-eh-**NOH**-mah) is a benign tumor of the pituitary gland that causes excess secretion of the adrenocorticotropic hormone. This hormone stimulates the excess production of cortisol, which causes most cases of Cushing's syndrome. See Pathology of the Adrenal Glands later in this chapter.

- A **prolactin-producing adenoma**, also known as a **prolactinoma** (proh-**lack**-tih-**NOH**-mah), is a benign tumor of the pituitary gland that causes it to produce too much prolactin. In females, this overproduction causes infertility and changes in menstruation. In males, it causes impotence.

Diabetes Insipidus

Diabetes insipidus (dye-ah-**BEE**-teez in-**SIP**-ih-dus) is caused by insufficient production of the antidiuretic hormone or by the inability of the kidneys to respond to this hormone. Either cause allows too much fluid to be excreted resulting in extreme polydipsia (excessive thirst) and polyuria (excessive urination). Diabetes insipidus is *not* similar to diabetes mellitus.

Treatment Procedures of the Pituitary Gland

- **Human growth hormone therapy**, also known as **recombinant GH**, is a synthetic version of the growth hormone. It is administered to stimulate growth when the natural supply of growth hormone is insufficient for normal development.

THE THYROID GLAND

The butterfly-shaped **thyroid gland** lies on either side of the larynx, just below the thyroid cartilage (Figure 13.1).

Functions of the Thyroid Gland

- One of the primary functions of the thyroid gland is to regulate the body's metabolism. The term *metab-*

olism describes all of the processes involved in the body's use of nutrients, including the rate at which they are utilized.

- Thyroid secretions also influence growth and the functioning of the nervous system.

Secretions of the Thyroid Gland

- **Thyroxine** (thigh-**ROCK**-sin) and **triiodothyronine** (try-**eye**-oh-doh-**THIGH**-roh-neen), which are the two primary thyroid hormones, influence the rate of metabolism. The secretion of these hormones is controlled by the thyroid-stimulating hormone.

- **Calcitonin** (**kal**-sih-**TOH**-nin), also known as **thyrocalcitonin**, works with the parathyroid hormone to regulate calcium levels in the blood and tissues. Calcitonin decreases blood levels by moving calcium into storage in the bones and teeth. Compare with the function of the *parathyroid hormone*.

Pathology of the Thyroid Gland

- **Hashimoto's thyroiditis** (hah-shee-**MOH**-tohz thigh-roi-**DYE**-tis) is an autoimmune disorder in which the immune system mistakenly attacks thyroid tissue. This begins an inflammatory process that can cause goiter or hypothyroidism, or progressively destroy the gland.

Insufficient Thyroid Secretion

- **Hypothyroidism** (**high**-poh-**THIGH**-roid-izm), also known as an **underactive thyroid**, is a deficiency of thyroid secretion (**hypo-** means deficient, **thyroid** means thyroid, and **-ism** means condition). Symptoms include fatigue, depression, sensitivity to cold, and a decreased metabolic rate.

- **Cretinism** (**CREE**-tin-izm) is a congenital form of hypothyroidism. If treatment is not started soon after birth, cretinism causes arrested physical and mental development.

- **Myxedema** (**mick**-seh-**DEE**-mah) is a severe form of adult hypothyroidism. Symptoms include an enlarged tongue and puffiness of the hands and face.

Excessive Thyroid Secretion

- **Hyperthyroidism** (**high**-per-**THIGH**-roid-izm) is a condition of excessive thyroid hormones in the bloodstream (**hyper-** means excessive, **thyroid** means thyroid, and **-ism** means condition).

Symptoms include an increased metabolic rate, sweating, nervousness, and weight loss.

- **Thyrotoxicosis** (**thy**-roh-**tock**-sih-**KOH**-sis), also known as **thyroid storm**, is a life-threatening condition resulting from the release of excessive quantities of the thyroid hormones into the bloodstream (**thyr/o** means thyroid, **toxic** means poison, and **-osis** means abnormal condition).

Graves' Disease

Graves' disease (**GRAYVZ** dih-**ZEEZ**) is an autoimmune disorder that is a form of hyperthyroidism characterized by goiter and/or exophthalmos.

- **Goiter** (**GOI**-ter), also known as **thyromegaly** (**thigh**-roh-**MEG**-ah-lee), is an abnormal enlargement of the thyroid gland that produces a swelling in the front of the neck (**thyr/o** means thyroid and **-megaly** means abnormal enlargement).

- **Exophthalmos** (**eck**-sof-**THAL**-mos) is an abnormal protrusion of the eyes.

Diagnostic and Treatment Procedures Related to the Thyroid Gland

- A **thyroid-stimulating hormone assay** is a diagnostic test to measure circulating blood levels of thyroid-stimulating hormone. This test is used to detect abnormal thyroid activity resulting from excessive pituitary stimulation.

- A **thyroid scan**, which measures thyroid function, is a form of nuclear medicine that is discussed in Chapter 15.

- An **antithyroid drug** is a medication administered to slow the ability of the thyroid gland to produce thyroid hormones.

- A **chemical thyroidectomy** (**thigh**-roi-**DECK**-toh-mee), also known as **radioactive iodine therapy**, is the administration of radioactive iodine to destroy thyroid cells. This procedure, which destroys at least part of the thyroid gland, is used to treat hyperthyroid disorders such as Graves' disease.

- A **lobectomy** (loh-**BECK**-toh-mee) is the surgical removal of one lobe of the thyroid gland. This term is also used to describe the removal of a lobe of the liver, brain, or lung.

- **Synthetic thyroid hormones** are administered to replace lost thyroid function.

THE PARATHYROID GLANDS

The four **parathyroid glands**, each of which is about the size of a grain of rice, are located within the thyroid gland (Figure 13.1).

Functions of the Parathyroid Glands

The primary function of the parathyroid glands is to regulate calcium levels throughout the body. These calcium levels are important to the smooth functioning of the muscular and nervous systems.

Secretions of the Parathyroid Glands

Parathyroid hormone, also known as or **parathormone**, works with calcitonin to regulate calcium levels in the blood and tissues. The parathyroid hormone *increases* calcium levels in the blood by mobilizing the release of calcium from storage in the bones and teeth. Compare with the function of the *calcitonin*.

Pathology of the Parathyroid Glands

Insufficient Parathyroid Secretion

- **Hypoparathyroidism** (**high**-poh-**par**-ah-**THIGH**-roid-izm) is caused by an insufficient or absent secretion of the parathyroid glands (**hypo-** means deficient, **parathyroid** means parathyroid, and **-ism** means condition). This condition is usually accompanied by hypocalcemia and, in severe cases, leads to tetany.

- **Hypocalcemia** (**high**-poh-kal-**SEE**-mee-ah) is characterized by abnormally low levels of calcium in the blood (**hypo-** means deficient, **calc** means calcium, and **-emia** means blood condition).

- Tetany (**TET**-ah-nee) is characterized by periodic painful muscle spasms and tremors.

Excessive Parathyroid Secretion

- **Hyperparathyroidism** (**high**-per-**par**-ah-**THIGH**-roid-izm) is the overproduction of the parathyroid hormone, PTH. This condition causes hypercalcemia that can lead to weakened bones and the formation of kidney stones.

- **Hypercalcemia** (**high**-per-kal-**SEE**-mee-ah) is characterized by abnormally high concentrations of calcium circulating in the blood instead of being stored in the bones (**hyper-** means excessive, **calc** means calcium, and **-emia** means blood condition).

- **Primary hyperparathyroidism** is caused by a diseased parathyroid gland. **Secondary hyperparathyroidism** is caused by a problem elsewhere in the body. For example, kidney failure causes secondary hyperparathyroidism by making the body resistant to the action of the parathyroid hormone.

Treatment Procedure of the Parathyroid Glands

A **parathyroidectomy** (**par**-ah-**thigh**-roi-**DECK**-toh-mee), which is the surgical removal of one or more of the parathyroid glands, is performed to control hyperparathyroidism.

THE ADRENAL GLANDS

The **adrenal glands**, also known as the **adrenals**, are located one on top of each kidney. Each adrenal gland is surrounded by an adrenal capsule and consists of two parts: the **adrenal cortex**, which is the outer portion, and the **adrenal medulla**, which is the middle portion (Figure 13.3).

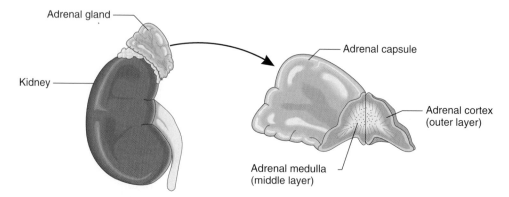

Adrenal gland

Kidney

Adrenal capsule

Adrenal cortex (outer layer)

Adrenal medulla (middle layer)

FIGURE 13.3 There is one adrenal gland on top of each kidney. Each adrenal gland consists of the adrenal cortex and the adrenal medulla surrounded by the adrenal capsule.

Functions of the Adrenal Glands

One of the primary functions of the adrenals is to control electrolyte levels within the body.

- **Electrolytes** (ee-**LECK**-troh-lytes) are mineral substances, such as sodium and potassium, which are normally found in the blood.

- Other important functions of the adrenal glands include helping to regulate metabolism and interacting with the sympathetic nervous system in response to stress.

Secretions of the Adrenal Cortex

Corticosteroid (**kor**-tih-koh-**STEHR**-oid) is the name given to any of the steroid hormones produced by the adrenal cortex and to their synthetic equivalents. These are described in three groups: mineralocorticoids, glucocorticoids, and gonadocorticoids.

- **Mineralocorticoids** regulate the mineral salts in the body. The primary mineralocorticoid is **aldosterone** (al-**DOSS**-ter-ohn), which regulates the salt and water levels in the body by increasing sodium reabsorption in the kidneys. *Reabsorption* means returning a substance to the bloodstream.

- **Glucocorticoids** regulate the metabolism of carbohydrates, fats, and proteins in the body. They also influence blood pressure and have an anti-inflammatory effect. The primary glucocorticoid is **cortisol** (**KOR**-tih-sol), which is also known as **hydrocortisone**.

- **Gonadocorticoids**, also known as **androgens** (**AN**-droh-jenz), are hormones that influence sex-related characteristics. Normally, in adults the production of androgens in the adrenal cortex is minimal; instead, these hormones are produced in the male and female gonads.

Secretions of the Adrenal Medulla

- **Epinephrine** (**ep**-ih-**NEF**-rin), also called **adrenaline** (ah-**DREN**-uh-lin), and **norepinephrine** (**nor**-ep-ih-**NEF**-rin) stimulate the sympathetic nervous system. This stimulation causes an increase in the heart rate and blood pressure. It also produces the other symptoms associated with severe stress. Norepinephrine also has a role as a neurotransmitter. See Chapter 10 for more about neurotransmitters.

Pathology of the Adrenal Glands

- **Adrenalitis** (ah-**dree**-nal-**EYE**-tis) is inflammation of the adrenal glands (**adrenal** means adrenal glands and -**itis** means inflammation).

Insufficient Adrenal Secretions

- **Addison's disease** (**AD**-ih-sonz) is a condition that occurs when the adrenal glands do not produce enough of the hormones cortisol or aldosterone. It is characterized by chronic, worsening fatigue and muscle weakness, loss of appetite, and weight loss.

Excessive Adrenal Secretions

- **Aldosteronism** (al-**DOSS**-teh-roh-**niz**-em *or* al-doh-**STER**-ohn-izm) is an abnormality of electrolyte balance caused by excessive secretion of aldosterone.

  Primary aldosteronism, also known as **Conn's syndrome**, is aldosteronism caused by disorders of the adrenal glands.

  Secondary aldosteronism is *not* caused by a disorder of the adrenal gland. It results from a disorder, such as a nephrotic syndrome, that occurs elsewhere in the body.

- A **pheochromocytoma** (fee-oh-**kroh**-moh-sigh-**TOH**-mah) is a benign tumor of the adrenal medulla that causes the gland to produce excess epinephrine (**phe/o** means dusky, **chrom/o** means dark, **cyt** means cell, and -**oma** means tumor).

Cushing's Syndrome

Cushing's syndrome (**KUSH**-ingz **SIN**-drohm) (**CS**), also known as **hypercortisolism**, is caused by prolonged exposure to high levels of cortisol. The symptoms include a rounded or "moon" face (Figure 13.4).

- CS may be caused by overproduction of cortisol by the body or by taking glucocorticoid hormone medications to treat inflammatory diseases such as asthma and rheumatoid arthritis.

Treatment Procedures of the Adrenal Glands

- A **laparoscopic adrenalectomy** (ah-**dree**-nal-**ECK**-toh-mee) is a minimally invasive procedure to surgically remove one or both adrenal glands (**adrenal** means adrenal gland and -**ectomy** means surgical removal).

- **Cortisone** (**KOR**-tih-sohn), also known as **hydrocortisone**, is the synthetic equivalent of corticosteroids

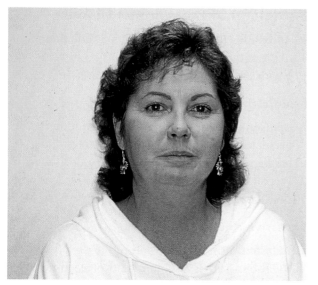

Figure 13.4 Cushing's syndrome causes a characteristic "moon" face. (*Courtesy of Matthew C. Leinung, MD, Acting Head, Division of Endocrinology, Albany Medical College, Albany NY.*)

produced by the body. Cortisone is administered to suppress inflammation and as an immunosuppressant.

- **Epinephrine** is a synthetic hormone used as a vasoconstrictor to treat conditions such as heart dysrhythmias and asthma attacks. A *vasoconstrictor* causes the blood vessels to contract.

THE PANCREATIC ISLETS

The **pancreas** (**PAN**-kree-as) is a feather-shaped organ located posterior to (behind) the stomach (see Figure 13.1). It primary functions primarily as part of the digestive system; these functions are discussed in Chapter 8.

- The **pancreatic islets** (**pan**-kree-**AT**-ick **EYE**-lets), also known as the **islets of Langerhans** (**EYE**-lets of **LAHNG**-er-hahnz), are cells within the pancreas that have an endocrine function.

Functions of the Pancreatic Islets

The functions of the islets are to control blood sugar levels and glucose metabolism throughout the body.

Secretions of the Pancreatic Islets

- **Glucagon** (**GLOO**-kah-gon) is a hormone secreted by the **alpha cells** of the pancreatic islets in response to low blood sugar levels. Glucagon increases the amount of glucose by stimulating the liver to convert glycogen into glucose for release into the bloodstream. *Glycogen* is the form in which the liver stores the excess glucose. *Glucose,* also known as blood sugar, is the basic form of energy used by the body.

- **Insulin** (**IN**-suh-lin) is secreted by the **beta cells** of the pancreatic islets in response to high blood sugar levels. It functions in two ways. First, insulin allows glucose to enter the cells for use as energy. When additional glucose is *not* needed, insulin stimulates the liver to convert glucose into glycogen for storage.

Pathology of the Pancreas

- **Hyperglycemia** (**high**-per-glye-**SEE**-mee-ah) is an abnormally high concentration of glucose in the blood (**hyper-** means excessive, **glyc** means sugar, and **-emia** means blood condition). Hyperglycemia is seen especially in patients with diabetes mellitus. The symptoms include polydipsia, polyphagia, and polyuria.

  Polydipsia (**pol**-ee-**DIP**-see-ah) is excessive thirst (**poly-** means many and **-dipsia** means thirst).

  Polyphagia (**pol**-ee-**FAY**-jee-ah) is excessive hunger (**poly-** means many and **-phagia** means eating).

  Polyuria (**pol**-ee-**YOU**-ree-ah) is excessive urination (**poly-** means many and **-uria** means urination).

- **Hyperinsulinism** (**high**-per-**IN**-suh-lin-izm) is a condition marked by excessive secretion of insulin (**hyper-** means excessive, **insulin** means insulin, and **-ism** means condition). Hyperinsulinism causes hypoglycemia.

- **Hypoglycemia** (**high**-poh-glye-**SEE**-mee-ah) is an abnormally low concentration of glucose (sugar) in the blood (**hypo-** means deficient, **glyc** means sugar, and **-emia** means blood condition).

- An **insulinoma** (**in**-suh-lin-**OH**-mah) is a benign tumor of the pancreas that causes hypoglycemia (**insulin** means insulin and **-oma** means tumor).

- **Pancreatalgia** (**pan**-kree-ah-**TAL**-jee-ah) is pain in the pancreas (**pancreat** means pancreas and **-algia** means pain).

- **Pancreatitis** (**pan**-kree-ah-**TYE**-tis) is an inflammation of the pancreas (**pancreat** means pancreas and **-itis** means inflammation).

Diabetes Mellitus

Diabetes mellitus (**dye**-ah-**BEE**-teez mel-**EYE**-tus *or* **MEL**-ih-tus) is a group of metabolic disorders characterized by hyperglycemia resulting from defects in insulin secretion, insulin action, or both.

- Although these are described as two distinct types, type 1 and type 2, many patients do not fit into a single category, and the treatment goals are to most effectively control the blood sugar levels and prevent diabetic complications.

Type 1 Diabetes

Type 1 diabetes, previously known as **insulin-dependent diabetes mellitus** or **juvenile diabetes**, is an autoimmune insulin deficiency disorder. Because this disorder involves the destruction of pancreatic islet beta cells, the body does not secrete insulin.

- Symptoms of type 1 diabetes include polydipsia, polyphagia, polyuria, weight loss, blurred vision, extreme fatigue, and slow healing.

- Type 1 diabetes is treated with carefully regulated insulin replacement therapy, diet, and exercise.

Type 2 Diabetes

Type 2 diabetes, previously known as **non-insulin-dependent diabetes mellitus**, is an insulin resistance disorder. Although insulin is being produced, the body does not use it effectively. In an attempt to compensate, the body secretes more insulin.

- With the rise in childhood obesity, type 2 diabetes is increasingly occurring in children and young adults.

- Type 2 diabetes may have no symptoms for years. When symptoms do occur, they include those of type 1 diabetes plus recurring infections, irritability, and a tingling sensation in the hands or feet.

- Type 2 diabetes is usually treated with diet, exercise, and medications.

- **Oral hypoglycemics** lower blood sugar by causing the body to release more insulin.

- **Glucophage** (metformin hydrochloride) and similar medications work within the cells to combat insulin resistance and to help insulin let blood sugar into the cells.

Gestational Diabetes Mellitus

Gestational diabetes mellitus (jes-**TAY**-shun-al **dye**-ah-**BEE**-teez mel-**EYE**-tus *or* **MEL**-ih-tus) is the form of diabetes that occurs during some pregnancies. This condition usually disappears after delivery; however, many of these women later develop type 2 diabetes.

Diabetes Mellitus Diagnostic Procedures

- A **fasting blood sugar test** measures the glucose (blood sugar) levels after the patient has not eaten for eight to 12 hours. This test is used to screen for, and to monitor treatment of, diabetes mellitus.

- An **oral glucose tolerance test** (**GLOO**-kohs) is performed to confirm a diagnosis of diabetes mellitus and to aid in diagnosing hypoglycemia.

- **Home blood glucose monitoring** measures the current blood sugar level. This test, which requires a drop of blood, is performed by the patient.

- The **fructosamine test** (fruck-**TOHS**-ah-meen) measures average glucose levels over the past three weeks. The fructosamine test is able to detect changes more rapidly than the HbA1c test.

- **Hemoglobin A1c testing**, also known as **HbA1c** and pronounced as "**H-B A-one-C**," is a blood test that measures the average blood glucose level over the previous three to four months. This test is used to evaluate how well blood sugar levels have been controlled during this time period. It may also be used as a screening test to detect diabetes mellitus.

Diabetic Emergencies

Diabetic emergencies are due to either too much, or too little blood sugar. Treatment depends on accurately diagnosing the cause of the emergency (Figure 13.5).

- **Insulin shock** is caused by very low blood sugar (hypoglycemia). A sugary substance that can quickly be absorbed into the bloodstream is administered to rapidly raise the blood sugar level.

- **Diabetic coma** is caused by very high blood sugar (hyperglycemia). Also known as **diabetic ketoacidosis** (**kee**-toh-**ass**-ih-**DOH**-sis), this condition is treated by the prompt administration of insulin.

Diabetic Complications

Most diabetic complications result from the damage to capillaries and other blood vessels due to long-term exposure to excessive blood sugar.

- **Heart disease** occurs because excess blood sugar makes the walls of the blood vessels sticky and rigid. This encourages hypertension and atherosclerosis. (See Chapter 5.)

- **Kidney disease** may lead to renal failure because damage to the blood vessel reduces blood flow through the kidneys. (See Chapter 9.)

- **Neuropathy** (new-**ROP**-ah-thee) is damage to the nerves. When this occurs in the hands and feet it is

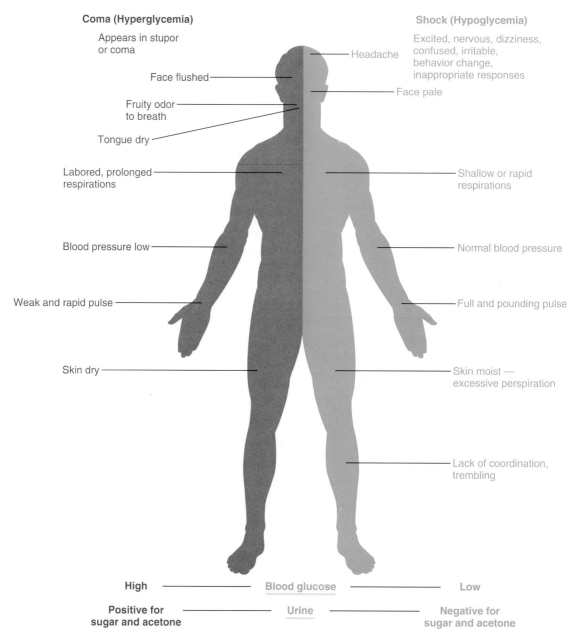

Coma (Hyperglycemia)	Shock (Hypoglycemia)
Appears in stupor or coma	Excited, nervous, dizziness, confused, irritable, behavior change, inappropriate responses
	Headache
Face flushed	
	Face pale
Fruity odor to breath	
Tongue dry	
Labored, prolonged respirations	Shallow or rapid respirations
Blood pressure low	Normal blood pressure
Weak and rapid pulse	Full and pounding pulse
Skin dry	Skin moist — excessive perspiration
	Lack of coordination, trembling

High ——— Blood glucose ——— **Low**

Positive for sugar and acetone ——— Urine ——— **Negative for sugar and acetone**

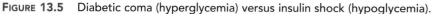

FIGURE 13.5 Diabetic coma (hyperglycemia) versus insulin shock (hypoglycemia).

known as *peripheral neuropathy* and causes pain, tingling, or numbness. (See Chapter 10.)

- **Diabetic retinopathy** (**ret**-ih-**NOP**-ah-thee) (**DR**) occurs when diabetes damages the tiny blood vessels in the retina of the eye. This can lead to blindness. *Retinopathy* means any disease of the retina (**retin/o** means retina and **-pathy** means disease). (See Chapter 11.)

Treatment Procedure of the Pancreas

- A **pancreatectomy** (**pan**-kree-ah-**TECK**-toh-mee) is the surgical removal of the pancreas (**pancreat**

means pancreas and **-ectomy** means surgical removal). This procedure, which is performed to treat pancreatic cancer, is referred to as a *total pancreatectomy*. This procedure involves the removal of the pancreas plus the attached organs (the spleen, gallbladder, common bile duct, and portions of the small intestine and stomach).

THE THYMUS

The **thymus** (**THIGH**-mus) is located near the midline in the anterior portion of the thoracic cavity. It is posterior to (behind) the sternum and slightly superior to (above) the heart (Figure 13.1).

Functions of the Thymus

The hormone secreted by the thymus plays an important role in the immune system.

Secretions of the Thymus

- **Thymosin** (**THIGH**-moh-sin) stimulates the maturation of lymphocytes into T cells of the immune system.

Pathology of the Thymus

- **Thymitis** (thigh-**MY**-tis) is an inflammation of the thymus gland (**thym** means thymus and **-itis** means inflammation).
- A **thymoma** (thigh-**MOH**-mah) is a usually benign tumor derived from the tissue of the thymus (**thym** means thymus and **-oma** means tumor).

Treatment Procedure of the Thymus

- A **thymectomy** (thigh-**MECK**-toh-mee) is the surgical removal of the thymus gland (**thym** means thymus and **-ectomy** means surgical removal).

THE PINEAL GLAND

The **pineal gland** (**PIN**-ee-al), which is very small and shaped something like a pine cone, is located in the central portion of the brain.

Functions of the Pineal Gland

- The function of the pineal gland is not clearly understood. However, the pineal gland is known to influence the sleep-wakefulness cycle.

Secretion of the Pineal Gland

- The hormone **melatonin** (**mel**-ah-**TOH**-nin) influences the sleep and wakefulness portions of the circadian cycle. The term *circadian cycle* refers to the biological functions that occur within a 24-hour period.

Pathology of the Pineal Gland

- **Pinealopathy** (pin-ee-ah-**LOP**-ah-thee) is any disorder of the pineal gland (**pineal/o** means pineal gland and **-pathy** means disease).

Treatment Procedures of the Pineal Gland

- A **pinealectomy** (**pin**-ee-al-**ECK**-toh-mee) is the surgical removal of the pineal body (**pineal** means pineal gland and **-ectomy** means surgical removal).

THE GONADS

The **gonads** (**GOH**-nadz), which are ovaries in females and testicles in males, are the gamete-producing glands.

- A **gamete** (**GAM**-eet) is a reproductive cell. This is the sperm in the male and ova (eggs) in the female.
- A **gonadotropic hormone** (gon-ah-doh-**TROHP**-ick), also known as **gonadotropin**, is any hormone that stimulates the gonads (**gonad/o** means gonad and **-tropin** means to stimulate).

Functions of the Gonads

- The gonads secrete the hormones that are responsible for the development and maintenance of the secondary sex characteristics that develop during puberty. The additional functions of these glands are discussed in Chapter 14.
- **Puberty** is the condition of first being capable of reproducing sexually. It is marked by maturing of the genital organs, development of secondary sex characteristics, and by the first occurrence of menstruation in the female. The average age at which puberty occurs is 14 in boys and 12 in girls.
- *Precocious puberty* is the early onset of the changes of puberty. This is before age 9 in females and before age 10 in males.

Secretions of the Testicles

- **Testosterone** (tes-**TOS**-teh-rohn), which is secreted by the testicles, stimulates the development of male secondary sex characteristics (Figure 13.6).

Secretions of the Ovaries

- **Estrogen** (**ES**-troh-jen) is important in the development and maintenance of the female secondary sex characteristics and in regulation of the menstrual cycle (Figure 13.7).
- **Progesterone** (proh-**JES**-ter-ohn) is the hormone released during the second half of the menstrual cycle by the corpus luteum in the ovary. Its function is to complete the preparations for pregnancy.

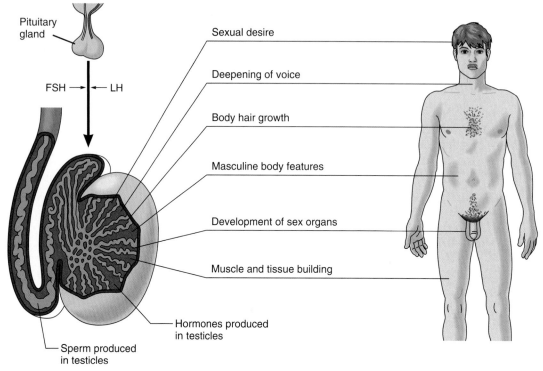

FIGURE 13.6   The secondary sex characteristics in the male produced by the secretion of testosterone.

- If pregnancy occurs, the placenta takes over the production of progesterone.
- If pregnancy does not occur, secretion of the hormone stops and is followed by the menstrual period.

The Placenta

During pregnancy the **placenta** secretes the hormone **human chorionic gonadotropin** (**kor**-ee-**ON**-ick **gon**-ah-doh-**TROH**-pin) to stimulate the corpus luteum to

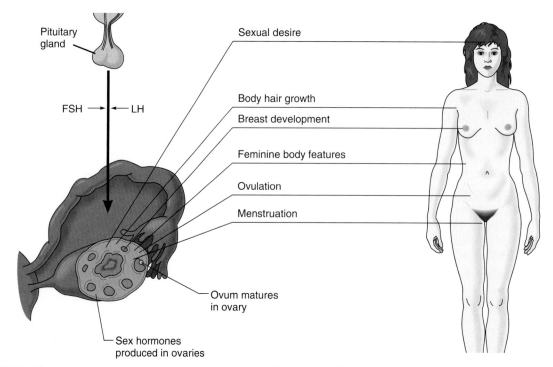

FIGURE 13.7   The secondary sex characteristics in the female produced by the secretion of estrogen.

continue producing the hormones required to maintain the pregnancy. It also stimulates the hormones required to stimulate lactation after childbirth. The corpus luteum and placenta are discussed in Chapter 14.

Pathology of the Gonads

- **Hypergonadism** (**high**-per-**GOH**-nad-izm) is the condition of excessive secretion of hormones by the sex glands (**hyper-** means excessive, **gonad** means sex gland, and **-ism** means condition).

- **Hypogonadism** (**high**-poh-**GOH**-nad-izm) is the condition of deficient secretion of hormones by the sex glands (**hypo-** means deficient, **gonad** means sex gland, and **-ism** means condition).

- **Gynecomastia** (**guy**-neh-koh-**MAS**-tee-ah) is the condition of excessive mammary development in

the male (**gynec/o** means female, **mast** means breast, and **-ia** means abnormal condition).

Treatment Procedures of the Gonads

Treatment procedures of the gonads are discussed in Chapter 14.

ABBREVIATIONS RELATED TO THE ENDOCRINE SYSTEM

Table 13.2 presents an overview of the abbreviations related to the terms introduced in this chapter. *Note:* To avoid errors or confusion, always be cautious when using abbreviations.

Table 13.2

ABBREVIATIONS RELATED TO THE ENDOCRINE SYSTEM

adrenocorticotropic hormone = ACTH	**ACTH** = adrenocorticotropic hormone
aldosterone = ALD	**ALD** = aldosterone
antidiuretic hormone = ADH	**ADH** = antidiuretic hormone
calcitonin = CAL	**CAL** = calcitonin
Cushing's syndrome = CS	**CS** = Cushing's syndrome
diabetes insipidus = DI	**DI** = diabetes insipidus
diabetes mellitus = DM	**DM** = diabetes mellitus
diabetic retinopathy = DR, DRP	**DR, DRP** = diabetic retinopathy
epinephrine = Epi, EPI	**Epi, EPI** = epinephrine
fasting blood sugar = FBS	**FBS** = fasting blood sugar
follicle-stimulating hormone = FSH	**FSH** = follicle-stimulating hormone
fructosamine test = FA	**FA** = fructosamine test
gestational diabetes mellitus = GDM	**GDM** = gestational diabetes mellitus
glucagon = GCG	**GCG** = glucagon
Graves' disease = GD	**GD** = Graves' disease
growth hormone = GH	**GH** = growth hormone

(continues)

Table 13.2 (continued)

ABBREVIATIONS RELATED TO THE ENDOCRINE SYSTEM

Hashimoto's thyroiditis = HT	**HT** = Hashimoto's thyroiditis
home blood glucose monitoring = HBGM	**HBGM** = home blood glucose monitoring
human chorionic gonadotropin = HCG	**HCG** = human chorionic gonadotropin
hyperparathyroidism = HP	**HP** = hyperparathyroidism
hypoglycemia = HG	**HG** = hypoglycemia
interstitial cell-stimulating hormone = ICSH	**ICSH** = interstitial cell-stimulating hormone
lactogenic hormone = LTH	**LTH** = lactogenic hormone
luteinizing hormone = LH	**LH** = luteinizing hormone
melanocyte-stimulating hormone = MSH	**MSH** = melanocyte-stimulating hormone
oral glucose tolerance test = OGTT	**OGTT** = oral glucose tolerance test
oxytocin = OXT	**OXT** = oxytocin
parathyroid hormone = PTH	**PTH** = parathyroid hormone
pheochromocytoma = PC	**PC** = pheochromocytoma
thyroid-stimulating hormone = TSH	**TSH** = thyroid-stimulating hormone
triiodothyronine = T_3	**T_3** = triiodothyronine
thyroxine = T_4	**T_4** = thyroxine

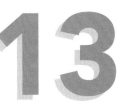
Learning Exercises

● Matching Word Parts 1

Write the correct answer in the middle column.

Definition	Correct Answer	Possible Answers
13.1. adrenal glands	_____	acr/o
13.2. extremities	_____	adren/o
13.3. ovaries or testicles	_____	crin/o
13.4. to secrete	_____	-dipsia
13.5. thirst	_____	gonad/o

● Matching Word Parts 2

Write the correct answer in the middle column.

Definition	Correct Answer	Possible Answers
13.6. pituitary	_____	-ism
13.7. pineal gland	_____	pancreat/o
13.8. pancreas	_____	parathyroid/o
13.9. parathyroid	_____	pineal/o
13.10. condition	_____	pituitar/o

● Matching Word Parts 3

Write the correct answer in the middle column.

Definition	Correct Answer	Possible Answers
13.11. to stimulate or act on	_____	poly-
13.12. thyroid gland	_____	somat/o
13.13. thymus, soul	_____	thym/o
13.14. many	_____	thyroid/o
13.15. body	_____	-tropin

● Definitions

Select the correct answer and write it on the line provided.

13.16. The hormone that stimulates ovulation is _____ .

      estrogen   follicle-stimulating hormone   luteinizing hormone   progesterone

13.17. The endocrine gland that secretes hormones that control the activity of the other endocrine glands is the

      _____ gland.

      adrenal   hypothalamus   pituitary   thymus

13.18. The growth and secretion of the adrenal cortex is stimulated by the _____ hormone.

    adrenocorticotropic   growth   melanocyte-stimulating   thyroid-stimulating

13.19. The _____ gland(s) also play(s) an important role in immune reactions.

      adrenal   parathyroid   pineal   thymus

13.20. The hormone that works with the parathyroid hormone to regulate calcium levels in the blood and

      tissues is _____ .

      aldosterone   calcitonin   glucagon   luteotropin

13.21. Cortisol is secreted by the _____ .

      adrenal cortex   pituitary gland   thymus   thyroid

13.22. The amount of glucose in the bloodstream is increased by the hormone _____ .

      adrenaline   glucagon   hydrocortisone   insulin

13.23. Norepinephrine is secreted by the _____ .

adrenal medulla   pancreatic islets   ovaries   testicles

13.24. Uterine contractions during childbirth are stimulated by the hormone _____ .

estrogen   lactogenic   oxytocin   thymosin

13.25. The development of the male secondary sex characteristics is stimulated by the hormone

_____ .

aldosterone   parathyroid   progesterone   testosterone

● Matching Structures

Write the correct answer in the middle column.

Definition	Correct Answer	Possible Answers
13.26. control blood sugar levels	_____	adrenal glands
13.27. influences the sleep- wakefulness cycle	_____	pancreatic islets
13.28. regulate electrolyte levels	_____	pineal gland
13.29. stimulates metabolism	_____	pituitary gland
13.30. controls the activity of other glands	_____	thyroid gland

---

● Which Word?

Select the correct answer and write it on the line provided.

13.31. Insufficient secretion of the parathyroid glands causes _____ .

hyperparathyroidism   hypoparathyroidism

13.32. The growth hormone is also known as _____ .

somatotropin   thyrotropin

13.33. The hormones that influence sex-related characteristics are known as _____ .

glucocorticoids   gonadocorticoids

13.34. Insulin replacement therapy is always used in _____ mellitus.

type 1 diabetes   type 2 diabetes

13.35. An insufficient production of ADH causes _____ .

diabetes insipidus   diabetes mellitus

● Spelling Counts

Find the misspelled word in each sentence. Then write that word, spelled correctly, on the line provided.

13.36. Metebolism is the rate at which the body uses energy and the speed at which body functions work.

_____

13.37. Diabetes melletus is a group of diseases characterized by defects in insulin production, use, or both.

_____

13.38. Hydrocortizone has an anti-inflammatory effect. _____

13.39. The hormone progestarone is released during the second half of the menstrual cycle.

_____

13.40. Thymosin is secreted by the thymos gland. _____

● Abbreviation Identification

In the space provided, write the words that each abbreviation stands for.

13.41. **ACTH**   _____

13.42. **ADH**   _____

13.43. **GDM**   _____

13.44. **OGTT**   _____

13.45. **FSH**   _____

● Term Selection

Select the correct answer and write it on the line provided.

13.46. A condition caused by excessive secretion of any gland is known as _____ .

    endocrinopathy   goiter   hypercrinism   hypocrinism

13.47. The life-threatening condition that results from the presence of excessive quantities of the thyroid

    hormones is known as _____ .

    aldosteronism   Cushing's syndrome   Graves' disease   thyrotoxicosis

13.48. The four endocrine glands that are about the size of a grain of rice are the _____ .

    adrenals   pancreatic islets   parathyroids   pineals

13.49. A prolactin-producing adenoma, also known as a/an _____ is a benign tumor of

    the pituitary gland.

    insuloma   pheochromocytoma   pituitary adenoma   prolactinoma

13.50. The average blood sugar over the past three weeks is measured by the _____ blood test.

    blood sugar monitoring   fructosamine   glucose tolerance   hemoglobin A1c

---

● Sentence Completion

Write the correct term on the line provided.

13.51. Substances, such as sodium and potassium, that are found in the blood are known as

    _____ .

13.52. Calcitonin and _____ are secreted by the thyroid gland.

13.53. Damage to the retina of the eye caused by diabetes mellitus is known as diabetic _____ .

13.54. The medical term that describes a severe form of adult hypothyroidism, with symptoms that include an

    enlarged tongue and puffiness of the hands and face is _____ .

13.55. Abnormal protrusion of the eyes associated with Graves' disease is known as

    _____ .

● Word Surgery

Divide each term into its component word parts. Write these word parts, in sequence, on the lines provided.

When necessary use a back slash (/) to indicate a combining vowel. (You may not need all of the lines provided.)

13.56. **Hyperpituitarism** is pathology that results in the excessive secretion by the anterior lobe of the pituitary gland.

_____   _____   _____   _____

13.57. **Hypoglycemia** is an abnormally low concentration of glucose (sugar) in the blood.

_____   _____   _____   _____

13.58. **Hyperinsulinism** is marked by excessive secretion of insulin that produces hypoglycemia.

_____   _____   _____   _____

13.59. **Gynecomastia** is excessive mammary development in the male.

_____   _____   _____   _____

13.60. **Hypocalcemia** is characterized by abnormally low levels of calcium in the blood.

_____   _____   _____   _____

● True/False

If the statement is true, write **T** on the line. If the statement is false, write **F** on the line.

13.61. _____ The alpha cells of the pancreatic islets secrete insulin.

13.62. _____ Precocious puberty is the early onset of the changes of puberty.

13.63. _____ Human chorionic gonadotropin (HCG) is secreted by the adrenal cortex.

13.64. _____ The growth hormone (GH) is secreted by the pineal gland.

13.65. _____ Goiter is also known as thyromegaly.

● Clinical Conditions

Write the correct answer on the line provided.

13.66. Grace McClelland was treated for a tumor derived from the tissue of the thymus. The medical term for this condition is a/an _____ .

13.67. Joseph Butler complains of being thirsty all the time. His doctor listed this excessive thirst on his chart as

_____ .

13.68. Carmella DeFillipo is being treated for _____ _____ , which

is an insulin resistance disorder.

13.69. Linda Thomas has a progressive disease that occurs when adrenal glands do not produce enough corti-

sol. This condition is known as _____ disease.

13.70. Patrick Edward has the autoimmune disorder Hashimoto's _____. In this condition

the immune system mistakenly attacks thyroid tissue and begins an inflammatory process that may pro-

gressively destroy the gland.

13.71. When "the champ" was training for the Olympics, he was tempted to use _____

steroids to increase his strength and muscle mass.

13.72. Leigh Franklin developed a condition that is characterized by extremely large hands and feet. The med-

ical term for this condition is _____ .

13.73. As a result of a congenital lack of thyroid secretion, the Vaugh-Eames child suffers from arrested physical

and mental development. The medical term for this condition is _____ .

13.74. Raymond Grovenor is excessively tall and large. This condition, which was caused by excessive function-

ing of the pituitary gland before puberty, is known as _____ .

13.75. Rose Liu required the surgical removal of her pancreas. The medical term for this procedure is a/an

_____ .

● **Which Is the Correct Medical Term?**

Select the correct answer and write it on the line provided.

13.76. Conn's syndrome is also known as _____ .

    hypercortisolism   hypothyroidism   primary aldosteronism   secondary aldosteronism

13.77. A benign tumor of the pituitary gland that causes the excess secretion of ACTH is known as a/an

_____ .

    hyperpituitarism   hypopituitarism   pituitary adenoma   prolactinoma

13.78. The autoimmune disorder that is characterized by exophthalmos is known as

_____ .

    Graves' disease   hypothyroidism   Hashimoto's thyroiditis   thyrotoxicosis

13.79. The diabetic emergency caused by very high blood sugar is _____ .

    diabetic coma   hypoglycemia   insulin shock   insuloma

13.80. The hormone _____ influences the sleep-wakefulness cycles.

    glucagon   melatonin   parathyroid   thymosin

● Challenge Word Building

These terms are *not* found in this chapter; however, they are made up of the following familiar word parts. You may want to look in the glossary or use a medical dictionary to check your answers.

endo-	adren/o	-emia
	crin/o	-itis
	insulin/o	-megaly
	pancreat/o	-ology
	pineal/o	-oma
	thym/o	-otomy
	thyroid/o	-pathy

13.81. The term meaning a surgical incision into the thyroid gland is a/an _____ .

13.82. The study of the endocrine glands and their secretions is known as _____ .

13.83. The term meaning enlargement of the adrenal glands is _____ .

13.84. The term meaning any disease of the thymus gland is _____ .

13.85. The term meaning an inflammation of the thyroid gland is _____ .

13.86. The term meaning a surgical incision into the pancreas is a/an _____ .

13.87. The term meaning any disease of the adrenal glands is _____ .

13.88. The term meaning a tumor of the pineal gland is a/an _____ .

13.89. The term meaning abnormally high levels of insulin in the blood is _____ .

13.90. The term meaning an inflammation of the adrenal glands is _____ .

● Labeling Exercises

Identify the numbered items on the accompanying figure.

13.91. _____ gland

13.92. _____ glands

13.93. _____ gland

13.94. _____ of the female

13.95. _____

13.96. _____ gland

13.97. _____ gland

13.98. _____ glands

13.99. _____ islets

13.100. _____ of the male

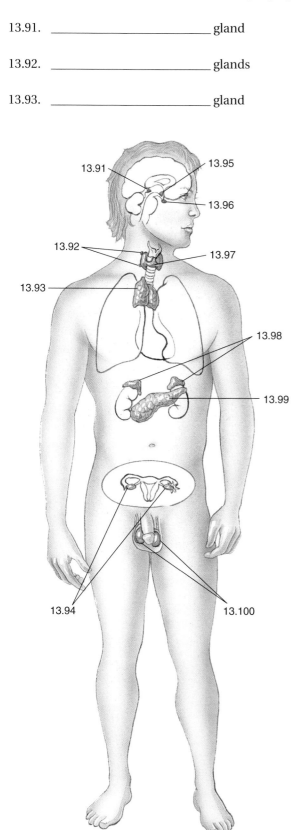

THE HUMAN TOUCH: CRITICAL THINKING EXERCISE

The following story and questions are designed to stimulate critical thinking through class discussion or as a brief essay response. There are no right or wrong answers to these questions.

By the time 14-year-old Jacob Tuls got home, he was sick enough for his mom to notice. He seemed shaky and confused and was sweaty even though the fall weather was cool. "Jake, let's get you a glass of juice right away," his mother said as calmly as she could. She was all too familiar with the symptoms of hypoglycemia brought on by Jake's type 1 diabetes. Ever since he was diagnosed at age six, she had carefully monitored his insulin, eating, and exercise. But now that he was in middle school, the ball was in his court, and it really worried her that he often seemed to mess up.

"Yeah, I know I shouldn't have gone so long without eating," Jake muttered once he was feeling better. "But you don't understand. I don't want to be different from the other kids." Before he could finish, his mom was on the telephone to the school nurse's office.

Jacob needed to inject himself with insulin three times a day. He knew what happened when his blood sugar got too high or if he didn't eat on schedule and it got too low. But when he was with his friends, he hated to go up to the chaperone on a field trip and say that he needed to eat something right away. And he hated it when some kid walked in while he was injecting. His mom had made arrangements with the school nurse for him to go to her office to get some privacy, but whenever he didn't show up between fourth and fifth period, she'd come into the classroom to get him as if he was some kind of sick "dweeb."

He was tired of having this disease, sick of shots, and angry that he couldn't sleep late and skip meals like other kids. He made a face at his mother as she talked on the telephone to the nurse, and slammed the back door on his way out to find his friend Joe.

Suggested Discussion Topics:

1. What could Jacob's parents do to help him get through this rough time of his life?
2. Why is it more difficult for Jacob to maintain his injection routine in middle school than it was in elementary school?
3. Knowing that missing an insulin injection could cause a diabetic coma and death, why wouldn't Jacob be more conscientious?
4. Do you think Jacob's schoolmates talk about him, or does he just think they do? Discuss both possibilities.
5. People with juvenile diabetes can live close to a normal life span if they follow a healthy routine. Discuss stages in their lives at which they might have the most difficulties with this disease.

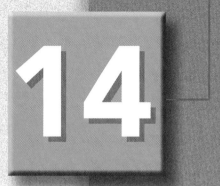

The Reproductive Systems

Overview of Structures, Combining Forms, and Functions of the Reproductive Systems

MAJOR STRUCTURES	RELATED COMBINING FORMS	PRIMARY FUNCTIONS
MALE		
Penis	pen/i, phalll/i	Used for sexual intercourse and urination.
Testicles, Testes	orch/o, orchid/o, test/i, test/o, testicul/o	Produce sperm and the male hormone testosterone.
FEMALE		
Ovaries	oophor/o, ovari/o	Produce ova (eggs) and female hormones.
Fallopian Tubes	salping/o	Catch mature ova, provide the site for fertilization, transport ova to uterus.
Uterus	hyster/o, metr/o, metri/o, uter/o	Protects and supports the developing child.
Vagina	vagin/o, colp/o	Used for sexual intercourse and also serves as channel for menstrual flow and birth.
Placenta	placent/o	Exchanges nutrients and waste between the mother and fetus during pregnancy.

● VOCABULARY   RELATED TO THE REPRODUCTIVE SYSTEMS

The items on this list have been identified as key word parts and terms for this chapter. However, all words in boldface in the text are also important and may be included in learning exercises and tests.

Word Parts

- [ ] cervic/o
- [ ] colp/o
- [ ] -gravida
- [ ] gynec/o
- [ ] hyster/o
- [ ] mamm/o
- [ ] men/o
- [ ] nulli-
- [ ] oophor/o
- [ ] orchid/o
- [ ] ov/o
- [ ] -para
- [ ] -pexy
- [ ] prostat/o
- [ ] salping/o

Medical Terms

- [ ] **ablation** (ab-**LAY**-shun)
- [ ] **abruptio placentae** (ab-**RUP**-shee-oh plah-**SEN**-tee)
- [ ] **amenorrhea** (ah-**men**-oh-**REE**-ah *or* ay-**men**-oh-**REE**-ah)
- [ ] **anorchism** (an-**OR**-kizm)
- [ ] **azoospermia** (ay-**zoh**-oh-**SPER**-mee-ah)
- [ ] **benign prostatic hypertrophy** (pros-**TAT**-ick high-**PER**-troh-fee)
- [ ] **bilateral hysterosalpingo-oophorectomy** (hiss-ter-oh-sal-**ping**-goh oh-**ahf**-oh-**RECK**-toh-mee)
- [ ] **cervical dysplasia** (**SER**-vih-kal dis-**PLAY**-see-ah)
- [ ] **cervicitis** (**ser**-vih-**SIGH**-tis)
- [ ] **chlamydia** (klah-**MID**-ee-ah)
- [ ] **colpopexy** (**KOL**-poh-**peck**-see)
- [ ] **colporrhaphy** (kol-**POR**-ah-fee)
- [ ] **colposcopy** (kol-**POS**-koh-pee)
- [ ] **dysmenorrhea** (**dis**-men-oh-**REE**-ah)
- [ ] **ectopic pregnancy** (eck-**TOP**-ick)
- [ ] **endocervicitis** (**en**-doh-**ser**-vih-**SIGH**-tis)
- [ ] **endometriosis** (**en**-doh-**mee**-tree-**OH**-sis)

- [ ] **epididymitis** (ep-ih-did-ih-**MY**-tis)
- [ ] **episiorrhaphy** (eh-**piz**-ee-**OR**-ah-fee)
- [ ] **episiotomy** (eh-**piz**-ee-**OT**-oh-mee)
- [ ] **fibrocystic breast disease** (**figh**-broh-**SIS**-tick)
- [ ] **galactorrhea** (gah-**lack**-toh-**REE**-ah)
- [ ] **gonorrhea** (**gon**-oh-**REE**-ah)
- [ ] **hydrocele** (**HIGH**-droh-seel)
- [ ] **hypomenorrhea** (**high**-poh-men-oh-**REE**-ah)
- [ ] **hysterectomy** (**hiss**-teh-**RECK**-toh-mee)
- [ ] **hysterosalpingography** (**hiss**-ter-oh-**sal**-pin-**GOG**-rah-fee)
- [ ] **hysteroscopy** (**hiss**-ter-**OSS**-koh-pee)
- [ ] **leukorrhea** (**loo**-koh-**REE**-ah)
- [ ] **mammography** (mam-**OG**-rah-fee)
- [ ] **mastalgia** (mass-**TAL**-jee-ah)
- [ ] **mastopexy** (**MAS**-toh-**peck**-see)
- [ ] **menarche** (meh-**NAR**-kee)
- [ ] **menometrorrhagia** (men-oh-**met**-roh-**RAY**-jee-ah)
- [ ] **metrorrhea** (mee-troh-**REE**-ah)
- [ ] **neonate** (**NEE**-oh-nayt)
- [ ] **nulligravida** (**null**-ih-**GRAV**-ih-dah)
- [ ] **nullipara** (nuh-**LIP**-ah-rah)
- [ ] **oligomenorrhea** (**ol**-ih-goh-**men**-oh-**REE**-ah)
- [ ] **oligospermia** (**ol**-ih-goh-**SPER**-mee-ah)
- [ ] **oophorectomy** (**oh**-ahf-oh-**RECK**-toh-mee)
- [ ] **oophoritis** (**oh**-ahf-oh-**RYE**-tis)
- [ ] **orchidectomy** (**or**-kih-**DECK**-toh-mee)
- [ ] **ovariorrhexis** (oh-**vay**-ree-oh-**RECK**-sis)
- [ ] **Papanicolaou test** (pap-ah-**nick**-oh-**LAY**-ooh)
- [ ] **perimenopause** (pehr-ih-**MEN**-oh-pawz)
- [ ] **placenta previa** (plah-**SEN**-tah **PREE**-vee-ah)
- [ ] **preeclampsia** (**pree**-ee-**KLAMP**-see-ah)
- [ ] **priapism** (**PRYE**-ah-**piz**-em)
- [ ] **primigravida** (**prye**-mih-**GRAV**-ih-dah)
- [ ] **primipara** (prye-**MIP**-ah-rah)
- [ ] **prostatectomy** (**pros**-tah-**TECK**-toh-mee)
- [ ] **prostatitis** (**pros**-tah-**TYE**-tis)
- [ ] **pruritus vulvae** (proo-**RYE**-tus **VUL**-vee)
- [ ] **salpingo-oophorectomy** (sal-**ping**-goh oh-**ahf**-oh-**RECK**-toh-mee)
- [ ] **syphilis** (**SIF**-ih-lis)
- [ ] **trichomonas** (**trick**-oh-**MOH**-nas)
- [ ] **varicocele** (**VAR**-ih-koh-**seel**)
- [ ] **vasovasostomy** (**vas**-oh-vah-**ZOS**-toh-mee *or* vay-zoh-vay-**ZOS**-toh-mee)
- [ ] **vulvodynia** (vul-voh-**DIN**-ee-ah)

On completion of this chapter, you should be able to:

1. Identify and describe the major functions and structures of the male reproductive system.

2. Recognize, define, spell, and pronounce the terms related to the pathology and the diagnostic and treatment procedures of the male reproductive system.

3. Name at least six sexually transmitted diseases.

4. Identify and describe the major functions and structures of the female reproductive system.

5. Recognize, define, spell, and pronounce the terms related to the pathology and the diagnostic and treatment procedures of the female reproductive system.

6. Recognize, define, spell, and pronounce the terms related to the pathology and the diagnostic and treatment procedures of the female during pregnancy, childbirth, and the postpartum period.

FUNCTIONS OF THE MALE REPRODUCTIVE SYSTEM

The primary function of the male reproductive system is to produce millions of sperm and deliver them into the female body where one sperm can unite with a single ovum (egg) to create a new life.

STRUCTURES OF THE MALE REPRODUCTIVE SYSTEM

Some of the structures of the male reproductive system also function as part of the urinary system. Urinary functions are discussed in Chapter 9.

The External Male Genitalia

The term **genitalia** (**jen**-ih-**TAY**-lee-ah) means reproductive organs. The external genitalia are those reproductive organs located outside of the body cavity.

● Major external male organs include the penis, scrotum, and two testicles, each with an attached coiled tube called the epididymis (Figure 14.1).

The Perineum

The **perineum** (pehr-ih-**NEE**-um) is the external region of the area covering the pelvic floor. In the male, the perineum is the region between the thighs that extends from the scrotum to the anus.

The Scrotum

The **scrotum** (**SKROH**-tum) encloses, protects, and supports the testicles. It is suspended from the pubic arch behind the penis and lies between the thighs (Figures 14.2).

The Testicles

The **testicles**, also known as **testes**, are the two small egg-shaped glands that produce the sperm, or spermatozoa (singular, **testis**) (Figure 14.2).

● The testicles develop within the abdomen of the male fetus and normally descend into the scrotum before, or soon after, birth.

● Sperm are formed within the **seminiferous tubules** located with each testicle (Figure 14.2).

● **Semen**, also called **ejaculate**, is a whitish fluid containing the sperm and various secretions that is ejaculated from the penis upon sexual climax, or orgasm. The term *ejaculate* also means to expel suddenly.

● The ideal temperature for semen formation is 93.2° F. In order to maintain this temperature, the scrotum adjusts how close the testicles are to the 98.6° F temperature of the body.

● The **epididymis** (ep-ih-**DID**-ih-mis) is a coiled tube at the upper part of each testicle. It runs down the length of the testicle then turns upward into the body, where it becomes a narrower tube called the vas deferens (plural, **epididymides**) (Figure 14.2).

The Penis

The **penis** (**PEE**-nis) is the male sex organ that transports the sperm into the female vagina. The penis is composed of three columns of erectile tissue (Figure 14.1).

● During sexual stimulation the erectile tissue fills with blood under high pressure. This causes the swelling, hardness, and stiffness known an *erection*.

a hormonal imbalance, may cause infertility, menstrual abnormalities, and the development of secondary male characteristics such as hair growth.

- **Ovariorrhexis** (oh-**vay**-ree-oh-**RECK**-sis) is the rupture of an ovary (**ovari/o** means ovary and -**rrhexis** means to rupture).

- **Pelvic inflammatory disease** is any inflammation of the female reproductive organs not associated with surgery or pregnancy. This condition, which frequently occurs as a complication of a sexually transmitted disease, can lead to infertility, tubal pregnancy, and other serious disorders.

- **Pyosalpinx** (**pye**-oh-**SAL**-pinks) is an accumulation of pus in the fallopian tube (**py/o** means pus and -**salpinx** means fallopian tube).

- **Salpingitis** (**sal**-pin-**JIGH**-tis) is an inflammation of a fallopian tube (**salping** means fallopian or eustachian tube and -**itis** means inflammation). *Caution*: This term also means inflammation of the eustachian tube of the middle ear.

The Uterus

- **Endometriosis** (**en**-doh-**mee**-tree-**OH**-sis) is a condition in which patches of endometrial tissue escape the uterus and become attached to other structures in the pelvic cavity, such as the ovaries (**endo-** means within, **metri** means uterus, and -**osis** means abnormal condition). It is a leading cause of infertility.

- A **fibroid**, also known as a **leiomyoma** (**lye**-oh-my-**OH**-mah), is a benign tumor composed of muscle and fibrous tissue that occurs in the wall of the uterus. Fibroids are a common phenomenon and are usually attributed to a rise in estrogen.

- **Metrorrhea** (**mee**-troh-**REE**-ah) is an abnormal discharge, such as mucus or pus, from the uterus (**metr/o** means uterus and -**rrhea** means flow or discharge).

- A **uterine prolapse** (proh-**LAPS**), also known as a **pelvic floor hernia**, is the condition in which the uterus sags from its normal position and moves part way, or all of the way, into the vagina (Figure 14.11). This is condition usually occurs after menopause, when reduced hormone levels weaken the ligaments. *Prolapse* means the falling or dropping down of an organ or internal part.

- **Uterine cancer** occurs most commonly after menopause. One of the earliest symptoms is abnormal bleeding from the uterus.

The Cervix

- **Cervical cancer** is the second most common cancer in women and usually affects women between the ages of 45 and 65. It can be detected early through routine Pap tests.

- **Cervical dysplasia** (**SER**-vih-kal dis-**PLAY**-see-ah), also known as **precancerous lesions**, is the abnormal growth of cells of the cervix that may be detected on a Pap smear. If not treated, these cells may become malignant. *Dysplasia* is abnormal tissue development.

- **Endocervicitis** (**en**-doh-**ser**-vih-**SIGH**-tis) is an inflammation of the mucous membrane lining the cervix (**endo-** means within, **cervic** means cervix, and -**itis** means inflammation).

The Vagina

- **Colporrhexis** (**kol**-poh-**RECK**-sis) means laceration (tearing) of the vaginal walls (**colp/o** means vagina and -**rrhexis** means to rupture).

- **Leukorrhea** (**loo**-koh-**REE**-ah) is a profuse whitish mucus discharge from the uterus and vagina (**leuk/o** means white and -**rrhea** means flow or discharge).

- **Vaginal candidiasis** (**kan**-dih-**DYE**-ah-sis), also known as **vaginal thrush** or as a **yeast infection**. This condition results from the yeast fungus *Candida albicans*, which often exists in the vagina, suddenly being allowed to grow rapidly, unimpeded by the bacteria that usually keeps it in check. Symptoms include burning, itching, and a "cottage cheese-like" vaginal discharge. A candidal infection in the mouth is called oral thrush.

- **Vaginitis** (**vaj**-ih-**NIGH**-tis), also known as **colpitis** (kol-**PYE**-tis), is an inflammation of the lining of the vagina (**vagin** and **colp** both mean vagina and -**itis** means inflammation). The most common causes of

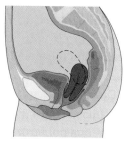

Figure 14.11 Uterine prolapse.

vaginal inflammation are bacterial vaginosis, trichomoniasis, and vaginal candidiasis.

The External Genitalia

- **Pruritus vulvae** (proo-**RYE**-tus **VUL**-vee) is a condition of severe itching of the external female genitalia. *Pruritus* means itching.
- **Vulvodynia** (vul-voh-**DIN**-ee-ah) is a nonspecific syndrome of unknown cause characterized by chronic burning, pain during sexual intercourse, itching, or stinging irritation of the vulva (**vulv/o** means vulva and **-dynia** means pain).
- **Vulvitis** (vul-**VYE**-tis) is an inflammation of the vulva (**vulv** means vulva and **-itis** means inflammation). Possible causes include fungal or bacterial infections, chafing, skin conditions, or allergies to products such as soaps and bubble bath.

The Breasts

- **Breast cancer** and its treatment are discussed in Chapter 6.
- **Fibrocystic breast disease** (**figh**-broh-**SIS**-tick) is the presence of single or multiple cysts in the breasts that are usually benign. A *cyst* is a closed sac containing fluid or semisolid material.
- **Fibroadenomas**, also known as **fibrous breast lumps**, are small, benign lumps of fibrous and glandular tissue. An *adenoma* is a benign tumor originating in a gland.
- **Galactorrhea** (gah-**lack**-toh-**REE**-ah) is the production of breast milk in women who are not breast feeding, due to a malfunction of the thyroid or pituitary gland (**galact/o** means milk and **-rrhea** means flow or discharge).
- **Mastalgia** (mass-**TAL**-jee-ah), also known as **mastodynia**, is pain in the breast, for example during the menstrual cycle (**mast** means breast and **-algia** means pain).
- **Mastitis** (mas-**TYE**-tis) is an inflammation of one or both breasts (**mast** means breast and **-itis** means inflammation). This condition is usually associated with the infection of a blocked milk duct during lactation; however, it also can occur for other reasons.

Menstrual Disorders

- **Amenorrhea** (ah-**men**-oh-**REE**-ah *or* ay-**men**-oh-**REE**-ah) is an absence of menstrual periods for three or more months (**a-** means without, **men/o** means menstruation, and **-rrhea** means flow or discharge). This condition is normal only before puberty, during pregnancy, while breast-feeding, and after menopause.
- **Dysmenorrhea** (**dis**-men-oh-**REE**-ah) is abdominal pain caused by uterine cramps during a menstrual period (**dys-** means bad, **men/o** means menstruation, and **-rrhea** means flow or discharge).
- **Hypomenorrhea** (**high**-poh-men-oh-**REE**-ah) is a small amount of menstrual flow during a shortened regular menstrual period (**hypo-** means deficient, **men/o** means menstruation, and **-rrhea** means flow or discharge).
- **Menorrhagia** (**men**-oh-**RAY**-jee-ah), also known as **hypermenorrhea**, is an excessive amount of menstrual flow or flow over a period of more than seven days (**men/o** means menstruation and **-rrhagia** means abnormal bleeding).
- **Menometrorrhagia** (**men**-oh-**met**-roh-**RAY**-jee-ah) is excessive uterine bleeding occurring both during the menses and at irregular intervals between periods (**men/o** means menstruation, **metr/o** means uterus, and **-rrhagia** means abnormal bleeding).
- **Oligomenorrhea** (**ol**-ih-goh-men-oh-**REE**-ah) means light or infrequent menstrual flow (**olig/o** means scanty, **men/o** means menstruation, and **-rrhea** means flow or discharge). Compare with *polymenorrhea*.
- **Polymenorrhea** (**pol**-ee-men-oh-**REE**-ah) means abnormally frequent menstruation (**poly-** means many, **men/o** means menstruation, and **-rrhea** means flow or discharge). Compare with *oligomenorrhea*.
- **Premature menopause** is a condition in which the ovaries cease functioning before age 40, causing infertility and often bringing on menopausal symptoms such as hot flashes and mood swings.
- **Premenstrual syndrome** is a group of symptoms experienced by some women within the two-week period before menstruation, possibly including bloating, edema, headaches, mood swings, and breast discomfort.
- **Premenstrual dysphoric disorder** is a condition associated with severe emotional and physical problems linked to the menstrual cycle.

DIAGNOSTIC PROCEDURES OF THE FEMALE REPRODUCTIVE SYSTEM

- **Colposcopy** (kol-**POS**-koh-pee) is the direct visual examination of the tissues of the cervix and vagina using a binocular magnifier called a *colposcope* (**colp/o** means vagina and **-scopy** means direct visual examination).

- **Endometrial biopsy** is a diagnostic test in which a small amount of the tissue lining the uterus is removed for microscopic examination, usually to determine the cause of abnormal vaginal bleeding.

- **Endovaginal ultrasound** (en-doh-**VAJ**-ih-nal) is a diagnostic test to determine the cause of abnormal vaginal bleeding with the use of an ultrasound transducer that is placed into the vagina so that the sound waves can create images of the uterus and ovaries.

- **Hysterosalpingography** (hiss-ter-oh-**sal**-pin-**GOG**-rah-fee) is a radiographic examination of the uterus and fallopian tubes following the instillation of radiopaque material into the uterine cavity and fallopian tubes (**hyster/o** means uterus, **salping/o** means tube, and **-graphy** means the process of producing a picture or record). *Instillation* means slowly pouring a liquid onto a body part or into a body cavity.

- **Hysteroscopy** (hiss-ter-**OSS**-koh-pee) is the direct visual examination of the interior of the uterus and fallopian tubes using the magnification of a *hysteroscope* (**hyster/o** means uterus and **-scopy** means direct visual examination) (Figure 15.19).

- A **Papanicolaou test** (pap-ah-**nick**-oh-**LAY**-ooh), also known as a **Pap smear**, is an exfoliative biopsy for the detection of conditions that may be early indicators of cervical cancer (Figure 14.12). As used here, *exfoliative* means that cells are scraped from the tissue and examined under a microscope.

- **Ultrasound** and **laparoscopy**, which are also used to diagnose disorders of the reproductive system, are discussed further in Chapter 15.

Diagnostic Procedures of the Breasts

- **Breast self-examination** is an important self-care procedure for the early detection of breast cancer. The focus of this self-examination is checking for any new lump, or a change in an existing lump, nipple shape, or the skin over the breast.

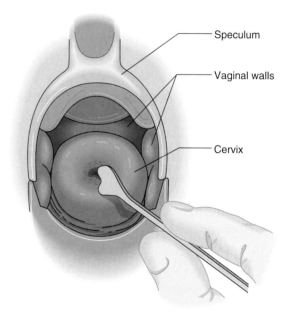

FIGURE 14.12   A Pap smear involves the use of a speculum to spread the vaginal walls so that a few cervical cells can be scraped away to be sent to a laboratory for examination.

- **Mammography** (mam-**OG**-rah-fee) is a radiographic examination of the breasts to detect the presence of tumors or precancerous cells (**mammo/o** means breast and **-graphy** means the process of producing a picture or record). The resulting record is a *mammogram* (Figures 14.13 and 14.14).

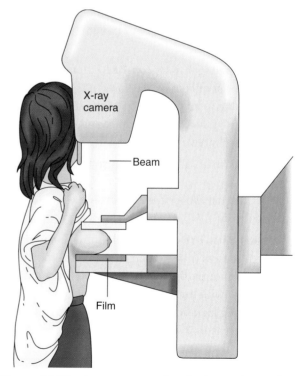

FIGURE 14.13   In mammography, the breast is gently flattened and then radiographed.

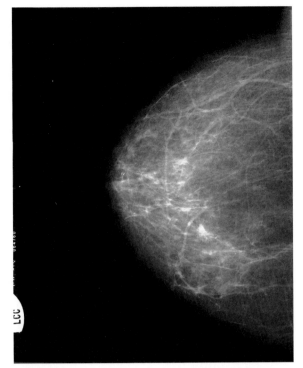

FIGURE 14.14   A normal mammogram in which no abnormal mass is visible.

- Ultrasound is used as one of the follow-up tests when an abnormality is found by mammography. Breast biopsies, which are an even more definitive test, are described in Chapter 6.

TREATMENT PROCEDURES OF THE FEMALE REPRODUCTIVE SYSTEM

Medications

- A **contraceptive** is a measure taken or device used to lessen the likelihood of conception and pregnancy. *Birth control pills* are a form of hormones that are administered as a contraceptive.
- An **intrauterine device**, also known as an **IUD**, is a molded plastic contraceptive inserted through the cervix into the uterus (**intra-** means within and **uterine** means uterus).
- **Hormone replacement therapy** is used when required to replace the estrogen and progesterone that are no longer produced during perimenopause and after menopause.

The Ovaries and Fallopian Tubes

- An **ovariectomy** (**oh**-vay-ree-**ECK**-toh-mee), also known as an **oophorectomy** (**oh**-ahf-oh-**RECK**-toh-

mee) is the surgical removal of an ovary (**ovari** and **oophor** both mean ovary and **-ectomy** means surgical removal).
- A **salpingectomy** (**sal**-pin-**JECK**-toh-mee) is the surgical removal of a fallopian tube (**salping** means tube and **-ectomy** means surgical removal).
- A **salpingo-oophorectomy** (sal-**ping**-goh oh-**ahf**-oh-**RECK**-toh-mee) (**SO**) is the surgical removal of a fallopian tube and ovary (**salping/o** means tube, **oophor** means ovary, and **-ectomy** means surgical removal). A *bilateral salpingo-oophorectomy* is the removal of both of the fallopian tubes and ovaries.
- **Tubal ligation** is a surgical procedure performed for purpose of female sterilization. Each fallopian tube is ligated and a section is removed to prevent the sperm from reaching the ovum. *Ligate* means to bind or tie (Figure 14.15).

The Uterus, Cervix, and Vagina

- A **colpopexy** (**KOL**-poh-**peck**-see) is the surgical fixation of the vagina to a surrounding structure (**colp/o** means vagina and **-pexy** means surgical fixation in place). This procedure is performed to repair a uterine prolapse.
- **Conization** (kon-ih-**ZAY**-shun *or* koh-nih-**ZAY**-shun), also known as a **cone biopsy**, is the surgical removal of a cone-shaped section of tissue from the

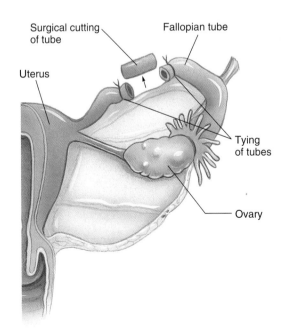

FIGURE 14.15   Tubal ligation is performed as a form of female sterilization.

cervix. This may be performed as a diagnostic procedure or to remove an abnormal area.

- **Colporrhaphy** (kol-**POR**-ah-fee) is the surgical suturing of a tear in the vagina (**colp/o** means vagina and -**rrhaphy** means surgical suturing).

- **Dilation and curettage** (dye-**LAY**-shun and **kyou**-reh-**TAHZH**), also known as a **D & C**, is the expansion of the opening of the cervix and the removal of material from the surface of the uterus. This may be performed as a diagnostic or treatment procedure (Figure 14.16). *Dilation* means the expansion of an opening. *Curettage*, which is the removal of material from the surface, may be accomplished by scraping with a *curette* or with the use of suction.

Hysterectomies

A **hysterectomy** (**hiss**-teh-**RECK**-toh-mee) is the surgical removal of the uterus that may, or may not, include removal of the cervix (**hyster** means uterus and -**ectomy** means surgical removal) (Figure 14.17).

- A *vaginal hysterectomy* is performed through the vagina (Figure 14.17A).

- An *abdominal hysterectomy* is performed through an incision in the abdomen. This procedure is sometimes performed laparoscopically through several small incisions.

- A *partial hysterectomy* is the removal of just the upper portion of the uterus, leaving the cervix intact.

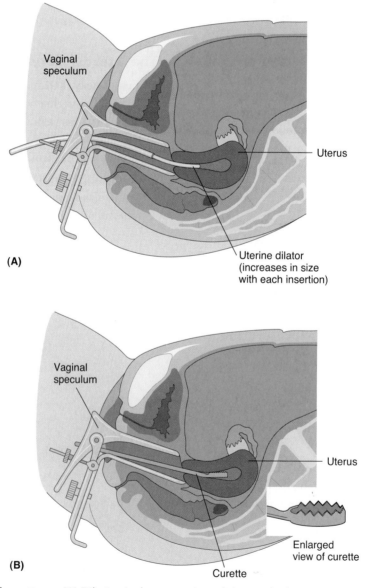

FIGURE 14.16 Dilation and curettage. (A) Dilation is the expansion of the cervical opening. (B) Curettage is the removal of material from the surface of the uterus.

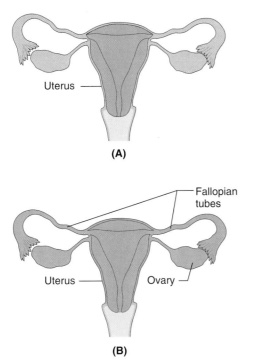

(A)

(B)

FIGURE 14.17 Types of hysterectomy. (A) In a vaginal hysterectomy only the uterus and cervix are removed. (B) In a bilateral hysterosalpingo-oophorectomy the cervix, uterus, fallopian tubes, and ovaries are removed.

- A *total hysterectomy*, also known as a *complete hysterectomy*, is the removal of the uterus and cervix.

- A **bilateral hysterosalpingo-oophorectomy** (**hiss**-ter-oh-sal-**ping**-goh oh-**ahf**-oh-**RECK**-toh-mee) is the surgical removal of the uterus and cervix, plus both fallopian tubes and ovaries (**hyster/o** means uterus, **salping/o** means tube, **oophor** means ovary, and -**ectomy** means surgical removal) (Figure 14.17B).

- A *radical hysterectomy*, also known as *panhysterectomy*, is the surgical removal of the cervix, uterus, fallopian tubes, ovaries, and related lymph nodes. This procedure is usually performed in the treatment of uterine cancer.

Breasts

- **Mastectomy** as treatment of breast cancer is discussed in Chapter 6.

- **Mammoplasty** (**MAM**-oh-**plas**-tee), also spelled **mammaplasty**, is the surgical repair or restructuring of the breast (**mamm/o** means breast and -**plasty** means surgical repair).

- **Breast augmentation** is mammoplasty that is performed to increase breast size. *Augmentation* means the process of adding to make larger. Compare with *breast reduction.*

- **Breast reduction** is mammoplasty performed to decrease and reshape excessively large, heavy breasts. Compare with *breast augmentation.*

- **Mastopexy** (**MAS**-toh-**peck**-see) is surgery to affix sagging breasts in a more elevated position (**mast/o** means breast and -**pexy** means surgical fixation).

PREGNANCY AND CHILDBIRTH

Ovulation

Ovulation (**ov**-you-**LAY**-shun) is the release of a mature egg from the follicle on the surface of the ovary.

- After the ovum is released, it is caught up by the fimbriae of the fallopian tube. There, wavelike peristaltic actions move the ovum down the fallopian tube toward the uterus.

- It usually takes an ovum about five days to pass through the fallopian tube. If sperm are present, fertilization occurs within the fallopian tube.

- After the ovum has been released, the ruptured follicle enlarges, takes on a yellow fatty substance, and becomes the corpus luteum.

- The **corpus luteum** (**KOR**-pus **LOO**-tee-um) secretes the hormone progesterone during the second half of the menstrual cycle. This maintains the growth of the uterine lining in preparation for the fertilized egg.

- If the ovum is not fertilized, the corpus luteum dies and the endometrium lining of the uterus sloughs off as the menstrual flow.

- If the ovum is fertilized, the corpus luteum continues to secrete the hormones required to maintain the pregnancy.

Fertilization

- During **coitus** (**KOH**-ih-tus), also known as **copulation** (kop-you-**LAY**-shun) or **sexual intercourse**, the male ejaculates approximately 100 million sperm cells into the female's vagina. The sperm travel upward through the vagina, into the uterus, and on into the fallopian tubes.

- When a sperm penetrates the descending ovum, **fertilization**, also known as **conception**, occurs and a new life begins.

- After fertilization occurs in the fallopian tube, the zygote travels to the uterus. A **zygote** (**ZYE**-goht) is a single cell formed by the union of the sperm and egg.

- **Implantation** is the embedding of the zygote into the lining of the uterus.

- From implantation through the eighth week of pregnancy, the developing child is known as an **embryo** (**EM**-bree-oh).

- A **fetus** (**FEE**-tus) is the developing child from the ninth week of pregnancy to the time of birth (**fet** means unborn child and **-us** is a singular noun ending) (Figure 14.18).

- The term **in utero** means within the uterus.

Multiple Births

If more than one egg is passing down the fallopian tube when sperm are present, the fertilization of more than one egg is possible.

- **Fraternal twins** result from the fertilization of separate ova by separate sperm cells. These develop into two separate embryos.

- **Multiple births** beyond twins (i.e., triplets, quadruplets, quintuplets) are almost always fraternal. The use of fertilization drugs and techniques increases the chances of multiple births.

- **Identical twins** are formed from the fertilization of a single egg cell by a single sperm. As the fertilized egg cell divides, it separates into two parts, with each part forming a separate embryo.

The Chorion and Placenta

- The **chorion** (**KOR**-ee-on) is the thin outer membrane that encloses the embryo. It contributes to the formation of the placenta (Figure 14.18).

- The **placenta** (plah-**SEN**-tah) is a temporary organ that forms within the uterus to allow the exchange of nutrients, oxygen, and waste products between the mother and fetus without allowing maternal

blood and fetal blood to mix (Figure 14.19). The placenta also produces hormones necessary to maintain the pregnancy. Hormones are discussed in Chapter 13.

- At delivery, the placenta is expelled as the **afterbirth**.

The Amniotic Sac

The **amniotic sac**, also known as the **amnion** (**AM**-nee-on) or the **bag of waters**, is the innermost of the membranes that surround the embryo in the uterus and form the **amniotic cavity** (**am**-nee-**OT**-ick) (Figure 14.18).

- **Amnionic fluid** (**am**-nee-**ON**-ick), also known as **amniotic fluid**, is the liquid in which the fetus floats and is protected (Figure 14.18).

The Umbilical Cord

The **umbilical cord** (um-**BILL**-ih-kal) is the structure that connects the fetus to the placenta (Figures 14.18 and 14.19).

- After birth, the **navel**, also known as the **belly button**, is formed where the umbilical cord was attached to the fetus.

- **Cord blood**, which is the blood present in the umbilical cord and placenta at the time of birth, is rich in stem cells. Some parents choose to donate this blood to a cord blood bank, or to freeze it so that their baby's own stem cells will be available for his or her future medical use. Stem cells are also discussed in Chapter 2.

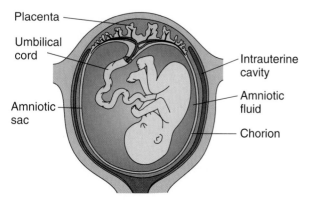

FIGURE 14.18 The anatomy of a pregnant uterus.

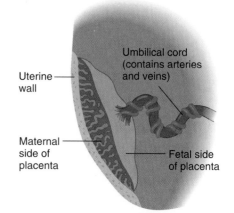

FIGURE 14.19 The placenta allows the exchange of nutrients and waste materials between mother and child without intermingling blood.

Gestation

Gestation (jes-**TAY**-shun), which lasts approximately 280 days, is the period of development of the child in the mother's uterus. Upon completion of this developmental time, the fetus is described as being *at term* and should be ready for birth.

- The term **pregnancy**, which is often used interchangeably with gestation, means the condition of having a developing child in the uterus.

- Pregnancy is described in terms of the number of weeks of gestation (40 total), or it may be divided into three **trimesters** of three months each (Figure 14.20).

The **due date**, or **estimated date of confinement**, is calculated from the first day of the **last menstrual period**. *Confinement* is an old-fashioned word for the lying-in period that used to follow childbirth.

- **Quickening** is the first movement of the fetus felt in the uterus. This usually occurs during the sixteenth to twentieth week of pregnancy.

- The fetus is **viable** when it is capable of living outside the mother. Viability depends on the developmental age, birth weight, and developmental stage of the lungs of the fetus.

The Mother

- A **nulligravida** (**null**-ih-**GRAV**-ih-dah) is a woman who has never been pregnant (**nulli**- means none and -**gravida** means pregnant). Compare with *nullipara*.

- A **primigravida** (**prye**-mih-**GRAV**-ih-dah) is a woman during her first pregnancy (**primi**- means first and -**gravida** means pregnant). A primigravida is also referred to as *Gravida I.* A *Gravida II* is in her second her pregnancy. Compare with *primipara*.

- A **nullipara** (nuh-**LIP**-ah-rah) is a woman who has never borne a viable child (**nulli**- means none and -**para** means to bring forth). Compare with *nulligravida*.

- A **primipara** (prye-**MIP**-ah-rah) is a woman who has borne one viable child (**primi**- means first and -**para** means to bring forth). A primipara is also referred to as *Para I.* Compare with *primigravida*.

- **Multiparous** (mul-**TIP**-ah-rus) means a woman who has given birth two or more times (**multi**- means many and -**parous** means having borne one or more children). A *Para II* has borne two viable children in separate pregnancies.

Antepartum

The term **antepartum** (an-tee-**PAHR**-tum) refers to the final stage of pregnancy, right before the onset of labor.

- **Braxton Hicks contractions**, which were named for John Braxton Hicks, a 19th century British gynecologist, are intermittent painless uterine contractions that are not true labor pains.

Childbirth

Parturition (par-tyou-**RISH**-un), also known as **labor** and **childbirth**, is the act of giving birth. **Labor and delivery (L & D)** occur in three stages: dilation, the

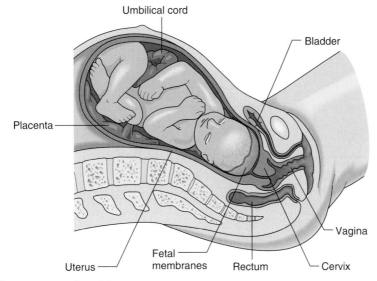

FIGURE 14.20   The fetus in normal position at term.

delivery of the baby, and the expulsion of the placenta and membranes (Figure 14.21).

- The first stage begins with contractions of the uterus and gradual dilatation (enlargement) of the cervix. *Effacement* (the thinning and shortening of the cervix) occurs during this stage. The amniotic sac ruptures either before or during this first stage.

- The second stage is the delivery of the infant. Then the uterine contractions become stronger and more frequent until the child is expelled through the vagina, or *birth canal.*

- *Presentation* is the term used to describe the portion of the fetus that can be touched by the examining finger during labor.

- Normally, the head presents first; the stage at which the head can be seen at the vaginal orifice is called *crowning.*

- The third stage is the expulsion of the placenta as the *afterbirth.* The term delivery includes the expulsion of the infant and afterbirth.

Postpartum

The term **postpartum** (pohst-**PAR**-tum) means after childbirth.

The Mother

- **Puerperium** (**pyou**-er-**PEE**-ree-um) is the period of three to six weeks after childbirth before the uterus returns to its normal size.

- **Uterine involution** is the return of the uterus to its normal size and former condition. *Involution* means the return of an enlarged organ to its normal size.

- **Colostrum** (kuh-**LOS**-trum) is the fluid secreted by the breasts during the first days postpartum. This fluid is rich in antibodies and confers passive immunity to the newborn.

- **Lactation** (lack-**TAY**-shun) is the process of forming and secreting milk from the breasts as nourishment for the infant.

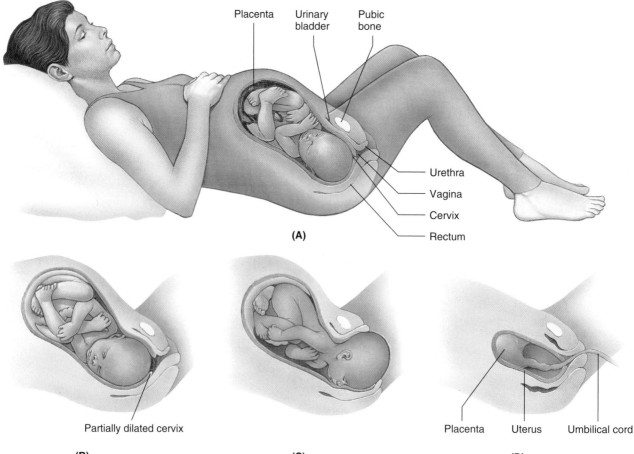

Placenta   Urinary bladder   Pubic bone

Urethra
Vagina
Cervix
Rectum

(A)

Partially dilated cervix

(B)   (C)   Placenta   Uterus   Umbilical cord

(D)

FIGURE 14.21   The stages of labor. (A) Position of the fetus before labor. (B) First state of labor, cervical dilation. (C) Second stage of labor, fetal delivery. (D) Third stage of labor, delivery of the placenta.

- **Lochia** (**LOH**-kee-ah) is the vaginal discharge during the first week or two after childbirth. It consists of blood, tissue, and mucus (**loch** means childbirth and **-ia** means pertaining to).

The Baby

The newborn infant is known as a **neonate** (**NEE**-oh-nayt) during the first four weeks after birth.

- **Vernix** (**VER**-nicks) is a greasy substance that protects the fetus in utero and may still be present at birth.
- **Meconium** (meh-**KOH**-nee-um) is a greenish material that collects in the intestine of a fetus and forms the first stools of a newborn.

ASSISTED REPRODUCTION

Infertility is the inability of a couple to achieve pregnancy after one year of regular, unprotected intercourse, or the inability of a woman to carry a pregnancy to a live birth.

- An infertile couple may seek the help of an **infertility specialist**, also known as a **fertility specialist**, who diagnoses and treats problems associated with conception and maintaining pregnancy.
- Table 14.2 summarizes the abbreviations and terms commonly associated with assisted reproduction.

MEDICAL SPECIALTIES RELATED TO CHILDBEARING AND CHILDREN

- An **obstetrician** (**ob**-steh-**TRISH**-un) specializes in providing medical care to women during pregnancy, childbirth, and immediately thereafter. This specialty is referred to as **obstetrics** (ob-**STET**-ricks).
- A **neonatologist** (**nee**-oh-nay-**TOL**-oh-jist) specializes in diagnosing and treating disorders of the newborn (**neo-** means new, **nat** means born, and **-ologist** means specialist).
- A **pediatrician** (**pee**-dee-ah-**TRISH**-un) specializes in diagnosing, treating, and preventing disorders and diseases of children. This specialty is known as **pediatrics** (**ped** means child and **-iatrics** means the medical practice of).

Table 14.2

ABBREVIATIONS AND TERMS RELATED TO ASSISTED FERTILIZATION

AMA	**Advanced maternal age** decreases the possibility of pregnancy. This term is applied to women in their late thirties to late forties.
AI	**Artificial insemination** is a technique in which sperm from a woman's partner or a donor are introduced into the vagina or uterus.
ART	**Assisted reproductive technology** is the term used to describe techniques used to aid an infertile couple in achieving a viable pregnancy.
GIFT	**Gamete intrafallopian transfer** is a procedure in which ovum and sperm are mixed outside of the body then transferred by laparoscopic surgery into the fallopian tube, where hopefully fertilization will occur.
ICSI	**Intra cytoplasmic sperm injection**, which is pronounced *icksy*, is used when the sperm are too weak or too few to fertilize an egg. Eggs are harvested and then fertilized in the laboratory by the direct injection of a single sperm into each egg. Three days later the eggs are transferred to the uterus.
IVF	**In vitro fertilization** is a procedure in which mature ova are removed from the mother and then fertilized. *In vitro* means in a glass or test tube. The resulting embryos are transferred into the uterus with the hope that they will implant and continue to develop as in a normal pregnancy.
ZIFT	**Zygote intrafallopian transfer** is a laparoscopic procedure in which a zygote, or fertilized egg, is placed in the fallopian tube, allowing it to travel down the tube to the uterus, where it implants.

PATHOLOGY OF PREGNANCY AND CHILDBIRTH

Pregnancy

- An **abortion** (ah-**BOR**-shun) is the interruption or termination of pregnancy before the fetus is viable. A *spontaneous abortion,* also known as a *miscarriage,* usually occurs early in the pregnancy because of a genetic disorder or abnormality.

- An *induced abortion,* caused by human intervention, is achieved through the use of drugs or suctioning. When done for medical purposes it is known as known as a *therapeutic abortion (TAB).*

- An **ectopic pregnancy** (eck-**TOP**-ick), also known as an **extrauterine pregnancy**, is a potentially dangerous condition in which a fertilized egg is implanted and begins to develop outside of the uterus. *Ectopic* means out of place.

- A *tubal pregnancy* is a form of ectopic pregnancy in which the embryo is implanted within the fallopian tube rather than the uterus.

- **Preeclampsia** (pree-ee-**KLAMP**-see-ah), also known as **pregnancy-induced hypertension** or **toxemia**, is a complication of pregnancy characterized by hypertension (high blood pressure), edema (swelling), and proteinuria (an abnormally high level of protein in the urine).

- **Eclampsia** (eh-**KLAMP**-see-ah), a more serious form of preeclampsia, is characterized by convulsions and sometimes coma.

The Rh Factor

When the mother's blood is **Rh negative (Rh–)**, and the father's is **Rh positive (Rh+)**, the baby may inherit the Rh+ factor from the father. The Rh factor is discussed further in Chapter 5.

- During labor or a miscarriage of a first pregnancy, some of the baby's Rh+ blood may enter the mother's Rh– blood circulation. This can cause the mother's body to develop Rh+ antibodies that may cause problems during subsequent pregnancies.

- Blood tests of the parents can identify this potential problem. If it exists, the mother is vaccinated with Rh immune globulin to prevent the development of these antibodies.

Childbirth

- **Abruptio placentae** (ab-**RUP**-shee-oh plah-**SEN**-tee) is an abnormal condition in which the placenta separates from the uterine wall prematurely before the birth of the fetus.

- **Breech presentation** is when the buttocks or feet of the fetus are presented first instead of the head.

- **Placenta previa** (plah-**SEN**-tah **PREE**-vee-ah) is the abnormal implantation of the placenta in the lower portion of the uterus. *Previa* means appearing before or in front of. Symptoms include painless sudden-onset bleeding during the third trimester.

- A **premature infant**, also known as a **preemie**, is a neonate born before the thirty-seventh week of gestation.

- **Stillbirth** is the birth of a fetus that died before, or during, delivery.

Diagnostic Procedures Related to Pregnancy and Childbirth

- A **pregnancy test** is performed on either a blood or urine specimen to determine the level of the human chorionic gonadotropin hormone. An unusually high level usually indicates pregnancy.

- **Fetal ultrasound** is a noninvasive procedure used to image and evaluate fetal development. Diagnostic ultrasound is discussed in Chapter 15.

- **First trimester screening** is a noninvasive blood test that, combined with a detailed ultrasound, can be performed as early as 11 weeks into a pregnancy to detect Down syndrome. This test is used to help determine which pregnant women should undergo more extensive testing for this genetic disorder.

- **Chorionic villus sampling** is the examination of chorionic cells retrieved from the edge of the placenta between the eighth and tenth weeks of pregnancy. These cells are used to test for genetic abnormalities in the developing child.

- **Amniocentesis** (am-nee-oh-sen-**TEE**-sis) is a surgical puncture with a needle to obtain a specimen of amniotic fluid (**amnio** means amnion and fetal membrane and **-centesis** means a surgical puncture to remove fluid). This specimen, which is obtained after the fourteenth week of pregnancy, is used to evaluate fetal health and to diagnose certain congenital disorders.

- **Pelvimetry** (pel-**VIM**-eh-tree) is a radiographic study to measure the dimensions of the pelvis to evaluate its capacity to allow passage of the fetus through the birth canal (**pelvi** means pelvis and **-metry** means to measure).

- **Fetal monitoring** is the use of an electronic device to record the fetal heart rate and the maternal uterine contractions during labor. Changes in fetal heart rate not caused by the contractions may indicate distress.

  Indirect fetal monitoring involves the placement of electrodes on the abdominal skin over the uterus.

  Direct fetal monitoring involves the placement of an electrode through the birth canal and onto the head of the fetus after the membranes have ruptured.

- An **Apgar score** is an evaluation of a newborn infant's physical status by assigning numerical values (0 to 2) to each of five criteria: (1) heart rate, (2) respiratory effort, (3) muscle tone, (4) response stimulation, and (5) skin color. The newborn is evaluated at one and five minutes after birth. A total score of 8 to 10 indicates the best possible condition.

TREATMENT PROCEDURES RELATED TO PREGNANCY AND CHILDBIRTH

- A **cesarean section** (seh-**ZEHR**-ee-un **SECK**-shun), also known as a **cesarean delivery** or a **C-section**, is the delivery of the child through an incision in the maternal abdominal and uterine walls. This is usually performed when a vaginal birth would be unsafe for either the mother or the baby.

- The vaginal delivery of a subsequent child after a cesarean birth is referred to as a *VBAC*.

- An **episiotomy** (eh-**piz**-ee-**OT**-oh-mee) is a surgical incision of the perineum and vagina to facilitate delivery and prevent laceration of the tissues (**episi** means vulva and **-otomy** means a surgical incision).

- An **episiorrhaphy** (eh-**piz**-ee-**OR**-ah-fee) is the surgical suturing to repair an episiotomy (**episi/o** means vulva and **-rrhaphy** means surgical suturing).

ABBREVIATIONS RELATED TO THE REPRODUCTIVE SYSTEMS

Table 14.3 presents an overview of the abbreviations related to the terms introduced in this chapter. *Note:* To avoid errors or confusion, always be cautious when using abbreviations.

Table 14.3

ABBREVIATIONS RELATED TO THE REPRODUCTIVE SYSTEMS	
abortion = AB	**AB** = abortion
abrupto placentae = AP	**AP** = abrupto placentae
amniocentesis = AMN	**AMN** = amniocentesis
amnion = Am	**Am** = amnion
amniotic fluid = AF	**AF** = amniotic fluid
bacterial vaginosis = BV	**BV** = bacterial vaginosis
benign prostatic hypertrophy = BPH	**BPH** = benign prostatic hypertrophy
breast self-examination = BSE	**BSE** = breast self-examination
chlamydia = C.	**C.** = chlamydia
chorionic villus sampling = CVS	**CVS** = chorionic villus sampling
circumcision = CIRC, circum	**CIRC, circum** = circumcision
digital rectal examination = DRE	**DRE** = digital rectal examination
dilation and curettage = D & C	**D & C** = dilation and curettage
ectopic pregnancy = EP	**EP** = ectopic pregnancy

(continues)

Table 14.3 (continued)

ABBREVIATIONS RELATED TO THE REPRODUCTIVE SYSTEMS

endometriosis = Endo	**Endo** = endometriosis
episiotomy = epis	**epis** = episiotomy
erectile dysfunction = ED	**ED** = erectile dysfunction
estimated date of confinement = EDC	**EDC** = estimated date of confinement
fetus = fet	**fet** = fetus
hormone replacement therapy = HRT	**HRT** = hormone replacement therapy
human papilloma virus = HPV	**HPV** = human papilloma virus
hysterosalpingography = HSG	**HSG** = hysterosalpingography
herpes simplex virus type 2 = HSV-2	**HSV-2** = herpes simplex virus type 2
hormone therapy = HT	**HT** = hormone therapy
hysteroscopy = HYS	**HYS** = hysteroscopy
labor and delivery = L & D	**L & D** = labor and delivery
last menstrual period = LMP	**LMP** = last menstrual period
menstruation = men	**men** = menstruation
pelvic inflammatory disease = PID	**PID** = pelvic inflammatory disease
placenta = pl	**pl** = placenta
placenta previa = PP	**PP** = placenta previa
polycystic ovary syndrome = PCOS	**PCOS** = polycystic ovary syndrome
preeclampsia = PE	**PE** = preeclampsia
premenstrual dysphoric disorder = PMDD	**PMDD** = premenstrual dysphoric disorder
premenstrual syndrome = PMS	**PMS** = premenstrual syndrome
pregnancy-induced hypertension = PIH	**PIH** = pregnancy-induced hypertension
prostate cancer = PC, PCA	**PC, PCA** = prostate cancer
prostate-specific antigen = PSA	**PSA** = prostate-specific antigen
radiation therapy = RT	**RT** = radiation therapy
sexually transmitted disease = STD	**STD** = sexually transmitted disease
testicular self-examination = TSE	**TSE** = testicular self-examination
trichomonas = Trich	**Trich** = trichomonas
vasectomy = VAS	**VAS** = vasectomy
venereal disease = VD	**VD** = venereal disease
zygote = zyg	**zyg** = zygote

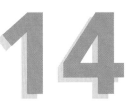
Learning Exercises

● Matching Word Parts 1

Write the correct answer in the middle column.

Definition	Correct Answer	Possible Answers
14.1. menstruation	_____	cervic/o
14.2. pregnant	_____	colp/o
14.3. female	_____	gynec/o
14.4. vagina	_____	men/o
14.5. cervix	_____	-gravida

● Matching Word Parts 2

Write the correct answer in the middle column.

Definition	Correct Answer	Possible Answers
14.6. egg	_____	hyster/o
14.7. ovary	_____	ov/o
14.8. prostate	_____	oophor/o
14.9. testicle	_____	orchid/o
14.10. uterus	_____	prostat/o

● Matching Word Parts 3

Write the correct answer in the middle column.

Definition	Correct Answer	Possible Answers
14.11. to bring forth	_____	nulli-
14.12. surgical fixation	_____	mamm/o
14.13. tube	_____	salping/o
14.14. breast	_____	-pexy
14.15. none	_____	-para

● Definitions

Select the correct answer and write it on the line provided.

14.16. The term that describes the inner layer of the uterus is _____ .

    corpus   endometrium   myometrium   perimetrium

14.17. The term describing the fertilized egg immediately after conception is _____ .

    embryo   fetus   gamete   zygote

14.18. Mucus to lubricate the vagina is produced by _____ glands.

    Bartholin's   bulbourethral   Cowper's   follicle

14.19. The finger-like structures of the fallopian tube that catch the ovum are the _____ .

    fimbriae   fundus   infundibulum   oviducts

14.20. Approximately between days 15 and 28, the _____ phase of the menstrual cycle occurs.

    menstrual   ovulatory   postmenstrual   premenstrual

14.21. An example of a yeast infection is _____ - _____ .

    colporrhea   leukorrhea   pruritus vulvae   vaginal candidiasis

14.22. The beginning of the menstrual function that begins during puberty is called _____ .

    menarche   menopause   menses   menstruation

14.23. The _____ runs down the length of the testicle and then turns upward into the

body, where it becomes a narrower tube called the vas deferens.

    ejaculatory duct   epididymis   seminal vesicle   urethra

14.24. The region between the vaginal orifice and the anus is known as the _____ .

    clitoris   mons pubis   perineum   vulva

14.25. The release of a mature egg by the ovary is known as _____ .

    coitus   sexual intercourse   implantation   ovulation

● Matching Structures

Write the correct answer in the middle column.

Definition	Correct Answer	Possible Answers
14.26. carry milk from the mammary glands	_____	clitoris
14.27. encloses the testicles	_____	lactiferous ducts
14.28. external female genitalia	_____	prepuce
14.29. protects the tip of the penis	_____	scrotum
14.30. sensitive tissue near the vaginal opening	_____	vulva

● Which Word?

Select the correct answer and write it on the line provided.

14.31. The term used to describe a woman during her first pregnancy is a _____ .

    primigravida   primipara

14.32. The fluid secreted by the breasts during the first days after giving birth is _____ .

    colostrum   meconium

14.33. The term meaning inflammation of the vulva is _____ .

    vulvodynia   vulvitis

14.34. The total absence of sperm in the semen is known as _____ .

azoospermia   oligospermia

14.35. A woman who has never borne a viable child is a _____ .

nulligravida   nullipara

● Spelling Counts

Find the misspelled word in each sentence. Then write that word, spelled correctly, on the line provided.

14.36. The prostrate gland secretes a thick fluid that aids the motility of the sperm. _____

14.37. The normal periodic discharge from the uterus is known as menstration. _____

14.38. The plasenta is also known as the afterbirth. _____

14.39. A Papanicola test is an exfoliative biopsy for the detection and diagnosis of conditions of the cervix and

surrounding tissues. _____

14.40. The surgical removal of the foreskin of the penis is known as cercumsion. _____

● Abbreviation Identification

In the space provided, write the words that each abbreviation stands for.

14.41. **AMA**   _____

14.42. **BPH**   _____

14.43. **PCOS**   _____

14.44. **PMDD**   _____

14.45. **STD**   _____

● Term Selection

Select the correct answer and write it on the line provided.

14.46. An accumulation of pus in the fallopian tube is known as _____ .

leiomyoma   pelvic inflammatory disease   pyosalpinx   salpingitis

14.47. A varicose vein of the testicles is known as _____ .

cryptorchidism   hydrocele   phimosis   varicocele

14.48. The direct visual examination of the tissues of the cervix and vagina using a specialized endoscope is

known as _____ .

colposcopy   endovaginal ultrasound   hysteroscopy   laparoscopy

14.49. A markedly reduced menstrual flow and abnormally infrequent menstruation is called

_____ .

amenorrhea   hypomenorrhea   oligomenorrhea   polymenorrhea

14.50. The diagnostic test that is usually performed between the eighth and tenth week of pregnancy is

_____ .

amniocentesis   chorionic villus sampling   fetal monitoring   pelvimetry

Sentence Completion

Write the correct term on the line provided.

14.51. The dark area surrounding the nipple is known as the _____ .

14.52. A hernia filled with fluid in the testicles or the tubes leading from the testicles is known as a/an

_____ .

14.53. The most serious form of toxemia of pregnancy is known as _____ .

14.54. The term meaning suturing the vagina is _____ .

14.55. The structure that connects the fetus to the placenta is known as the _____ cord.

Word Surgery

Divide each term into its component word parts. Write these word parts, in sequence, on the lines provided.

When necessary use a back slash (/) to indicate a combining vowel. (You may not need all of the lines provided.)

14.56. **Endocervicitis** is an inflammation of the mucous membrane lining of the cervix.

_____   _____   _____   _____

14.57. **Menometrorrhagia** is excessive uterine bleeding occurring both during the menses and at irregular intervals.

_____   _____   _____   _____

14.58. **Hysterosalpingography** is a specialized radiographic examination of the uterus and fallopian tubes.

_____   _____   _____   _____

14.59. **Anorchism** is the congenital absence of one or both testicles.

_____   _____   _____   _____

14.60. **Oligospermia** is also known as a low sperm count.

_____   _____   _____   _____

● **True/False**

If the statement is true, write **T** on the line. If the statement is false, write **F** on the line.

14.61. _____ Dilation is the expansion of an opening.

14.62. _____ A PSA test is used to determine the number of sperm in a semen specimen.

14.63. _____ An Apgar score is an evaluation of a newborn infant's physical status.

14.64. _____ Hysterosalpingography is the use of ultrasound to image the uterus and fallopian tubes.

14.65. _____ An ectopic pregnancy may occur in a fallopian tube.

● **Clinical Conditions**

Write the correct answer on the line provided.

14.66. Mr. Romer's surgeon performed a radical _____. In this procedure, which was performed through the abdomen, the entire prostate gland, the seminal vesicles, and some surrounding tissues were removed.

14.67. Mary Smith required the delivery of her baby through an incision in the maternal abdominal and uterine wall. The full medical term for this procedure is a/an _____ section.

14.68. Daniel Grossman was treated for a urethral discharge coming from the prostate gland. The medical term for this condition is _____ .

14.69. Rita Chen, who is 25, is concerned because her menstrual periods have stopped and she knows that she

is not pregnant. Her doctor described this condition as _____ .

14.70. To prevent laceration of the tissues during the delivery of Barbara Klein's baby, her doctor performed

a/an _____ .

14.71. Early in her pregnancy, Maria Jimenez suffered a miscarriage. The medical term for this condition is a

spontaneous _____ .

14.72. Harriet Ingram was diagnosed as having a leiomyoma, which is a benign tumor derived from the smooth

muscle of the uterus. This condition is also known as a/an _____ .

14.73. Harry Belcher's doctor removed a portion of each vas deferens. The medical term for this sterilization

procedure is a/an _____ .

14.74. There were complications in Jane Marsall's pregnancy caused by the abnormal implantation of the

placenta in the lower portion of the uterus. The medical term for this condition is

_____ _____ .

14.75. Immediately after birth, the Reicher baby was described as being a newborn or a/an

_____ .

● Which Is the Correct Medical Term?

Select the correct answer and write it on the line provided.

14.76. The vaginal discharge during the first week or two after childbirth is known as _____ .

colostrum   involution   lochia   meconium

14.77. Abdominal pain caused by uterine cramps during a menstrual period is known as _____ .

dysmenorrhea   menorrhagia   menometrorrhagia   polymenorrhea

14.78. The term that describes an inflammation of the glans penis is _____ .

anorchism   balanitis   epididymitis   orchitis

14.79. An inflammation of the lining of the vagina is known as _____ .

cervical dysplasia   cervicitis   colporrhexis   vaginitis

14.80. Which term means a profuse white mucus discharge from the uterus and vagina? _____

endocervicitis   leukorrhea   pruritus vulvae   vaginitis

● Challenge Word Building

These terms are *not* found in this chapter; however, they are made up of the following familiar word parts. You may want to look in the textbook glossary or use a medical dictionary to check your answers.

endo-	hyster/o	-cele
	mast/o	-dynia
	metr/i	-itis
	oophor/o	-plasty
	vagin/o	-pexy
	vulv/o	-rrhaphy
		-rrhexis

14.81. The term meaning a hernia protruding into the vagina is _____ .

14.82. The term meaning pain in the breast is _____ .

14.83. The term meaning an inflammation of the endometrium is _____ .

14.84. The term meaning the surgical repair of an ovary is a/an _____ .

14.85. The term meaning pain in the vagina is _____ .

11.86. The term meaning surgical suturing of the uterus is _____ .

14.87. The term meaning a hernia of the uterus, particularly during pregnancy, is a/an _____ .

14.88. The term meaning the surgical fixation of a displaced ovary is _____ .

14.89. The term meaning the rupture of the uterus, particularly during pregnancy, is _____ .

14.90. The term meaning an inflammation of the vulva and the vagina is _____ .

● Labeling Exercises

Identify the numbered items on these accompanying figures.

14.91. _____ bladder

14.92. _____ gland

14.93. _____

14.94. _____

14.95. _____

14.96. _____ tube

14.97. _____

14.98. _____ bladder

14.99. _____

14.100. _____

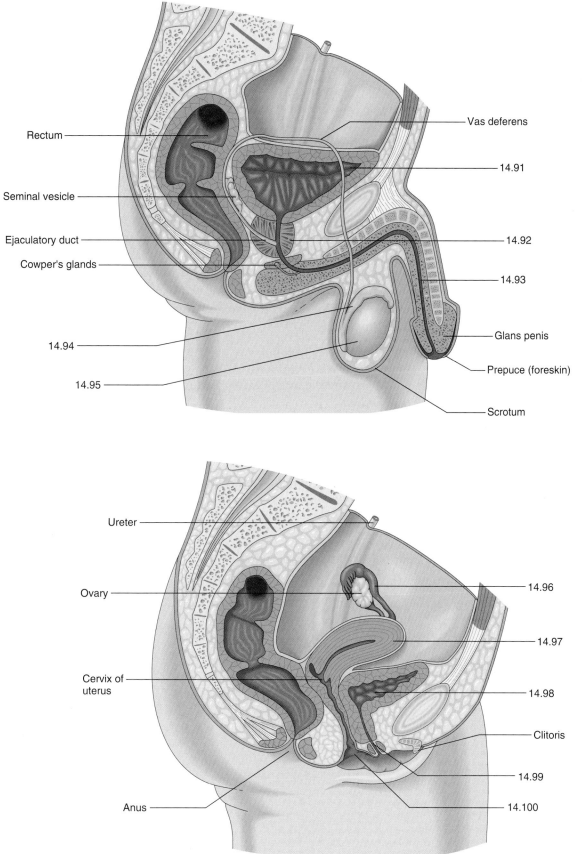

Rectum

Seminal vesicle

Ejaculatory duct

Cowper's glands

14.94

14.95

Vas deferens

14.91

14.92

14.93

Glans penis

Prepuce (foreskin)

Scrotum

Ureter

Ovary

Cervix of uterus

Anus

14.96

14.97

14.98

Clitoris

14.99

14.100

THE HUMAN TOUCH: CRITICAL THINKING EXERCISE

The following story and questions are designed to stimulate critical thinking through class discussion or as a brief essay response. There are no right or wrong answers to these questions.

"But Sam, you promised!" Jamie Chu began.

"Please do not get so upset," her husband interrupted. "I know I agreed to a vasectomy, but Grandmother may have a point. I do not have a son. Our family name has to be considered. I just feel that we should think about this."

"But Sam, we already discussed it. You're scheduled for the procedure." It seemed to Jamie that they had already spent plenty of time considering the number of children they wanted and talking about various contraceptive methods. Jamie had problems taking the pill and Sam didn't like using a condom. A tubal ligation could have been the answer, but Jamie had a fear of not waking up from the anesthesia. Besides, she had been the one to go through two pregnancies and childbirths. Sam had reluctantly agreed that it was his turn to take responsibility for family planning.

Their two daughters, 2-year-old Nanyn and her big sister Nadya, made the perfect size family, Jamie thought. She had grown up in a large family. A lot of her childhood was spent taking care of her brothers and sisters, and she rarely had her mother's undivided attention. She didn't want that for her children.

Sam's story was different. Before his parents immigrated to America they had had four daughters. His father was so proud when Sam was born, a son to carry on the family tradition.

It had taken quite a long time to convince Sam that a family of only daughters could be considered complete. And now Grandmother was questioning that decision.

Suggested Discussion Topics:

1. Which partner is responsible for birth control and why?
2. If a couple cannot agree about family size or birth control methods, what should they do?
3. Compare large families to small families. Discuss the good and bad points of each.
4. Discuss how cultural differences and religious beliefs influence choices like family size and birth control.
5. Why do some cultures value male children over female children?

Diagnostic Procedures and Pharmacology

Overview of Diagnostic Procedures and Pharmacology

Basic Diagnostic Procedures	Vital signs
	Auscultation
	Palpation and percussion
	Basic examination instruments
	Basic examination positions
Laboratory Tests	Blood tests
	Urinalysis
Endoscopy	Visual examination
	Endoscopic surgery
Imaging Techniques	Radiography (x-ray)
	Computerized tomography (CT)
	Magnetic resonance imaging (MRI)
	Fluoroscopy
	Diagnostic ultrasound
Nuclear Medicine	Nuclear medicine
Radiographic Projections and Positioning	Projections
	Positioning
	Basic radiographic projections
Pharmacology	Terms related to pharmacology
	Routes of administration

● VOCABULARY   RELATED TO DIAGNOSTIC PROCEDURES AND PHARMACOLOGY

The items on this list have been identified as key word parts and terms for this chapter. However, all words in boldface in the text are also important and may be included in learning exercises and tests.

Word Parts

- [ ] albumin/o
- [ ] calc/i
- [ ] fluor/o
- [ ] glycos/o
- [ ] -graph
- [ ] -graphy
- [ ] hemat/o
- [ ] lapar/o
- [ ] -ous
- [ ] per-
- [ ] phleb/o
- [ ] radi/o
- [ ] -scope
- [ ] -scopy
- [ ] -uria

Medical Terms

- [ ] **abdominocentesis** (ab-**dom**-ih-noh-sen-**TEE**-sis)
- [ ] **agglutination tests** (ah-**gloo**-tih-**NAY**-shun)
- [ ] **albuminuria** (**al**-byou-mih-**NEW**-ree-ah)
- [ ] **arthrocentesis** (**ar**-throh-sen-**TEE**-sis)
- [ ] **auscultation** (**aws**-kul-**TAY**-shun)
- [ ] **bacteriuria** (back-**tee**-ree-**YOU**-ree-ah)
- [ ] **bruit** (**BREW**-ee *or* **BROOT**)
- [ ] **calciuria** (**kal**-sih-**YOU**-ree-ah)
- [ ] **computerized tomography** (toh-**MOG**-rah-fee)
- [ ] **contraindication**
- [ ] **creatinuria** (kree-**at**-ih-**NEW**-ree-ah)
- [ ] **endoscope** (**EN**-doh-**skope**)
- [ ] **fluoroscopy** (**floo**-or-**OS**-koh-pee)
- [ ] **glycosuria** (**glye**-koh-**SOO**-ree-ah)
- [ ] **hematocrit test** (hee-**MAT**-oh-krit)
- [ ] **hematuria** (**hee**-mah-**TOO**-ree-ah *or* hem-ah-**TOO**-ree-ah)
- [ ] **hyperthermia** (**high**-per-**THER**-mee-ah)
- [ ] **hypothermia** (**high**-poh-**THER**-mee-ah)
- [ ] **idiosyncratic reaction** (**id**-ee-oh-sin-**KRAT**-ick)
- [ ] **immunofluorescence** (**im**-you-noh-**floo**-oh-**RES**-ens)

- [ ] **intradermal injection**
- [ ] **intramuscular injection**
- [ ] **intravenous injection**
- [ ] **ketonuria** (kee-toh-**NEW**-ree-ah)
- [ ] **laparoscopy** (**lap**-ah-**ROS**-koh-pee)
- [ ] **lithotomy position** (lih-**THOT**-oh-mee)
- [ ] **magnetic resonance imaging**
- [ ] **ophthalmoscope** (ahf-**THAL**-moh-skope)
- [ ] **otoscope** (**OH**-toh-skope)
- [ ] **palliative** (**PAL**-ee-**ay**-tiv *or* **PAL**-ee-ah-tiv)
- [ ] **palpation** (pal-**PAY**-shun)
- [ ] **parenteral** (pah-**REN**-ter-al)
- [ ] **percussion** (per-**KUSH**-un)
- [ ] **percutaneous treatment** (**per**-kyou-**TAY**-nee-us)
- [ ] **pericardiocentesis** (**pehr**-ih-**kar**-dee-oh-sen-**TEE**-sis)
- [ ] **phlebotomist** (fleh-**BOT**-oh-mist)
- [ ] **phlebotomy** (fleh-**BOT**-oh-mee)
- [ ] **placebo** (plah-**SEE**-boh)
- [ ] **positron emission tomography**
- [ ] **potentiation** (poh-**ten**-shee-**AY**-shun)
- [ ] **prone position**
- [ ] **proteinuria** (**proh**-tee-in-**YOU**-ree-ah)
- [ ] **pyuria** (pye-**YOU**-ree-ah)
- [ ] **radioimmunoassay** (**ray**-dee-oh-**im**-you-noh-**ASS**-ay)
- [ ] **radiolucent** (**ray**-dee-oh-**LOO**-sent)
- [ ] **radiopaque** (**ray**-dee-oh-**PAYK**)
- [ ] **rale** (**RAHL**)
- [ ] **rhonchus** (**RONG**-kus)
- [ ] **Sims' position**
- [ ] **single photon emission computerized tomography**
- [ ] **speculum** (**SPECK**-you-lum)
- [ ] **sphygmomanometer** (**sfig**-moh-mah-**NOM**-eh-ter)
- [ ] **stethoscope** (**STETH**-oh-skope)
- [ ] **stridor** (**STRYE**-dor)
- [ ] **subcutaneous injection**
- [ ] **supine position** (**SUE**-pine)
- [ ] **transesophageal echocardiography** (**trans**-eh-**sof**-ah-**JEE**-al **eck**-oh-**kar**-dee-**OG**-rah-fee)
- [ ] **ultrasonography** (**ul**-trah-son-**OG**-rah-fee)
- [ ] **urinalysis** (**you**-rih-**NAL**-ih-sis)
- [ ] **venipuncture** (**VEN**-ih-**punk**-tyour)

BASIC EXAMINATION PROCEDURES

Basic examination procedures are performed during the assessment of the patient's condition. As used in medicine, **assessment** means the evaluation or appraisal of a condition. This information is used in reaching a diagnosis and in formulating a patient care plan.

Vital Signs

Four vital signs are recorded for most patient visits. These are temperature, pulse, respiration, and blood pressure. In some settings pain is measured as a fifth vital sign.

Temperature

An average normal temperature is 98.6° F (Fahrenheit) or 37.0° C (Celsius) (Figure 15.1).

- Temperature readings are named for the location in which they are taken: **oral** (in the mouth), **aural** (in the ear), **axillary** (under the arm), and **rectally**. Caution: *oral* and *aural* sound alike; however, they require different equipment and are taken in different locations.

- Temperature readings vary depending upon the location where they are taken.

- **Hypothermia** (**high**-poh-**THER**-mee-ah) is an abnormally low body temperature (**hypo-** means deficient, **therm** means heat, and **-ia** means pertaining to).

- **Hyperthermia** (**high**-per-**THER**-mee-ah) is an extremely high fever (**hyper-** means excessive, **therm** means heat, and **-ia** means pertaining to).

Pulse

The **pulse** is the rhythmic pressure against the walls of an artery caused by the contraction of the heart. The pulse rate reflects the number of times the heart beats each minute and is recorded as **bpm**. As shown in Figure 15.2, the pulse may be measured at different points on the body.

- Normal resting pulse rates differ by age group. In adults, normal is from 50 to 80 bpm. In contrast, the normal rate for a newborn is from 130 to 160 bpm.

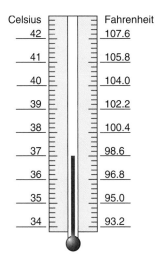

FIGURE 15.1   The average normal temperature is 37.0° C (Celsius) or 98.6° F (Fahrenheit).

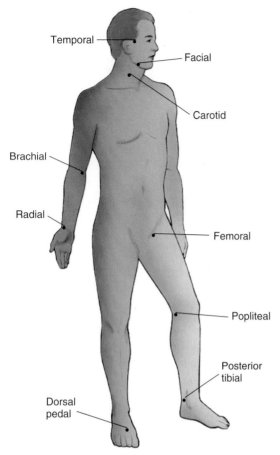

FIGURE 15.2   Major sites where arterial pulses can be detected.

Respiration

Respirations, also known as **respiratory rate**, are the number of complete respirations per minute. A *respiration* is one inhalation and one exhalation. The normal respiratory rate for adults ranges from 10 to 20 respirations per minute.

Blood Pressure

- A **sphygmomanometer** (**sfig**-moh-mah-**NOM**-eh-ter) and a stethoscope are the instrument used to measure **blood pressure** (Figure 15.3).

- Blood pressure is recorded with the **systolic** over the **diastolic** reading. For example, 120/80. Systolic (the first beat heard) and diastolic (the last beat heard) are explained in Chapter 5. *Memory aid: SSSS-systolic* is like steam going up. *DDDD-diastolic* as in going down (Figure 15.4).

Pain

Pain, which is considered to be the fifth vital sign in certain settings, is a subjective symptom and cannot be measured objectively. Therefore, this must be determined as reported by the patient.

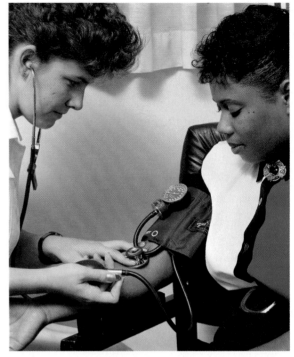

FIGURE 15.3   A sphygmomanometer and stethoscope are being used to measure blood pressure.

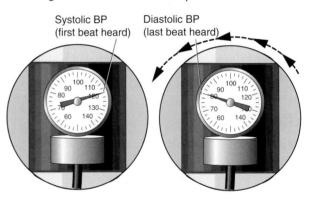

FIGURE 15.4   Systolic pressure is the first sound heard. Diastolic pressure is the last beat heard.

- Using the **pain verbal rating scale**, the patient is asked to measure his or her pain on a scale of 1 to 10 with 10 being unbearable pain and 1 being little or no pain.

Auscultation

The term **auscultation** (**aws**-kul-**TAY**-shun) means listening through a stethoscope for respiratory, heart, and abdominal sounds within the body (**auscult/a** means to listen and **-tion** means the process of).

Respiratory Sounds

Respiratory sounds heard through a stethoscope provide information about the condition of the lungs and pleura.

- A **rale** (**RAHL**), also known as a **crackle**, is an abnormal rattle or crackle-like respiratory sound heard during inspiration (breathing in). *Memory aid:* Rale is a "rattley" sound.

- **Rhonchus** (**RONG**-kus), also known as **wheezing**, is an added musical sound occurring during inspiration or expiration that is caused by a partially obstructed airway (plural, **rhonchi**). *Memory aid*: Rhonchus is a musical sound.

- **Stridor** (**STRYE**-dor) is an abnormal, high-pitched, harsh or crowing sound heard during inspiration that results from a partial blockage of the pharynx, larynx, and trachea. *Memory aid*: Stridor is a harsh sound.

Heart Sounds

The heartbeat heard through a stethoscope has two distinct sounds. These are called the "lubb dupp" or "lub dub" sounds.

- The **lubb sound** is heard first. This is caused by the tricuspid and mitral valves closing between the atria and the ventricles.

- The **dupp sound**, which is shorter and higher pitched, is heard next. It is caused by the closing of the semilunar valves in the aorta and pulmonary arteries as blood is pumped out of the heart.

- A **bruit** (**BREW**-ee) is an abnormal intermittent musical sound heard in auscultation of a vein or artery. This sound may be heard as blood flows through a partially blocked carotid artery or as blood flows through an aneurysm. *Memory aid*: A **bruit** sounds "murmury."

- A **heart murmur** is a swishing or a whistling sound that may be heard in addition to the normal sounds. A murmur can be a harmless sound made by a healthy heart or it can be an indication of a septal or a valvular problem.

Abdominal Sounds

Auscultation of the abdomen is performed to evaluate bowel sounds and to detect bruits that may be present (Figure 15.5). *Bowel sounds,* which originate from the movement of air and fluid through the intestine, are described as being *normal, hypoactive,* or *hyperactive.*

Palpation and Percussion

- **Palpation** (pal-**PAY**-shun) is an examination technique in which the examiner's hands are used to feel the texture, size, consistency, and location of certain body parts (Figure 15.6).

- **Percussion** (per-**KUSH**-un) is a diagnostic procedure to determine the density of a body area that uses the sound produced by tapping the surface with the finger or an instrument (Figure 15.7).

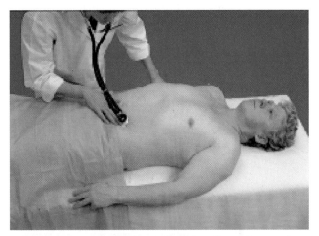

FIGURE 15.5 Auscultation is listening through a stethoscope to sounds within the body.

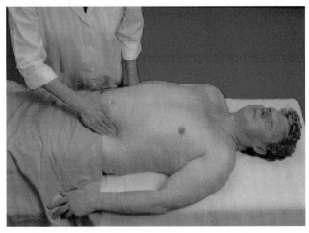

FIGURE 15.6 Palpation is an examination technique in which the examiner's hands are used to feel the texture, size, consistency, and location of certain body parts.

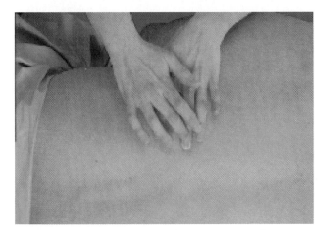

FIGURE 15.7 Percussion is a diagnostic procedure to determine the density of a body area.

Additional Instruments and Examination Procedures

- An **ophthalmoscope** (ahf-**THAL**-moh-skope) is used to examine the interior of the eye (**ophthalm/o** means eye and **-scope** means instrument for visual examination) (Figure 15.8).

- **PERRLA** is an abbreviation meaning **P**upils are **E**qual, **R**ound, **R**esponsive to **L**ight and **A**ccommodation. This is a diagnostic observation; any abnormality might indicate a head injury or damage to the brain

- An **otoscope** (**OH**-toh-skope) is used to visually examine the external ear canal and tympanic membrane (**ot/o** means ear and **-scope** means instrument for visual examination) (Figure 15.9).

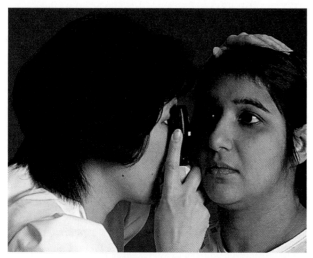

FIGURE 15.8   An ophthalmoscope is used to examine the interior of the eye.

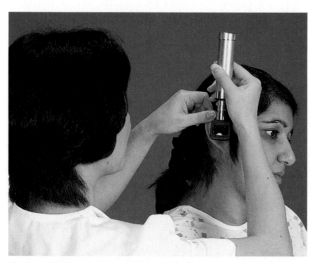

FIGURE 15.9   An otoscope is used to examine the ear canal and tympanic membrane.

- A **speculum** (**SPECK**-you-lum) is used to enlarge the opening of any canal or cavity to facilitate inspection of its interior (Figure 15.10).

- A **stethoscope** (**STETH**-oh-skope) is used to listen to sounds within the body and during the measurement of blood pressure (**steth/o** means chest and **-scope** means instrument for visual examination) (Figures 15.3 and 15.5).

BASIC EXAMINATION POSITIONS

Specific examination positions are used to examine different areas of the body.

Recumbent Position

The term **recumbent** (ree-**KUM**-bent) may be used to describe any position in which the patient is lying down on the back, front, or side.

- The term **decubitus** (dee-**KYOU**-bih-tus) also means the act of lying down or the position assumed in lying down.

- In radiography, the term **decubitus** describes the position of the patient when lying in a recumbent position. However *decubitus* is most commonly used to describe a decubitus ulcer, which is also known as a bedsore. (See Chapter 12.)

Prone Position

In a **prone position** the patient is lying on the belly with the *face down*. The arms may be placed under the head for comfort (Figure 15.11). This position is used for the examination and treatment of the back and buttocks.

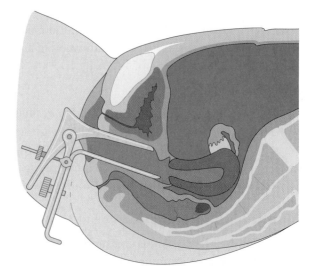

FIGURE 15.10   A speculum in place for inspection of the vagina.

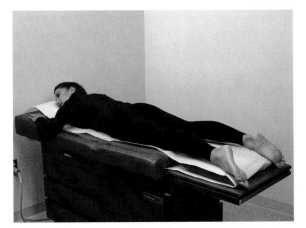

FIGURE 15.11   The prone position.

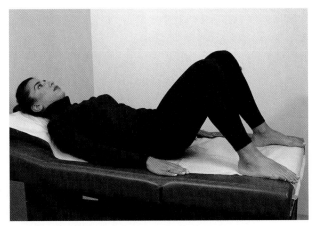

FIGURE 15.13   The dorsal recumbent position.

Supine Position

In the **supine position** (**SUE**-pine), also known as the **horizontal recumbent position**, the patient is lying on the back with the *face up* (Figure 15.12). This position is used for examination and treatment of the anterior surface of the body and for x-rays. *Memory aid:* Without the letter *u* in supine it spells *spine*. In this position, the patient is lying on his or her spine.

Dorsal Recumbent Position

In the **dorsal recumbent position**, the patient is supine (lying on the back) with the knees bent (Figure 15.13). This position is used for the examination and treatment of the abdominal area and for vaginal or rectal examinations.

Sims' Position

In the **Sims' position** the patient is lying on the left side with the right knee and thigh drawn up and with the left arm placed along the back (Figure 15.14). This

position is used in the examination and treatment of the rectal area. This position was named for James Marion Sims, an American physician who lived from 1813 to 1883. The name of this position is spelled properly either as shown here or as *Sims position*.

Knee-Chest Position

In the **knee-chest position**, the patient is lying face down with the hips flexed (bent) so the knees and chest rest on the table (Figure 15.15). This position is used for rectal examinations.

Lithotomy Position

In the **lithotomy position** (lih-**THOT**-oh-mee) the patient is supine with the feet and legs raised and supported in stirrups (Figure 15.16). This position is used for vaginal and rectal examinations.

- *Lithotomy* also means a surgical incision for the removal of a stone, usually from the urinary bladder. This is discussed in Chapter 9.

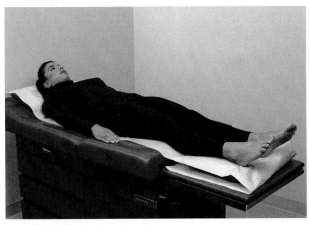

FIGURE 15.12   The horizontal recumbent (supine) position.

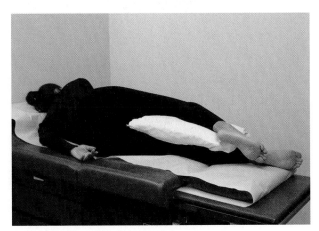

FIGURE 15.14   The Sims' position.

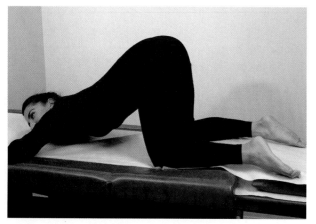

FIGURE 15.15 The knee-chest position.

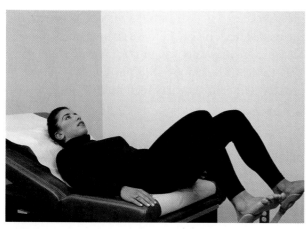

FIGURE 15.16 The lithotomy position.

Trendelenburg Position

In the **Trendelenburg position** the patient is lying on the back with the pelvis higher than the head with the knees slightly bent and the legs hanging off the end of the table (Figure 15.17). This position is used for pelvic surgery and for some radiographic examinations.

- The *modified Trendelenburg position*, which is not shown here, is used in the treatment of shock. The

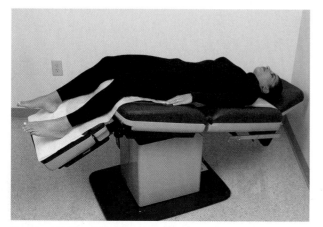

FIGURE 15.17 The Trendelenburg position.

patient is positioned lying flat on the back with the legs elevated 12 to 16 inches above the head in an effort to improve the blood flow to the brain.

LABORATORY TESTS

When a laboratory test is ordered **stat** the results are needed immediately, and the tests have top priority in the laboratory. *Stat* comes from the Latin word meaning immediately.

Blood Tests

When used in regard to laboratory tests, the term **profile** means tests that are frequently performed as a group on automated multichannel laboratory testing equipment.

Obtaining Specimens

- **Phlebotomy** (fleh-**BOT**-oh-mee) is the puncture of a vein for the purpose of drawing blood (**phleb** means vein and **-otomy** means a surgical incision). This is also known as **venipuncture** (**VEN**-ih-**punk**-tyour).

- A **phlebotomist** (fleh-**BOT**-oh-mist) is an individual trained and skilled in phlebotomy.

- A **capillary puncture** is the technique used when only a small amount of blood is needed as a specimen for a blood test. Named for where it is performed, a capillary puncture can be a fingerstick, heel stick, or an earlobe stick.

Complete Blood Cell Counts

A **complete blood cell count** is a series of tests performed as a group to evaluate several blood conditions.

- **Erythrocyte sedimentation rate** (eh-**RITH**-roh-site), also known as a **sed rate**, is a test based on the rate at which the red blood cells separate from the plasma and settle to the bottom of the container. An elevated sed rate indicates the presence of inflammation in the body.

- A **hematocrit test** (hee-**MAT**-oh-krit) measures the percentage, by volume, of packed red blood cells in a whole blood sample (**hemat/o** means blood and **-crit** means to separate). This test is used to diagnose abnormal states of *hydration* (fluid level in the body), *polycythemia* (excess red blood cells), and *anemia* (deficient red blood cells).

- A **platelet count**, which measures the number of platelets in a specified amount of blood, is a screening test to evaluate platelet function. It is also used to monitor thrombocytosis or thrombocytopenia associated with chemotherapy and radiation therapy. *Thrombocytosis* is an abnormal increase in the number of platelets in the circulating blood. *Thrombocytopenia* is an abnormally small number of platelets in the circulating blood.

- A **red blood cell count** is a determination of the number of erythrocytes in the blood. A depressed count may indicate anemia or a hemorrhage lasting more than 24 hours.

- A **total hemoglobin test** measures the amount of hemoglobin found in whole blood (**hem/o** means blood and **-globin** means protein). This test is used to measure the severity of anemia or polycythemia and monitor the response to therapy. *Anemia* is a lower-than-normal level of red cells in the blood. *Polycythemia* is a higher-than-normal in the number of red cells in the blood.

- A **white blood cell count** is a determination of the number of leukocytes in the blood. An elevated count may be an indication of infection or inflammation.

- A **white blood cell differential test** determines what percentage of the total count is composed of each of the five types of leukocyte. This test provides information about the patient's immune system, detects certain types of leukemia, and determines the severity of infection.

Additional Blood Tests

- **Agglutination tests** (ah-**gloo**-tih-**NAY**-shun) are blood tests that involve the clumping together of cells or particles when mixed with incompatible serum. These tests are performed to determine the patient's blood type and to check compatibility of donor and recipient blood before a transfusion.

- **Blood urea nitrogen** (you-**REE**-ah) is the amount of urea present in the blood. This test is a rough indicator of kidney function. *Urea* is the major end product of protein metabolism found in urine and blood.

- **CRP**, which stands for **C-reactive protein**, is a blood test that detects coronary-artery inflammation that could signal an increased risk of heart attack. A score below one is considered to be ideal. A score of three or higher indicates a higher risk.

- **Lipid tests**, also known as a **lipid panel**, measure the amounts of total cholesterol, high-density lipoprotein (HDL), low-density lipoprotein (LDL), and triglycerides in a blood sample.

- **Prothrombin time** (proh-**THROM**-bin), also known as **pro time**, is a test used to diagnose conditions associated with abnormal bleeding and to monitor anticoagulant therapy.

- **Serum enzyme tests** are used to measure the blood enzymes. These tests are useful as evidence of a myocardial infarction.

- The **serum bilirubin test** measures how well red blood cells are being broken down. Elevated levels of bilirubin, which cause jaundice, may indicate liver problems or gallstones.

- A **thyroid-stimulating hormone assay** measures circulating blood levels of thyroid-stimulating hormone that may indicate abnormal thyroid activity.

Urinalysis

Urinalysis (**you**-rih-**NAL**-ih-sis) is the examination of the physical and chemical properties of urine to determine the presence of abnormal elements.

- **Routine urinalysis** is performed to screen for urinary and systemic disorders. This test utilizes a **dipstick**, which is a plastic strip impregnated with chemicals that react with substances in the urine and change color when abnormalities are present (Figure 15.18).

- **Microscopic examination** of the specimen is performed when more detailed testing of the specimen is necessary, for example, to identify casts. **Casts** are fibrous or protein materials, such as pus and fats, that are thrown off into the urine in kidney disease.

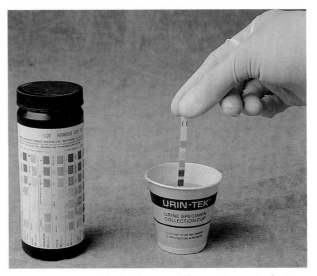

FIGURE 15.18   A dipstick is used for routine urinalysis.

pH Values of Urine

The average normal **pH** range of urine is from 4.5 to 8.0. (The abbreviation **pH** describes the degree of acidity or alkalinity of a substance. A pH of 7 is neutral, that is, neither acid nor alkaline. Maximum acidity is pH 0, and maximum alkalinity is pH 14.)

- A pH value *below* 7 indicates acid urine and is an indication of acidosis.

- A pH value *above* 7 indicates alkaline urine and may indicate conditions including a urinary tract infection.

Specific Gravity

The **specific gravity** of urine reflects the amount of wastes, minerals, and solids that are present.

- **Low specific gravity** (dilute urine) is characteristic of diabetes insipidus.

- **High specific gravity** (concentrated urine) occurs in conditions such as dehydration, liver failure, and shock.

Conditions Identified Through Urinalysis

- **Acetone** (**ASS**-eh-tohn), which has a sweet fruity odor, is found in small quantities in normal urine and in larger amounts in diabetic urine.

- **Albuminuria** (**al**-byou-mih-**NEW**-ree-ah) is the presence of the protein albumin in the urine and is a sign of impaired kidney function (**albumin** means albumin or protein and **-uria** means urine). *Albumin* is a form of protein found in most body tissues.

- **Bacteriuria** (back-**tee**-ree-**YOU**-ree-ah) is the presence of bacteria in the urine (**bacteri** means bacteria and **-uria** means urine).

- **Calciuria** (**kal**-sih-**YOU**-ree-ah) is the presence of calcium in the urine (**calci** means calcium and **-uria** means urine). Abnormally high levels may be diagnostic for hyperparathyroidism, as described in Chapter 13. Lower-than-normal levels may indicate osteomalacia, which is discussed in Chapter 3.

- **Creatinuria** (kree-**at**-ih-**NEW**-ree-ah) is an increased concentration of creatine in the urine (**creatin** means creatinine and **-uria** means urine). *Creatinine* is a waste product of muscle metabolism that is normally removed by the kidneys. The presence of excess creatine is an indication of increased muscle breakdown or a disruption of kidney function.

- A **drug screening** urine test is a rapid method of identifying the presence in the body of one or more abuse drugs such as cocaine, heroin, and marijuana.

- **Glycosuria** (**glye**-koh-**SOO**-ree-ah), which is the presence of glucose in the urine, is most commonly caused by diabetes (**glycos** means glucose and **-uria** means urine).

- **Hematuria** (**hee**-mah-**TOO**-ree-ah *or* **hem**-ah-**TOO**-ree-ah) is the presence of blood in the urine (**hemat** means blood and **-uria** means urine). This condition may be caused by kidney stones, infection, damage to the kidney, or bladder cancer.

- In **gross hematuria** the urine may look pink, brown, or bright red, and the presence of blood can be detected without magnification. In **microscopic hematuria** the urine is clear, but blood cells can be seen under a microscope.

- **Ketonuria** (**kee**-toh-**NEW**-ree-ah) is the presence of ketones in the urine (**keton** means ketones and **-uria** means urine). *Ketones* are formed when the body breaks down fat. Their presence in urine may indicate starvation or uncontrolled diabetes.

- **Proteinuria** (**proh**-tee-in-**YOU**-ree-ah), which is the presence of an abnormal amount of protein in the urine, is usually a sign of kidney disease (**protein** means protein and **-uria** means urine).

- **Pyuria** (pye-**YOU**-ree-ah) is the presence of pus in the urine (**py** means pus and **-uria** means urine).

- **Urine culture and sensitivity** is an additional laboratory test to identify the cause of a urinary tract infection and to determine which antibiotic would be the most effective treatment.

ENDOSCOPY

Endoscopy (en-**DOS**-koh-pee) is the visual examination of the interior of a body cavity (**endo-** means within and **-scopy** means visual examination). These procedures are usually named for the organs involved.

The term **endoscopic surgery** describes a surgical procedure that is performed through very small incisions with the use of an endoscope. These procedures are named for the body parts involved, for example arthroscopic surgery, which is discussed in Chapter 3.

Endoscopes

An **endoscope** (**EN**-doh-**skope**) is the fiber optic instrument that is used for endoscopy and is named for the body parts involved. For example, a hysteroscope is used to examine the interior of the uterus (Figure 15.19).

Laparoscopic Procedures

Laparoscopy (**lap**-ah-**ROS**-koh-pee) is the visual examination of the interior of the abdomen with the use of a laparoscope passed through the abdominal wall (**lapar/o** means abdomen and **-scopy** means visual examination).

Laparoscopic surgery involves the use of a laparoscope plus instruments inserted into the abdomen through small incisions (Figure 15.19). A laparoscope is used to:

- Explore and examine the interior of the abdomen.
- Take specimens to be biopsied.
- Perform surgical procedures.

CENTESIS

Centesis (sen-**TEE**-sis) is a surgical puncture to remove fluid for diagnostic purposes or to remove excess fluid.

- **Abdominocentesis** (ab-**dom**-ih-noh-sen-**TEE**-sis) is the surgical puncture of the abdominal cavity to remove fluid (**abdomin/o** means abdomen and **-centesis** means a surgical puncture to remove fluid).

- **Arthrocentesis** (**ar**-throh-sen-**TEE**-sis) is a surgical puncture of the joint space to remove synovial fluid for analysis to determine the cause of pain or swelling in a joint (**arthr/o** means joint and **-centesis** means a surgical puncture to remove fluid).

- **Cardiocentesis** (**kar**-dee-oh-sen-**TEE**-sis), also known as **cardiopuncture**, is the puncture of a chamber of the heart for diagnosis or therapy (**cardi/o** means heart and **-centesis** means a surgical puncture to remove fluid).

- **Pericardiocentesis** (**pehr**-ih-**kar**-dee-oh-sen-**TEE**-sis) is the drawing of fluid from the pericardial sac for diagnostic purposes or to relieve pressure on the heart (**peri-** means surrounding, **cardi/o** means heart, and **-centesis** means a surgical puncture to remove fluid).

- **Tympanocentesis** (**tim**-pah-noh-sen-**TEE**-sis) is the surgical puncture of the tympanic membrane with a needle to remove fluid from the middle ear (**tympan/o** means eardrum and **-centesis** means a surgical puncture to remove fluid).

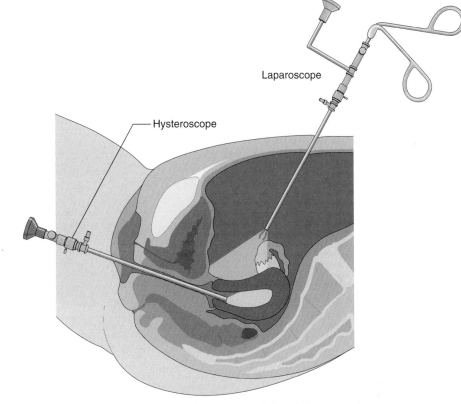

Figure 15.19   A laparoscope is used to examine the interior of the abdomen. A hysteroscope is used to examine the interior of the uterus.

IMAGING TECHNIQUES

Imaging techniques are used to visualize and examine internal body structures. The three most commonly used techniques are compared in Table 15.1. Two of these techniques are compared in Figure 15.20.

Two of these techniques involve the use of ionizing radiation, commonly known as **x-rays**. This radiation is invisible, has no odor, and cannot be felt. But, although this radiation is beneficial in producing images and in treating cancer, excessive exposure is dangerous and can cause death.

Contrast Medium

A **radiographic contrast medium** is a substance used to make visible structures that are otherwise hard to see. These substances may be administered by swallowing, enema, or intravenously.

- A **radiopaque contrast medium** (**ray**-dee-oh-**PAYK**), such as barium, *does not allow* x-rays to pass through and appears white or light gray on the resulting film. Compare with *radiolucent*.

- A **radiolucent contrast medium** (**ray**-dee-oh-**LOO**-sent), such as air or nitrogen gas, *does allow* x-rays to pass through and appears black or dark gray on the resulting film. Compare with *radiopaque*.

- An **intravenous contrast medium** is injected into a vein to make the flow of blood through blood vessels and organs visible. This technique, which is usually named for the vessels or organs involved, is illustrated in Chapter 5 (Figure 5.20).

Barium

Barium is a radiopaque contrast medium used primarily to visualize the gastrointestinal tract (Figure 15.21). It is administered orally as a *barium swallow* for an upper GI study. It is administered rectally as a *barium enema (BE)* for a lower GI study. X-rays and fluoroscopy are used to trace the flow of the barium.

Table 15.1

IMAGING SYSTEMS COMPARED

Method	How It Works
Conventional radiography (x-ray)	Uses radiation (x-rays) passing through the patient to expose a film that shows the body in profile. Hard tissues are light, soft tissues appear as shades of gray, and air is black.
Computerized tomography (CT)	Uses radiation (x-rays) with computer assistance to produce multiple cross-sectional views of the body. Hard tissues are light, and soft tissues appear as shades of gray.
Magnetic resonance imaging (MRI)	Uses a combination of radio waves and a strong magnetic field to produce images. Hard tissues are dark, and soft tissues appear as shades of gray.

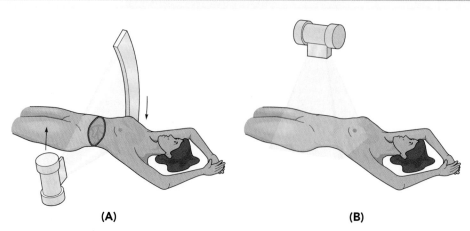

(A)   (B)

FIGURE **15.20**   (A) Computerized tomography provides cross-sectional images. (B) Conventional x-rays superimpose anatomy and can capture images in only one plane.

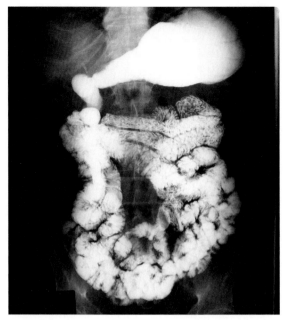

FIGURE 15.21   A radiograph after a barium swallow. The stomach and a portion of the small intestine are visible.

RADIOLOGY

- A **radiologist** (**ray**-dee-**OL**-oh-jist) is a physician who specializes in diagnosing and treating diseases and disorders with x-rays and other forms of radiant energy (**radi** means radiation and **-ologist** means specialist).

- In conventional **radiology**, also known as **x-ray** or **radiography**, an image of hard tissue internal structures is created by the exposure of sensitized film to x-radiation (**radi/o** means radiation and **-graphy** means the process of recording). The resulting film is known as an **x-ray** or **radiograph** (**radi/o** means radiation and **-graph** means the resulting record).

- Radiographs are made up of shades of gray. Radiopaque hard tissues, such as bone and tooth enamel, appear white or light gray on the radiograph. Radiolucent soft tissues appear as shades of gray to black on the radiograph (Figure 15.22).

Radiographic Positioning

The term **radiographic positioning** describes the body placement and the part of the body closest to the x-ray film. For example, in a left lateral position, the left side of the body is placed nearest the film. Compare with *radiographic projections*.

Radiographic Projections

The term **radiographic projection** describes the path that the x-ray beam follows through the body from

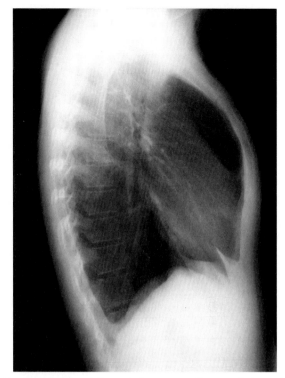

FIGURE 15.22   A lateral chest x-ray. Bones of the spine are white and the soft tissues are shades of gray.

entrance to exit. Compare with *radiographic positioning*.

- The basic projections described in the next section may be used for most body parts (Figure 15.23). These projections may be exposed with the patient in a standing or recumbent position.

- When the name of the projection combines two terms into a single word, the term listed first is the one that the x-ray penetrates first. For example, in a posteroanterior projection, the x-rays travel through the body from the posterior (back) toward the anterior (front) to expose the film (Figure 15.23).

Basic Radiographic Projections

- An **anteroposterior projection** has the patient positioned with the back parallel to the film (**anter/o** means front, **poster** means back, and **-ior** means pertaining to). The x-ray beam travels from anterior (front) to posterior (back).

- A **posteroanterior projection** has the patient positioned facing the film and parallel to it (**poster/o** means back, **anter** means front, and **-ior** means pertaining to). The x-ray beam travels through the body from posterior to anterior.

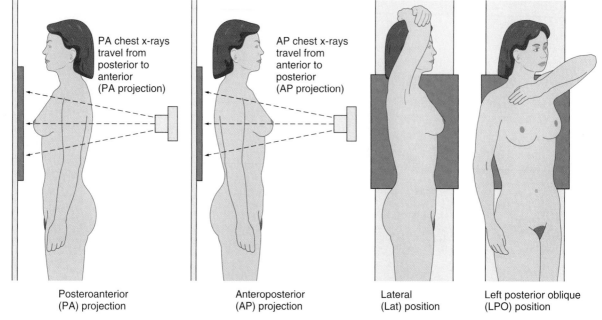

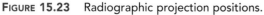

| Posteroanterior (PA) projection | Anteroposterior (AP) projection | Lateral (Lat) position | Left posterior oblique (LPO) position |

FIGURE 15.23 Radiographic projection positions.

- A **lateral projection**, also known as a **side view**, has the patient positioned at right angles to the film. This view is named for the side of the body nearest the film.

- An **oblique projection** has the patient positioned so the body is slanted sideways to the film. This is halfway between a parallel and a right angle position. This view is named for the side of the body nearest the film. *Oblique* means slanted sideways.

Dental Radiography

Specialized techniques and equipment are used in obtaining dental radiographs.

Extraoral Radiography

Extraoral radiography, as used in dentistry, means that the film is placed outside of the mouth. Figure 15.24 is a **panoramic radiograph**, which is also known as a **Panorex**. This film shows all of the structures in both dental arches.

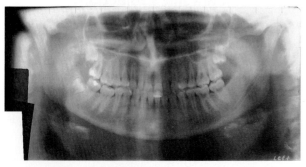

FIGURE 15.24 A Panorex radiograph shows all of the teeth and surrounding structures of the upper and lower dental arches on a single film.

Intraoral Radiography

Intraoral radiography, as used in dentistry, means that the film is placed within the mouth with the camera positioned next to the cheek (Figure 15.25).

- **Periapical radiographs**, which show the entire tooth and some surrounding tissue, are used to detect abnormalities, such as an abscess at the tip

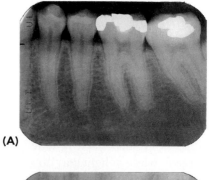

(A)

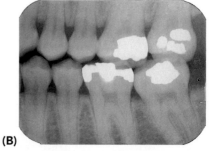

(B)

FIGURE 15.25 Intraoral dental radiographs. (A) A periapical film shows the entire length of a tooth and some of the tissues surrounding the root. (B) A bitewing film shows the crowns of the upper and lower teeth in one area of both jaws. The white areas on these teeth are amalgam (silver) fillings.

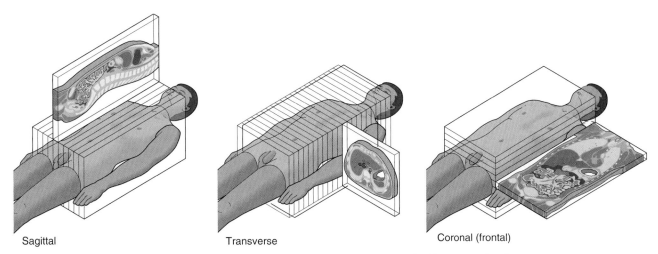

Sagittal   Transverse   Coronal (frontal)

FIGURE 15.26 Computerized tomography provides cross-sectional views of different body planes.

of the root (**peri-** means surrounding, **apic** means apex, and **-al** means pertaining to).

- **Bitewing radiographs**, which show the crowns of teeth in both arches, are used primarily to detect dental decay (cavities) between the teeth.

COMPUTERIZED TOMOGRAPHY

Computerized tomography (toh-**MOG**-rah-fee) uses a thin fan-shaped x-ray beam that rotates around the patient to produce multiple cross-sectional views of the body (**tom/o** means to cut, section, or slice and **-graphy** means the process of recording a picture or record) (Figure 15.26).

- Information gathered by radiation detectors is downloaded to a computer, analyzed, and converted into gray-scale images corresponding to anatomic slices of the body (Figure 15.27). These

images are viewed on a monitor or printed as hard copy (films).

MAGNETIC RESONANCE IMAGING

Magnetic resonance imaging (MRI) uses a combination of radio waves and a strong magnetic field to create signals that are sent to a computer and converted into images of any plane through the body. MRI is used for the study of the heart, blood vessels, brain, spinal cord, joints, muscles, and internal organs. In these images, hard tissues appear dark and soft tissues are bright (Figure 15.28).

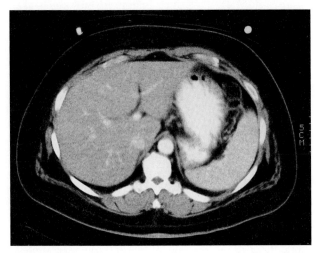

FIGURE 15.27 An abdominal CT scan in which the liver is predominant in the upper left and the stomach is visible in the upper right.

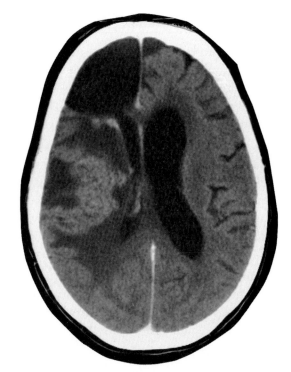

FIGURE 15.28 An MRI of the brain with a tumor visible in the upper left.

- In **closed architecture MRI**, also known as **high-field MRI**, patients may be uncomfortable because of the noise generated by the machine and the feeling of being closed in. In **open architecture MRI**, the design of the equipment is less confining and more comfortable for some patients.

- **Magnetic Resonance Angiography**, also known as **MRA** or **magnetic resonance angio**, combines MRI with the use of a contrast medium to locate problems with blood vessels throughout the body. MRA is frequently used as an alternative to conventional angiography, which is described in Chapter 5.

FLUOROSCOPY

Fluoroscopy (**floo**-or-**OS**-koh-pee) is the visualization of body parts in motion by projecting x-ray images on a luminous fluorescent screen (**fluor/o** means glowing and **-scopy** means visual examination). *Luminous* means glowing.

- **Cineradiography** (**sin**-eh-**ray**-dee-**OG**-rah-fee) is the recording of images as they appear in motion on a fluorescent screen (**cine-** means relationship to movement, **radi/o** means radiation, and **-graphy** means process of recording a picture or record).

- Fluoroscopy may also be used in conjunction with conventional x-ray techniques to capture a record of parts of the examination.

DIAGNOSTIC ULTRASOUND

Diagnostic ultrasound, also known as **ultrasonography** (**ul**-trah-son-**OG**-rah-fee), is imaging of deep body structures by recording the echoes of pulses of sound waves above the range of human hearing. The resulting record is called a **sonogram** (**SOH**-noh-gram).

- Commonly referred to as **ultrasound**, this technique is most effective for viewing solid organs of the abdomen and soft tissues where the signal is not stopped by intervening bone or air. Common uses of ultrasound include evaluating fetal development, detecting the presence of gallstones, or confirming the presence of a mass found on a mammogram.

- **Carotid ultrasonography** is the use of sound waves to image the carotid artery to detect an obstruction that could cause an ischemic stroke, which is described in Chapter 10.

- **Echocardiography** (**eck**-oh-**kar**-dee-**OG**-rah-fee) is an ultrasonic diagnostic procedure used to evaluate the structures and motion of the heart (**ech/o** means sound, **cardi/o** means heart, and **-graphy** means the process of recording a picture or record). The resulting record is an **echocardiogram**.

- A **Doppler echocardiogram** is performed in the same way as an echocardiogram; however, this procedure measures the speed and direction of the blood flow within the heart. Shown in Figure 15.29 is a Doppler echocardiogram enhanced with color.

- **Transesophageal echocardiography** (**trans**-eh-**sof**-ah-**JEE**-al **eck**-oh-**kar**-dee-**OG**-rah-fee), which is an ultrasonic imaging technique used to evaluate heart structures, is performed from inside the esophagus. Because the esophagus is so close to the heart, this technique produces clearer images than those obtained with echocardiography.

NUCLEAR MEDICINE

Nuclear medicine (**NM**) utilizes radioactive substances known as **radiopharmaceuticals** for both diagnosis and treatment purposes.

- Each radiopharmaceutical contains a **radionuclide tracer**, also known as a **radioactive tracer**, which is specific to the body system being examined.

- Radiopharmaceuticals emit gamma rays that are detected by a **gamma-ray camera** attached to a computer. This data is used to generate an image showing the pattern of absorption that indicates pathology.

- When used for diagnostic purposes, NM is referred to as **nuclear imaging**. The images that are pro-

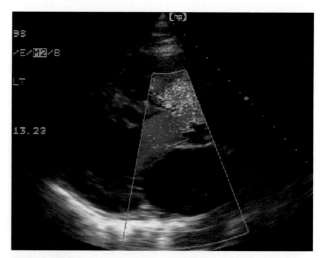

Figure 15.29   A Doppler echocardiogram. The large area of red shows the flow of blood through an abnormal opening between the aorta and right atrium.

duced document the structure and function of the organ or organs being examined.

Nuclear Scans

A **nuclear scan**, also known as a **scintigram** (**SIN**-tih-gram), is a diagnostic procedure that uses nuclear medicine technology to gather information about the structure and function of organs or systems that cannot be seen on conventional x-rays.

Bone Scans

In a **bone scan** the radionuclide tracer is injected into the bloodstream; the patient then waits while the material travels through the body tissues. Only pathology in the bones absorbs the radionuclide, and these are visible as dark areas on the scan (Figure 15.30).

Thyroid Scans

For a **thyroid scan**, a radiopharmaceutical containing radioactive iodine is administered. The rate of iodine uptake by the thyroid is an indicator of thyroid function.

Single Photon Emission Computerized Tomography

Single photon emission computerized tomography, also known as **SPECT**, is a nuclear imaging technique in which pictures are taken by one to three gamma cameras after a radionuclide tracer has been injected into the blood. *Emission* means the process of giving off or throwing forth.

- During SPECT, these **gamma cameras**, also known as **detectors**, rotate around the patient's body collecting data and producing images on a variety of planes.

- This technique is used to study myocardial perfusion. **Perfusion** (per-**FYOU**-zuhn) is the flow of blood through an organ.

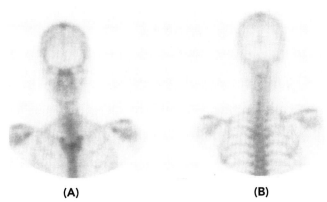

(A)   **(B)**

FIGURE 15.30   A bone scan of the head, shoulders, and upper spine. (A) Anterior view. (B) Posterior view.

Positron Emission Tomography

Positron emission tomography combines tomography with radionuclide tracers to produce enhanced images of selected body organs or areas. This imagining technique is used to determine cardiac or cerebral perfusion and for brain imaging to aid in the diagnosis of epilepsy, dementia, and recurrent brain tumors.

RADIOIMMUNOASSAY

Radioimmunoassay (**ray**-dee-oh-**im**-you-noh-**ASS**-ay) (**RIA**), also known as **radioassay**, is a laboratory technique in which a radioactively labeled substance is mixed with a blood specimen.

- *Assay* means to determine the amount of a particular substance in a mixture. These techniques can be used to evaluate function of the pituitary and thyroid glands.

- **Immunofluorescence** (**im**-you-noh-**floo**-oh-**RES**-ens) is a method of tagging antibodies with a fluorescent dye to detect or localize antigen-antibody combinations.

PHARMACOLOGY

Pharmacology is the study of the nature, uses, and effects of drugs for medical purposes. A **pharmacist** is a specialist who is licensed to formulate and dispense prescribed medications.

- A **prescription** is an order for medication, therapy, or a therapeutic device. This order is given by one authorized person to another authorized person to properly dispense or perform the order. Abbreviations commonly used in relation to prescriptions and drug administration are shown in Table 15.2.

Prescription and Over-the-Counter Drugs

- A **prescription drug** is a medication that may be dispensed only with a prescription from an appropriately licensed professional, such as a physician or dentist.

- An **over-the-counter drug**, also known as an **O-T-C**, is a medication that may be dispensed without a written prescription.

Generic and Brand Name Drugs

- A **generic drug** is usually named for its chemical structure and is not protected by a brand name or

Table 15.2

FREQUENTLY USED DRUG ADMINISTRATION ABBREVIATIONS AND SYMBOLS

Abbreviation	Meaning	Abbreviation	Meaning
@	at	q.i.d.	four times a day
ac	before meals	↑	increase
ad lib	as desired	↓	decrease
amt	amount	>	greater than
b.i.d., bid	twice a day	≥	greater than or equal to
c̄	with	<	less than
NPO	nothing by mouth	≤	less than or equal to
p.c.	after meals	Rx	prescription
p.o.	by mouth	sig	let it be labeled
p.r.n.	as needed	t.i.d.	three times a day
q.d.	every day	♀	female
q.h.	every hour	♂	male

trademark. For example, *diazepam* is the generic name of a drug frequently used as a muscle relaxant.

- A **brand name** drug is sold under the name given the drug by the manufacturer. A brand name is always spelled with a capital letter. For example, *Valium* is a brand name for diazepam.

Terminology Related to Pharmacology

- **Addiction** is compulsive, uncontrollable dependence on a substance, habit, or practice to the degree that stopping causes severe emotional, mental, or physiologic reactions.
- An **adverse drug reaction**, also known as a **side effect** or an **adverse drug event**, is an undesirable drug response that accompanies the principal response for which the drug was taken.
- **Compliance** is the patient's consistency and accuracy in following the regimen prescribed by a physician or other health care professional. As used here, **regimen** (**REJ**-ih-men) means directions or rules.

- A **contraindication** is a factor in the patient's condition that makes the use of a drug dangerous or ill advised.
- A **drug interaction** changes the effect of one drug when it is administered at the same time as another drug.
- An **idiosyncratic reaction** (**id**-ee-oh-sin-**KRAT**-ick) is an unexpected reaction to a drug.
- A **palliative** (**PAL**-ee-**ay**-tiv *or* **PAL**-ee-ah-tiv) is a substance that eases the pain or severity of a disease but does not cure it.
- A **paradoxical drug reaction** is an induced effect that is the exact opposite of that which was therapeutically intended. *Paradoxical* means not being normal or the usual kind.
- A **placebo** (plah-**SEE**-boh) is a substance containing no active ingredients that is given for its suggestive effects. In research, a placebo identical in appearance with the material being tested is administered to distinguish between drug action and suggestive effect of the material under study.

- **Potentiation** (poh-**ten**-shee-**AY**-shun), also known as **synergism** (**SIN**-er-jizm), is a drug interaction that occurs when the effect of one drug is potentiated (increased) by another drug.

Routes of Drug Administration

- **Inhalation administration** refers to vapor and gases taken in through the nose or mouth and absorbed into the bloodstream through the lungs. For example, the gases used for general anesthesia are administered by inhalation.

- **Oral administration** refers to drugs taken by mouth to be absorbed from the stomach or small intestine. These drugs may be in forms such as liquids, pills, or capsules. An *enteric coating* is applied to some tablets or capsules to prevent the release and absorption of their contents until they reach the small intestine.

- **Percutaneous treatment** (**per**-kyou-**TAY**-nee-us) is a procedure that is performed through the skin (**per**- means through, **cutane** means skin, and -**ous** means pertaining to). See Chapters 3 and 5 for examples of percutaneous treatment.

- **Rectal administration** is the insertion of medication in the rectum by use of either suppositories or liquid solutions. A *suppository* is medication in a semisolid form that is introduced into the rectum. The suppository melts at body temperature and the medication is absorbed through the surrounding tissues.

- With **sublingual administration**, the medication is placed under the tongue and allowed to dissolve slowly (**sub**- means under, **lingu** means tongue, and

-**al** means pertaining to). Once dissolved, the medication is quickly absorbed through the sublingual tissue directly into the bloodstream.

- **Topical and transdermal administration** are discussed in Chapter 12.

Parenteral Administration

- **Parenteral administration** (pah-**REN**-ter-al) is the administration of medication by injection through a **hypodermic syringe** (**high**-poh-**DER**-mick) (Figure 15.31).

- A **subcutaneous injection** is made into the fatty layer just below the skin.

- An **intradermal injection** is made into the middle layers of the skin.

- An **intramuscular injection** is made directly into muscle tissue.

- An **intravenous injection** is made directly into a vein.

- A **bolus** (**BOH**-lus), also known as a **bolus infusion**, is a single dose of drug usually injected into a blood vessel over a short period of time. The term *bolus* is also used in relation to the digestive system in Chapter 8.

ABBREVIATIONS RELATED TO THE DIAGNOSTIC PROCEDURES AND PHARMACOLOGY

Table 15.3 presents an overview of the abbreviations related to the terms introduced in this chapter. *Note:* To avoid errors or confusion, always be cautious when using abbreviations.

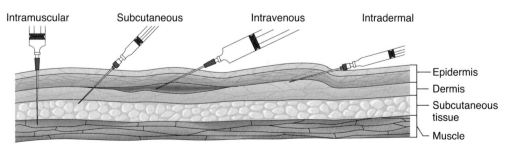

FIGURE 15.31   Types of injections.

Table 15.3

ABBREVIATIONS RELATED TO THE DIAGNOSTIC PROCEDURES AND PHARMACOLOGY

adverse drug reaction = ADR	**ADR** = adverse drug reaction
anteroposterior = AP	**AP** = anteroposterior
auscultation = A	**A** = auscultation
barium = Ba	**Ba** = barium
beats per minute = bpm	**bpm** = beats per minute
blood pressure = BP	**BP** = blood pressure
blood urea nitrogen = BUN	**BUN** = blood urea nitrogen
bruit = B	**B** = bruit
complete blood count = CBC	**CBC** = complete blood count
computerized tomography = CT	**CT** = computerized tomography
echocardiography = ECHO	**ECHO** = echocardiography
endoscopy = endo	**endo** = endoscopy
erythrocyte sedimentation rate = ESR	**ESR** = erythrocyte sedimentation rate
fluoroscopy = Flour	**Flour** = fluoroscopy
hematuria = HEM	**HEM** = hematuria
hematocrit = Hct, hct, hemat, hmt	**Hct, hct, hemat, hmt** = hematocrit
intradermal = ID	**ID** = intradermal
intramuscular = IM	**IM** = intramuscular
immunofluorescence = IMI	**IMI** = immunofluorescence
intravenous = IV	**IV** = intravenous
laparoscopy = LAP	**LAP** = laparoscopy
lateral = lat	**lat** = lateral
magnetic resonance angiography = MRA	**MRA** = magnetic resonance angiography
magnetic resonance imaging = MRI	**MRI** = magnetic resonance imaging
nuclear imaging = NI	**NI** = nuclear imaging
nuclear medicine = NM	**NM** = nuclear medicine
oblique = obl	**obl** = oblique

Table 15.3 (continued)

ABBREVIATIONS RELATED TO THE DIAGNOSTIC PROCEDURES AND PHARMACOLOGY

percussion, pulse = P	**P** = percussion, pulse
platelet count = PLC	**PLC** = platelet count
posteroanterior = PA	**PA** = posteroanterior
positron emission tomography = PET	**PET** = positron emission tomography
prothrombin time = PT	**PT** = prothrombin time
radioimmunoassay = RIA	**RIA** = radioimmunoassay
radiopharmaceuticals = RP	**RP** = radiopharmaceuticals
red blood count = RBC	**RBC** = red blood count
respiratory rate = RR	**RR** = respiratory rate
subcutaneous = SC	**SC** = subcutaneous
single photon emission computerized tomography = SPECT	**SPECT** = single photon emission computerized tomography
temperature = T	**T** = temperature
temperature, pulse, respiration = TPR	**TPR** = temperature, pulse, respiration
transesophageal echocardiography = TEE	**TEE** = transesophageal echocardiography
urinalysis = UA, U/A	**UA, U/A** = urinalysis
white blood count = WBC	**WBC** = white blood count

Learning Exercises

Matching Word Parts 1

Write the correct answer in the middle column.

Definition	Correct Answer	Possible Answers
15.1. abdomen	_____	**albumin/o**
15.2. glowing	_____	**calc/i**
15.3. sugar	_____	**lapar/o**
15.4. albumin, protein	_____	**fluor/o**
15.5. calcium	_____	**glycos/o**

Matching Word Parts 2

Write the correct answer in the middle column.

Definition	Correct Answer	Possible Answers
15.6. blood	_____	**-graph**
15.7. pertaining to	_____	**-graphy**
15.8. the process of producing a picture or record	_____	**hemat/o**
15.9. a picture or record	_____	**-ous**
15.10. through	_____	**per-**

● **Matching Word Parts 3**

Write the correct answer in the middle column.

Definition	Correct Answer	Possible Answers
15.11. visual examination instrument	_____	**phleb/o**
15.12. urine	_____	**radi/o**
15.13. vein	_____	**-scope**
15.14. visual examination	_____	**-scopy**
15.15. radiation	_____	**-uria**

● **Definitions**

Select the correct answer and write it on the line provided.

15.16. The _____ projection has the patient positioned at right angles to the film.

    anteroposterior   lateral   oblique   posteroanterior

15.17. A/An _____ is used to enlarge the opening of any canal or cavity to facilitate inspection of its interior.

    endoscope   otoscope   speculum   sphygmomanometer

15.18. The imaging technique that produces multiple cross-sectional images using x-radiation is

_____ .

    conventional x-ray   computerized tomography   magnetic resonance imaging   ultrasound

15.19. The blood test used to indicate the presence of inflammation in the body is commonly known as a/an

_____ test.

    agglutination   CRP   lipid   sed rate

15.20. The diagnostic technique that uses the echoes of sound waves to image deep structures of the body is

_____ .

    cineradiography   fluoroscopy   magnetic resonance imaging   ultrasound

15.21. The term _____ describes the presence of calcium in the urine.

    albuminuria   calciuria   creatinuria   glycosuria

15.22. The _____ _____ test is used to monitor anticoagulant therapy.

      lipid panel   prothrombin time   sedimentation rate   serum enzyme

15.23. The _____ test measures the percentage by volume of packed red blood cells in a

      whole blood sample.

      hematocrit   hemoglobin   red blood cell count   white blood cell count

15.24. An abnormal "rattley" respiratory sound heard while listening to the chest while the patient is breathing

      in is known as a _____ .

      bruit   rale   rhonchus   stridor

15.25. The substance, which has a sweet fruity odor, that is found in small quantities in normal urine and in

      larger amount in diabetic urine is _____ .

      acetone   creatinine   ketone   urea

● Matching Techniques

Write the correct answer in the middle column.

Definition	Correct Answer	Possible Answers
15.26. uses powerful magnets	_____	centesis
15.27. uses a glowing screen	_____	CT
15.28. provides cross-sectional views	_____	x-rays
15.29. removal of fluid for diagnostic purposes	_____	fluoroscopy
15.30. shows hard tissues as white	_____	MRI

● Which Word?

Select the correct answer and write it on the line provided.

15.31. The term meaning an unexpected reaction to a drug is _____ .

      idiosyncratic   palliative

15.32. The technology that combines tomography with radionuclide traces is called _____ .

      PET   radioimmunoassay

15.33. A substance that does not allow x-rays to pass through is said to be _____ .

     radiolucent   radiopaque

15.34. A periapical film is an example of an _____ dental radiograph.

     extraoral   intraoral

15.35. The name of a _____ drug is always spelled with a capital letter.

     brand name   generic

● Spelling Counts

Find the misspelled word in each sentence. Then write that word, spelled correctly, on the line provided.

15.36. Listening through a stethoscope for sounds within the body to determine the condition of the lungs, pleura, heart, and abdomen is known as asultation. _____

15.37. A sphygnomanometer is used to measure blood pressure. _____

15.38. The technique used to visualize body parts in motion is known as fluroscopy. _____

15.39. The clumping together of cells or particles when mixed with incompatible blood is called agelutination.

_____

15.40. An opthalmoscope is used to examine the interior of the eye. _____

● Abbreviation Identification

In the space provided, write the words that each abbreviation stands for.

15.41. **ad lib**   _____

15.42. **IV**   _____

15.43. **NPO**   _____

15.44. **q.i.d.**   _____

15.45. **sig**   _____

● **Term Selection**

Select the correct answer and write it on the line provided.

15.46. The term meaning drawing of fluid from the sac surrounding the heart is _____ .

    abdominocentesis   cardiocentesis   pericardiocentesis   tympanocentesis

15.47. The term meaning the abnormal presence of blood in the urine is _____ .

    albuminuria   creatinuria   hematuria   ketonuria

15.48. The term meaning a projection in which the patient is positioned with his or her back parallel to the film

    is a/an _____ projection.

    anteroposterior   lateral   oblique   posteroanterior

15.49. The term _____ describes a laboratory technique in which a radioactively labeled

    substance is mixed with a blood specimen.

    nuclear scan   perfusion   radioactive tracer   radioimmunoassay

15.50. The term meaning the administration of a medication by injection is _____ .

    parenteral   percutaneous   transcutaneous   transdermal

● **Sentence Completion**

Write the correct term on the line provided.

15.51. The path that the x-ray beam follows through the body from entrance to exit is known as the

    _____ .

15.52. When a factor in the patient's condition makes the use of a drug dangerous or ill-advised, this is known

    as a/an _____ .

15.53. The respiratory sound that is also known as wheezing is _____ . This sound occurs

    during inspiration or expiration and is caused by a partially obstructed airway.

15.54. The instrument used to visually examine the external ear and the eardrum is a/an

    _____ .

15.55. A compulsive, uncontrollable dependence on a substance or drug is known as a/an

    _____ .

● Word Surgery

Divide each term into its component word parts. Write these word parts, in sequence, on the lines provided.

When necessary use a back slash (/) to indicate a combining vowel. (You may not need all of the lines provided.)

15.56. **Tympanocentesis** is the surgical puncture of the tympanic membrane with a needle to remove fluid from

the middle ear.

_____   _____   _____   _____

15.57. **Cineradiography** is the recording of images as they appear in motion on a fluorescent screen.

_____   _____   _____   _____

15.58. **Echocardiography** is an ultrasonic diagnostic procedure used to evaluate the structures and motion of

the heart.

_____   _____   _____   _____

15.59. **Bacteriuria** is the presence of bacteria in the urine.

_____   _____   _____   _____

15.60. **Auscultation** is listening through a stethoscope for respiratory, heart, and abdominal sounds within the

body.

_____   _____   _____   _____

● True/False

If the statement is true, write **T** on the line. If the statement is false, write **F** on the line.

15.61. _____ For an oblique projection, the patient's body is positioned parallel to the film.

15.62. _____ Casts are fibrous or protein materials, such as pus and fats, that are thrown off into the urine in

kidney disease.

15.63. _____ A placebo has the potential to cure a disease.

15.64. _____ An MRI creates images by combining high-frequency ultrasonic waves and strong magnets.

15.65. _____ Compliance means that the patient has accurately followed instructions.

● **Clinical Conditions**

Write the correct answer on the line provided.

15.66. The urinalysis for Selma LaPinta showed the presence of pus. The medical term for this condition is

_____ .

15.67. For the rectal examination, Mr. Johnson was placed in the _____-_____

position, with his face down, his hips flexed, and his knees and chest resting on the table.

15.68. Kelly Harrison was extremely cold after being stranded in a snowstorm. When rescued, the medics said

she was suffering from _____ .

15.69. During her examination of the patient, Dr. Wong used _____ to feel the texture,

size, consistency, and location of certain body parts.

15.70. Dr. McDowell ordered a blood _____ _____ (BUN) test for

his patient because this test is a rough indicator of kidney function.

15.71. In preparation for his upper GI series, Dwight Oshone swallowed a liquid containing the contrast

medium _____.

15.72. Maria Martinez required _____ echocardiography (TEE) to evaluate the structures

of her heart.

15.73. For the examination, Scott Cunningham was placed lying on his belly with his face down. This is a/an

_____ position.

15.74. The urinalysis for Kathleen McCaffee showed the presence of glucose in the urine. The medical term for

this condition is _____ .

15.75. During the examination, Dr. Roberts used _____ . This involves tapping the sur-

face of the body with a finger or instrument.

● **Which Is the Correct Medical Term?**

Select the correct answer and write it on the line provided.

15.76. The term meaning an undesirable drug response is a/an _____ response.

adverse drug   idiosyncratic   potentiation   synergism

15.77. The examination position that is also used for the treatment of shock is the _____

position.

      lithotomy   recumbent   Sims'   Trendelenburg

15.78. The type of dental radiograph that shows the entire tooth and some of the surrounding tissue is a/an

_____ film.

      bite-wing   extraoral   periapical   survey

15.79. The imaging technique that uses one to three gamma cameras to capture images is

_____ .

      MRI   PET   radioimmunoassay   SPECT

15.80. The examination position that has the patient in a supine position with the feet and legs supported in

stirrups is the _____ position.

      decubitus   dorsal recumbent   lithotomy   Sims'

● Challenge Word Building

These terms are *not* found in this chapter; however, they are made up of the following familiar word parts. You

may want to look in the textbook glossary or use a medical dictionary to check your answers.

hyper-	**albumin/o**	**-centesis**
hypo-	**angi/o**	**-emia**
	arthr/o	**-gram**
	calc/i	**-ology**
	cyst/o	**-scope**
	glycos/o	**-scopy**
	protein/o	**-uria**
	py/o	
	radi/o	

15.81. The term meaning the visual examination of the interior of a joint is _____ .

15.82. The term meaning an abnormally high level of albumin in the blood is _____ .

15.83. The term meaning the presence of excess sugar in the urine is _____ .

15.84. The instrument used to visually examine the interior of the urinary bladder is a/an

_____ .

15.85. The term meaning the study of the use of radiant energy and radioactive substances in medicine is

_____ .

15.86. The term meaning a surgical puncture to remove fluid from the interior of a joint is

_____ .

15.87. The term meaning an abnormally low level of calcium in the circulating blood is

_____ .

15.88. The term meaning the record produced by a radiographic study of blood vessels is a/an

_____ .

15.89. The term meaning the presence of pus-forming organisms in the blood is _____ .

15.90. The term meaning the presence of excess protein in the urine is _____ .

● Labeling Exercises

Identify the numbered items on the accompanying figures.

15.91. This is the _____ position.

15.92. This is the _____ recumbent position.

15.93. This is the _____ position.

15.94. This is the _____ recumbent position.

15.95. This is the _____ position.

15.96. This is the _____ position.

15.97. This is a/an _____ injection.

15.98. This is a/an _____ injection.

15.99. This is a/an _____ injection.

15.100. This is a/an _____ injection.

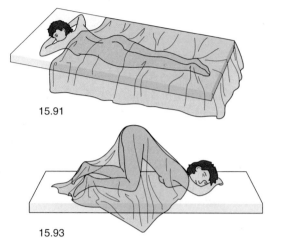

15.91

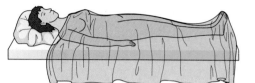

15.92

15.93

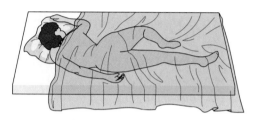

15.94

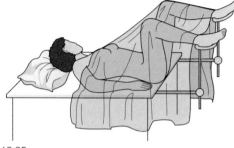

15.95

15.96

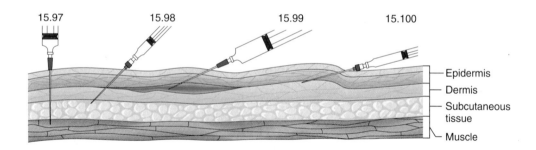

15.97   15.98   15.99   15.100

Epidermis
Dermis
Subcutaneous tissue
Muscle

THE HUMAN TOUCH: CRITICAL THINKING EXERCISE

The following story and questions are designed to stimulate critical thinking through class discussion or as a brief essay response. There are no right or wrong answers to these questions.

Terrance Ortega had finally made it. Sitting behind the counter of the pharmacy at SuperDrug, he thought back on his years at pharmacology school. He had studied hard, and it paid off when he landed this job.

A young man approached the counter, "I'm James Tirendale, and I'm here to pick up my mom Ginny's prescription for MS Contin." He flashed a handwritten scrawled note from his mom. "Sure thing James, let me just find that for you."

Terrance headed to the counter where filled prescriptions were kept and grabbed the one marked Ginny Tirendale. Sure enough, there was a prescription for MS Contin; a palliative usually prescribed for pain.

He explained to James the adverse affects that this drug could have, that it was to be administered orally, and that it was not to be crushed or cut. James paid cash and headed out of the store in a hurry.

Later that day a woman came up to the pharmacy counter on crutches. She explained that her name was Ginny Tirendale and that she needed to pick up some pain medication because she'd just had knee surgery. A confused look came over Terrance's face. "Your son already picked that up, Ms. Tirendale," he explained. "Oh no!" Ginny replied, "I knew I shouldn't have told him I was coming here this afternoon. He must have realized which drug I was prescribed and got here before me."

Suddenly Terrance realized that he should have looked at the note more closely or called Ms. Tirendale before giving out a prescription for a drug with such a high "street value." It occurred to him that potentiation would occur if MS Contin was taken with alcohol, and it could easily lead to psychological and physical dependence if abused. What if her son didn't know that and died, or sold it to someone else who abused it?

Suggested Discussion Topics:

1. Could Terrance have his pharmacology license suspended for giving a prescription to the wrong person?

2. If James suffers harm from the drug, should Terrance be held responsible?

3. What can pharmacists do to help prevent situations such as this from happening?

4. If Ms. Tirendale suspects her son is abusing MS Contin or other prescription drugs, what steps could she take to help him?

5. Imagine that you are in Terrance's situation. How would you deal with telling the young man that he could not pick up the prescription?

Comprehensive Medical Terminology Review

Overview of Comprehensive Medical Terminology Review

Study Tips	Hints to help you review more effectively.
Review Section	A 100-question multiple-choice practice session with an answer key to help you determine where you need more study emphasis. The Review Session Test may be taken repeatedly; however, be aware that none of these questions is from the actual final test.
Confirming Mastery	A 100-question multiple-choice "mock" final test with an answer key to help you evaluate your progress. The Confirming Mastery Test may be taken repeatedly; however, be aware that none of these questions is from the actual final test.

Vocabulary Review List

The items on this list have been selected from the first 15 chapters of this book. However, all words on chapter vocabulary list and terms in boldface in the text are also important and may be included in review exercises and tests.

Word Parts

- [ ] angi/o
- [ ] aort/o
- [ ] arteri/o
- [ ] ather/o
- [ ] brady-
- [ ] cardi/o
- [ ] coron/o
- [ ] -emia
- [ ] erythr/o
- [ ] hem/o, hemat/o
- [ ] leuk/o
- [ ] phleb/o
- [ ] tachy-
- [ ] thromb/o
- [ ] ven/o

Medical Terms

- [ ] **acromegaly** (**ack**-roh-**MEG**-ah-lee)
- [ ] **acronym** (**ACK**-roh-nim)
- [ ] **adhesion** (ad-**HEE**-zhun)
- [ ] **Alzheimer's disease** (**ALTZ**-high-merz)
- [ ] **anaphylaxis** (**an**-ah-fih-**LACK**-sis)
- [ ] **aneurysm** (**AN**-you-rizm)
- [ ] **auscultation** (**aws**-kul-**TAY**-shun)
- [ ] **blepharoplasty** (**BLEF**-ah-roh-**plas**-tee)
- [ ] **catheterization** (**kath**-eh-ter-eye-**ZAY**-shun)
- [ ] **cholecystitis** (**koh**-lee-sis-**TYE**-tis)
- [ ] **cirrhosis** (sih-**ROH**-sis)
- [ ] **Cushing's syndrome** (**KUSH**-ingz **SIN**-drohm)
- [ ] **decubitus ulcer** (dee-**KYOU**-bih-tus)
- [ ] **diabetes mellitus** (**dye**-ah-**BEE**-teez mel-**EYE**-tus *or* **MEL**-ih-tus)
- [ ] **diphtheria** (dif-**THEE**-ree-ah)
- [ ] **electromyography** (ee-**leck**-troh-my-**OG**-rah-fee)
- [ ] **embolus** (**EM**-boh-lus)
- [ ] **endoscopy** (en-**DOS**-koh-pee)

- [ ] **eponym** (**EP**-oh-nim)
- [ ] **esophagogastroduodenoscopy** (eh-**sof**-ah-goh-**gas**-troh-**dew**-oh-deh-**NOS**-koh-pee)
- [ ] **factious disorder** (fack-**TISH**-us)
- [ ] **hemodialysis** (**hee**-moh-dye-**AL**-ih-sis)
- [ ] **hepatitis** (**hep**-ah-**TYE**-tis)
- [ ] **hydrocephalus** (high-droh-**SEF**-ah-lus)
- [ ] **hypercapnia** (**high**-per-**KAP**-nee-ah)
- [ ] **hyperopia** (**high**-per-**OH**-pee-ah)
- [ ] **idiopathic disease** (id-ee-oh-**PATH**-ick)
- [ ] **kinesiology** (kih-**nee**-see-**OL**-oh-jee)
- [ ] **kyphosis** (kye-**FOH**-sis)
- [ ] **metastasis** (meh-**TAS**-tah-sis)
- [ ] **metastasize** (meh-**TAS**-tah-sighz)
- [ ] **myocardial infarction** (**my**-oh-**KAR**-dee-al in-**FARK**-shun)
- [ ] **myopia** (my-**OH**-pee-ah)
- [ ] **necrotizing fasciitis** (**fas**-ee-**EYE**-tis)
- [ ] **nosocomial infection** (**nos**-oh-**KOH**-mee-al)
- [ ] **osteopenia** (**oss**-tee-oh-**PEE**-nee-ah)
- [ ] **Papanicolaou test** (**pap**-ah-**nick**-oh-**LAY**-ooh)
- [ ] **Parkinson's disease**
- [ ] **perimenopause** (pehr-ih-**MEN**-oh-pawz)
- [ ] **peritoneal dialysis** (**pehr**-ih-toh-**NEE**-al dye-**AL**-ih-sis)
- [ ] **phlebotomy** (fleh-**BOT**-oh-mee)
- [ ] **polycystic kidney disease** (**pol**-ee-**SIS**-tick)
- [ ] **presbyopia** (**pres**-bee-**OH**-pee-ah)
- [ ] **rheumatism** (**ROO**-mah-tizm)
- [ ] **sarcoma** (sar-**KOH**-mah)
- [ ] **sarcopenia** (**sar**-koh-**PEE**-nee-ah)
- [ ] **scoliosis** (**skoh**-lee-**OH**-sis)
- [ ] **sphygmomanometer** (**sfig**-moh-mah-**NOM**-eh-ter)
- [ ] **spina bifida** (**SPY**-nah **BIF**-ih-dah)
- [ ] **syndrome** (**SIN**-drohm)
- [ ] **syphilis** (**SIF**-ih-lis)
- [ ] **thrombosis** (throm-**BOH**-sis)
- [ ] **thyrotoxicosis** (**thy**-roh-**tock**-sih-**KOH**-sis)
- [ ] **tinnitus** (tih-**NIGH**-tus)
- [ ] **tracheostomy** (**tray**-kee-**OS**-toh-mee)
- [ ] **tracheotomy** (**tray**-kee-**OT**-oh-mee)
- [ ] **trauma** (**TRAW**-mah)
- [ ] **triage** (tree-**AHZH**)
- [ ] **vertigo** (**VER**-tih-go)
- [ ] **xeroderma** (zee-roh-**DER**-mah)

● O B J E C T I V E S

On completion of this chapter, you should be able to:

1. Recognize, define, spell, and pronounce the terms on the vocabulary lists from the first 15 chapters.

2. Recognize and define the word parts from the flash cards.

3. Recognize, define, spell, and pronounce the medical terms in Appendix C.

STUDY TIPS

Use Your Vocabulary Lists

- After you have added any terms suggested by your instructor, photocopy the vocabulary list for each chapter in your textbook. These sheets are easy to carry with you for additional review whenever you have a free minute.

- Review the terms on each list. When you have mastered a term, put a check in the box next to it. If you cannot spell and define a term, highlight it for further study.

- Look up the meanings of the highlighted terms in the textbook and work on mastering them.

- When using a list isn't convenient, consider listening to the **Audio CD** that accompanies this text.

- *Caution:* Do not limit your studying to these lists. Although they contain important terms, there are many additional important words in each chapter that you need to know.

Use Your Flash Cards

- Use the flash cards from the back of this book.

- As you go through them, remove from the stack all those word parts you can define.

- Keep working until you have mastered all of these word parts.

Appendix C

- Appendix C contains all of the pathology and treatment terms from the textbook, including the challenge word-building terms you created at the end of each chapter.

- Review the terms in this appendix. Put a check mark next to the terms you know. Highlight terms you have not mastered and next time through, concentrate on these terms.

Make Your Own Study List

- By now you should have greatly reduced the number of terms still to be mastered. Make a list of these terms and word parts and concentrate on them.

Help Someone Else

- One of the greatest ways to really learn something is to teach it! If a classmate is having trouble, tutoring that person will help both of you learn the material.

REVIEW SECTION

Create an answer sheet by numbering a paper from RS.1 to RS.100 and write the letters of your answers on this sheet. When you have finished, check your answers against the answer key.

This section contains exercises that bring together information from all of the chapters. A wrong answer means you need more work on that area! All answer choices are medical terms that you should be able to define. If you are not sure of a meaning, look the term up in the glossary or in your medical dictionary.

Review Questions

RS.1. Which term describes an abnormally rapid rate of respiration of more than 20 breaths per minute?

    a. bradypnea

    b. eupnea

    c. hyperventilation

    d. tachypnea

RS.2. Which condition is a pounding or racing heart with or without irregularity in rhythm?

    a. bradycardia

    b. dysrhythmia

    c. palpitation

    d. tachycardia

RS.3. Which suffix means surgical fixation?

    a. **-desis**

    b. **-lysis**

    c. **-pexy**

    d. **-ptosis**

RS.4. Which term means toward or nearer the midline?

    a. distal

    b. dorsal

    c. medial

    d. ventral

RS.5. The condition that causes a progressive loss of lung function due to a decrease in the total number of alveoli is

    a. emphysema.

    b. atelectasis.

    c. diphtheria.

    d. pertussis.

RS.6. Which term means the surgical removal of a joint?

    a. angiectomy

    b. arteriectomy

    c. atherectomy

    d. arthrectomy

RS.7. Which term means the abnormal development or growth of cells?

    a. dyscrasia

    b. dyslexia

    c. dysmenorrhea

    d. dysplasia

RS.8. Which form of anemia is a genetic disorder?

    a. aplastic anemia

    b. hemolytic anemia

    c. megaloblastic anemia

    d. sickle cell anemia

RS.9. Which medical term describes the condition commonly known as brown lung disease?

    a. anthracosis

    b. byssinosis

    c. pneumoconiosis

    d. silicosis

RS.10. Which condition is characterized by rapidly worsening muscle weakness that may lead to temporary paralysis?

    a. Becker's muscular dystrophy

    b. Bell's palsy

    c. Guillain-Barré syndrome

    d. Raynaud's phenomenon

RS.11. Which blood test is used to assess the cause of excess bleeding or the effects of chemotherapy and radiation therapy?

    a. hematocrit test

    b. platelet count (PLC)

    c. red blood cell (RBC) count

    d. total hemoglobin (Hb) test

RS.12. Which suffix means blood or blood condition?

    a. **-emia**

    b. **-oma**

    c. **-pnea**

    d. **-uria**

RS.13. Which term means the surgical removal of part of the stomach and upper portion of the small intestine?

    a. esophagogastrectomy

    b. esophagoplasty

    c. gastroduodenostomy

    d. gastrostomy

RS.14. Which term describes an added respiratory sound that is also known as wheezing?

    a. bruit

    b. rale

    c. rhonchus

    d. stridor

RS.15. Which term means abnormal enlargement of the liver?

    a. hepatitis

    b. hepatomalacia

c. hepatomegaly

d. hepatorrhexis

RS.16. Which term means bleeding from the bladder?

    a. cystoptosis

    b. cystorrhagia

    c. cystorrhaphy

    d. cystorrhexis

RS.17. Which condition is commonly known as a bruise?

    a. ecchymosis

    b. embolus

    c. emesis

    d. epistaxis

RS.18. Which respiratory condition in children and infants is characterized by obstruction of the larynx, hoarseness, and a barking cough?

    a. asthma

    b. croup

    c. diphtheria

    d. pneumonia

RS.19. Which autoimmune disorder progressively destroys the thyroid gland?

    a. Conn's disease

    b. Hashimoto's thyroiditis

    c. Lou Gehrig's disease

    d. Grave's disease

RS.20. Which of these sexually transmitted diseases is caused by a spirochete?

    a. chlamydia

    b. gonorrhea

    c. syphilis

    d. trichomonas

RS.21. Which term describes a blood clot attached to the interior wall of a vein or artery?

    a. embolism

    b. embolus

    c. thrombosis

    d. thrombus

RS.22. Which term means the removal or destruction of the function of a body part?

    a. ablation

    b. abrasion

c. cryosurgery

d. exfoliative cytology

RS.23. Which term describes the twisting of the intestine on itself that causes an obstruction?

    a. ileus

    b. intestinal adhesions

    c. intussusception

    d. volvulus

RS.24. Which term means a woman who has delivered one child?

    a. nulligravida

    b. nullipara

    c. primigravida

    d. primipara

RS.25. Which term means inflammation of the pancreas?

    a. pancreatalgia

    b. pancreatectomy

    c. pancreatitis

    d. pancreatotomy

RS.26. Which term means an abnormally increased amount of cerebrospinal fluid within the brain?

    a. hydrocele

    b. hydrocephalus

    c. hydronephrosis

    d. hydroureter

RS.27. Which term means the surgical repair of the vagina?

    a. colpopexy

    b. colporrhaphy

    c. vaginoplasty

    d. valvoplasty

RS.28. Which combining form means vagina?

    a. **cervic/o**

    b. **colp/o**

    c. **men/o**

    d. **metr/o**

RS.29. Which statement is accurate regarding cystic fibrosis (CF)?

    a. CF causes abnormal hemoglobin and is also known as iron overload disease.

    b. CF is a congenital disorder in which an essential digestive enzyme is missing.

c. CF is a genetic disorder that affects the lungs and digestive system.

d. CF is characterized by short-lived red blood cells.

RS.30. Which condition is characterized by abnormal softening of bone tissue?

a. osteomalacia

b. osteopenia

c. osteoporosis

d. osteosclerosis

RS.31. A specialist who provides medical care to women during pregnancy, childbirth, and immediately thereafter is a/an

a. gerontologist.

b. gynecologist.

c. neonatologist.

d. obstetrician.

RS.32. Which of these conditions is an autoimmune disorder characterized by exophthalmos?

a. Conn's syndrome

b. Graves' disease

c. Hashimoto's thyroiditis

d. Huntington's disease

RS.33. Which hormone stimulates uterine contractions during childbirth?

a. estrogen

b. oxytocin

c. progesterone

d. testosterone

RS.34. An induced effect that is exactly the opposite of what was therapeutically intended is known as

a. an addictive drug reaction.

b. an idiosyncratic drug reaction.

c. a palliative drug reaction.

d. a paradoxical drug reaction.

RS.35. Which term means the freeing of a kidney from adhesions?

a. nephrolithiasis

b. nephrolysis

c. nephropyosis

d. pyelitis

RS.36. Which term means the tissue death of an artery or arteries?

a. arterionecrosis

b. arthrosclerosis

c. atherosclerosis

d. atherostenosis

RS.37. Which plane divides the body vertically into unequal left and right portions?

a. coronal

b. frontal

c. sagittal

d. transverse

RS.38. Which term means toward or nearer the midline?

a. distal

b. dorsal

c. medial

d. ventral

RS.39. Alice Wilkinson has a family history of osteoporosis. To determine if she has indications of this condition, Alice's doctor ordered a/an

a. bone scan test.

b. DXA test.

c. fluoroscopic test.

d. MRI test.

RS.40. Which term means movement away from the midline of the body?

a. abduction

b. adduction

c. extension

d. flexion

RS.41. When he fell, Manuel tore the posterior femoral muscles in his left leg. This is known as a/an

a. Achilles tendon injury.

b. hamstring injury.

c. myofascial injury.

d. shin splint injury.

RS.42. Mrs. Valladares has a bacterial infection of the lining of her heart. This condition is known as bacterial

a. endocarditis.

b. myocarditis.

c. pericarditis.

d. valvulitis.

RS.43. The dental condition commonly known as tooth decay or a cavity is

    a. dental caries.

    b. dental plaque.

    c. gingivitis.

    d. periodontal disease.

RS.44. Enrique was diagnosed as having an inflammation of the bone marrow. Which term describes this condition?

    a. encephalitis

    b. meningitis

    c. myelitis

    d. myelosis

RS.45. Which term describes a disorder characterized by the unnatural and irresistible urge to pull out one's own hair?

    a. acrophobia

    b. agoraphobia

    c. kleptomania

    d. trichotillomania

RS.46. The term describing an adhesion that binds the iris to an adjacent structure is

    a. blepharoptosis.

    b. dacryocystitis.

    c. scleritis.

    d. synechia.

RS.47. Which combining form means old age?

    a. **percuss/o**

    b. **presby/o**

    c. **prurit/o**

    d. **pseud/o**

RS.48. Mr. Ramirez had a heart attack. His physician recorded this as a/an

    a. myocardial angina.

    b. myocardial infarction.

    c. myocardial infraction.

    d. myocardial ischemia.

RS.49. The term unguis means the

    a. fibrous protein found in hair.

    b. fingernails and toenails.

    c. narrow band of epidermis attached to the surface of a fingernail or toenail.

    d. pale half-moon-shaped region at the nail root.

RS.50. Psoriasis is a skin condition

    a. characterized by a red, scaly rash on the face and upper trunk.

    b. characterized by erythema, papules, and possibly itching.

    c. characterized by red papules covered with silvery scales.

    d. that produces redness, tiny pimples, and broken blood vessels.

RS.51. The group of disorders associated with degenerative changes in the brain structure is known as

    a. Reye's syndrome.

    b. persistent vegetative state.

    c. deliriums tremens.

    d. Alzheimer's disease.

RS.52. A specialist in the diagnosis and treatment of diseases characterized by inflammation in the connective tissues is a/an

    a. chiropractor.

    b. internist.

    c. orthopedist.

    d. rheumatologist.

RS.53. Acute respiratory distress syndrome (ARDS) is

    a. a form of sudden onset severe lung dysfunction affecting most of both lungs.

    b. an accumulation of fluid in lung tissues.

    c. an accumulation of pus in the pleural cavity.

    d. the abnormal escape of fluid into the pleural cavity.

RS.54. Which term means slight paralysis of one side of the body?

    a. hemiparesis

    b. hemiplegia

    c. myoparesis

    d. quadriplegia

RS.55. Which type of cells play an important role in the clotting of blood?

    a. basophils

    b. erythrocytes

    c. leukocytes

    d. thrombocytes

RS.56. Which term describes a benign tumor made up of newly formed blood vessels?

a. hemangioma

b. hematemesis

c. hematoma

d. hematuria

RS.57. Which structure receives the sound vibrations and relays them to the auditory nerve fibers?

a. cochlea

b. eustachian tube

c. organ of Corti

d. semicircular canal

RS.58. Which condition is a skin infection caused by an infestation with the itch mite?

a. pediculosis capitis

b. pediculosis corpus

c. pediculosis pubis

d. scabies

RS.59. Baby Hagachi was treated for a congenital deformity in which his foot turned inward. The family referred to this as a clubfoot; however, the medical term for this condition is

a. hallux valgus.

b. rickets.

c. spasmodic torticollis.

d. talipes.

RS.60. Which term describes the bulging deposit that forms around the area of the break during the healing of a fractured bone?

a. callus

b. cicatrix

c. crepitus

d. keloid

RS.61. Which of these structures is commonly known as the collar bone?

a. clavicle

b. olecranon

c. patella

d. sternum

RS.62. Which type of bacteria are spiral-shaped, have flexible walls, and are capable of movement?

a. bacilli

b. spirochetes

c. staphylococcus

d. streptococcus

RS.63. Which of the following is a hard tissue sarcoma?

a. adenocarcinoma

b. myosarcoma

c. neurosarcoma

d. osteosarcoma

RS.64. The West Nile virus

a. causes a dry hacking cough.

b. causes a fine, rapidly spreading rash.

c. is transmitted by human-to-human contact.

d. is transmitted to humans by mosquito or tick bites.

RS.65. Which term means abnormally decreased motor function or activity?

a. hyperkinesia

b. hypertonia

c. hypokinesia

d. hypotonia

RS.66. Which skin condition, usually caused by a staphylococcal infection, is commonly known as a boil?

a. abscess

b. carbuncle

c. furuncle

d. pustule

RS.67. Which of these medications is a barbiturate administered as a sedative and as an anticonvulsant?

a. anticonvulsant

b. hypnotic

c. phenobarbital

d. sedative

RS.68. Mr. Kuebler suffers from fine muscle tremors, has a masklike facial expression, and walks with a shuffling gait. The medical term for his progressive condition is

a. multiple sclerosis.

b. muscular dystrophy.

c. myasthenia gravis.

d. Parkinson's disease.

RS.69. Which term describes the condition that is commonly known as a bruise?

a. cicatrix

b. ecchymosis

c. keloid

d. lesion

RS.70. Ruth is pregnant and has the skin condition that is commonly known as the mask of pregnancy. What is the medical term for this condition?

a. chloasma

b. albinism

c. melanosis

d. vitiligo

RS.71. The autoimmune disorder in which there are well-defined bald areas is known as alopecia

a. areata.

b. capitis.

c. totalis.

d. universalis.

RS.72. Tony Oliveri was diagnosed as having a fracture in which the ends of the bones were crushed together. Which type of fracture is this?

a. comminuted

b. compound

c. compression

d. spiral

RS.73. Which combining form means vertebra or vertebral column?

a. **synovi/o**

b. **spondyl/o**

c. **scoli/o**

d. **splen/o**

RS.74. Which heart chamber receives oxygen-poor blood from all tissues, except the lungs?

a. left atrium

b. left ventricle

c. right atrium

d. right ventricle

RS.75. Which substance is commonly known as good cholesterol?

a. high-density lipoprotein cholesterol

b. homocysteine

c. low-density lipoprotein cholesterol

d. triglycerides

RS.76. Which symbol means less than?

a. >

b. ≥

c. <

d. ≤

RS.77. In which administration method is the medication placed under the tongue and allowed to dissolve slowly?

a. oral

b. parenteral

c. sublingual

d. topical

RS.78. Which examination technique is used to visualize body parts in motion by projecting x-ray images on a luminous screen?

a. cineradiography

b. computerized tomography

c. fluoroscopy

d. magnetic resonance imaging (MRI)

RS.79. Which of these medications are also known as antianxiety drugs?

a. antidepressant drugs

b. antipsychotic drugs

c. anxiolytic drugs

d. psychotropic drugs

RS.80. Which of these terms describes a surgical puncture of the eardrum?

a. abdominocentesis

b. arthrocentesis

c. thoracentesis

d. tympanocentesis

RS.81. Which term means inflammation of the gallbladder?

a. cholecystectomy

b. cholecystitis

c. cholecystotomy

d. cholelithiasis

RS.82. Which term means vomiting?

a. emesis

b. nausea

c. reflux

d. singultus

RS.83. Which term describes a bluish discoloration of the skin caused by a lack of adequate oxygen?

a. cyanosis

b. erythema

c. jaundice

d. pallor

RS.84. Which of these conditions is a form of aldosteronism caused by disorders of the adrenal glands?

a. Conn's syndrome

b. Crohn's disease

c. Ewing's sarcoma

d. Raynaud's phenomenon

RS.85. Which statement is accurate regarding lymphedema?

a. Primary lymphedema is an autoimmune disorder.

b. Primary lymphedema may be caused by cancer treatment, burns, or trauma.

c. Secondary lymphedema is a hereditary disorder that may appear at any time in life.

d. Secondary lymphedema is caused by cancer treatment, burns, or trauma.

RS.86. Which of the following is a condition characterized by hemorrhage into the skin that causes spontaneous bruising?

a. dermatosis

b. pruritus

c. purpura

d. suppuration

RS.87. Which of these conditions is also known as Lou Gehrig's disease?

a. amyotrophic lateral sclerosis

b. tic douloureux

c. trigeminal neuralgia

d. spasmodic torticollis

RS.88. A band of fibrous tissue that holds structures together abnormally is a/an

a. adhesion.

b. ankylosis.

c. contracture.

d. ligation.

RS.89. Which procedure is used in the treatment of spider veins?

a. blepharoplasty

b. Botox

c. liposuction

d. sclerotherapy

RS.90. Which instrument is used to view the interior of the ear canal?

a. anoscope

b. ophthalmoscope

c. otoscope

d. speculum

RS.91. Which of the following accounts for the majority of all breast cancers?

a. ductal carcinoma in situ

b. infiltrating lobular carcinoma

c. invasive ductal carcinoma

d. invasive lobular carcinoma

RS.92. Which of the following are enlarged and swollen veins at the lower end of the esophagus?

a. esophageal aneurisms

b. esophageal varices

c. hemorrhoids

d. varicose veins

RS.93. Which of these conditions is a progressive autoimmune disorder characterized by scattered patches of demyelination of nerve fibers of the brain and spinal cord?

a. lupus erythematosus

b. multiple sclerosis

c. muscular dystrophy

d. spina bifida

RS.94. Which abdominal region is located below the stomach?

a. epigastric region

b. hypogastric region

c. left hypochondriac region

d. umbilical region

RS.95. Which sexually transmitted disease is a bacterial infection?

a. genital herpes

b. gonorrhea

c. human immunodeficiency virus (HIV)

d. trichomonas

RS.96. Which term describes a narrowing of the opening of the foreskin so it cannot be retracted to expose the glans penis?

a. penitis

b. phallitis

c. phimosis

d. priapism

RS.97. Which procedure is an exfoliative screening biopsy for the detection and diagnosis of conditions of the cervix and surrounding tissues?

a. Papanicolaou test

b. sentinel node biopsy

c. lymph node dissection

d. endometrial biopsy

RS.98. In the field of assisted fertilization, the abbreviation AMA stands for

a. advanced maternal age.

b. against medical advice.

c. American Medical Association.

d. American Mother's Association.

RS.99. Which term means turning the palm upward or forward?

a. circumduction

b. pronation

c. rotation

d. supination

RS.100. Which term means inflammation of a vein?

a. angiitis

b. arthritis

c. phlebitis

d. phlebostenosis

● Review Section Answer Key

RS.1	D	RS.26	B	RS.51	D	RS.76	C
RS.2	C	RS.27	C	RS.52	D	RS.77	C
RS.3	C	RS.28	B	RS.53	A	RS.78	C
RS.4	C	RS.29	C	RS.54	A	RS.79	C
RS.5	A	RS.30	A	RS.55	D	RS.80	D
RS.6	D	RS.31	D	RS.56	A	RS.81	B
RS.7	D	RS.32	B	RS.57	C	RS.82	A
RS.8	D	RS.33	B	RS.58	D	RS.83	A
RS.9	B	RS.34	D	RS.59	D	RS.84	A
RS.10	C	RS.35	B	RS.60	A	RS.85	D
RS.11	B	RS.36	A	RS.61	A	RS.86	C
RS.12	A	RS.37	C	RS.62	B	RS.87	A
RS.13	C	RS.38	C	RS.63	D	RS.88	A
RS.14	C	RS.39	B	RS.64	D	RS.89	D
RS.15	C	RS.40	A	RS.65	C	RS.90	C
RS.16	B	RS.41	B	RS.66	C	RS.91	C
RS.17	A	RS.42	A	RS.67	C	RS.92	B
RS.18	B	RS.43	A	RS.68	D	RS.93	B
RS.19	B	RS.44	C	RS.69	B	RS.94	B
RS.20	C	RS.45	D	RS.70	A	RS.95	B
RS.21	D	RS.46	D	RS.71	A	RS.96	B
RS.22	A	RS.47	B	RS.72	A	RS.97	A
RS.23	D	RS.48	B	RS.73	B	RS.98	A
RS.24	D	RS.49	B	RS.74	C	RS.99	D
RS.25	C	RS.50	C	RS.75	A	RS.100	C

CONFIRMING MASTERY

Create an answer sheet by numbering a paper from FT.1 to FT.100 and write the letters of your answers on this sheet. When you have finished, check your answers against the answer key.

A wrong answer identifies an area where you need more work. All answer choices are medical terms that you should be able to define. If you are not sure of a meaning, look the term up in the glossary or in your medical dictionary.

● Simulated Final Test

FT.1. Which medical term describes a torn or ragged wound?

   a. fissure

   b. fistula

   c. laceration

   d. lesion

FT.2. The term cystopexy means

   a. drooping of the urinary bladder.

   b. inflammation of the gallbladder.

   c. laparoscopic examination of the gallbladder.

   d. surgical fixation of the urinary bladder.

FT.3. Which medical term is commonly known as a heart attack?

   a. arthrostenosis

   b. myocardial infarction

   c. transient ischemic attack

   d. ventricular fibrillation

FT.4. Which term means inflammation of the connective tissues that enclose the spinal cord and brain?

   a. encephalitis

   b. encephalopathy

   c. meningitis

   d. myelopathy

FT.5. Which disease is also known as osteitis deformans?

   a. Crohn's disease

   b. Ewing's sarcoma

   c. Paget's disease

   d. Raynaud's phenomenon

FT.6. The term myorrhexis means

   a. bleeding from the spinal cord.

   b. rupture of a muscle.

   c. rupture of the spinal cord.

   d. to suture a muscle.

FT.7. Which term means abnormal softening of the kidney?

   a. nephromalacia

   b. nephrosclerosis

   c. neuromalacia

   d. neurosclerosis

FT.8. Which of the following is a life-threatening complication of uncontrolled diabetes mellitus?

   a. an embolism

   b. a thrombus

   c. convulsions

   d. diabetic ketoacidosis

FT.9. A carotid endarterectomy is performed to

   a. prevent a heart attack.

   b. prevent a stroke.

   c. relieve angina symptoms.

   d. treat hypertension.

FT.10. Which medical term means the flow of pus from the ear?

   a. otopyorrhea

   b. otorrhagia

   c. pyoderma

   d. pyosalpinx

FT.11. Which term is commonly known as itching?

   a. perfusion

   b. pruritus

   c. purpura

   d. suppuration

FT.12. Which term means spasmodic choking pain due to interference with the oxygen supply to the heart muscle?

   a. angina pectoris

   b. claudication

   c. cyanosis

   d. myocardial infarction

FT.13. Which condition is also known as trigeminal neuralgia?

a. Hodgkin's disease

b. Lou Gehrig's disease

c. tic douloureux

d. spasmodic torticollis

FT.14. Which term means an unexpected reaction to a drug?

a. adverse

b. idiosyncratic

c. placebo

d. palliative

FT.15. Which term means a prediction of the probable course and outcome of a disease or disorder?

a. differential diagnosis

b. diagnosis

c. prognosis

d. syndrome

FT.16. Which term means blue discoloration of the skin caused by a lack of adequate oxygen?

a. cyanosis

b. erythroderma

c. leukoplakia

d. melanosis

FT.17. A Colles' fracture is associated with which bone disease?

a. osteomalacia

b. osteomyelitis

c. osteoporosis

d. otosclerosis

FT.18. Which medical term is commonly known as bed-wetting?

a. nocturnal myoclonus

b. nocturnal enuresis

c. nocturia

d. urinary incontinence

FT.19. Which term describes any benign skin condition in which there is overgrowth and thickening of the epidermis?

a. epithelioma

b. keratosis

c. melanoma

d. papilloma

FT.20. Which term means inflammation of the lymph nodes?

a. adenoiditis

b. angiitis

c. lymphadenitis

d. lymphangioma

FT.21. Which term describes a sudden, involuntary contraction of a muscle?

a. adhesion

b. contracture

c. spasm

d. stricture

FT.22. Which respiratory disease is commonly known as whooping cough?

a. croup

b. diphtheria

c. emphysema

d. pertussis

FT.23. Which body system is affected by the autoimmune disorder Crohn's disease?

a. digestive

b. endocrine

c. nervous

d. reproductive

FT.24. Which condition is commonly known as low back pain?

a. kyphosis

b. lordosis

c. lumbago

d. scoliosis

FT.25. Which term means the surgical creation of an opening between the small intestine and the body surface?

a. colostomy

b. enteropexy

c. gastroptosis

d. ileostomy

FT.26. Which visualization technique is used to examine body parts in motion?

a. computed tomography

b. fluoroscopy

c. magnetic resonance imaging

d. radiography

FT.27. Which term means bleeding from the pharynx?

a. epistaxis

b. pharyngoplegia

c. pharyngorrhagia

d. pharyngorrhea

FT.28. Which autoimmune disease gradually destroys thyroid tissue?

a. Cushing's syndrome

b. goiter

c. Hashimoto's

d. Parkinson's disease

FT.29. What condition is an accumulation of pus in the fallopian tube?

a. leukorrhea

b. metrorrhea

c. pyosalpinx

d. salpingitis

FT.30. Which syndrome is characterized by sudden, severe, sharp headache usually present only on one side?

a. cephalagia

b. migraine headache

c. Bell's palsy

d. tic douloureux

FT.31. Which term means vomiting blood?

a. epistaxis

b. hemarthrosis

c. hematemesis

d. hyperemesis

FT.32. Which term describes the condition commonly known as a bruise?

a. ecchymosis

b. exophthalmos

c. hematoma

d. hemangioma

FT.33. Which term means abnormally rapid, deep breathing resulting in decreased levels of carbon dioxide at the cellular level?

a. apnea

b. dyspnea

c. hyperventilation

d. hypoventilation

FT.34. Which term means difficult or painful urination?

a. dyskinesia

b. dyspepsia

c. dysphagia

d. dysuria

FT.35. Which term means a false personal belief that is maintained despite obvious proof to the contrary?

a. delirium

b. delusion

c. dementia

d. hallucination

FT.36. Which type of heartbeat is known as tachycardia?

a. extremely rapid

b. fluttering

c. pounding

d. very slow

FT.37. Which eye condition is characterized by increased intraocular pressure?

a. cataracts

b. glaucoma

c. macular degeneration

d. monochromatism

FT.38. Which diagnostic tool is commonly used to image the brain and spinal cord?

a. echoencephalography

b. electroencephalography

c. magnetic resonance imaging

d. ultrasound

FT.39. Which vision condition is commonly known as nearsightedness?

a. hyperopia

b. myopia

c. presbyopia

d. strabismus

FT.40. Which body cavity protects the brain?

a. anterior

b. cranial

c. superior

d. ventral

FT.41. Which condition is a hernia of the bladder through the vaginal wall?

a. cystocele

b. cystopexy

c. vaginocele

d. vesicovaginal fistula

FT.42. Which term means a violent shaking up or jarring of the brain caused by a direct blow or explosion?

a. cerebral concussion

b. cerebral contusion

c. intracerebral hematoma

d. subdural hematoma

FT.43. Which term means a ringing sound in the ears?

a. presbycusis

b. syncope

c. tinnitus

d. vertigo

FT.44. Which term means a sudden and widespread outbreak of a disease within a population group or area?

a. endemic

b. epidemic

c. pandemic

d. syndrome

FT.45. Which condition is an excessive flow of gastric secretions?

a. ascites

b. aerophagia

c. gastrorrhea

d. gastrorrhexis

FT.46. Which structure is a small, flat, discolored lesion such as a freckle?

a. macule

b. papule

c. plaque

d. vesicle

FT.47. The Western blot test is used to

a. confirm an HIV infection.

b. detect hepatitis B.

c. diagnose Kaposi's sarcoma.

d. test for tuberculosis.

FT.48. Which term means excessive uterine bleeding occurring both during the menses and at irregular intervals?

a. dysmenorrhea

b. menometrorrhagia

c. menorrhagia

d. hypermenorrhea

FT.49. Which term describes an injury that does not break the skin and is characterized by swelling, discoloration, and pain?

a. concussion

b. contusion

c. laceration

d. lesion

FT.50. Which term describes an abnormal rattle or crackle-like respiratory sound heard during inspiration?

a. bruit

b. rale

c. rhonchus

d. stridor

FT.51. Which condition is commonly known as wear-and-tear arthritis?

a. gouty arthritis

b. osteoarthritis

c. rheumatoid arthritis

d. spondylosis

FT.52. Which term means to free a tendon from adhesions?

a. tenodesis

b. tenolysis

c. tenorrhaphy

d. tenotomy

FT.53. Hodgkin's lymphoma is

a. a type of leukemia.

b. an autoimmune disorder.

c. distinguished by the presence of Reed-Sternberg cells.

d. staged as low-grade, intermediate-grade, and high-grade.

FT.54. Which term describes a progressive degenerative disease characterized by disturbance of structure and function of the liver?

a. cirrhosis

b. hepatitis A

c. hepatitis E

d. jaundice

FT.55. Which procedure removes waste products directly from the blood of patients whose kidneys no longer function?

a. diuresis

b. epispadias

c. hemodialysis

d. peritoneal dialysis

FT.56. Which condition is commonly known as fainting?

a. comatose

b. narcolepsy

c. stupor

d. syncope

FT.57. Which term means a deficiency of blood supply due to the constriction or obstruction of a blood vessel?

a. embolism

b. infarction

c. ischemia

d. thrombosis

FT.58. Which term means an accumulation of blood in the pleural cavity?

a. hemophilia

b. hemoptysis

c. hemostasis

d. hemothorax

FT.59. Which term means the return of swallowed food into the mouth?

a. emesis

b. nausea

c. reflux

d. regurgitation

FT.60. Which condition is caused by prolonged exposure to high levels of cortisol?

a. Addison's disease

b. Cushing's syndrome

c. Huntington's disease

d. Parkinson's disease

FT.61. Which term describes a yellow discoloration of the skin caused by abnormal amounts of bilirubin in the blood?

a. cyanosis

b. ileus

c. jaundice

d. volvulus

FT.62. Which term means excessive urination?

a. anuria

b. oliguria

c. polyuria

d. pyuria

FT.63. Which term means the surgical removal of the gallbladder?

a. cholecystectomy

b. cholecystostomy

c. cholecystotomy

d. choledocholithotomy

FT.64. Which blood test is used to detect the presence of inflammation in the body?

a. agglutination

b. a platelet count

c. complete blood cell count

d. erythrocyte sedimentation rate

FT.65. Which term means a closed sac or pouch containing fluid or semisolid material?

a. abscess

b. cyst

c. pustule

d. ulcer

FT.66. Which type of injection is administered within the substance of a muscle?

a. intradermal

b. intramuscular

c. intravenous

d. subcutaneous

FT.67. Which structure has roles in both the immune and endocrine systems?

a. pancreas

b. pituitary gland

c. spleen

d. thymus

FT.68. Which term means inflammation of the brain?

    a. encephalitis

    b. mastitis

    c. meningitis

    d. myelitis

FT.69. Which term means a spasm or twitching of a muscle or group of muscles?

    a. contractures

    b. myoclonus

    c. seizures

    d. tremors

FT.70. Which term describes the condition when the heart is unable to pump enough blood to meet the body's needs?

    a. congestive heart failure

    b. hypoperfusion

    c. myocarditis

    d. mitral valve prolapse

FT.71. Which term describes a hospital-acquired infection?

    a. functional

    b. iatrogenic

    c. idiopathic

    d. nosocomial

FT.72. Which term means a malignant tumor that arises from connective tissue?

    a. carcinoma

    b. malignant melanoma

    c. metastasis

    d. sarcoma

FT.73. Which term describes the eye disorder that may develop as a complication of diabetes?

    a. diabetic neuropathy

    b. diabetic retinopathy

    c. papilledema

    d. retinal detachment

FT.74. Which term describes an eating disorder characterized by refusing to maintain a minimally normal body weight and an intense fear of gaining weight?

    a. anorexia nervosa

    b. bulimia nervosa

    c. hypochondriasis

    d. pica

FT.75. Which term means the presence of blood in the urine?

    a. albuminuria

    b. blood urea nitrogen

    c. hematuria

    d. proteinuria

FT.76. Which term describes the condition caused when a blood vessel in the brain leaks or ruptures?

    a. cerebral hematoma

    b. embolism

    c. hemorrhagic stroke

    d. ischemic stroke

FT.77. Which term describes the condition characterized by enlargement of the hands and feet caused by excessive secretion of the growth hormone *after* puberty?

    a. acromegaly

    b. acrophobia

    c. cretinism

    d. gigantism

FT.78. Which terms means an ingrown toenail?

    a. cryptorchidism

    b. onychocryptosis

    c. onychophagia

    d. oophoropexy

FT.79. An otoscope is used to examine the

    a. adnexa of the eye.

    b. auditory canal and tympanic membrane.

    c. eustachian tube.

    d. retina and optic nerve of the eye.

FT.80. Which term means protrusion of part of the stomach through the esophageal opening in the diaphragm?

    a. esophageal hernia

    b. esophageal varices

    c. hiatal hernia

    d. hiatal varices

FT.81. Which term means a surgical incision of the vulva to facilitate delivery of a baby?

a. episiorrhaphy

b. episiotomy

c. epispadias

d. epistaxis

FT.82. Which term describes a condition of severe itching of the external female genitalia?

a. colpitis

b. leukorrhea

c. pruritus vulvae

d. vaginal candidiasis

FT.83. Which term describes an infestation commonly known as head lice?

a. pediculosis capitis

b. pediculosis pubis

c. tinea capitis

d. tinea pedis

FT.84. Which instrument is used to enlarge the opening of a canal or body cavity to make it possible to inspect its interior?

a. endoscope

b. speculum

c. sphygmomanometer

d. stethoscope

FT.85. Cellulitis is a

a. diffuse infection of connective tissue.

b. dry patch made up of excess dead epidermal cells.

c. groove or crack-like sore.

d. localized collection of pus.

FT.86. Which condition is a malignant tumor composed of cells derived from hemopoietic tissues of the bone marrow?

a. mycosis

b. myelitis

c. myeloma

d. myelosis

FT.87. Which term means an inflammation of the lungs in which the air sacs fill with pus and other liquid?

a. pneumoconiosis

b. pneumonia

c. pneumonitis

d. pneumothorax

FT.88. Which term means ankylosis of the bones of the middle ear resulting in a conductive hearing loss?

a. labyrinthitis

b. mastoiditis

c. osteosclerosis

d. otosclerosis

FT.89. Which term means to free a tendon from adhesions?

a. arthrodesis

b. arthrolysis

c. tenodesis

d. tenolysis

FT.90. Which term means to suture the vagina?

a. colporrhaphy

b. cystorrhaphy

c. hepatorrhaphy

d. hysterorrhaphy

FT.91. Which term means the surgical removal of plaque from the interior lining of an artery?

a. angiectomy

b. arteriectomy

c. atherectomy

d. arthrectomy

FT.92. Which term means abnormally increased motor function or activity?

a. bradykinesia

b. dyskinesia

c. hyperkinesia

d. hypokinesia

FT.93. Which term means difficulty in swallowing?

a. dyspepsia

b. dysphagia

c. dysphonia

d. dysplasia

FT.94. Which term means the process of recording electrical brain wave activity?

a. echoencephalography

b. electroencephalography

c. electromyography

d. electroneuromyography

FT.95. Which term means a woman who has never been pregnant?

a. nulligravida

b. nullipara

c. primigravida

d. primipara

FT.96. Which eye condition causes the loss of central vision but not total blindness?

a. cataracts

b. glaucoma

c. macular degeneration

d. presbyopia

FT.97. Which term means the surgical removal of excess skin for the elimination of wrinkles?

a. ablation

b. blepharoplasty

c. rhytidectomy

d. sclerotherapy

FT.98. Which term means a group of inherited muscle disorders that cause muscle weakness without affecting the nervous system?

a. multiple sclerosis

b. muscular dystrophy

c. myasthenia gravis

d. Parkinson's disease

FT.99. Which term describes the process by which cancer spreads from one place to another?

a. metabolism

b. metastasis

c. metastasize

d. staging

FT.100. Which term means a collection of blood trapped within tissues?

a. hemangioma

b. hematemesis

c. hematoma

d. hematuria

● Final Test Answer Key

FT.1	C	FT.26	B	FT.51	B	FT.76	C
FT.2	D	FT.27	C	FT.52	B	FT.77	A
FT.3	B	FT.28	C	FT.53	C	FT.78	B
FT.4	C	FT.29	C	FT.54	A	FT.79	B
FT.5	C	FT.30	B	FT.55	C	FT.80	C
FT.6	B	FT.31	C	FT.56	D	FT.81	B
FT.7	A	FT.32	A	FT.57	C	FT.82	C
FT.8	D	FT.33	C	FT.58	D	FT.83	A
FT.9	B	FT.34	D	FT.59	D	FT.84	B
FT.10	A	FT.35	B	FT.60	B	FT.85	A
FT.11	B	FT.36	A	FT.61	C	FT.86	C
FT.12	A	FT.37	B	FT.62	C	FT.87	B
FT.13	C	FT.38	C	FT.63	A	FT.88	D
FT.14	B	FT.39	B	FT.64	D	FT.89	D
FT.15	C	FT.40	B	FT.65	B	FT.90	A
FT.16	A	FT.41	A	FT.66	B	FT.91	C
FT.17	C	FT.42	A	FT.67	D	FT.92	C
FT.18	B	FT.43	C	FT.68	A	FT.93	B
FT.19	B	FT.44	B	FT.69	B	FT.94	B
FT.20	C	FT.45	C	FT.70	A	FT.95	A
FT.21	C	FT.46	A	FT.71	D	FT.96	C
FT.22	D	FT.47	A	FT.72	D	FT.97	C
FT.23	A	FT.48	B	FT.73	B	FT.98	B
FT.24	C	FT.49	B	FT.74	A	FT.99	C
FT.25	D	FT.50	B	FT.75	C	FT.100	C

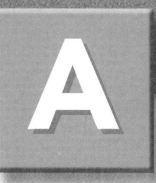

Appendix A
Prefixes, Combining Forms, and Suffixes

Pertaining to

-ac	pertaining to
-al	pertaining to
-ar	pertaining to
-ary	pertaining to
-eal	pertaining to
-ical	pertaining to
-ial	pertaining to
-ic	pertaining to
-ine	pertaining to
-ior	pertaining to
-ory	pertaining to
-ous	pertaining to
-tic	pertaining to

Abnormal Conditions

-ago	abnormal condition, disease
-esis	abnormal condition, disease
-ia	abnormal condition, disease
-iasis	abnormal condition, disease
-ion	condition
-ism	condition, state of
-osis	abnormal condition, disease

Noun Endings

-a	noun ending
-e	noun ending
-um	singular noun ending
-us	singular noun ending
-y	noun ending

A

a-	no, not, without, away from, negative
-a	noun ending
ab-	away from, negative, absent
abdomin/o	abdomen
-able	capable of, able to
abort/o	premature expulsion of a nonviable fetus
abrad/o, abras/o	rub or scrape off
abrupt/o	broken away from
abs-	away from
abscess/o	collection of pus, going away
absorpt/o	suck up, suck in
-ac	pertaining to
acanth/o	spiny, thorny
acetabul/o	acetabulum (hip socket)
-acious	characterized by
acne/o	point or peak
acous/o, acoust/o	hearing, sound
acquir/o	get, obtain
acr/o	extremities (hands and feet), top, extreme point
acromi/o	acromion, point of shoulder blade
actin/o	light
acu/o	sharp, severe, sudden
acuit/o, acut/o	sharp, sharpness
acust/o, -acusia, -acusis	hearing, sense of hearing
ad-	toward, to, in the direction of
aden/o	gland
adenoid/o	adenoids
adhes/o	stick to, cling to
adip/o	fat
adnex/o	bound to
adren/o, adrenal/o	adrenal glands
aer/o	air, gas
aesthet/o	sensation, sense of perception
af-	toward, to
affect/o	exert influence on
agglutin/o	clumping, stick together
aggress/o	attack, step forward
-ago	abnormal condition, disease
agor/a	marketplace
-agra	excessive pain, seizure, attack of severe pain
-aise	comfort, ease

-al	pertaining to
alb/i, alb/o, albin/o	white
albumin/o	albumin, protein
alg/e, algi/o, alg/o, algesi/o	relationship to pain
-algesia, -algesic	painful, pain sense
-algia	pain, painful condition
align/o	bring into line or correct position
aliment/o	to nourish
all/o, all-	other, different from normal, reversal
alopec/o	baldness, mangy
alveol/o	alveolus, air sac, small sac
ambi-	both sides, around or about, double
ambly/o	dull, dim
ambul/o, ambulat/o	walk
ametr/o	out of proportion
-amine	nitrogen compound
amni/o	amnion, fetal membrane
amph-	around, on both sides, doubly
amput/o, amputat/o	cut away, cut off a part of the body
amyl/o	starch
an-	no, not, without
an-, ana-	up, apart, backward, excessive
an/o	anus, ring
-an	characteristic of, pertaining to
-ancy	state of
andr/o	relationship to the male
aneurysm/o	aneurysm
angi/o	blood or lymph vessels
angin/o	angina, choking, strangling
anis/o	unequal
ankyl/o	crooked, bent, stiff
anomal/o	irregularity
ante-	before, in front of
anter/o	before, front
anthrac/o	coal, coal dust
anti-	against
anxi/o, anxiet/o	anxiety, anxious, uneasy
aort/o	aorta
ap-	toward, to
ap-, apo-	separation, away from, opposed, detached
-apheresis	removal
aphth/o	ulcer
apic/o	apex

aplast/o	defective development, lack of development
aponeur/o	aponeurosis (type of tendon)
apoplect/o	a stroke
append/o, appendic/o	appendix
aqu/i, aqu/o, aque/o	water
-ar	pertaining to
arachn/o	spider web, spider
arc/o	bow, arc or arch
-arche	beginning
areat/o	occurring in patches or circum- scribed areas
areol/o	little open space
-aria	connected with
arrect/o	upright, lifted up, raised
arter/o, arteri/o	artery
arthr/o	joint
articul/o	joint
-ary	pertaining to
as-	toward, to
asbest/o	asbestos
-ase	enzyme
aspir/o, aspirat/o	to breathe in
asthen-, -asthenia	weakness, lack of strength
asthmat/o	gasping, choking
astr/o	star, start shaped
at-	toward, to
atel/o	incomplete, imperfect
ather/o	plaque, fatty substance
athet/o	uncontrolled
atop/o	strange, out of place
atres/i	without an opening
atri/o	atrium
attenuat/o	diluted, weakened
aud-, audi/o, audit/o	ear, hearing, the sense of hearing
aur/i, aur/o	ear, hearing
auscult/a, auscult/o	listen
aut/o	self
-ax	noun ending
ax/o	axis, main stem
axill/o	armpit
azot/o	urea, nitrogen

B

bacill/o	rod-shaped bacterium (plural, *bacteria*)

bacteri/o	bacteria (singular, *bacterium*)
balan/o	glans penis
bar/o	pressure, weight
bartholin/o	Bartholin's gland
bas/o	base, opposite of acid
bi-	twice, double, two
bi/o	life
bifid/o	split, divided into two parts
bifurcat/o	divide or fork into two branches
bil/i	bile, gall
bilirubin/o	bilirubin
bin-	two by two
-blast	embryonic, immature, formative element
blephar/o	eyelid
borborygm/o	rumbling sound
brachi/o	arm
brachy-	short
brady-	slow
brev/i, brev/o	short
bronch/i, bronchi/o, bronch/o	bronchial tube, bronchus
bronchiol/o	bronchiole, bronchiolus
brux/o	grind
bucc/o	cheek
burs/o	bursa, sac of fluid near joint
byssin/o	cotton dust

C

cadaver/o	dead body, corpse
calc/i	calcium, lime, the heel
calcane/o	calcaneus, heel bone
calci-, calc/o	calcium
calcul/o	stone, little stone
cali/o, calic/o	cup, calyx
call/i, callos/o	hard, hardened and thickened
calor/i	heat
canalicul/o	little canal or duct
canth/o	corner of the eye
capill/o	hair
capit/o	head
capn/o	carbon dioxide, sooty or smoky appearance
capsul/o	little box
carb/o	carbon
carbuncl/o	carbuncle
carcin/o	cancerous
cardi/o, card/o	heart

cari/o	rottenness, decay
carot/o	stupor, sleep
carp/o	wrist bones
cartilag/o	cartilage, gristle
caruncul/o	bit of flesh
cat-, cata-, cath-	down, lower, under, downward
catabol/o	a breaking down
cathart/o	cleansing, purging
cathet/o	insert, send down
caud/o	lower part of body, tail
caus/o, caust/o	burning, burn
cauter/o, caut/o	heat, burn
cav/i, cav/o	hollow, cave
cavern/o	containing hollow spaces
cec/o	cecum
-cele	hernia, tumor, swelling
celi/o, cel/o	abdomen, belly
cement/o	cementum, a rough stone
cent-	hundred
-centesis	surgical puncture to remove fluid
cephal/o, -ceps	head
cera-	wax
cerebell/o	cerebellum
cerebr/o	cerebrum, brain
cerumin/o	cerumen, earwax
cervic/o	neck, cervix (neck of uterus)
cheil/o	lip
cheir/o	hand
chem/i, chem/o, chemic/o	drug, chemical
chir/o	hand
chlor/o	green
chlorhydr/o	hydrochloric acid
chol/e	bile, gall
cholangi/o	bile duct
cholecyst/o	gallbladder
choledoch/o	common bile duct
cholesterol/o	cholesterol
chondr/i, chondr/o	cartilage
chord/o	spinal cord, cord
chore/o	dance
chori/o, chorion/o	chorion, membrane
choroid/o	choroid layer of eye
chrom/o, chromat/o	color
chron/o	time
chym/o	to pour, juice
cib/o	meal
cicatric/o	scar
-cidal	pertaining to killing
-cide	causing death
cili/o	eyelashes, microscopic hairlike projections
cine-	relationship to movement
circ/i	ring or circle
circulat/o	circulate, go around in a circle
circum-	around, about
circumcis/o	cutting around
circumscrib/o	confined, limited in space
cirrh/o	orange-yellow, tawny
cis/o	cut
clasis, -clast	break down
claudicat/o	limping
claustr/o	barrier
clav/i	key
clavicul/o, cleid/o	clavicle, collar bone
climacter/o	crisis, rung of a ladder
clitor/o	clitoris
-clonus	violent action
clus/o	shut or close
-clysis	irrigation, washing
co-	together, with
coagul/o, coagulat/o	clotting, coagulation
coarct/o, coarctat/o	press together, narrow
cocc/i, cocc/o, -coccus	spherical bacteria
coccyg/o	coccyx, tailbone
cochle/o	spiral, snail, snail shell
coher/o, cohes/o	cling, stick together
coit/o	a coming together
col/o	colon, large intestine
coll/a	glue
colon/o	colon, large intestine
colp/o	vagina
column/o	pillar
com-	together, with
comat/o	deep sleep
comminut/o	break into pieces
communic/o	share, to make common
compatibil/o	sympathize with
con-	together, with
concav/o	hollow
concentr/o	condense, intensify, remove excess water
concept/o	become pregnant
conch/o	shell

concuss/o	shaken together, violently agitated
condyl/o	knuckle, knob
confus/o	confusion, disorder
coni/o	dust
conjunctiv/o	conjunctiva, joined together, connected
consci/o	aware, awareness
consolid/o	become firm or solid
constipat/o	pressed together, crowded together
constrict/o	draw tightly together
-constriction	narrowing
contact/o	touched, infected
contagi/o	infection, unclean, touching of something
contaminat/o	render unclean by contact, pollute
contine/o, continent/o	keep in, contain, hold back, restrain
contra-	against, counter, opposite
contracept/o	prevention of conception
contus/o	bruise
convalesc/o	recover, become strong
convex/o	arched, vaulted
convolut/o	coiled, twisted
convuls/o	pull together
copi/o	plentiful
copulat/o	joining together, linking
cor/o	pupil
cord/o	cord, spinal cord
cordi/o	heart
core/o, cor/o	pupil
cori/o	skin, leather
corne/o	cornea
coron/o	coronary, crown
corp/u, corpor/o	body
corpuscul/o	little body
cort-	covering
cortic/o	cortex, outer region
cost/o	rib
cox/o	hip, hip joint
crani/o	skull
-crasia	a mixture or blending
creatin/o	creatine
crepit/o, crepitat/o	crackling, rattling
crin/o, -crine	secrete
cris/o, critic/o	turning point
-crit	to separate
cry/o	cold
crypt/o	hidden

cubit/o	elbow
cuboid/o	cubelike
culd/o	cul-de-sac, blind pouch
cult/o	cultivate
-cusis	hearing
cusp/i	point, pointed flap
cutane/o	skin
cyan/o	blue
cycl/o	ciliary body of eye, cycle
-cyesis	pregnancy
cyst-, -cyst	bladder, bag
cyst/o	urinary bladder, cyst, sac of fluid
cyt/o, -cyte	cell
-cytic	pertaining to a cell
- cytosis	condition of cells

D

dacry/o	tear, lacrimal duct (tear duct)
dacryocyst/o	lacrimal sac (tear sac)
dactyl/o	fingers, toes
de-	down, lack of, from, not, removal
debrid/e	open a wound
deca-, deci-	ten, tenth
decidu/o	shedding, falling off
decubit/o	lying down
defec/o, defecat/o	free from waste, clear
defer/o	carrying down or out
degenerat/o	gradual impairment, breakdown, diminished function
deglutit/o	swallow
dehisc/o	burst open, split
deliri/o	wandering in the mind
delt/o	Greek letter delta, triangular shape
delus/o	delude, mock, cheat
dem/o	people, population
-dema	swelling (fluid)
demi-	half
dendr/o	branching, resembling a tree
dent/i, dent/o	tooth, teeth
depilat/o	hair removal
depress/o	press down, lower, pressed or sunk down
derma-, dermat/o, derm/o	skin
desic/o	drying
-desis	surgical fixation of bone or joint, to bind, tie together

deteriorat/o	worsening or gradual impairment
dextr/o	right side
di-	twice, twofold, double
dia-	through, between, apart, complete
diaphor/o	sweat
diaphragmat/o	diaphragm, wall across
diastol/o	standing apart, expansion
didym/o	testes, twins, double
diffus/o	pour out, spread apart
digest/o	divide, distribute
digit/o	finger or toe
dilat/o, dilatat/o	spread out, expand
-dilation	widening, stretching, expanding
dilut/o	dissolve, separate
diphther/o	membrane
dipl/o	double
dips/o, -dipsia	thirst
dis-	negative, apart, absence of
dislocat/o	displacement
dissect/o	cutting apart
disseminat/o	widely scattered
dist/o	far
distend/o, distent/o	stretch apart, expand
diur/o, diuret/o	tending to increase urine output
divert/i	turning aside
domin/o	controlling, ruling
don/o	give
dors/i, dors/o	back of body
-dote	what is given
-drome	to run, running
-duct	opening
duct/o	to lead, carry
duoden/i, duoden/o	duodenum, first part of small intestine
-dural	pertaining to dura mater
-dynia	pain
dys-	bad, difficult, painful

E

e-	out of, from
-e	noun ending
-eal	pertaining to
ec-	out, outside
ecchym/o	pouring out of juice
ech/o	sound

eclamps/o, eclampt/o	flashing or shining forth
ectasia, -ectasis	stretching, dilation, enlargement
ecto-	out, outside
-ectomy	surgical removal, cutting out, excision
-ectopy	displacement
eczemat/o	eruption
-edema	swelling
edem-, edemat/o	swelling, fluid, tumor
edentul/o	without teeth
ef-	out
effect/o	bring about a response, activate
effus/o	pouring out
ejaculat/o	throw or hurl out
electr/o	electricity, electric
eliminat/o	expel from the body
em-	in
emaciat/o	wasted by disease
embol/o	something inserted or thrown in
embry/o	fertilized ovum, embryo
-emesis	vomiting
emet/o	vomit
-emia	blood, blood condition
emmetr/o	in proper measure
emolli/o	make soft, soften
en-	in, within, into
encephal/o	brain
end-, endo-	in, within, inside
endocrin/o	secrete within
enem/o	end in, inject
enter/o	small intestine
ento-	within
eosin/o	red, rosy
epi-	above, upon, on
epidemi/o	among the people, an epidemic
epididym/o	epididymis
epiglott/o	epiglottis
episi/o	vulva
epithel/i, epitheli/o	epithelium
equin/o	pertaining to a horse
-er	one who
erect/o	upright
erg/o, -ergy	work
erot/o	sexual love
eruct/o, eructat/o	belch forth
erupt/o	break out, burst forth
erythem/o, erythemat/o	flushed, redness

erythr/o	red
es-	out of, outside, away from
-esis	abnormal condition, disease
eso-	inward
esophag/o	esophagus
-esthesia, esthesi/o	sensation, feeling
esthet/o	feeling, nervous sensation, sense of perception
estr/o	female
ethm/o	sieve
eti/o	cause
eu-	good, normal, well, easy
-eurysm	widening
evacu/o, evacuat/o	empty out
ex-	out of, outside, away from
exacerbat/o	aggravate, irritate
exanthemat/o	rash
excis/o	cutting out
excori/o, excoriat/o	abrade or scratch
excret/o	separate, discharge
excruciat/o	intense pain, agony
exhal/o, exhalat/o	breathe out
exo-	out of, outside, away from
exocrin/o	secrete out of
expector/o	cough up
expir/o, expirat/o	breathe out
exstroph/o	turned or twisted out
extern/o	outside, outer
extra-	on the outside, beyond, outside
extrem/o, extremit/o	extremity, outermost
extrins/o	from the outside, contained outside
exud/o, exudat/o	to sweat out

F

faci/o	face, form
-facient	making, producing
fasci/o	fascia, fibrous band
fascicul/o	little bundle
fatal/o	pertaining to fate, death
fauc/i	narrow pass, throat
febr/i	fever
fec/i, fec/o	dregs, sediment, waste
femor/o	femur, thigh bone
fenestr/o	window
fer/o	bear, carry
-ferent	carrying

-ferous	bearing, carrying, producing
fertil/o	fertile, fruitful, productive
fet/i, fet/o	fetus, unborn child
fibr/o	fiber
fibrill/o	muscular twitching
fibrin/o	fibrin, fibers, threads of a clot
fibros/o	fibrous connective tissue
fibul/o	fibula
-fic, fic/o	making, producing, forming
-fication	process of making
-fida	split
filtr/o, filtrat/o	filter, to strain through
fimbri/o	fringe
fiss/o, fissur/o	crack, split, cleft
fistul/o	tube or pipe
flamme/o	flame colored
flat/o	flatus, breaking wind, rectal gas
flex/o	bend
flu/o	flow
fluor/o	glowing, luminous
foc/o	focus, point
foll/i	bag, sac
follicul/o	follicle, small sac
foramin/o	opening, foramen
fore-	before, in front of
-form, form/o	resembling, in the shape of
fornic/o	arch, vault, brothel
foss/o	ditch, shallow depression
fove/o	pit
fract/o	break, broken
fren/o	device that limits movement
frigid/o	cold
front/o	forehead, brow
-fuge	to drive away
funct/o, function/o	perform, function
fund/o	bottom, base, ground
fung/i	fungus
furc/o	forking, branching
furuncul/o	furunculus, a boil, an infection
-fusion	pour

G

galact/o	milk
gamet/o	wife or husband, egg or sperm
gangli/o, ganglion/o	ganglion
gangren/o	eating sore, gangrene
gastr/o	stomach, belly

gastrocnemi/o	gastrocnemius, calf muscle
gemin/o	twin, double
gen-, gen/o, -gen	producing, forming
-gene	production, origin, formation
-genic, -genesis	creation, reproduction
genit/o	produced by, birth, reproductive organs
-genous	producing
ger/i	old age
germin/o	bud, sprout, germ
geront/o	old age
gest/o, gestat/o	bear, carry young or offspring
gigant/o	giant, very large
gingiv/o	gingival tissue, gums
glauc/o	gray
glen/o	socket or pit
gli/o	neurologic tissue, supportive tissue of nervous system
globin/o, -globulin	protein
globul/o	little ball
glomerul/o	glomerulus
gloss/o	tongue
glott/i, glott/o	back of the tongue
gluc/o	glucose, sugar
glute/o	buttocks
glyc/o, glycos/o	glucose, sugar
glycer/o	sweet
glycogen/o	glycogen, animal starch
gnath/o	jaw
-gnosia	knowledge, to know
-gog, -gogue	make flow
goitr/o	goiter, enlargement of the thyroid gland
gon/e, gon/o	seed
gonad/o	gonad, sex glands
goni/o	angle
gracil/o	slender
grad/i	move, go, step, walk
-grade	go
-gram	a picture or record
granul/o	granule(s)
-graph	a picture or record, machine for recording record
-graphy	the process of producing a picture or record
gravid/o	pregnancy
-gravida	pregnant
gynec/o	woman, female
gyr/o	turning, folding

H

hal/o, halit/o	breath
halluc/o	great or large toe
hallucin/o	hallucination, to wander in the mind
hem/e	deep red iron-containing pigment
hem/o, hemat/o	blood, relating to the blood
hemangi/o	blood vessel
hemi-	half
hemoglobin/o	hemoglobin
hepat/o	liver
hered/o, heredit/o	inherited, inheritance
herni/o	hernia
herpet/o	creeping
heter/o	other, different
-hexia	habit
hiat/o	opening
hidr/o	sweat
hil/o	hilum, notch or opening from a body part
hirsut/o	hairy, rough
hist/o, histi/o	tissue
holo-	all
hom/o	same, like, alike
home/o	sameness, unchanging, constant
hormon/o	hormone
humer/o	humerus (upper arm bone)
hydr/o, hydra-	relating to water
hygien/o	healthful
hymen/o	hymen, a membrane
hyp-	deficient, decreased
hyper-	excessive, increased
hypn/o	sleep
hypo-	deficient, decreased
hyster/o	uterus

I

-ia	abnormal condition, disease, plural of -ium
-ial	pertaining to
-ian	specialist
-iasis	abnormal condition, disease
iatr/o	physician, treatment
-iatrics	field of medicine, healing
-iatrist	specialist
-iatry	field of medicine
-ible	capable of, able to
-ic	pertaining to

ichthy/o	dry, scaly
-ician	specialist
icter/o	jaundice
idi/o	peculiar to the individual or organ, one, distinct
-iferous	bearing, carrying, producing
-ific	making, producing
-iform	shaped or formed like, resembling
-igo	attack, diseased condition
-ile	capable of
ile/o	ileum, small intestine
ili/o	ilium, hip bone
illusi/o	deception
im-	not
immun/o	immune, protection, safe
impact/o	pushed against, wedged against, packed
impress/o	pressing into
impuls/o	pressure or pushing force, drive, urging on
in-	in, into, not, without
incis/o	cutting into
incubat/o	incubation, hatching
indurat/o	hardened
-ine	pertaining to
infarct/o	filled in, stuffed
infect/o	infected, tainted
infer/o	below, beneath
infest/o	attack, assail, molest
inflammat/o	flame within, set on fire
infra-	below, beneath, inferior to
infundibul/o	funnel
ingest/o	carry or pour in
inguin/o	groin
inhal/o, inhalat/o	breathe in
inject/o	to force or throw in
innominat/o	unnamed, nameless
inocul/o	implant, introduce
insipid/o	tasteless
inspir/o, inspirat/o	breathe in
insul/o	island
insulin/o	insulin
intact/o	untouched, whole
inter-	between, among
intermitt/o	not continuous
intern/o	within, inner
interstiti/o	the space between things
intestin/o	intestine
intim/o	innermost
intoxic/o	put poison in

intra-	within, inside
intrins/o	contained within
intro-	within, into, inside
introit/o	entrance or passage
intussuscept/o	take up or receive within
involut/o	rolled up, curled inward
iod/o	iodine
-ion	action, process, state or condition
ion/o	ion, to wander
-ior	pertaining to
ipsi-	same
ir-	in
ir/i, ir/o, irid/o, irit/o	iris, colored part of eye
-is	noun ending
is/o	same, equal
isch/o	to hold back
ischi/o	ischium
-ism	condition, state of
iso-	equal
-ist	a person who practices, specialist
-isy	noun ending
-itis	inflammation
-ium	structure, tissue
-ive	performs, tends toward
-ize	to make, to treat

J

jejun/o	jejunum
jugul/o	throat
juxta-	beside, near, nearby

K

kal/i	potassium
kary/o	nucleus, nut
kata-, kath-	down
kel/o	growth, tumor
kera-	horn, hardness
kerat/o	horny, hard, cornea
ket/o, keton/o	ketones, acetones
kines/o, kinesi/o, -kinesia	movement
-kinesis	motion
klept/o	to steal
koil/o	hollow or concave
kraur/o	dry
kyph/o	bent, hump

L

labi/o	lip
labyrinth/o	maze, labyrinth, the inner ear
lacer/o, lacerat/o	torn, mangled
lacrim/o	tear, tear duct, lacrimal duct
lact/i, lact/o	milk
lactat/o	secrete milk
lamin/o	lamina
lapar/o	abdomen, abdominal wall
laps/o	slip, fall, slide
-lapse	to slide, fall, sag
laryng/o	larynx, throat
lat/i, lat/o	broad
later/o	side
lav/o, lavat/o	wash, bathe
lax/o, laxat/o	loosen, relax
leiomy/o	smooth (visceral) muscle
lemm/o	husk, peel, bark
-lemma	sheath, covering
lent/i	the lens of the eye
lenticul/o	shaped like a lens, pertaining to a lens
-lepsy	seizure
lept/o	thin, slender
-leptic	to seize, take hold of
lepto-	small, soft
letharg/o	drowsiness, oblivion
leuk/o	white
lev/o, levat/o	raise, lift up
lex/o, -lexia	word, phrase
libid/o, libidin/o	sexual drive, desire, passion
ligament/o	ligament
ligat/o	binding or tying off
lingu/o	tongue
lipid/o, lip/o	fat, lipid
-listhesis	slipping
lith/o, -lith	stone, calculus
lithiasis	presence of stones
lob/i, lob/o	lobe, well-defined part of an organ
loc/o	place
loch/i	childbirth, confinement
-logy	study of
longev/o	long-lived, long life
lord/o	curve, swayback bent
lumb/o	lower back, loin
lumin/o	light
lun/o, lunat/o	moon

lunul/o	crescent
lup/i, lup/o	wolf
lute/o	yellow
lux/o	to slide
lymph/o	lymph, lymphatic tissue
lymphaden/o	lymph gland
lymphangi/o	lymph vessel
-lysis	breakdown, separation, setting free, destruction, loosening
-lyst	agent that causes lysis or loosening
-lytic	to reduce, destroy

M

macro-	large, abnormal size or length, long
macul/o	spot
magn/o	great, large
major/o	larger
mal-	bad, poor, evil
-malacia	abnormal softening
malign/o	bad, evil
malle/o	malleus, hammer
malleol/o	malleolus, little hammer
mamm/o	breast
man/i	madness, rage
man/i, man/o	hand
mandibul/o	mandible, lower jaw
-mania	obsessive preoccupation
manipul/o	use of hands
manubri/o	handle
masset/o	chew
mast/o	breast
mastic/o, masticat/o	chew
mastoid/o	mastoid process
matern/o	maternal, of a mother
matur/o	ripe
maxill/o	maxilla (upper jaw)
maxim/o	largest, greatest
meat/o	opening or passageway
medi/o	middle
mediastin/o	mediastinum, middle
medic/o	medicine, physician, healing
medicat/o	medication, healing
medull/o	medulla (inner section), middle, soft, marrow
mega-, megal/o	large, great
-megaly	enlargement

mei/o	less, meiosis
melan/o	black, dark
mellit/o	honey, honeyed
membran/o	membrane, thin skin
men/o	menstruation, menses
mening/o, meningi/o	membranes, meninges
menisc/o	meniscus, crescent
mens/o	menstruate, menstruation, menses
menstru/o, menstruat/o	occurring monthly
ment/o	mind, chin
mes-	middle
mesenter/o	mesentery
mesi/o	middle, median plane
meso-	middle
meta-	change, beyond, subsequent to, behind, after or next
metabol/o	change
metacarp/o	metacarpals, bones of the hand
metatars/o	bones of the foot between the tarsus and toes
-meter	measure, instrument used to measure
metr/i, metr/o, metri/o	uterus
-metrist	one who measures
-metry	to measure
micr/o, micro-	small
mictur/o, micturit/o	urinate
mid-	middle
midsagitt/o	from front to back, at the middle
milli-	one-thousandth
-mimetic	mimic, copy
mineral/o	mineral
minim/o	smallest, least
minor/o	smaller
mio-	smaller, less
-mission	to send
mit/o	a thread
mitr/o	a miter having two points on top
mobil/o	capable of moving
monil/i	string of beads, genus of parasitic mold or fungus
mono-	one, single
morbid/o	disease, sickness
moribund/o	dying
morph/o	shape, form

mort/i, mort/o, mort/u	death, dead
mortal/i	pertaining to death, subject to death
mot/o, motil/o	motion, movement
mu/o	close, shut
muc/o, mucos/o	mucus
multi-	many, much
muscul/o	muscle
mut/a	genetic change
mut/o	unable to speak, inarticulate
mutagen/o	causing genetic change
my/o	muscle
myc/e, myc/o	fungus
mydri/o	wide
mydrias/i	dilation of the pupil
myel/o	spinal cord, bone marrow
myocardi/o	myocardium, heart muscle
myom/o	muscle tumor
myos/o	muscle
myring/o	tympanic membrane, eardrum
myx/o, myxa-	mucus

N

nar/i	nostril
narc/o	numbness, stupor
nas/i, nas/o	nose
nat/i	birth
natr/o	sodium
nause/o	nausea, seasickness
necr/o	death
-necrosis	tissue death
neo-, ne/o	new, strange
nephr/o	kidney
nerv/o, neur/i, neur/o	nerve, nerve tissue
neutr/o	neither, neutral
nev/o	birthmark, mole
nid/o	next
niter-, nitro-	nitrogen
noct/i	night
nod/o	knot, swelling
nodul/o	little knot
nom/o	law, control
non-	no
nor-	chemical compound
norm/o	normal or usual
nuch/o	the nape
nucle/o	nucleus

nucleol/o	little nucleus, nucleolus
nulli-	none
numer/o	number, count
nunci/o	messenger
nutri/o, nutrit/o	nourishment, food, nourish, feed
nyct/o, nyctal/o	night

O

ob-	against
obes/o	obese, extremely fat
obliqu/o	slanted, sideways
oblongat/o	oblong, elongated
obstetr/i, obstetr/o	midwife, one who stands to receive
occipit/o	back of the skull, occiput
occlud/o, occlus/o	shut, close up
occult/o	hidden, concealed
ocul/o	eye
odont/o	tooth
-oid	like, resembling
-ole	little, small
olecran/o	elbow, olecranon
olfact/o	smell, sense of smell
olig/o	scanty, few
-ologist	specialist
-ology	the science or study of
om/o	shoulder
-oma	tumor, neoplasm
oment/o	omentum, fat
omphal/o	umbilical cord, the navel
onc/o	tumor
-one	hormone
onych/o	fingernail or toenail
o/o, oo/o	egg
oophor/o	ovary
opac/o, opacit/o	shaded, dark, impenetrable to light
-opaque	obscure
oper/o, operat/o	perform, operate, work
opercul/o	cover or lid
ophthalm/o	eye, vision
-opia	vision condition
opisth/o	backward
-opsia, -opsis, -opsy	vision, view of
opt/i, opt/o, optic/o	eye, vision
or/o	mouth, oral cavity
orbit/o	orbit, bony cavity or socket

orch/o, orchid/o, orchi/o	testicles, testis, testes
-orexia	appetite
organ/o	organ
orgasm/o	swell, be excited
orth/o	straight, normal, correct
-ory	pertaining to
os-	mouth, bone
-ose	full of, pertaining to, sugar
-osis	abnormal condition, disease
osm/o	pushing, thrusting
-osmia	smell, odor
oss/e, oss/i	bone
ossicul/o	ossicle (small bone)
ost/o, oste/o	bone
-ostomy	surgically creating an opening
-ostosis	condition of bone
ot/o	ear, hearing
-otia	ear condition
-otomy	cutting, surgical incision
ov/i, ov/o	egg, ovum
ovari/o	ovary
ovul/o	egg
ox/i, ox/o, ox/y	oxygen
-oxia	oxygen condition
oxid/o	containing oxygen
oxy/o	the presence of oxygen in a compound

P

pachy-	heavy, thick
palat/o	palate, roof of mouth
pall/o, pallid/o	pale, lacking or drained of color
palliat/o	cloaked, hidden
palm/o	palm of the hand
palpat/o	touch, feel, stroke
palpebr/o	eyelid
palpit/o	throbbing, quivering
pan-	all, entire, every
pancreat/o	pancreas
papill/i, papill/o	nipple-like
papul/o	pimple
par-, para-	beside, near, beyond, abnormal, apart from, opposite, along side of
par/o	to bear, bring forth, labor
-para	to give birth
paralys/o, paralyt/o	disable

parasit/o	parasite
parathyroid/o	parathyroid glands
pares/i	to disable
-paresi	partial or incomplete paralysis
paret/o	to disable
-pareunia	sexual intercourse
pariet/o	wall
parotid/o	parotid gland
-parous	having borne one or more children
paroxysm/o	sudden attack
-partum, parturit/o	childbirth, labor
patell/a, patell/o	patella, kneecap
path/o, -pathy	disease, suffering, feeling, emotion
paus/o	cessation, stopping
-pause	stopping
pector/o	chest
ped/o	child, foot
pedi/a	child
pedicul/o	louse (singular), lice (plural)
pelv/i, pelv/o	pelvic bone, pelvic cavity, hip
pen/i	penis
pend/o	to hang
-penia	deficiency, lack, too few
peps/i, -pepsia, pept/o	digest, digestion
per-	excessive, through
percept/o	become aware, perceive
percuss/o	strike, tap, beat
peri-	surrounding, around
perine/o	perineum
peristals/o, peristalt/o	constrict around
peritone/o	peritoneum
perme/o	to pass or go through
pernici/o	destructive, harmful
perone/o	fibula
perspir/o	perspiration
pertuss/i	intensive cough
petechi/o	skin spot
-pexy	surgical fixation
phac/o	lens of eye
phag/o	eat, swallow
-phage	a cell that destroys, eat, swallow
-phagia	eating, swallowing
phak/o	lens of eye
phalang/o	phalanges, finger and toe
phall/o	penis

pharmac/o, pharmaceut/o	drug
pharyng/o	throat, pharynx
phas/o	speech
-phasia	speak or speech
phe/o	dusky
pher/o	to bear or carry
-pheresis	removal
phil/o, -phila, -philia	attraction to, like, love
phleb/o	vein
phlegm/o	thick mucus
phob/o, -phobia	abnormal fear
phon/o, -phonia	sound, voice
phor/o	carry, bear, movement
-phoresis	carrying, transmission
-phoria	to bear, carry, feeling, mental state
phot/o	light
phren/o	diaphragm, mind
-phthisis	wasting away
-phylactic	protective, preventive
-phylaxis	protection
physi/o, physic/o	nature
-physis	to grow
phyt/o, -phyte	plant
pigment/o	pigment, color
pil/i, pil/o	hair
pineal/o	pineal gland
pinn/i	external ear, auricle
pituit/o, pituitar/o	pituitary gland
plac/o	flat plate or patch
placent/o	placenta, round flat cake
plak/o, -plakia	plaque, plate, thin flat layer or scale
plan/o	flat
plant/i, plant/o	sole of foot
plas/i, plas/o, -plasia	development, growth, formation
-plasm	formative material of cells
plasm/o	something molded or formed
-plastic	pertaining to formation
-plasty	surgical repair
ple/o	more, many
-plegia	paralysis, stroke
-plegic	one affected with paralysis
pleur/o	pleura, side of the body
plex/o	plexus, network
plic/o	fold or ridge
pne/o-	breath, breathing

-pnea	breathing
-pneic	pertaining to breathing
pneum/o, pneumon/o	lung, air
pod/o	foot
-poiesis	formation, to make
poikil/o	varied, irregular
pol/o	extreme
poli/o	gray matter of brain and spinal cord
pollic/o	thumb
poly-	many
polyp/o	polyp, small growth
pont/o	pons (a part of the brain), bridge
poplit/o	back of the knee
por/o	pore, small opening
-porosis	lessening in density, porous condition
port/i	gate, door
post-	after, behind
poster/o	behind, toward the back
potent/o	powerful
pract/i, practic/o	practice, pursue an occupation
prandi/o, -prandial	meal
-praxia	action, condition concerning the performance of movements
-praxis	act, activity, practice use
pre-	before, in front of
precoc/i	early, premature
pregn/o	pregnant, full of
prematur/o	too early, untimely
preputi/o	foreskin, prepuce
presby/o	old age
press/o	press, draw
priap/o	penis
primi-	first
pro-	before, in behalf of
process/o	going forth
procident/o	fall down or forward
procreat/o	reproduce
proct/o	anus and rectum
prodrom/o	running ahead, precursor
product/o	lead forward, yield, produce
prolaps/o	fall downward, slide forward
prolifer/o	reproduce, bear offspring
pron/o, pronat/o	bent forward
pros-	before
prostat/o	prostate gland
prosth/o, prosthet/o	addition, appendage

prot/o, prote/o	first
protein/o	protein
proxim/o	near
prurit/o	itching
pseud/o	false
psor/i, psor/o	itch, itching
psych/o	mind
ptomat/o	a fall
-ptosis	droop, sag, prolapse, fall
-ptyal/o	saliva
-ptysis	spitting
pub/o	pubis, part of hip bone
pubert/o	ripe age, adult
pudend/o	pudendum
puerper/i	childbearing, labor
pulm/o, pulmon/o	lung
pulpos/o	fleshy, pulpy
puls/o	beat, beating, striking
punct/o	sting, prick, puncture
pupill/o	pupil
pur/o	pus
purpur/o	purple
purul/o	pus-filled
pustul/o	infected pimple
py/o	pus
pyel/o	renal pelvis, bowl of kidney
pylor/o	pylorus, pyloric sphincter
pyr/o, pyret/o	fever, fire
pyramid/o	pyramid shaped

Q

quadr/i, quadr/o	four

R

rabi/o	madness, rage
rachi/o	spinal column, vertebrae
radi/o	radiation, x-rays, radius (lateral lower arm bone)
radiat/o	giving off rays or radiant energy
radicul/o	nerve root
raph/o	seam, suture
re-	back, again
recept/o	receive, receiver
recipi/o	receive, take to oneself
rect/o	rectum, straight
recticul/o	network
recuperat/o	recover, regain health
reduct/o	bring back together
refract/o	bend back, turn aside

regurgit/o	flood or gush back
remiss/o	give up, let go, relax
ren/o	kidney
restor/o	rebuild, put back, restore
resuscit/o	revive
retent/o	hold back
reticul/o	network
retin/o	retina, net
retract/o	draw back or in
retro-	behind, backward, back of
rhabd/o	rod, rod shaped
rhabdomy/o	striated muscle
rheum/o, rheumat/o	watery flow, subject to flow
rhin/o	nose
rhiz/o	root
rhonc/o	snore, snoring
rhythm/o	rhythm
rhytid/o	wrinkle
rigid/o	stiff
ris/o	laugh
roentgen/o	x-ray
rotat/o	rotate, revolve
-rrhage, -rrhagia	bleeding, abnormal excessive fluid discharge
-rrhaphy	surgical suturing
-rrhea	flow or discharge
-rrhexis	rupture
rube-	red
rug/o	wrinkle, fold

S

sacc/i, sacc/o	sac
sacchar/o	sugar
sacr/o	sacrum
saliv/o	saliva
salping/o	uterine (fallopian) tube, auditory (eustachian) tube
-salpinx	uterine (fallopian) tube
san/o	sound, healthy, sane
sangu/i, sanguin/o	blood
sanit/o	soundness, health
saphen/o	clear, apparent, manifest
sapr/o	decaying, rotten
sarc/o	flesh, connective tissue
scalp/o	carve, scrape
scapul/o	scapula, shoulder blade
schiz/o	division, split
scintill/o	spark

scirrh/o	hard
scler/o	sclera, white of eye, hard
-sclerosis	abnormal hardening
scoli/o	curved, bent
-scope	instrument for visual examination
-scopic	pertaining to visual examination
-scopy	visual examination
scot/o	darkness
scrib/o, script/o	write
scrot/o	bag or pouch
seb/o	sebum
secret/o	produce, separate out
sect/o, secti/o	cut, cutting
segment/o	pieces
sell/o	saddle
semi-	half
semin/i	semen, seed, sperm
sen/i	old
senesc/o	grow old
senil/o	old age
sens/i	feeling, sensation
sensitiv/o	sensitive to, affected by
seps/o	infection
sept/o	infection, partition
ser/o	serum
seros/o	serous
sial/o	saliva
sialaden/o	salivary gland
sider/o	iron
sigm/o	Greek letter sigma
sigmoid/o	sigmoid colon
silic/o	glass
sin/o, sin/u	hollow, sinus
sinistr/o	left, left side
sinus/o	sinus
-sis	abnormal condition, disease
sit/u	place
skelet/o	skeleton
soci/o	companion, fellow being
-sol	solution
solut/o, solv/o	loosened, dissolved
soma-, somat/o	body
somn/i, somn/o	sleep
son/o	sound
sopor/o	sleep
spad/o	draw off, draw
-spasm, spasmod/o	sudden involuntary contraction, tightening or cramping
spec/i	look at, a kind or sort

specul/o	mirror
sperm/o, spermat/o	sperm, spermatozoa, seed
sphen/o	sphenoid bone, wedge
spher/o	round, sphere, ball
sphincter/o	tight band
sphygm/o	pulse
spin/o	spine, backbone
spir/o	to breathe
spirill/o	little coil
spirochet/o	coiled microorganism
splen/o	spleen
spondyl/o	vertebrae, vertebral column, back bone
spontane/o	unexplained, of one's own accord
spor/o	seed, spore
sput/o	sputum, spit
squam/o	scale
-stalsis	contraction, constriction
staped/o, stapedi/o	stapes (middle ear bone)
staphyl/o	clusters, bunch of grapes
-stasis, -static	control, maintenance of a constant level
steat/o	fat, lipid, sebum
sten/o	narrowing, contracted
-stenosis	abnormal narrowing
ster/o	solid structure
stere/o	solid, three-dimensional
steril/i	sterile
stern/o	sternum, the breastbone
stert/o	snore, snoring
steth/o	chest
-sthenia	strength
stigmat/o	point, spot
stimul/o	goad, prick, incite
stol/o	send or place
stomat/o	mouth
-stomosis, -stomy	furnish with a mouth or outlet, new opening
strab/i	squint, squint-eyed
strat/i	layer
strept/o	twisted chain
striat/o	stripe, furrow, groove
stric-	narrowing
strict/o	draw tightly together, bind or tie
strid/o	harsh sound
stup/e	benumbed, stunned
styl/o	pen, pointed instrument
sub-	under, less, below
subluxat/o	partial dislocation
sucr/o	sugar
sudor/i	sweat
suffoc/o, suffocat/o	choke, strangle
sulc/o	furrow, groove
super-, super/o	above, excessive, higher than
superflu/o	overflowing, excessive
supin/o	lying on the back
supinat/o	bend backward, place on the back
suppress/o	press down
suppur/o, suppurat/o	to form pus
supra-	above, upper, excessive
supraren/o	above or on the kidney, suprarenal gland
-surgery	operative procedure
sutur/o	stitch, seam
sym-	with, together, joined together
symptomat/o	falling together, symptom
syn-	together, with, union, association
synaps/o, synapt/o	point of contact
syncop/o	to cut short, cut off
-syndesis	surgical fixation of vertebrae
syndesm/o	ligament
syndrom/o	running together
synovi/o, synov/o	synovial membrane, synovial fluid
syphil/i, syphil/o	syphilis
syring/o	tube
system/o, systemat/o	body system
systol/o	contraction

T

tachy-	fast, rapid
tact/i	touch
talip/o	foot and ankle deformity
tars/o	tarsus (ankle bone), instep, edge of the eyelid
tax/o	coordination, order
techn/o, techni/o	skill
tectori/o	covering, rooflike
tele/o	distant, far
tempor/o	temporal bone, temple
ten/o, tend/o	tendon, stretch out, extend, strain
tenac/i	holding fast, sticky
tendin/o	tendon
tens/o	stretch out, extend, strain
terat/o	malformed fetus

termin/o	end, limit
test/i, test/o, testicul/o	testis, testicle
tetan/o	rigid, tense
tetra-	four
thalam/o	thalamus, inner room
thalass/o	sea
thanas/o, thanat/o	death
the/o	put, place
thec/o	sheath
thel/o	nipple
therap/o, therapeut/o	treatment
therm/o	heat
thio-	sulfur
thora/o, thorac/o	chest
-thorax	chest, pleural cavity
thromb/o	clot
thym/o	thymus gland, soul
-thymia	a state of mind
-thymic	pertaining to the mind, relating to the thymus gland
thyr/o, thyroid/o	thyroid gland
tibi/o	tibia (shin bone)
-tic	pertaining to
tine/o	gnawing worm, ringworm
tinnit/o	ringing, buzzing, tinkling
-tion	process, state or quality of
toc/o, -tocia, -tocin	labor, birth
tom/o	cut, section, slice
-tome	instrument to cut
-tomy	process of cutting
ton/o	tension, tone, stretching
tone/o	to stretch
tonsill/o	tonsil, throat
top/o	place, position, location
tors/o	twist, rotate
tort/i	twisted
tox/o, toxic/o	poison, poisonous
trabecul/o	little beam marked with cross bars or beams
trache/i, trache/o	trachea, windpipe
trachel-	neck
tract/o	draw, pull, path, bundle of nerve fibers
tranquil/o	quiet, calm, tranquil
trans-	across, through
transfus/o	pour across, transfer
transit/o	changing
transvers/o	across, crosswise
traumat/o	injury
trem/o	shaking, trembling
tremul/o	fine tremor or shaking
treponem/o	coiled, turning microbe
tri-	three
trich/o	hair
trigon/o	trigone
-tripsy	to crush
-trite	instrument for crushing
trop/o, -tropia	turn, change
troph/o, -trophy	development, nourishment
-tropic	turning
-tropin	to stimulate, act on
tub/i, tub/o	tube, pipe
tubercul/o	little knot, swelling
tunic/o	covering, cloak, sheath
turbinat/o	coiled, spiral shaped
tuss/i	cough
tympan/o	tympanic membrane, eardrum
-type	classification, picture

U

-ula	small, little
-ule	small one
ulcer/o	sore, ulcer
uln/o	ulna (medial lower arm bone)
ultra-	beyond, excess
-um	singular noun ending
umbilic/o	navel
un-	not
ungu/o	nail
uni-	one
ur/o	urine, urinary tract
-uresis	urination
ureter/o	ureter
urethr/o	urethra
urg/o	press, push
-uria	urination, urine
urin/o	urine or urinary organs
urtic/o	nettle, rash, hives
-us	thing, singular noun ending
uter/i, uter/o	uterus
uve/o	iris, choroid, ciliary body, uveal tract
uvul/o	uvula, little grape

V

vaccin/i, vaccin/o	vaccine
vacu/o	empty

vag/o	vagus nerve, wandering
vagin/o	vagina
valg/o	bent or twisted outward
valv/o, valvul/o	valve
var/o	bent or twisted inward
varic/o	varicose veins, swollen or dilated vein
vas/o	vas deferens, vessel
vascul/o	blood vessel, little vessel
vast/o	vast, great, extensive
vect/o	carry, convey
ven/o	vein
vener/o	sexual intercourse
venter-	abdomen
ventilat/o	expose to air, fan
ventr/o	in front, belly side of body
ventricul/o	ventricle of brain or heart, small chamber
venul/o	venule, small vein
verg/o	twist, incline
verm/i	worm
verruc/o	wart
-verse, -version	to turn
vers/o, vert/o	turn
vertebr/o	vertebra, backbone
vertig/o, vertigin/o	whirling round
vesic/o	urinary bladder
vesicul/o	seminal vesicle, blister, little bladder
vestibul/o	entrance, vestibule
vi/o	force

vill/i	shaggy hair, tuft of hair
vir/o	poison, virus
viril/o	masculine, manly
vis/o	seeing, sight
visc/o	sticky
viscer/o	viscera, internal organ
viscos/o	sticky
vit/a, vit/o	life
viti/o	blemish, defect
vitre/o	glassy, made of glass
voc/i	voice
vol/o	palm or sole
volv/o	roll, turn
vulgar/i	common
vulv/o	vulva, covering

X

xanth/o	yellow
xen/o	strange, foreign
xer/o	dry
xiph/i, xiph/o	sword

Y

-y	noun ending

Z

zo/o	animal life
zygomat/o	cheek bone, yoke
zygot/o	joined together

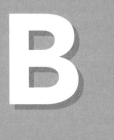

Appendix B
Abbreviations and Their Meanings

Reminder about abbreviations: (1) An abbreviation can have several meanings. (2) A term can have several abbreviations. When in doubt, always verify the meaning.

A

A	abnormal; adult; age; allergy; anaphylaxis; anesthesia; anterior; antibody; auscultation
A2 or A_2	aortic valve closure
a	accommodation; acid
aa	amino acid
AA	alopecia areata; asthma; asthmatic
AAA	abdominal aortic aneurysm
AAL	anterior axillary line
AAV	adeno-associated virus
A&B	apnea and bradycardia
A/B	acid-base ratio
AB, Ab, ab	abortion
AB, Abnl, abn	abnormal
Ab	antibody
ABC	aspiration; biopsy; cytology
Abd, Abdo	abdomen
ABE	acute bacterial endocarditis
ABG	arterial blood gases
ABP	arterial blood pressure
ABR	auditory brainstem response

abx	antibiotics
AC, ac	anticoagulant; before meals
ac	acute
acc	accident; accommodation
ACD	absolute cardiac dullness; acid-citrate-dextrose; anterior chest diameter; area of cardiac disease
ACE	acute care of the elderly; aerobic chair exercises; angiotensin-converting enzyme
ACG	angiocardiogram; angiocardiography; apex cardiogram
ACH	adrenocortical hormone
ACL	anterior cruciate ligament
ACLS	advanced cardiac life support
ACT	activated coagulation time; anticoagulant therapy
ACTH	adrenocorticotropic hormone
ACU	acute care unit; ambulatory care unit
ACVD	acute cardiovascular disease
AD	admitting diagnosis; advanced directive; after discharge; Alzheimer's disease; right ear
ADC	AIDS dementia complex
ADD	attention deficit disorder
ADE	acute disseminated encephalitis; adverse drug event
ADH	adhesion; antidiuretic hormone
ADHD	attention deficit hyperactivity disorder
ADL	activities of daily life; activities of daily living

ad lib	as desired
adm	admission
ADR	adverse drug reaction
ADS	antibody deficiency syndrome
ADT	admission, discharge, transfer
AE, A/E	above elbow
AED	automated external defibrillation
AF	acid-fast; amniotic fluid; atrial flutter
AF, A fib, AFib	atrial fibrillation
AFB	acid-fast bacilli
AFP	alpha-fetoprotein
AG, Ag	antigen
AH	abdominal hysterectomy
AHD	antihypertensive drug; arteriosclerotic heart disease; autoimmune hemolytic disease
AI	accidentally incurred; aortic insufficiency; atherogenic index
AID	acute infectious disease; artificial insemination donor
AIDS	acquired immunodeficiency syndrome
AIH	artificial insemination by husband
AIHA	autoimmune hemolytic anemia
AJ, aj	ankle jerk
AK	above knee
AKA	above-knee amputation
alb	albumin
ALD	aldosterone
alk	alkaline
ALL	acute lymphoblastic leukemia; acute lymphocytic leukemia
ALND	axillary lymph node dissection
ALP	acute lupus pericarditis; alkaline phosphatase
ALS	advanced life support; amyotrophic lateral sclerosis; antilymphocytic serum
ALT, alt	alternative; altitude
alt dieb	alternate days; every other day
alt hor	alternate hours
alt noct	alternate nights
Am	amnion
AMA	advanced maternal age; against medical advice; American Medical Association
amb	ambulance; ambulatory
AMD	age-related macular degeneration
AMI	acute myocardial infarction
AML	acute myeloblastic leukemia; acute myelocytic leukemia; amyotrophic lateral sclerosis

AMN	amniocentesis
amp	amplification; ampule; amputate
AMS	altered mental status; automated multiphasic screening
amt	amount
AN	aneurysm; anorexia nervosa
ANA	antinuclear antibodies
ANAS	anastomosis
anat	anatomy
anes, anesth	anesthesia; anesthetic
ANLL	acute nonlymphocytic leukemia
ANS	anterior nasal spine; autonomic nervous system
ant, ANT	anterior
ANUG	acute necrotizing ulcerative gingivitis
AOD	arterial occlusive disease
AODM	adult-onset diabetes mellitus
AOM	acute otitis media
A & P	anatomy and physiology; anterior and posterior; auscultation and percussion
AP	abruptio placenta; angina pectoris; antero-posterior; anterior-posterior; appendectomy; appendicitis
APAP	acetaminophen
Aph	aphasia
APLD	aspiration percutaneous lumbar diskectomy
aPTT	activated partial thromboplastin time
aq	aqueous; water
AR	abnormal record; achievement ration; alarm reaction; artificial respiration
ARD	acute respiratory disease
ARDS	acute respiratory distress syndrome; adult respiratory distress syndrome
ARF	acute renal failure; acute respiratory failure
ARI	acute respiratory infection
ARM	artificial rupture of membranes
ART	arthritis; assisted reproductive technology
AS	ankylosing spondylitis; aortic stenosis; astigmatism; left ear
ASA	acetylsalicylic acid (aspirin)
ASAP	as soon as possible
ASCVD	arteriosclerotic cardiovascular disease
ASD	atrial septal defect
ASH	asymmetrical septal hypertrophy
ASHD	arteriosclerotic heart disease
ASO	administrative services only; arteriosclerosis obliterans
ASS	anterior superior spine

AST	Aphasia Screening Test; aspartate aminotransferase
As tol	as tolerated
AT	Achilles tendon
ATP	adenosine triphosphate
atr	atrophy
AU	aures unitas; both ears
AUL	acute undifferentiated leukemia
aus, ausc, auscul	auscultation
A-V, AV	aortic valve; artificial ventilation; arterio-venous; atrioventricular
AVM	arteriovenous malfunction
AVN	atrioventricular node
AVR	aortic valve replacement
A & W	alive and well
Ax, ax	axilla; axillary
AZT	Aschheim-Zondek test

B

B	bruit
B/A	backache
BA	bronchial asthma
Ba	barium
BAC	blood alcohol concentration
BACT, Bact bact	bacteria; bacterium
BaE	barium enema
BAO	basal acid output
bas	basophils
BBB	blood-brain barrier; bundle branch block
BBT	basal body temperature
BC	bone conduction
BCC	basal cell carcinoma
BD	bronchodilator
BDT	bone density testing
BE	barium enema; below elbow
BEAM	brain electrical activity map
BED	binge eating disorder
BFP	biologic false positive
BID	brought in dead
bid, b.i.d.	bis in die; twice a day
BIL, bil, bili	bilirubin
bil	bilateral
BIN, bin	twice a night
BJ	Bence Jones
BK	below knee
BKA	below-knee amputation

Bld	blood
BM	bone marrow; bowel movement
BMB	bone marrow biopsy
BMD	Becker's muscular dystrophy; bone mineral density
BMI	body mass index
BMR	basal metabolic rate
BMT	barium meal test; bone marrow transplant
BNO	bladder neck obstruction
BNR	bladder neck resection
BOM	bilateral otitis media
BP	Bell's palsy; bedpan; bathroom privileges; blood pressure
BPD	borderline personality disorder
BPH	benign prostatic hyperplasia; benign prostatic hypertrophy
BPM	breaths per minute
bpm	beats per minute
BP&P	blood pressure and pulse
BPPV	benign paroxysmal positional vertigo
BR, Br	bed rest; bronchitis
BRBPR	bright red blood per rectum
BRO, Bronch	bronchoscope; bronchoscopy
BRP	bathroom privileges
BS	blood sugar; bowel sounds; breath sounds
BSE	breast self-examination
BSO	bilateral salpingo-oophorectomy
BT	bleeding time
BUN	blood urea nitrogen
BV	bacterial vaginosis; blood volume
Bx, bx	biopsy

C

C_1 through C_7	cervical vertebrae
C	centigrade; Celsius; cholesterol; convergence; cyanosis
C.	chlamydia
c	centimeter
$\bar{c}$	with
$\underline{c}$	without
Ca	calcium
CA, Ca	cancer; cardiac arrest; carcinoma; chronological age
CAB	coronary artery bypass
CABG	coronary artery bypass graft

CAD	computer-assisted diagnosis; coronary artery disease
CAL	calcitonin
cal	calorie
cap, **caps**	capsule
CAPD	continuous ambulatory peritoneal dialysis
card cath	cardiac catheterization
CAT	cataract
cath	catheter; catheterization; catheterize
caut	cauterization
CAVH	continuous arteriovenous hemofiltration
CBC, **cbc**	complete blood count
CBF	capillary blood flow; coronary blood flow
CBI	continuous bladder irrigation
CBR	complete bedrest
CBS	chronic brain syndrome
CC	chief complaint; colony count; cardiac cycle; cardiac cauterization; creatinine clearance
cc	cubic centimeter (1/1000 liter)
CCA	circumflex coronary artery
CCCR	closed chest cardiopulmonary resuscitation
CCE	cholecystectomy
CCPD	continuous cycle peritoneal dialysis
CCr	creatinine clearance
CCT	computerized cranial tomography
CCU	coronary care unit
CD	communicable disease; contact dermatitis; Crohn's disease
CDC	calculated date (day) of confinement; Centers for Disease Control and Prevention
CDE	common duct exploration
CDH	congenital dislocation of the hip
CEA	carotid endarterectomy
CEPH	cephalic
CF	complete fixation; counting fingers; cystic fibrosis
CFS	chronic fatigue syndrome
CGL	chronic granulomatous leukemia
C gl	with correction; with glasses
CH	chromosome
CHB	complete heart block
CHD	congenital heart defects; coronary heart disease
CHF	congestive heart failure
CHO	carbohydrate
chol	cholesterol
chole	cholecystectomy

chr	chromosome; chronic
CI	conjunctivitis; coronary insufficiency
cib	food
CID	cytomegalic inclusion disease
CIR, **CIRR**	cirrhosis
CIRC, **circum**	circumcision
CIS	carcinoma in situ
CIT	conventional insulin treatment
CK	creatine kinase
ck	check
CL	cholelithiasis; chronic leukemia; cirrhosis of the liver; cleft lip; corpus luteum
Cl, **cl**	clinic; chloride
CLD	chronic liver disease
CLL	chronic lymphocytic leukemia
cl liq	clear liquid
cm	centimeter (1/100 meter)
cm³	cubic centimeter
CME	cystoid macular edema
CMG	cystometrogram
CML	chronic myelocytic leukemia
CMM	cutaneous malignant melanoma
CMV	controlled mechanical ventilation; cytomegalovirus
CNS	central nervous system; cutaneous nerve stimulation
C/O, **c/o**	complains of
CO	carbon monoxide; coronary occlusion; coronary output
CO₂	carbon dioxide
COD	cause of death
COH	carbohydrate
COL	colonoscopy
COLD	chronic obstructive lung disease
comp	compound
cond	condition
contra	against
COPD	chronic obstructive pulmonary disease
CP	cardiopulmonary; cerebral palsy
CPA	carotid phonoangiograph
CPAP	continuous positive airway pressure
CPC	clinicopathologic conference
CPD	cephalopelvic disproportion
CPE	cardio-pulmonary edema
CPK	creatine phosphokinase
CPN	chronic pyelonephritis
CPPB	continuous positive-pressure breathing
CPR	cardiopulmonary resuscitation
CPS	cycles per second

CR	closed reduction; complete response; conditioned reflex
CRC	colorectal carcinoma
CRD	chronic respiratory disease
creat	creatinine
CRF	chronic renal failure
CRP	C-reactive protein
CRPS	complex regional pain syndrome
CRYO	cryosurgery
C & S	culture and sensitivity
CS	central supply; complete stroke; conditioned stimulus; Cushing's syndrome
CSAP	cryosurgical ablation of the prostate
CSB	Cheyne-Stokes breathing
c sect, **c section,** **C-section,** **CS**	cesarian section
CSF	cerebrospinal fluid
CSO	craniostenosis
CSR	central supply room; Cheyne-Stokes respiration
CT	computerized tomography
CTCL	cutaneous T-cell lymphoma
CTD	cumulative trauma disorders
CTR	carpal tunnel release
CTS	carpal tunnel syndrome
cu	cubic
CUC	chronic ulcerative colitis
CUG	cystourethrogram
CV	cardiovascular
CVA	cardiovascular accident; cerebrovascular accident
CVD	cardiovascular disease
CVL	central venous line
CVP	central venous pressure; Cytoxan, vincristine, prednisone
CVS	chorionic villus sampling
CWP	childbirth without pain; coal workers' pneumoconiosis
Cx	cervix
CX, CXR	chest x-ray film
cysto	cystoscopic examination; cystoscopy
cyt	cytology; cytoplasm

D

D	diopter; dorsal
d	day

DAT	diet as tolerated
db, dB	decibel
D&C	dilation and curettage
D/C, d/c	diarrhea/constipation
DCC	direct-current cardioversion
DCIS	ductal carcinoma in situ
DCR	direct cortical response
D/D, DD, **DDx, Ddx**	differential diagnosis
D & E	dilation and evacuation
debr	debridement
del	delivery
DES	diethylstilbestrol
DEXA	dual energy x-ray absorptiometry
DF	dorsiflexion
DG, dg	diagnosis
DGE	delayed gastric emptying
DHFS	dengue hemorrhagic fever shock syndrome
DI	diabetes insipidus
Diag, diag	diagnosis
DIC	diffuse intravascular coagulation
D/D, DD, **DDx, diff**	differential
diopt, Dptr	diopter
DIP	distal interphalangeal
diph	diphtheria
disch	discharge
DJD	degenerative joint disease
DKA	diabetic ketoacidosis
DL	danger list
DLE	discoid lupus erythematosus
DM	dermatomyositis; diabetes mellitus; diastolic murmur
DMD	Duchenne's muscular dystrophy
DNA	deoxyribonucleic acid
DNR	do not resuscitate
DNS	deviated nasal septum
DOA	dead on arrival
DOB	date of birth
DOC	date of conception
DOE	dyspnea on exertion
DOMS	delayed-onset muscle soreness
DOT	directly observed therapy
DPT	diphtheria-pertussis-tetanus
DQ	developmental quotient
DR	diabetic retinopathy; digital radiography; doctor
dr	dram; dressing
DRD	developmental reading disorder

DRE	digital rectal exam
DRG	diagnosis-related group
DRP	diabetic retinopathy
D/S	dextrose in saline
DS	Down syndrome
DSA	digital subtraction angiography
DSD	dry sterile dressing
dsg	dressing
DT	diphtheria and tetanus toxoids
DT, DT's, DTs	delirium tremens
DTP	diphtheria, tetanus toxoids, and pertussis vaccine
DTR	deep tendon reflex
du	decubitus ulcer
DUB	dysfunctional uterine bleeding
DVA	distance visual acuity
DVI	digital vascular imaging
DVT	deep vein thrombosis
D/W	dextrose in water
DX, Dx	diagnosis
DXA	dual x-ray absorptiometry

E

E	encephalitis; enema; etiology
e	epinephrine; estrogen
EBL	estimated blood loss
EBP	epidural blood patch
EBV	Epstein-Barr virus
ECC	endocervical curettage; extracorporeal circulation
ECCE	extracapsular cataract extraction
ECG	electrocardiogram; electrocardiography
ECHO	echocardiogram; echocardiography
E coli	*Escherichia coli*
ECT	electroconvulsive therapy
ED	effective dose; emergency department; epidural; erythema dose; erectile dysfunction
EDA	epidural anesthesia
EDC	estimated date (day) of confinement
EDD	end-diastolic dimension
EDS	Ehlers-Danlos syndrome
EDV	end-diastolic volume
EECG	electroencephalography
EEE	eastern equine encephalomyelitis
EEG	electroencephalogram; electro-encephalography
EENT	eye, ear; nose, and throat
EFM	electronic fetal monitor

EGD	esophagogastroduodenoscopy
EIA	enzyme immunoassay
EIB	exercise-induced bronchospasm
Ej	elbow jerk
EKG	electrocardiogram; electrocardiography
ELISA	enzyme-linked immunosorbent assay
elix	elixir
EM	electron microscope; emmetropia, erythema multiforme
emb	embolism
EMG	electromyogram; electromyography
EMP	emphysema
EMR	educable mentally retarded; electronic medical record; eye movement record
EMS	early morning specimen; electromagnetic spectrum
EN, endo	endoscopy
Endo	endometriosis
ENG	electronystagmography
ENT	ear, nose, and throat
EOG	electro-oculogram
EOM	extraocular muscles; extraocular movement
Eos, eosins	eosinophils
EP	ectopic pregnancy; evoked potential
EPF	early pregnancy factor; exophthalmos-producing factor
Epi, EPI	epinephrine
epi, epil	epilepsy
epid	epidemic
epis	episiotomy
EPO	erythropoietin
EPR	electron paramagnetic resonance; emergency physical restraint
EPS	extrapyramidal symptoms; exophthalmos-producing substance
ER	emergency room; epigastric region
ERCP	endoscopic retrograde cholangio-pancreatography
ERPF	effective renal plasma flow
ERT	estrogen replacement therapy; external radiation therapy
ERV	expiratory reserve volume
ESD	end-systolic dimension
ESPF	end-stage pulmonary fibrosis
ESR	erythrocyte sedimentation rate
ESRD	end-stage renal disease
EST	electric shock therapy
ESV	end-systolic volume

ESWL	extracorporeal shock-wave lithotripsy
ET	embryo transfer; enterically transmitted; esotropia; eustachian tube
et	and
ETF	eustachian tube function
ETI	endotracheal intubation
etiol	etiology
ETT	endotracheal tube; exercise tolerance test
EU	Ehrlich units; emergency unit; etiology unknown
EV	esophageal varices
EWB	estrogen withdrawal bleeding
ex	excision; exercise
exam	examination
exp	expiration
ext	extraction; external
Ez	eczema

F

F	Fahrenheit
FA	fluorescein angiography; fluorescent antibody; fructosamine test
FAS	fetal alcohol syndrome
FB	foreign body
FBS	fasting blood sugar
FCD	fibrocystic disease
FDP	fibrin-fibrinogen degradation products
FECG	fetal electrocardiogram
FEF	forced expiratory flow
FESS	functional endoscopic sinus surgery
fet	fetus
FEV	forced expiratory volume
FFA	free fatty acids
FH	family history
FHR	fetal heart rate
FHS	fetal heart sounds
FHT	fetal heart tones
FIA	fluorescent immunoassay; fluoro-immunoassay
Flour	fluoroscopy
FME	full mouth extractions
fMRI	functional magnetic resonance imaging
FMS	fibromyalgia syndrome
FNA	fine-needle aspiration
FOBT	fecal occult blood test
FPG	fasting plasma glucose
fr	French (catheter size)
FRC	functional residual capacity
FROM	full range of motion

FS	frozen section
FSH	follicle-stimulating hormone
FSP	fibrin-fibrinogen split products
FSS	functional endoscopic sinus surgery
FT	family therapy
FTND	full-term normal delivery
FTT	failure to thrive
FU, F/U	follow-up; follow up
FUO	fever of unknown origin
FX, Fx	fracture

G

G	gingiva; glaucoma; glycogen
g	gram
g$_1$	gravida (pregnancy)
GA	gastric analysis; general anesthesia
ga	gallium
GAD	generalized anxiety disorder
GB	gallbladder
GBM	glomerular basement membrane
GBS	gallbladder series; Guillain-Barré syndrome
G-Cs	glucocorticoids
GC	gonorrhea
GCG	glucagon
G&D	growth and development
GD	Graves' disease
GDM	gestational diabetes mellitus
GE	gastroenteritis
GER	gastroesophageal reflux
GERD	gastroesophageal reflux disease
GFR	glomerular filtration rate
GG	gamma globulin
GGT	gamma-glutamyl transferase
GH	growth hormone
GHb	glycohemoglobin
GI	gastrointestinal
GIFT	gamete intrafallopian transfer
GIT	gastrointestinal tract
glau, glc	glaucoma
GLTT	glucose tolerance test
gm	gram
GN	glomerulonephritis
GP	general practice
gr	grain
grav I	pregnancy one; primigravida
GS	general surgery
GSW	gunshot wound
GT	glucose tolerance

GTT	glucose tolerance test
gtt	drops
GU	genitourinary
GVHD	graft-versus-host disease
GxT	graded exercise test
GYN, Gyn	gynecology

H

H	hydrogen; hypodermic; hyperopia
h	hour
H & H	hemoglobin and hematocrit
HA	hemolytic anemia; histamine
HAA	hepatitis associated antigen; hepatitis Australia antigen
halluc	hallucination
HASHD	hypertensive arteriosclerotic heart disease
HAV	hepatitis A virus
HB	heart block; hemoglobin; hepatitis B; His bundle
Hb	hemoglobin
HBE	His bundle electrocardiogram
HbF	fetal hemoglobin
HBGM	home blood glucose monitoring
HBP	high blood pressure
HbS	sickle cell hemoglobin
HBV	hepatitis B virus
HC	Huntington's cholera
HCD	heavy-chain disease
HCG	human chorionic gonadotropin
HCl	hydrochloric acid
HCL	hairy cell leukemia
HCT, Hct, hct	hematocrit
HCV	hepatitis C virus
HCVD	hypertensive cardiovascular disease
HD	hearing distance; heart disease; hemodialysis; hip disarticulation; Hodgkin's disease; Huntington's disease
HDL	high-density lipoproteins
HDN	hemolytic disease of the newborn
HDS	herniated disk syndrome
HE	hereditary elliptocytosis; hyperextension
He	helium; hemorrhage
HEENT	head, eyes, ears, nose, throat
HEM	hematuria
HEM, hemo	hemophilia; hemodialysis
hemat	hematocrit
hemi	hemiplegia

HF	heart failure
HG	hypoglycemia
Hg	mercury
HgA1c	glycohemoglobin test
Hgb	hemoglobin
HGE	human granulocytic Ehrlichiosis
HH	hiatal hernia
HIE	hypoxic ischemic encephalopathy
Hi, hist	histamine
HIS, Histo, histol	histology
HIV	human immunodeficiency virus
H & L	heart and lungs
HL	Hodgkin's lymphoma
HLA	human leukocyte antigen
HLR	heart-lung resuscitation
HM	hand motion; Holter monitor
HMD	hyaline membrane disease
HMO	health maintenance organization
hmt	hematocrit
HNP	herniated nucleus pulposus
HO	hyperbaric oxygen
HOB	head of bed
H & P	history and physical
HP	hemipelvectomy; hyperparathyroidism
HPN	hypertension
HPO	hypothalamic-pituitary-ovarian
HPS	hantavirus pulmonary syndrome
HPV	human papilloma virus
HR	heart rate
hr	hour
HRT	hormone replacement therapy
HS	hamstring; heavy smoker; herpes simplex; hospital stay
hs, h.s.	at bedtime; hour of sleep
HSG	hysterosalpingogram; hystero-salpingography
HSV	herpes simplex virus
HSV-1	oral herpes simplex virus type 1
HSV-2	herpes simplex virus type 2
HT	Hashimoto's thyroiditis; hormone therapy
ht	height; hematocrit
HTO	high tibial osteotomy
HV	hallux valgus; hospital visit
HVD	hypertensive vascular disease
HVT	hyperventilation
Hx	history
hypo	hypodermic
HYS	hysteroscopy

HZ	herpes zoster
Hz	hertz

I

I	intensity of magnetism; iodine
IABP	intra-aortic balloon pump
IACP	intra-aortic counterpulsation
IADH	inappropriate antidiuretic hormone
IASD	interatrial septal defect
IBC	iron-binding capacity
IBD	inflammatory bowel disease
IBS	irritable bowel syndrome
IC	inspiratory capacity; intermittent claudication; interstitial cystitis
ICCE	intracapsular lens extraction
ICCU	intensive coronary care unit
ICD	implantable cardioverter defibrillator
ICF	intracellular fluid
ICP	intracranial pressure
ICS	ileocecal sphincter; intercostal space
ICSH	interstitial cell-stimulating hormone
ICSI	intracytoplasmic sperm injection
ICT	indirect Coombs' test; insulin coma therapy
ict ind	icterus index
ICU	intensive care unit
I & D	incision and drainage
ID	infectious disease; intradermal
IDC	infiltrating ductal carcinoma; invasive ductal carcinoma
IDD	insulin-dependent diabetes
IDDM	insulin-dependent diabetes mellitus
IDK	internal derangement of the knee
IDS	immunity deficiency state
I/E	inspiratory-expiratory ratio
IEMG	integrated electromyogram
IF	interferon; interstitial fluid
IFG	impaired fasting glucose
Ig	immunoglobulin
IgA	immunoglobulin A
IgD	immunoglobulin D
IgE	immunoglobulin E
IgG	immunoglobulin G
IgM	immunoglobulin M
IGT	impaired glucose tolerance
IH	infectious hepatitis; inguinal hernia
IHD	ischemic heart disease
IL	interleukin
ILC	infiltrating lobar carcinoma; invasive lobular carcinoma
ILD	interstitial lung diseases
IM	infectious mononucleosis; intramuscular
IMAG	internal mammary artery graft
IMF	idiopathic myelofibrosis
IMI	immunofluorescence
IMV	intermittent mandatory ventilation
inf	inferior; infusion
Inflam, Inflamm	inflammation
I & O	intake and output
IO	intestinal obstruction; intraocular
IOD	iron-overload disease (hemochromatosis)
IOL	intraocular lens
IOP	intraocular pressure
IPF	idiopathic pulmonary fibrosis
IPG	impedance plethysmography
IPPB	intermittent positive-pressure breathing
IQ	intelligence quotient
irrig	irrigation
IS	impingement syndrome; intercostal space
ISG	immune serum globulin
isol	isolation
IT	immunotherapy
ITP	idiopathic thrombocytopenic purpura
IU	international unit
IUD	intrauterine device
IUP	intrauterine pressure
IV	intravenous; intravenously
IVC	inferior vena cava
IVCP	inferior vena cava pressure
IVD	intervertebral disk
IVDA	intravenous drug abuse
IVF	in vitro fertilization
IVFA	intravenous fluorescein angiography
IVP	intravenous pyelogram
IVSD	interventricular septal defect
IVU	intravenous urogram

J

j, jaund	jaundice
jct	junctions
JOD	juvenile-onset diabetes
JRA	juvenile rheumatoid arthritis
Jt	joint
JVP	jugular venous pressure; jugular venous pulse

K

K	potassium
KB	ketone bodies
KCF	key clinical findings
KCl	potassium chloride
KD	knee disarticulation
KE	kinetic energy
kg	kilogram
kj	knee jerk
KO	keep open
KOH	potassium hydrochloride
KS	Kaposi's sarcoma
KUB	kidneys, ureters, bladder
KVO	keep vein open

L

l	liter
L_1 through L_5	lumbar vertebrae
L & A	light and accommodation
LA	left atrium
lab	laboratory
lac	laceration
LAD	left anterior descending
LAP	laparoscopy; leucine aminopeptidase
lap	laparotomy
lar	larynx
laryn	laryngitis; laryngoscopy
laser	light amplification by stimulated emission of radiation
LASIK	laser in situ keratomileusis
lat	lateral
LAVH	laparoscopically assisted vaginal hysterectomy
LB	large bowel; low back
lb	pound
LBBB	left bundle branch block
LBBX	left breast biopsy and examination
LBP	low back pain
LBW	low birth weight
LCIS	lobular carcinoma in situ
L & D	labor and delivery
LDD	light-dark discrimination
LDL	low-density lipoproteins
LE	left eye; life expectancy; lower extremity; lupus erythematosus; lymphedema
LES	lower esophageal sphincter
lg	large
LH	luteinizing hormone

LHBD	left heart bypass device
LHF	left-sided heart failure
lig	ligament
liq	liquid
litho	lithotripsy
LLE	lower left extremity
LLL	left lower lobe
LLQ	left lower quadrant
LLSB	left lower sternal border
L/min	liters per minute
LMP	last menstrual period
LNMP	last normal menstrual period
LOC	level of consciousness; loss of consciousness
LOM	limitation of motion; loss of motion
LOS	length of stay
LP	light perception; lumbar puncture; lumboperitoneal
LPF	low-power field
LPS	lipase
LR	light reaction
LRDKT	living related donor kidney transplant
LRT	lower respiratory tract
LSB	left sternal border
lt	left
LTB	laryngotracheobronchitis
LTC	long-term care
LTH	lactogenic hormone; luteotropic hormone
LUE	left upper extremity
LUL	left upper lobe
LUQ	left upper quadrant
LV	left ventricle
LVH	left ventricle hypertrophy
lx	larynx
lymphs	lymphocytes

M

M	meter; murmur; myopia
MABS	monoclonal antibodies
MAO	maximal acid output; monoamine oxidase
MAR	multiple antibiotic resistant
MBC	maximal breathing capacity
MBD	minimal brain damage
mc	millicurie
mcg	microgram
MCH	mean corpuscular hemoglobin
MCHC	mean corpuscular hemoglobin concentration

MCT	mean circulation time
MCV	mean corpuscular volume
MD	macular degeneration; medical doctor; muscular dystrophy
MDS	myelodysplastic syndrome
MDR-TB	multidrug-resistant tuberculosis
MDS	myelodysplastic syndrome
ME	middle ear
MED	minimal effective dose; minimal erythema dose
men	menstruation
men, mgtis	meningitis
mEq	milliequivalent
MET	metastasis
met	metastasize
M & F	mother and father
MFT	muscle function test
mg	milligram
MG	myasthenia gravis
mgm	milligram
MH	malignant hyperpyrexia; malignant hyperthermia; marital history
MHC	mental health care
MI	mitral insufficiency; myocardial infarction
MICU	medical intensive care unit; mobile intensive care unit
MID	multi-infarct dementia
MIDCAB	minimally invasive direct coronary artery bypass
MIP	maximal inspiratory pressure
ml, mL	milliliter
MLD	median lethal dose
MM	multiple myeloma; malignant melanoma
mm	millimeter
mm Hg	millimeters of mercury
MND	motor neuron disease
MNT	medical nutrition therapy
MO	morbid obesity
MODY	maturity-onset diabetes of the young
MOM	milk of magnesia
mono	monocytes
MP	metacarpal-phalangeal
MPD	myofascial pain dysfunction
MR	mental retardation; metabolic rate; mitral regurgitation
MRA	magnetic resonance angiography
MRD	medical record department
MRI	magnetic resonance imaging
MS	mitral stenosis; multiple sclerosis; musculoskeletal

MSH	melanocyte-simulating hormone
MTD	right eardrum
MTS	left eardrum
MTX	methotrexate
MV	mitral valve
MVP	mitral valve prolapse
MY, Myop	myopia
myel	myelogram
myop	myopia

N

N & T	nose and throat
NA	not applicable; numerical aperture
Na	sodium
NaCl	sodium chloride
NAD	no acute disease; no apparent distress
NB	newborn
N/C	no complaints
NCV	nerve conduction velocity
NED	no evidence of disease
NEG, neg	negative
Neph	nephron
neuro	neurology
NF	National Formulary; necrotizing fasciitis; neurofibromatosis
N/G	nasogastric (tube)
ng	*Neisseria gonorrhoeae*
NGF	nerve growth factor
NGU	nongonococcal urethritis
NHL	non-Hodgkin's lymphoma
NI	nuclear imaging
NICU	neurologic intensive care unit
NIDDM	non-insulin-dependent diabetes mellitus
NK cell	natural killer cell
NKA	no known allergies
NLP	neurolinguistic programming
N & M	nerves and muscles; night and morning
NM	nuclear medicine
nm	neuromuscular
NMR	nuclear magnetic resonance
No	number
noc, noct	night
NOFTT	nonorganic failure to thrive
NP	nasopharynx
NPC	no point of convergence
NPO	nothing by mouth
NR	no response
NREM	no rapid eye movements

NS	nephrotic syndrome; normal saline; not stated; not sufficient
NSAID	nonsteroidal anti-inflammatory drug
NSR	normal sinus rhythm
nst	nystagmus
NSU	nonspecific urethritis
Nt	neutralization
NTD	neural tube defect
NTG	nitroglycerin
N & V	nausea and vomiting
NVA	near visual acuity
NVD	nausea, vomiting, and diarrhea; neck vein distention
NVS	neural vital signs
NYD	not yet diagnosed
ny, nst	nystagmus

O

OA	osteoarthritis
OAB	overactive bladder
OB	obstetrics
OB-GYN	obstetrics and gynecology
obl	oblique
OBS	organic brain syndrome
Obs	obstetrics
OC	office call; oral contraceptive
OCC	occasional
OCD	obsessive compulsive disorder; oral cholecystogram
OCT	oral contraceptive therapy
OD	overdose; right eye (oculus dexter)
od	once a day
OGN	obstetric-gynecologic-neonatal
OGTT	oral glucose tolerance test
oint	ointment
OJD	osteoarthritic joint disease
OM	otitis media
OME	otitis media with effusion
OMR	optic mark recognition
OOB	out of bed
O & P	ova and parasites
OP	oropharynx; osteoporosis; outpatient
OPA	oropharyngeal airway
OPD	outpatient department
OPG	oculoplethysmography
Ophth	ophthalmic
OPT	outpatient
OPV	oral poliovirus vaccine
OR	operating room

ORIF	open reduction internal fixation
ORT	oral rehydration therapy
Orth	orthopedics
OS	left eye (oculus sinister)
os	mouth
OSA	obstructive sleep apnea
OT	occupational therapy; old tuberculin
OTC	over-the-counter
Oto	otology
OU	each eye (oculus unitas)
OXT	oxytocin
oz	ounce

P

P	percussion; phosphorous; physiology; posterior; presbyopia; progesterone; prolactin; pulse
P & A	percussion and auscultation
PA	pernicious anemia; physician's assistant; polyarteritis; posteroanterior; pulmonary artery
PA, pa	pathology
PAC	premature atrial contraction
PACAB	port-access coronary artery bypass
PADP	pulmonary artery diastolic pressure
PAMP	pulmonary arterial mean pressure
Pap	Papanicolaou smear
PAR	perennial allergic rhinitis; postanesthetic recovery
PARA (P_1)	full-term infants delivered
paren	parenterally
PASP	pulmonary artery systolic pressure
PAT	paroxysmal atrial tachycardia
Path	pathology
Pb	presbyopia
PBC	primary biliary cirrhosis
PBI	protein-bound iodine
PBP	progressive bulbar palsy
PBT$_4$	protein-bound thyroxine
PC	pheochromocytoma; prostate cancer
p.c.	after meals
PCA	prostate cancer
PCKD	polycystic kidney disease
PCNL	percutaneous nephrolithotomy
PCO, PCOS	polycystic ovary syndrome
PCP	*Pneumocystis carinii* pneumonia
PCT	plasmacrit time
PCU	progressive care unit
PCV	packed cell volume

PD	interpupillary distance; Parkinson's disease; peritoneal dialysis; postural drainage
PDA	patent ductus arteriosus
PDD	pervasive developmental disorder
PDL	periodontal ligament
PE	physical examination; preeclampsia
PEA	pulseless electrical activity
Peds	pediatrics
PEEP	positive end-expiratory pressure
PEF	peak expiratory flow rate
PEG	pneumoencephalogram; pneumo-encephalography
PEL	permissible exposure limit
per	by; through
PERLA	pupils equally reactive (responsive) to light and accommodation
PERRLA	pupils equal, round, react (respond) to light and accommodation
PET	positron emission tomography; preeclamptic toxemia
PFT	pulmonary function test
PG	pregnant; prostaglandin
PGH	pituitary growth hormone
PGL	persistent generalized lymphadenopathy
PH	past history; personal history; public health
pH	acidity; hydrogen ion concentration
PHN	postherpetic neuralgia
PI	present illness
PICU	pulmonary intensive care unit
PID	pelvic inflammatory disease
PIF	peak inspiratory flow
PIH	pregnancy-induced hypertension
PK	pyruvate kinase; pyruvate kinase deficiency
PKD	polycystic kidney disease
PKR	partial knee replacement
PKU	phenylketonuria
PL	light perception
pl	placenta
PLC	platelet count
PLMS	periodic limb movements in sleep
PLS	primary lateral sclerosis
PLTS	platelets
PM	evening or afternoon; physical medicine; polymyositis; postmortem
PMA	progressive muscular atrophy
PMDD	premenstrual dysphoric disorder

PMH	past medical history
PMI	point of maximal impulse
PMN	polymorphonuclear neutrophils
PMP	past menstrual period; previous menstrual period
PMR	physical medicine and rehabilitation; polymyalgia rheumatica
PMS	premenstrual syndrome
PMT	premenstrual tension
PMVS	prolapsed mitral valve syndrome
PN	peripheral neuropathy; postnatal
PN, Pn, PNA, pneu, pneum	pneumonia
PND	paroxysmal nocturnal dyspnea; postnasal drip
PNH	prenatal headache
Pno	pneumothorax
PNP	peripheral neuropathy
PNS	parasympathetic nervous system; peripheral nervous system
PO, p.o.	by mouth; orally; phone order; post-operative
POC	products of conception
polys	polymorphonuclear leukocytes
POMR	problem-oriented medical record
POS	polycystic ovary syndrome
pos	positive
post-op	postoperatively
PP	placenta previa; postpartum; post-prandial (after meals); pulse pressure
ppb	parts per billion
PPBS	postprandial blood sugar
PPD	purified protein derivative
ppm	parts per million
PPS	postperfusion syndrome; postpolio syndrome; progressive systemic sclerosis
PPT	partial prothrombin time
PPV	positive-pressure ventilation
PR	peripheral resistance; pulse rate
Pr	presbyopia; prism
pr	by rectum
PRA	plasma renin activity
PRC	packed red cells
PRE	progressive restrictive exercise
preg	pregnant
preop	preoperative

prep	prepare
PRK	photo-refractive keratectomy
p.r.n.	as needed
proct	proctology
prog, **progn**	prognosis
PROM	passive range of motion; premature rupture of membranes
pro time	prothrombin time
PRRE	pupils round, regular, and equal
Prx	prognosis
PS, Ps	psoriasis
PSA	prostate-specific antigen
PSS	progressive systemic sclerosis; physiologic saline solution
psych	psychiatry
PT	paroxysmal tachycardia; physical therapy; prothrombin time
pt	patient; pint
PTA	percutaneous transluminal angioplasty
PTC	percutaneous transhepatic cholangiography
PTCA	percutaneous transluminal coronary angioplasty
PTD	permanent and total disability
PTE	parathyroid extract; pulmonary thromboembolism
PTH	parathyroid hormone; parathormone
PTSD	posttraumatic stress disorder
PTT	partial thromboplastin time; prothrombin time
PU	peptic ulcer; pregnancy urine; prostatic urethra
PUD	peptic ulcer disease; pulmonary disease
pul	pulmonary
P & V	pyloroplasty and vagotomy
PV	peripheral vascular; plasma volume; polycythemia vera
PVC	premature ventricular contraction
PVD	peripheral vascular disease
PVE	prosthetic valve endocarditis
PVOD	peripheral vascular occlusive disease
PVS	persistent vegetative state
PVT	paroxysmal ventricular tachycardia
pvt	private
PWB	partial weight-bearing
PWP	pulmonary wedge pressure
Px	prognosis

Q

q	every
qd, q.d.	every day
qh, q.h.	every hour
q 2 h	every 2 hours
QID, qid, **q.i.d.**	four times a day
qm	every morning
qn	every night
qns	quantity not sufficient
qod	every other day
qoh	every other hour
QOL	quality of life
q.q.	each
qs	quantity sufficient
qt	quart; quiet
quad	quadrant; quadriplegia; quadriplegic

R

R	rectal; respiration; right
RA	refractory anemia; rheumatoid arthritis; right arm; right atrium
rad	radiation absorbed dose
RAF	rheumatoid arthritis factor
RAI	radioactive iodine
RAIU	radioactive iodine uptake determination
RAS	reticular activating system
RAST	radioallergosorbent
RAT	radiation therapy
RBBB	right bundle branch block
RBC	red blood cell; red blood count
RBCV	red blood cell volume
RBE	relative biologic effects
RCA	right coronary artery
RD	respiratory distress; retinal detachment
RDA	recommended daily allowance
RDS	respiratory distress syndrome
RE	right eye
reg	regular
rehab	rehabilitation
rem	roentgen-equivalent-man
REM sleep	rapid eye movement sleep
RER	renal excretion rate
resp	respiration
RF	renal failure; respiratory failure; rheumatoid factor; rheumatic fever
RFS	renal function study
RH	right hand

RHD	rheumatic heart disease
Rh neg	Rhesus factor negative
Rh pos	Rhesus factor positive
RIA	radioimmunoassay
RICE	rest, ice, compression, elevate
Rick	rickettsia
RIST	radioimmunosorbent
RK	radial keratotomy
RL	right leg
RLC	residual lung capacity
RLD	related living donor
RLE	right lower extremity
RLL	right lower lobe
RLQ	right lower quadrant
RLS	restless legs syndrome
RM	respiratory movement
RMD	repetitive motion disorder
RML	right mediolateral
RMSF	Rocky Mountain spotted fever
RNA	ribonucleic acid
RND	radical neck dissection
R/O	rule out
ROA	radiopaque agents
ROM	range of motion; rupture of membranes
ROP	retinopathy of prematurity
ROPS	roll over protection structures
ROS	review of systems
ROT	right occipitis transverse
RP	radiopharmaceuticals; relapsing polychondritis; retrograde pyelogram
RPF	renal plasma flow
RPG	retrograde pyelogram
rpm	revolutions per minute
RPO	right posterior oblique
RPR	rapid plasma reagin
RQ	respiratory quotient
R & R	rate and rhythm
RR	recovery room; respiratory rate
RSD	repetitive stress disorder
RSDS	reflex sympathetic dystrophy syndrome
RSHF	right-sided heart failure
RSI	repetitive stress injuries
RSR	regular sinus rhythm
RSV	right subclavian vein
RT	radiation therapy; renal transplantation; respiratory therapy
rt	right; routine
RTA	renal tubular acidosis
rtd	retarded
rt lat	right lateral

RU	roentgen unit; routine urinalysis
RUE	right upper extremity
RUL	right upper lobe
RUQ	right upper quadrant
RV	residual volume; right ventricle
RVG	radionuclide ventriculogram
RVH	right ventricular hypertrophy
RVS	relative value schedule
RW	ragweed
Rx	prescription; take; therapy; treatment

S

s	without
S-A	sinoatrial node
S & A	sugar and acetone
SA	salicylic acid; sinoatrial; sperm analysis; surgeon's assistant
SAAT	serum aspartate aminotransferase
SAB	spontaneous abortion
SACH	self-assessed change in health
SAD	seasonal affective disorder
SAH	subarachnoid hemorrhage
SAL	sensorineural activity level; sterility assurance level; suction-assisted lipectomy
Sal, Salm	*Salmonella*
SALP	salpingectomy; salpingography; serum alkaline phosphatase
Salpx	salpingectomy
SAM	self-administered medication program
SARS	severe acute respiratory syndrome
SAS	short arm splint; sleep apnea syndrome; social adjustment scale; subarachnoid space
SB	small bowel; spina bifida; stillbirth; suction biopsy
SBE	subacute bacterial endocarditis
SBO	small bowel obstruction
SC, sc	subcutaneous
SC	Snellen chart; spinal cord
SCA	sickle cell anemia
SCC	squamous cell carcinoma
SCD	sudden cardiac death
schiz	schizophrenia
SCI	spinal cord injury
SCID	severe combined immune deficiency
SCT	sickle cell trait

SD	septal defect; shoulder disarticulation; spontaneous delivery; standard deviation; sudden death
SDAT	senile dementia of Alzheimer's type
SDM	standard deviation of the mean
SDS	sudden death syndrome
sec	second
SED	sub-erythema dose
sed rate	sedimentation rate
seg	segmented neutrophils
SEM	scanning electron microscopy
semi	half
SES	subcutaneous electric stimulation
sev	sever; severed
SF	scarlet fever; spinal fluid
SG	serum globulin; skin graft
SGA	small for gestational age
SH	serum hepatitis; sex hormone; social history
sh	shoulder
SI	saturation index
SICU	surgical intensive care unit
SIDS	sudden infant death syndrome
sig	let it be labeled
SIRS	systemic inflammatory response syndrome
SIS	saline infusion sonohysterography
SISI	short increment sensitivity index
SLE	St. Louis encephalitis; systemic lupus erythematosus
SLND	sentinel lymph node dissection
SLPS	serum lipase
SM	simple mastectomy
sm	small
SMA	sequential multiple analysis
SMAC	sequential multiple analysis computer
SMG	senile macular degeneration
SMR	submucous resection
SMRR	submucous resection and rhinoplasty
SNR	signal-to-noise ratio
SNRI	serotonin and norepinephrine reuptake inhibitor
SNS	sensory nervous system; sympathetic nervous system
SO	salpingo-oophorectomy
SOAP	symptoms, observations, assessments, plan; subjective, objective, assessment, plan
SOB	shortness of breath
SOM	serous otitis media
SONO	sonography
SOP	standard operating procedure

sos	if necessary
spec	specimen
SPECT	single photon emission computerized tomography
SPF	skin protective factor; sun protection factor
sp gr	specific gravity
SPP	suprapubic prostatectomy
SPR	scanned projection radiography
SQ	subcutaneous
SR	sedimentation rate; stimulus response; system review
SRS	smoker's respiratory syndrome
SS	signs and symptoms; Sjögren's syndrome; soap solution
ss	half
SSE	soap suds enema
SSRI	selective serotonin reuptake inhibitor
SSU	sterile supply unit
ST	esotropia; sclerotherapy
staph	staphylococcus
stat	immediately
STD	sexually transmitted disease; skin test dose
STH	somatotropic hormone
STK	streptokinase
strab	strabismus
strep	streptococcus
STS	serologic test for syphilis
STSG	split thickness skin graft
subcu, sub-Q	subcutaneous
SUI	stress urinary incontinence
supp	suppository
surg	surgical; surgery
SVC	superior vena cava
SVD	spontaneous vaginal delivery
SVG	saphenous vein graft
SVN	small volume nebulizer
SX	symptom reduction
Sx	symptoms
Sz	seizure

T

T	temperature; thrombosis
T$_1$ through T$_{12}$	thoracic vertebrae
T3	triiodothyronine
T4	thyroxine
T & A	tonsillectomy and adenoidectomy
TA, TAB	therapeutic abortion

tab	tablet
TACT	target air-enema computed tomography
TAF	tumor angiogenesis factor
TAH	total abdominal hysterectomy
TAH-BSO	total abdominal hysterectomy with bilateral salpingo-oophorectomy
TAO	thromboangiitis obliterans
TB	tuberculosis
TBD	total body density
TBF	total body fat
TBG	thyroxine-binding globulin
TBI	thyroxine-binding index
TBW	total body weight
TCD	transcranial doppler
TCDB	turn, cough, deep breathe
TCP	time care profile
TD	total disability; transdermal
TDM	therapeutic drug monitoring
TDT	tone decay test
TE	tetanus; tonsillectomy
TEE	transesophageal echocardiography
temp	temperature
TEN	toxic epidermal necrolysis
TENS	transcutaneous electrical nerve stimulation
TES	treadmill exercise score
TF	tactile fremitus
TFS	thyroid function studies
TGA	transposition of great arteries
THA	total hip arthroplasty
THR	total hip replacement
TIA	transient ischemic attack
TIA-IR	transient ischemic attack incomplete recovery
TIBC	total iron-binding capacity
TID, tid, t.i.d.	times interval difference; three times a day
tinct	tincture
TJA	total joint arthroplasty
TKA	total knee arthroplasty
TKO	to keep open
TKR	total knee replacement
TLC	tender loving care; total lung capacity
TLE	temporal lobe epilepsy
TM	temporomandibular; tympanic membrane
TMD	temporomandibular disease; temporo-mandibular disorder
TMJ	temporomandibular joint
TMs	tympanic membranes
Tn	normal intraocular tension
TND	term normal delivery
TNF	tumor necrosis factor
TNI	total nodal irradiation
TNM	tumor, nodes, metastases
TO	telephone order
top	topically
TP	testosterone propionate; total protein
TPA, tPA	tissue plasminogen activator; *Treponema pallidum* agglutination
TPBF	total pulmonary blood flow
TPI	*Treponema pallidum* immobilization
TPN	total parenteral nutrition
TPR	temperature, pulse, respiration
TPUR	transperineal urethral resection
TR	tuberculin residue
tr	tincture
trach	trachea; tracheostomy
TRBF	total renal blood flow
TRH	thyrotropin-releasing hormone
Trich	trichomonas
TS	Tourette syndrome
TSD	Tay-Sachs disease
TSE	testicular self-examination
TSH	thyroid-stimulating hormone
TSP	total serum protein
TSS	toxic shock syndrome
TST	thallium stress test; tuberculin skin test
TT	thrombin time
TTH	thyrotropic hormone
TULIP	transurethral ultrasound-guided laser-induced proctectomy
TUMT	transurethral microwave therapy
TUR	transurethral resection
TURP	transurethral resection of prostate; prostatectomy
TV	tidal volume; tricuspid valve
TVH	total vaginal hysterectomy
TW	tap water
TWE	tap water enema
Tx	traction; treatment

U

U	units
U/A, UA	urinalysis
UB	urinary bladder
UC	ulcerative colitis; urine culture; uterine contractions
UCD	usual childhood diseases
UCG	urinary chorionic gonadotropin; uterine chorionic gonadotropin
UCR	unconditioned reflex
UE	upper extremity

UFR	uroflowmeter; uroflowmetry
UG	upper gastrointestinal; urogenital
UGI	upper gastrointestinal
UK	unknown
UL	upper lobe
ULQ	upper left quadrant
umb	umbilical; umbilicus
UN	urea nitrogen
ung	ointment
UOQ	upper outer quadrant
UPP	urethral pressure profile
UR	upper respiratory
ur	urine
URD	upper respiratory disease
URI	upper respiratory infection
urol	urology
URQ	upper right quadrant
URT	upper respiratory tract
US	ultrasonic; ultrasonography
USP	United States Pharmacopeia
UTI	urinary tract infection
UV	ultraviolet
UVJ	ureterovesical junction

V

V	ventral; visual acuity
VA	vacuum aspiration; visual acuity
vag	vaginal
VAS	vasectomy
VB	viable birth
VBAC	vaginal birth after cesarean
VBP	ventricular premature beat
VC	acuity of color vision; vena cava; vital capacity
VCUG	voiding cystourethrogram
VD	venereal disease
VDG	venereal disease, gonorrhea
VDH	valvular disease of heart
VDRL	Venereal Disease Research Laboratory
VDS	venereal disease, syphilis
VE	visual efficiency
vent, ventr	ventral
VEP	visual evoked potential
VER	visual evoked response
VF	ventricular fibrillation; visual field; vocal fremitus
V fib	ventricular fibrillation
VG	ventricular gallop
VH	vaginal hysterectomy

VHD	valvular heart disease; ventricular heart disease
VI	volume index
vit cap	vital capacity
VLDL	very-low-density lipoprotein
VP	venipuncture; venous pressure
VPC	ventricular premature contraction
VPRC	volume of packed red cells
VS, vs	vital signs
VSD	ventricular septal defect
VTAs	vascular targeting agents
VV	varicose veins
VVF	vesicovaginal fistula
VZV	varicella-zoster virus (chickenpox)

W

W	water
WA	while awake
WB	weight-bearing; whole blood
WBC	white blood cell; white blood count
W/C, w/c	wheelchair
WD, w/d	well-developed
wd	wound
WDWN	well-developed, well-nourished
wf	white female
w/n	well nourished
WNL	within normal limits
w/o	without
WR, W.r.	Wassermann reaction
wt	weight
w/v	weight by volume

X

X	xerophthalmia
x	multiplied by; times
XDP	xeroderma pigmentosum
XM	cross-match
XR	x-ray
XT	exotropia
XU	excretory urogram

Y

y/o	year(s) old
YOB	year of birth
yr	year

Z

Z	atomic number; no effect; zero
zyg	zygote

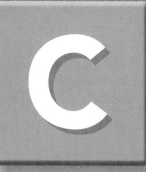

Appendix C
Glossary of Pathology and Procedures

A

abdominocentesis (ab-**dom**-ih-noh-sen-**TEE**-sis): The surgical puncture of the abdominal cavity to remove fluid.

ablation (ab-**LAY**-shun): The removal of a body part or the destruction of its function.

abortion (ah-**BOR**-shun): The interruption or termination of pregnancy before the fetus is viable.

abrasion (ah-**BRAY**-zhun): An injury in which superficial layers of skin are scraped or rubbed away.

abruptio placentae (ab-**RUP**-shee-oh plah-**SEN**-tee): An abnormal condition in which the placenta separates from the uterine wall prematurely before the birth of the fetus.

abscess (**AB**-sess): A closed pocket containing pus caused by a purulent bacterial infection.

ACE inhibitors: Medications administered to treat hypertension and congestive heart failure.

acetaminophen (ah-**seet**-ah-**MIN**-oh-fen): Medication that controls pain without the side effects of NSAIDs.

Achilles tendinitis (**ten**-dih-**NIGH**-tis): Inflammation of the Achilles tendon caused by excessive stress.

acid blockers: Medications taken before eating to block the effects of histamine that signals the stomach to produce acid.

acne vulgaris (**ACK**-nee vul-**GAY**-ris): A chronic inflammatory disease that is caused by an over-production of sebum and is characterized by pustular eruptions of the skin.

acquired immunodeficiency syndrome: The advanced stage of an HIV infection; also known as AIDS.

acromegaly (**ack**-roh-**MEG**-ah-lee): Enlargement of the extremities caused by excessive secretion of growth hormone *after* puberty.

acrophobia (**ack**-roh-**FOH**-bee-ah): An excessive fear of being in high places.

actinic keratosis (ack-**TIN**-ick **kerr**-ah-**TOH**-sis): A skin lesion caused by excessive exposure to the sun.

acute nasopharyngitis (**nay**-zoh-**far**-in-**JIGH**-tis): A term used to describe the common cold; also known as an upper respiratory infection.

acute necrotizing ulcerative gingivitis: An abnormal growth of bacteria in the mouth that usually occurs in teens or young adults; also known as trench mouth.

acute renal failure: Sudden onset of kidney failure that may be caused by many factors including a drop in blood volume or blood pressure due to injury or surgery.

acute respiratory distress syndrome: The sudden onset of severe lung dysfunction that affects both lungs and makes breathing extremely difficult.

addiction: Compulsive, uncontrollable dependence on a substance, habit, or practice to the degree that stopping causes severe emotional, mental, or physiologic reactions.

Addison's disease (**AD**-ih-sonz): A condition that occurs when the adrenal glands do not produce enough cortisol or aldosterone.

adenectomy (**ad**-eh-**NECK**-toh-mee): Surgical removal of a gland.

adenitis (**ad**-eh-**NIGH**-tis): Inflammation of a gland.

adenocarcinoma (**ad**-eh-noh-**kar**-sih-**NOH**-mah): Carcinoma derived from glandular tissue.

adenoidectomy (**ad**-eh-noid-**ECK**-toh-mee *or* **ad**-eh-noy-**DECK**-toh-mee): Surgical removal of the adenoids.

adenoma (**ad**-eh-**NOH**-mah): A benign tumor of glandular origin.

adenomalacia (**ad**-eh-noh-mah-**LAY**-shee-ah): Abnormal softening of a gland.

adenosclerosis (**ad**-eh-noh-skleh-**ROH**-sis): Abnormal hardening of a gland.

adenosis (**ad**-eh-**NOH**-sis): Any disease condition of a gland.

adhesion (ad-**HEE**-zhun): A band of fibrous tissue that holds structures together abnormally and can form in muscles or internal organs as the result of an injury or surgery.

adrenalitis (ah-**dree**-nal-**EYE**-tis): Inflammation of the adrenal glands; also known as adrenitis.

adrenitis (**ad**-reh-**NIGH**-tis): Inflammation of the adrenal glands; also known as adrenalitis.

adrenomegaly (ah-**dree**-noh-**MEG**-ah-lee): Enlargement of the adrenal glands.

adrenopathy (**ad**-ren-**OP**-ah-thee): Any disease of the adrenal glands.

adverse drug reaction: An undesirable drug response that accompanies the principal response for which the drug was taken; also known as a side effect or an adverse drug event.

aerophagia (**ay**-er-oh-**FAY**-jee-ah): Excessive swallowing of air while eating or drinking.

agglutination tests (ah-**gloo**-tih-**NAY**-shun): Blood tests performed to determine the patient's blood type and to check compatibility of donor and recipient blood before a transfusion.

agoraphobia (**ag**-oh-rah-**FOH**-bee-ah): An excessive fear of situations in which having a panic attack seems likely.

AIDS dementia complex: A degenerative neurological condition that is a central nervous system complication of an HIV infection.

albinism (**AL**-bih-niz-um): An inherited deficiency or absence of pigment in the skin, hair, and irises due to a missing enzyme necessary for the production of melanin.

albuminuria (**al**-byou-mih-**NEW**-ree-ah): The presence of the protein albumin in the urine that is a sign of impaired kidney function.

alcoholism (**AL**-koh-hol-izm): Chronic alcohol dependence with specific signs and symptoms upon withdrawal.

aldosteronism (al-**DOSS**-teh-roh-**niz**-em *or* **al**-doh-**STER**-ohn-izm): An abnormality of electrolyte balance caused by excessive secretion of aldosterone.

aldosteronism, primary: An abnormality of electrolyte balance caused by disorders of the adrenal glands; also known as Conn's syndrome.

aldosteronism, secondary: An abnormality of electrolyte balance that is not caused by a disorder of the adrenal gland.

allergen (**AL**-er-jen): An antigen capable of inducing an allergic response.

allergic rhinitis (rye-**NIGH**-tis): An allergic reaction to airborne allergens.

allergy: An overreaction by the body to a particular antigen; also known as hypersensitivity.

allogenic bone marrow transplant (**al**-oh-**JEN**-ick): A transplant in which the recipient receives bone marrow from a donor.

alopecia (**al**-oh-**PEE**-shee-ah): The partial, or complete, loss of hair most commonly on the scalp; also known as baldness.

Alzheimer's disease (**ALTZ**-high-merz): Disorders associated with degenerative changes in the brain structure that lead to progressive memory loss, impaired cognition, and personality changes.

amblyopia (**am**-blee-**OH**-pee-ah): Dimness of vision or the partial loss of sight, especially in one eye, without detectable disease of the eye.

amebic dysentery (ah-**MEE**-bik **DIS**-en-**ter**-ee): Frequent, watery stools often with blood and mucus caused by the parasite *Entamoeba histolytica*.

amenorrhea (ah-**men**-oh-**REE**-ah *or* ay-**men**-oh-**REE**-ah): The absence of menstrual periods for three months or more.

ametropia (**am**-eh-**TROH**-pee-ah): Any error of refraction in which images do not focus properly on the retina.

amnesia (am-**NEE**-zee-ah): A disturbance in the memory marked by a total or partial inability to recall past experiences.

amniocentesis (**am**-nee-oh-sen-**TEE**-sis): A surgical puncture to remove amniotic fluid to evaluate fetal health and to diagnose certain congenital disorders.

amobarbital (**am**-oh-**BAR**-bih-tal): A barbiturate medication that is administered as a sedative and hypnotic.

amyotrophic lateral sclerosis (ah-**my**-oh-**TROH**-fick): A degenerative disease in which patients become progressively weaker until they are completely paralyzed; also known as Lou Gehrig's disease.

anal fissure: A small tear in the skin of the anus that can cause severe pain during a bowel movement.

analgesic (**an**-al-**JEE**-zick): A medication that relieves pain without affecting consciousness.

anaphylaxis (**an**-ah-fih-**LACK**-sis): A severe response to a foreign substance such as a drug, food, insect venom, or chemical.

anaplasia (**an**-ah-**PLAY**-zee-ah): A change in the structure of cells and in their orientation to each other.

anastomosis (ah-**nas**-toh-**MOH**-sis): A surgical connection between two hollow or tubular structures (plural, anastomoses).

anemia (ah-**NEE**-mee-ah): A disorder characterized by lower than normal levels of red blood cells in the blood.

anesthesia (**an**-es-**THEE**-zee-ah): The absence of normal sensation, especially sensitivity to pain.

anesthetic (**an**-es-**THET**-ick): Medication used to induce anesthesia.

aneurysm (**AN**-you-rizm): A localized weak spot or balloon-like enlargement of the wall of an artery.

aneurysmectomy (**an**-you-riz-**MECK**-toh-mee): The surgical removal of an aneurysm.

aneurysmorrhaphy (**an**-you-riz-**MOR**-ah-fee): Surgical suturing of an aneurysm.

angiectomy (**an**-jee-**ECK**-toh-mee): Surgical removal of a blood vessel.

angiitis (**an**-jee-**EYE**-tis): Inflammation of a blood or lymph vessel; also known as vasculitis (alternative spelling, *angitis*).

angina pectoris (an-**JIGH**-nah *or* **AN**-jih-nuh **PECK**-toh-riss): Episodes of severe chest pain due to inadequate blood flow to the myocardium; also known as angina.

angiogenesis (**an**-jee-oh-**JEN**-eh-sis): The process through which the tumor supports its growth by creating its own blood supply.

angiogram (**AN**-jee-oh-**gram**): The film produced by angiography.

angiography (**an**-jee-**OG**-rah-fee): A radiographic study of the blood vessels after the injection of a contrast medium.

angionecrosis (**an**-jee-oh-neh-**KROH**-sis): Death of the walls of blood vessels.

angiorrhaphy (**an**-jee-**OR**-ah-fee): Surgical suturing of any vessel, especially of a blood vessel.

angiosclerosis (**an**-jee-oh-skleh-**ROH**-sis): Abnormal hardening of the walls of blood vessels.

angiospasm (**AN**-jee-oh-**spazm**): A spasmodic contraction of the blood vessels.

angiostenosis (**an**-jee-oh-steh-**NOH**-sis): Abnormal narrowing of a blood vessel.

anhidrosis (**an**-high-**DROH**-sis): The abnormal condition of lacking sweat in response to heat.

anisocoria (**an**-ih-so-**KOH**-ree-ah): A condition in which the pupils are unequal in size.

ankylosing spondylitis (**ang**-kih-**LOH**-sing **spon**-dih-**LYE**-tis): A form of rheumatoid arthritis characterized by the progressive fusion of the vertebral bodies.

ankylosis (**ang**-kih-**LOH**-sis): The loss or absence of mobility in a joint due to disease, injury, or a surgical procedure.

anomaly (ah-**NOM**-ah-lee): A deviation from what is regarded as normal.

anorchism (an-**OR**-kizm): The congenital absence of one or both testicles.

anorexia (**an**-oh-**RECK**-see-ah): The loss of appetite for food, especially when caused by disease.

anorexia nervosa (**an**-oh-**RECK**-see-ah): An eating disorder characterized by a false perception of body appearance that leads to a refusal to maintain a normal body weight.

anoscopy (ah-**NOS**-koh-pee): The visual examination of the anal canal and lower rectum using a short speculum called an anoscope.

anovulation (**an**-ov-you-**LAY**-shun): The failure to ovulate.

anoxia (ah-**NOCK**-see-ah): The absence of oxygen from the blood gases or tissues.

antacids: Medications to relieve indigestion or help peptic ulcers heal by neutralizing stomach acids.

anthracosis (**an**-thrah-**KOH**-sis): The form of pneumoconiosis caused by coal dust in the lungs; also known as black lung disease.

antiangiogenesis: Cancer treatment that disrupts the blood supply to the tumor.

antiarrhythmic (**an**-tih-ah-**RITH**-mick): Medication administered to control irregularities of the heartbeat.

antibiotics: Chemical substances capable of inhibiting growth or killing pathogenic microorganisms that are used to combat bacterial infections.

anticholinergic (**an**-tih-**koh**-lin-**ER**-jik): Medication administered to control spasmodic activity of smooth muscles, such as those of the intestine; also known as an antispasmodic.

anticoagulant (**an**-tih-koh-**AG**-you-lant): Medication that slows coagulation and prevents new clots from forming; also known as a thrombolytic or clot-busting drug.

anticonvulsant (**an**-tih-kon-**VUL**-sant): Medication that prevents seizures and convulsions.

antidepressant: Medications administered to prevent or relieve depression.

antiemetic (**an**-tih-ee-**MET**-ick): Medication administered to prevent or relieve nausea.

antihistamines: Medications administered to block and control allergic reactions.

antihypertensive (**an**-tih-**high**-per-**TEN**-siv): Medication administered to lower blood pressure.

anti-inflammatory: Medication administered to relieve inflammation and pain.

antineoplastic (**an**-tih-nee-oh-**PLAS**-tick): Medication administered to block the development, growth, or proliferation of malignant cells.

antipsychotic (**an**-tih-sigh-**KOT**-ick): Medications administered to treat symptoms of severe disorders of thinking and mood.

antipyretic (**an**-tih-pye-**RET**-ick): Medication administered to reduce fever.

antispasmodic: Medication administered to control spasmodic activity of smooth muscles, such as those of the intestine; also known as an anticholinergic drug.

antitussive (**an**-tih-**TUSS**-iv): Medication administered to prevent or relieve coughing.

antiviral drug (**an**-tih-**VYE**-ral): Medication administered to treat viral infections or to provide temporary immunity.

anuria (ah-**NEW**-ree-ah): The absence of urine formation by the kidneys.

anxiety disorders: Mental conditions characterized by anxiety or fear out of proportion to the real danger in a situation.

anxiolytic (**ang**-zee-oh-**LIT**-ick): Medication administered to temporarily suppress anxiety; also known as antianxiety drugs or tranquilizers.

Apgar score: An evaluation of a newborn infant's physical status by assigning numerical values to five criteria.

aphasia (ah-**FAY**-zee-ah): Loss of the ability to speak, write, and/or comprehend the written or spoken word.

aphonia (ah-**FOH**-nee-ah): The loss of the ability of the larynx to produce normal speech sounds.

aphthous ulcers (**AF**-thus): Grey-white pits with a red border in the soft tissues lining the mouth; also known as canker sores or mouth ulcers.

aplasia (ah-**PLAY**-zee-ah): The defective development or congenital absence of an organ or tissue.

aplastic anemia (ay-**PLAS**-tick ah-**NEE**-mee-ah): A condition marked by the absence of all formed blood elements.

apnea (**AP**-nee-ah *or* ap-**NEE**-ah): The absence of spontaneous respiration.

appendectomy (**ap**-en-**DECK**-toh-mee): Surgical removal of the appendix.

appendicitis (ah-**pen**-dih-**SIGH**-tis): Inflammation of the appendix.

arrhythmia (ah-**RITH**-mee-ah): A change in the rhythm of the heartbeat; also known as cardiac arrhythmia or dysrhythmia.

arteriectomy (**ar**-teh-ree-**ECK**-toh-mee): Surgical removal of part of an artery.

arteriomalacia (ar-**tee**-ree-oh-mah-**LAY**-shee-ah): Abnormal softening of the walls of an artery or arteries.

arterionecrosis (ar-**tee**-ree-oh-neh-**KROH**-sis): Tissue death of an artery or arteries.

arterioplasty (ar-**tee**-ree-oh-**PLAS**-tee): The surgical repair of an artery.

arteriosclerosis (ar-**tee**-ree-oh-skleh-**ROH**-sis): Abnormal hardening of the walls of an artery or arteries.

arteriostenosis (ar-**tee**-ree-oh-steh-**NOH**-sis): Abnormal narrowing of an artery or arteries.

arteritis (**ar**-teh-**RYE**-tis): Inflammation of an artery or arteries.

arthralgia (ar-**THRAL**-jee-ah): Pain in a joint or joints.

arthrectomy (ar-**THRECK**-toh-mee): The surgical removal of a joint.

arthritis (ar-**THRIGH**-tis): An inflammatory condition of one or more joints (plural, arthritides).

arthrocentesis (**ar**-throh-sen-**TEE**-sis): Surgical puncture of the joint space to remove synovial fluid for analysis.

arthrodesis (**ar**-throh-**DEE**-sis): A surgical procedure to stiffen a joint; also known as fusion or surgical ankylosis.

arthrolysis (ar-**THROL**-ih-sis): Surgical loosening of an ankylosed joint.

arthroplasty (**AR**-throh-**plas**-tee): Surgical repair of a damaged joint; also the surgical replacement of a joint with an artificial joint.

arthrosclerosis (**ar**-throh-skleh-**ROH**-sis): Stiffness of the joints, especially in the elderly.

arthroscopic surgery (**ar**-throh-**SKOP**-ick): A minimally invasive procedure for the treatment of the interior of a joint.

arthroscopy (ar-**THROS**-koh-pee): Visual examination and treatment of the internal structure of a joint using an arthroscope.

arthrotomy (ar-**THROT**-oh-mee): A surgical incision into a joint.

asbestosis (**ass**-beh-**STOH**-sis): The form of pneumoconiosis caused by asbestos particles in the lungs.

ascites (ah-**SIGH**-teez): An abnormal accumulation of serous fluid in the peritoneal cavity.

aspergillosis (**ass**-per-jil-**OH**-sis): An infection caused by the fungus of the genus *Aspergillus*.

asphyxia (ass-**FICK**-see-ah): The condition that occurs when the body cannot get the air it needs to function.

asphyxiation (ass-**fick**-see-**AY**-shun): Any interruption of breathing resulting in asphyxia; also known as suffocation.

aspiration pneumonia (**ass**-pih-**RAY**-shun): Pneumonia caused by a foreign substance, such as vomit, being inhaled into the lungs.

asthma (**AZ**-mah): A chronic allergic disorder characterized by episodes of severe breathing difficulty, coughing, and wheezing.

astigmatism (ah-**STIG**-mah-tizm): A condition in which the eye does not focus properly because of uneven curvatures of the cornea.

ataxia (ah-**TACK**-see-ah): The inability to coordinate muscle activity during voluntary movement.

atelectasis (at-ee-**LEK**-tah-sis): A condition in which the lung fails to expand completely due to shallow breathing or because the air passages are blocked.

atherectomy (**ath**-er-**ECK**-toh-mee): Surgical removal of plaque from the interior lining of an artery.

atheroma (**ath**-er-**OH**-mah): A deposit of fatty plaque within the arterial wall that is characteristic of atherosclerosis.

atherosclerosis (**ath**-er-oh-skleh-**ROH**-sis): Hardening and narrowing of the arteries due to a buildup of cholesterol plaques.

atonic (ah-**TON**-ick): Lacking normal muscle tone or strength.

atrial fibrillation: Rapid irregular twitching of the muscular wall of the atria; also known as a fib.

atrophy (**AT**-roh-fee): Weakness or wearing away of body tissues and structures caused by pathology or by disuse over a long period of time.

atropine (**AT**-roh-peen): An antispasmodic medication that may be administered preoperatively to relax smooth muscles.

attention deficit disorder: A condition characterized by a short attention span and impulsive behavior inappropriate for the child's developmental age.

audiometry (**aw**-dee-**OM**-eh-tree): The use of an audiometer to measure hearing acuity.

auscultation (**aws**-kul-**TAY**-shun): Listening through a stethoscope for respiratory, heart, and abdominal sounds within the body.

autism (**AW**-tizm): A condition in which a young child cannot develop normal social relationships, compulsively follows repetitive routines, and frequently has poor communication skills; also known as autistic disorder.

autoimmune disorder (**aw**-toh-ih-**MYOUN**): A condition in which the immune system reacts incorrectly to normal antigens and creates antibodies against the body's own tissues.

autologous bone marrow transplant (aw-**TOL**-uh-guss): A transplant utilizing the patient's own bone marrow that was harvested before treatment began.

automated external defibrillator (dee-**fib**-rih-**LAY**-ter): Electronic equipment that externally shocks the heart to restore a normal cardiac rhythm.

azoospermia (ay-**zoh**-oh-**SPER**-mee-ah): The absence of sperm in the semen.

B

bacterial endocarditis: Inflammation of the lining or valves of the heart caused by bacteria in the bloodstream.

bacterial pneumonia: Pneumonia caused by *Streptococcus pneumoniae*.

bacterial vaginosis (**vaj**-ih-**NOH**-sis): A sexually transmitted bacterial infection of the vagina.

bacteriuria (back-**tee**-ree-**YOU**-ree-ah): The presence of bacteria in the urine.

balanitis (**bal**-ah-**NIGH**-tis): Inflammation of the glans penis and the foreskin often associated with phimosis.

balloon angioplasty (**AN**-jee-oh-**plas**-tee): A treatment procedure to open a partially blocked coronary artery by flattening the plaque deposit and stretching the lumen; also called percutaneous transluminal coronary angioplasty.

barbiturates (bar-**BIT**-you-raytz): A class of drugs whose major action is a calming or depressed effect on the central nervous system.

barium: A radiopaque contrast medium used primarily to visualize the gastrointestinal tract.

barotrauma (**bar**-oh-**TRAW**-mah): Pressure-related ear discomfort often cause by changes in pressure when the eustachian tube is blocked.

basal cell carcinoma: A malignant tumor of the basal cell layer of the epidermis.

Becker's muscular dystrophy (**BECK**-urz): A form of muscular dystrophy that does not appear until early adolescence or adulthood.

behavioral therapy: Treatment of mental disorders that focuses on changing behavior by identifying problem behaviors, replacing them with appropriate behaviors, and using rewards or other consequences to make the changes.

Bell's palsy: Temporary paralysis of the seventh cranial nerve that causes drooping only on the affected side of the face.

benign: Something that is not life-threatening and does not recur.

benign prostatic hypertrophy (high-**PER**-troh-fee): Abnormal enlargement of the prostate gland often found in men over 50; also known as prostatomegaly.

beta-blockers: Medications administered to reduce blood pressure by slowing the heartbeat.

bilateral hysterosalpingo-oophorectomy (**hiss**-ter-oh-sal-**ping**-goh oh-**ahf**-oh-**RECK**-toh-mee): Surgical removal of the uterus and cervix, plus both fallopian tubes and both ovaries.

biopsy (**BYE**-op-see): The removal of a small piece of living tissue for examination to confirm or establish a diagnosis.

bipolar disorders: Mental conditions that are characterized by the occurrence of manic or hypomanic episodes sometimes alternating with depressive episodes.

bitewing radiographs: Dental x-rays that show the crowns of teeth in both arches.

blepharedema (**blef**-ahr-eh-**DEE**-mah): Swelling of the eyelid.

blepharitis (**blef**-ah-**RYE**-tis): Inflammation of the eyelid.

blepharoplasty (**BLEF**-ah-roh-**plas**-tee): Surgical reduction of the upper and lower eyelids; also known as a lid lift.

blepharoptosis (**blef**-ah-roh-**TOH**-sis *or* **blef**-ah-rop-**TOH**-sis): Drooping of the upper eyelid usually due to paralysis.

blindness: The inability to see.

blood urea nitrogen (you-**REE**-ah): A blood test performed to determine the amount of urea present in the blood.

bolus infusion (**BOH**-lus): A single dose of a drug usually injected into a blood vessel over a short period of time.

bone density testing: A diagnostic test to determine losses or changes in bone density.

bone marrow biopsy: A diagnostic test to determine why blood cells are abnormal or to find a donor match for a bone marrow transplant.

bone marrow transplant: Cancer treatment in which abnormal bone marrow is destroyed and replaced with new stem cells; also known a a stem cell transplant.

bone scan: A specialized nuclear scan to detect pathology in the bones.

Botox: A formulation of botulinum toxin type A that is administered by injection to temporarily improve the appearance of moderate to severe frown lines between the eyebrows.

botulism (**BOT**-you-lizm): Food poisoning characterized by paralysis, and often death, that is caused by the bacterium *Clostridium botulinum*.

bowel incontinence (in-**KON**-tih-nents): The inability to control the excretion of feces.

brachytherapy (**brack**-ee-**THER**-ah-pee): The use of radioactive materials in contact with, or implanted into, the tissues to be treated.

bradycardia (brad-ee-**KAR**-dee-ah): An abnormally slow heartbeat, usually at a rate of less than 60 beats per minute.

bradykinesia (**brad**-ee-kih-**NEE**-zee-ah *or* **brad**-ee-kih-**NEE**-zhuh): Extreme slowness in movement.

bradypnea (**brad**-ihp-**NEE**-ah *or* **brad**-ee-**NEE**-ah): An abnormally slow rate of respiration, usually of less than 10 breaths per minute.

brain tumor: An abnormal growth within the brain that may be either benign or malignant.

brand name: Medication sold under the name given the drug by the manufacturer.

Braxton Hicks contractions: Intermittent painless uterine contractions that are not true labor pains.

breast augmentation: Mammoplasty performed to increase breast size.

breast reduction: Mammoplasty performed to decrease and reshape excessively large, heavy breasts.

breast self-examination: A self-care procedure for the early detection of breast cancer.

breech presentation: A birth complication in which the buttocks or feet of the fetus are presented first instead of the head.

bronchiectasis (**brong**-kee-**ECK**-tah-sis): Chronic, irreversible enlargement of bronchi or bronchioles.

bronchitis (brong-**KYE**-tis): Inflammation of the bronchial walls.

bronchodilator (**brong**-koh-dye-**LAY**-tor): An agent that expands the opening of the passages into the lungs.

bronchoplasty (**BRONG**-koh-**plas**-tee): Surgical repair of a bronchial defect.

bronchoplegia (**brong**-koh-**PLEE**-jee-ah): Paralysis of the walls of the bronchi.

bronchopneumonia (**brong**-koh-new-**MOH**-nee-ah): The form of pneumonia that affects patches of the bronchioles throughout both lungs.

bronchorrhea (**brong**-koh-**REE**-ah): An excessive discharge of mucus from the bronchi.

bronchoscopy (brong-**KOS**-koh-pee): The visual examination of the bronchi using a bronchoscope.

bruit (**BREW**-ee): An abnormal intermittent musical sound heard in auscultation of a vein or artery.

bruxism (**BRUCK**-sizm): Involuntary grinding or clenching of the teeth that usually occurs during sleep.

bulimia nervosa (byou-**LIM**-ee-ah *or* boo-**LEE**-mee-ah): An eating disorder characterized by episodes of binge eating followed by compensatory behaviors, such as self-induced vomiting.

bulla (**BULL**-ah): A large blister that is usually *more than* 0.5 cm in diameter (plural, bullae).

burn: An injury to body tissues caused by heat, flame, electricity, sun, chemicals, or radiation.

burn, first-degree: A burn in which there are no blisters and only slight damage to the epidermis; also known as a superficial burn.

burn, second-degree: A burn in which there are blisters and damage to both the epidermis and the dermis; also known as a partial-thickness burn.

burn, third-degree: A burn in which there is damage to the epidermis, dermis, subcutaneous layers, and possibly also the muscle below; also known as a full-thickness burn.

bursectomy (ber-**SECK**-toh-mee): The surgical removal of a bursa.

bursitis (ber-**SIGH**-tis): Inflammation of a bursa.

byssinosis (**biss**-ih-**NOH**-sis): The form of pneumoconiosis caused by inhaling cotton dust into the lungs; also known as brown lung disease.

C

calcium channel blockers: Medications administered to treat hypertension, angina, and arrhythmia by reducing the contraction of the muscles that squeeze blood vessels tight.

calciuria (**kal**-sih-**YOU**-ree-ah): The abnormal presence of calcium in the urine.

calculus (**KAL**-kyou-luhs): An abnormal mineral deposit; also known as a stone (plural, calculi); also the hardened deposit that forms on the teeth.

callus (**KAL**-us): A bulging deposit that forms around the area of the break in a bone; also a thickening the skin that is caused by repeated rubbing.

carbuncle (**KAR**-bung-kul): A cluster of connected furuncles (boils).

carcinoma (**kar**-sih-**NOH**-mah): A malignant tumor that occurs in epithelial tissue.

carcinoma in situ: A malignant tumor in its original position that has not yet disturbed or invaded the surrounding tissues.

cardiac arrhythmia (ah-**RITH**-mee-ah): A change in the rhythm of the heartbeat; also known as cardiac arrhythmia or dysrhythmia.

cardiac catheterization (**KAR**-dee-ack **kath**-eh-ter-eye-**ZAY**-shun): A diagnostic procedure in which a catheter is passed into a vein or artery and guided into the heart.

cardiocentesis (**kar**-dee-oh-sen-**TEE**-sis): The puncture of a chamber of the heart for diagnosis or therapy; also known as cardiopuncture.

cardiomegaly (**kar**-dee-oh-**MEG**-ah-lee): Abnormal enlargement of the heart.

cardioplegia (**kar**-dee-oh-**PLEE**-jee-ah): Paralysis of the muscles of the heart.

cardiopulmonary resuscitation: An emergency procedure for life support consisting of artificial respiration and manual external cardiac compression; also known as CPR.

cardiorrhaphy (**kar**-dee-**OR**-ah-fee): Surgical suturing of the wall of the heart.

cardiorrhexis (**kar**-dee-oh-**RECK**-sis): Rupture of the heart.

cardiotomy (**kar**-dee-**OT**-oh-mee): A surgical incision into the heart.

cardioversion (**kar**-dee-oh-**VER**-zhun): The use of electrical shock to restore the heart's normal rhythm; also known as defibrillation.

carditis (kar-**DYE**-tis): An inflammation of the heart.

carotid endarterectomy (**end**-ar-ter-**ECK**-toh-mee): Surgical removal of the lining of a portion of a clogged carotid artery.

carotid ultrasonography: An ultrasound study of the carotid artery that is performed to predict or diagnose an ischemic stroke.

carpal tunnel release: The surgical enlargement of the carpal tunnel, or cutting of the carpal ligament, to relieve nerve pressure.

carpal tunnel syndrome: Swelling that creates pressure on the median nerve as it passes through the carpal tunnel.

castration (kas-**TRAY**-shun): Surgical removal or destruction of both testicles; also known as bilateral orchidectomy.

cataract (**KAT**-ah-rakt): The loss of transparency of the lens of the eye.

catatonic behavior (**kat**-ah-**TON**-ick): Marked by a lack of responsiveness, stupor, and a tendency to remain in a fixed posture.

catheterization, urinary: The withdrawal of urine from the urinary bladder to obtain a sterile specimen for diagnostic purposes, the withdrawal of urine to control incontinence, or the placement of fluid, such as a chemotherapy solution, into the bladder.

causalgia (kaw-**ZAL**-jee-ah): Persistent, severe, burning pain that usually follows an injury to a sensory nerve.

cauterization (**kaw**-ter-eye-**ZAY**-zhun): The destruction of tissue by burning.

cellulitis (**sell**-you-**LYE**-tis): An acute, rapidly spreading infection within the connective tissues of the skin.

centesis (sen-**TEE**-sis): A surgical puncture to remove fluid for diagnostic purposes or to remove excess fluid.

cephalalgia (**sef**-ah-**LAL**-jee-ah): Pain in the head; also known as a headache.

cerebral contusion (kon-**TOO**-zhun): Bruising of brain tissue as the result of a head injury that may also cause swelling of the brain.

cerebral palsy (**SER**-eh-bral *or* seh-**REE**-bral **PAWL**-zee): A congenital condition characterized by poor muscle control, spasticity, speech defects, and other neurologic deficiencies.

cerebrovascular accident (**ser**-eh-broh-**VAS**-kyou-lar): Damage to the brain that occurs when the blood flow to the brain is disrupted; also known as a stroke.

cervical dysplasia (**SER**-vih-kal dis-**PLAY**-see-ah): The abnormal growth of cells of the cervix; also known as precancerous lesions.

cervical radiculopathy (rah-**dick**-you-**LOP**-ah-thee): Nerve pain caused by pressure on the spinal nerve roots in the neck region.

cervicitis (**ser**-vih-**SIGH**-tis): Inflammation of the cervix.

cesarean section (seh-**ZEHR**-ee-un **SECK**-shun): The delivery of the child through an incision in the maternal abdominal and uterine walls; also known as a cesarean delivery or a C-section.

chalazion (kah-**LAY**-zee-on): A localized swelling inside the eyelid resulting from obstruction of one of the sebaceous glands; also known as an internal stye.

chemabrasion (keem-ah-**BRAY**-shun): The use of chemicals to remove the outer layers of skin to treat acne scaring, fine wrinkling, and general keratoses; also known chemical peel.

chemical thyroidectomy (**thigh**-roi-**DECK**-toh-mee): The administration of radioactive iodine to destroy thyroid cells to treat hyperthyroid disorders; also known as radioactive iodine therapy.

chemotherapy: The use of chemical agents and drugs in combinations selected to destroy malignant cells and tissues.

Cheyne-Stokes respiration (**CHAYN**-**STOHKS**): A pattern of alternating periods of hypopnea, or apnea, followed by hyperpnea.

chlamydia (klah-**MID**-ee-ah): A sexually transmitted disease caused by the bacterium *Chlamydia trachomatis*.

chloasma (kloh-**AZ**-mah): A pigmentation disorder characterized by brownish spots on the face; also known as melasma or the mask of pregnancy.

cholecystalgia (**koh**-lee-sis-**TAL**-jee-ah): Pain in the gallbladder.

cholecystitis (**koh**-lee-sis-**TYE**-tis): Inflammation of the gallbladder that is usually associated with gallstones.

choledocholithotomy (koh-**led**-oh-koh-lih-**THOT**-oh-mee): An incision in the common bile duct for the removal of gallstones.

cholelithiasis (**koh**-lee-lih-**THIGH**-ah-sis): The presence of gallstones in the gallbladder or bile ducts.

cholera (**KOL**-er-ah): Severe diarrhea, vomiting, and dehydration caused by the bacterium *Vibrio cholerae*.

cholesterol (koh-**LES**-ter-ol): A waxy fatlike substance that travels in the blood in packages called lipoproteins.

cholesterol-lowering drugs: Medications, such as statins, that are administered to reduce the undesirable cholesterol levels in the blood.

chondroma (kon-**DROH**-mah): A slow-growing benign tumor derived from cartilage cells.

chondromalacia (**kon**-droh-mah-**LAY**-shee-ah): Abnormal softening of the cartilage.

chondropathy (kon-**DROP**-ah-thee): A disease of the cartilage.

chondroplasty (**KON**-droh-**plas**-tee): Surgical repair of damaged cartilage.

chorionic villus sampling: A diagnostic test performed between the eighth to tenth weeks of pregnancy to detect genetic abnormalities in the developing child.

chronic obstructive pulmonary disease: A group of irreversible respiratory conditions characterized by chronic airflow limitations.

chronic renal failure: The progressive loss of renal function due to a variety of conditions.

cicatrix (sick-**AY**-tricks): A normal scar resulting from the healing of a wound (plural, cicatrices).

cineradiography (**sin**-eh-**ray**-dee-**OG**-rah-fee): The recording of images as they appear in motion on a fluorescent screen.

circumcision (**ser**-kum-**SIZH**-un): Surgical removal of the foreskin of the penis that is usually performed a few days after birth.

cirrhosis (sih-**ROH**-sis): A progressive degenerative disease of the liver in which scar tissue replaces normal tissue.

claustrophobia (**klaws**-troh-**FOH**-bee-ah): Abnormal fear of being in narrow or enclosed spaces.

cleft lip: A developmental defect resulting in a deep fissure of the lip running upward to the nose; also known as a harelip.

cleft palate: Failure of the palate to close during the early development of the fetus that involves the upper lip, hard palate, and/or soft palate.

closed fracture: A fracture in which the bone is broken but there is no open wound in the skin; also known as a simple or complete fracture.

clubbing: Abnormal curving of the nails that is often accompanied by enlargement of the fingertips.

cluster headaches: Episodes of concentrated pain on one side of the head that that are less common than migraines, but are more painful, and often occur one or more times daily for weeks or months.

cochlear implant (**KOCK**-lee-ar): An electronic device that allows individuals with severe-to-profound hearing loss to perceive sound.

cognitive therapy: Treatment that focuses on changing problematic beliefs, cognitions, or thoughts.

colectomy (koh-**LECK**-toh-mee): Surgical removal of all or part of the colon.

collagen replacement therapy: A form of soft-tissue augmentation used to soften facial lines or scars, or to make lips appear fuller.

Colles' fracture: A fracture at the lower end of the radius that occurs when a person tries to break a fall by landing on his or her hands.

colonoscopy (**koh**-lun-**OSS**-koh-pee): Direct visual examination of the inner surface of the colon from the rectum to the cecum.

colorectal carcinoma: A common form of cancer that often first manifests itself in polyps in the colon.

colostomy (koh-**LAHS**-toh-mee): The surgical creation of an artificial excretory opening between the colon and the body surface.

colotomy (koh-**LOT**-oh-mee): A surgical incision into the colon.

colpitis (kol-**PYE**-tis): Inflammation of the lining of the vagina; also known as vaginitis.

colpopexy (**KOL**-poh-**peck**-see): Surgical fixation of the vagina to a surrounding structure.

colporrhaphy (kol-**POR**-ah-fee): Surgical suturing of a tear in the vagina.

colporrhexis (**kol**-poh-**RECK**-sis): The laceration of the vaginal walls.

colposcopy (kol-**POS**-koh-pee): Direct visual examination of the tissues of the cervix and vagina using a binocular magnifier called a colposcope.

coma (**KOH**-mah): A deep state of unconsciousness marked by the absence of spontaneous eye movements, no response to painful stimuli, and no vocalization.

comatose (**KOH**-mah-tohs): The state of a person who is in a coma.

comedo (**KOM**-eh-doh): A noninfected lesion formed by the buildup of sebum and keratin in a hair follicle (plural, comedones).

comminuted fracture (**KOM**-ih-**newt**-ed): A fracture in which the bone is splintered or crushed.

complete blood cell count: A series of blood tests performed as a group to evaluate several blood conditions.

complex regional pain syndrome: A form of causalgia caused by either an identifiable injury to a sensory nerve or an injury to a body part such as the arms or legs; also known as reflex sympathetic dystrophy syndrome.

compression fracture: A fracture in which the bone is compressed on itself.

computerized tomography (toh-**MOG**-rah-fee): An imaging technique that uses a thin, fan-shaped x-ray beam to produce multiple cross-sectional views of the body.

concussion (kon-**KUSH**-un): A violent shaking up or jarring of the brain that may result in a temporary loss of awareness and function.

conductive hearing loss: A hearing loss in which the tiny bones in the middle ear do not conduct sound vibrations normally.

congenital disorder (kon-**JEN**-ih-tahl): An abnormal condition that exists at the time of birth.

congestive heart failure: A syndrome in which the heart is unable to pump enough blood to meet the needs of the body for oxygen and nutrients.

conization (**kon**-ih-**ZAY**-shun *or* **koh**-nih-**ZAY**-shun): Surgical removal of a cone-shaped section of tissue from the cervix; also known as a cone biopsy.

conjunctivitis (kon-**junk**-tih-**VYE**-tis): Inflammation of the conjunctiva, usually caused by an infection or allergy; also known as pinkeye.

conjunctivoplasty (**kon**-junk-**TYE**-voh-**plas**-tee): Surgical repair of the conjunctiva.

Conn's syndrome: An abnormality of electrolyte balance caused by disorders of the adrenal glands; also known as primary aldosteronism.

conscious: Being awake, aware, and responding appropriately; also known as alert.

constipation: A decrease in frequency in the passage of stools or difficulty in passing hard, dry stools.

contact dermatitis: A localized allergic response caused by contact with an irritant or allergen.

contraceptive: A measure taken, or a device used, to lessen the likelihood of pregnancy.

contracture (kon-**TRACK**-chur): The permanent tightening of fascia, muscles, tendons, ligaments, or skin that occurs when normally elastic connective tissues are replaced with nonelastic fibrous tissues.

contraindication: A factor in the patient's condition that makes the use of a drug dangerous or ill advised.

contrast medium: A substance used to make visible structures that are otherwise hard to see.

contusion (kon-**TOO**-zhun): An injury that does not break the skin and is characterized by discoloration and pain; also known as a bruise.

conversion disorder: A condition characterized by a serious temporary or ongoing change in function, such as paralysis or blindness, triggered by psychological factors rather than any physical cause.

convulsion: A disturbance in the brain that can be caused by extreme high fever or by brain injury or lesions; also known as a seizure.

Cooley's anemia: A diverse group of genetic blood diseases characterized by absent or decreased production of normal hemoglobin; also known as thalassemia.

corneal abrasion: An injury, such as a scratch or irritation, to the outer layers of the cornea.

corneal ulcer: A pitting of the cornea of the eye caused by an infection or injury.

coronary artery bypass graft: A surgical procedure in which a piece of vein from the leg is implanted on the heart to replace a blocked coronary artery; also known as bypass surgery.

coronary artery disease: Atherosclerosis of the coronary arteries that may cause angina pectoris, myocardial infarction, and/or sudden death.

coronary thrombosis (**KOR**-uh-**nerr**-ee throm-**BOH**-sis): Damage to the heart muscle caused by a thrombus blocking a coronary artery.

corticosteroid drug: A hormone-like preparation used primarily as an anti-inflammatory and as an immunosuppressant.

cortisone (**KOR**-tih-sohn): The synthetic equivalent of natural corticosteroids that are administered to suppress inflammation and to act as an immunosuppressant; also known as hydrocortisone.

costectomy (kos-**TECK**-toh-mee): Surgical removal of a rib or ribs.

costotomy (kos-**TOT**-oh-mee): A surgical incision or division of a rib or ribs.

COX-2 inhibitors: Medications that control the pain and inflammation of osteoarthritis and rheumatoid arthritis with fewer side effects than with NSAIDs.

cramp: A localized muscle spasm named for its cause, such as a heat cramp or writer's cramp.

cranial hematoma (**hee**-mah-**TOH**-mah *or* **hem**-ah-**TOH**-mah): A collection of blood trapped in the tissues of the brain.

craniectomy (**kray**-nee-**EK**-toh-mee): Surgical removal of a portion of the skull.

craniocele (**KRAY**-nee-oh-**seel**): The congenital protrusion of brain substance through a gap in the skull; also known as an encephalocele

craniomalacia (**kray**-nee-oh-mah-**LAY**-shee-ah): Abnormal softening of the skull.

cranioplasty (**KRAY**-nee-oh-**plas**-tee): Surgical repair of the skull.

craniostenosis (**kray**-nee-oh-steh-**NOH**-sis): A malformation of the skull due to the premature closure of the cranial sutures.

craniotomy (**kray**-nee-**OT**-oh-mee): A surgical incision or opening into the skull; also known as a bone flap.

creatinuria (**kree**-at-ih-**NEW**-ree-ah): An increased concentration of creatine in the urine.

crepitation (**krep**-ih-**TAY**-shun): The crackling sound heard when the ends of a broken bone move together; also the sound heard in lungs affected with pneumonia and with the noisy discharge of gas from the intestine; also known as crepitus.

crepitus (**KREP**-ih-tus): The crackling sound heard when the ends of a broken bone move together; also the sound heard in lungs affected with pneumonia and with the noisy discharge of gas from the intestine; also known as crepitation.

cretinism (**CREE**-tin-izm): A congenital form of hypothyroidism that, if not treated early in life, causes arrested physical and mental development.

Crohn's disease: A chronic autoimmune disorder that can occur anywhere in the digestive tract; however, it is most often found in the ileum and in the colon.

croup (**KROOP**): An acute respiratory syndrome in children and infants characterized by obstruction of the larynx, hoarseness, and a barking cough.

CRP (C-reactive protein): A blood test that detects coronary-artery inflammation that could signal increased risk of heart attack.

crust: A collection of dried serum and cellular debris; also known as a scab.

cryosurgery: The destruction or elimination of abnormal tissue cells, such as warts or tumors, through the application of extreme cold, often by using liquid nitrogen.

cryptorchidism (krip-**TOR**-kih-dizm): A developmental defect in which one or both testicles fail to descend into the scrotum; also known as an undescended testis.

curettage (**kyou**-reh-**TAHZH**): The removal of material from the surface by scraping.

Cushing's syndrome (**KUSH**-ingz **SIN**-drohm): A condition caused by overproduction of cortisol by the body or by taking glucocorticoid hormone medications to treat inflammatory diseases such as asthma and rheumatoid arthritis; also known as hypercortisolism.

cyanosis (**sigh**-ah-**NOH**-sis): Blue discoloration of the skin caused by a lack of adequate oxygen.

cyst: A deep closed sac just under the skin containing soft or semisolid material.

cystalgia (sis-**TAL**-jee-ah): Pain in the urinary bladder.

cystectomy (sis-**TECK**-toh-mee): The surgical removal of all or part of the urinary bladder.

cystic fibrosis (**SIS**-tick figh-**BROH**-sis): A genetic disorder in which the lungs and pancreas are clogged with large quantities of abnormally thick mucus.

cystitis (sis-**TYE**-tis): Inflammation of the bladder.

cystocele (**SIS**-toh-seel): A hernia of the bladder through the vaginal wall; also called a fallen bladder.

cystodynia (**sis**-toh-**DIN**-ee-ah): Pain in the urinary bladder.

cystography (sis-**TOG**-rah-fee): A radiographic examination of the bladder after instillation of a contrast medium via a urethral catheter.

cystolith (**SIS**-toh-lith): A stone located in the urinary bladder.

cystopexy (**sis**-toh-**peck**-see): The surgical fixation of the bladder to the abdominal wall.

cystoplasty (**SIS**-toh-**plas**-tee): Surgical repair of the bladder.

cystoptosis (**sis**-top-**TOH**-sis *or* **sis**-toh-**TOH**-sis): Prolapse of the bladder into the urethra.

cystorrhaphy (sis-**TOR**-ah-fee): Surgical suturing of the bladder.

cystorrhexis (**sis**-toh-**RECK**-sis): Rupture of the bladder.

cystoscope (**SIS**-toh-**skope**): A specialized endoscope used to examine and treat the interior of the urinary bladder.

cystoscopy (sis-**TOS**-koh-pee): The visual examination of the urinary bladder using a cystoscope; also known as cysto.

cystostomy (sis-**TOS**-toh-mee): The creation of an artificial opening between the urinary bladder and the exterior of the body.

cytomegalovirus (**sigh**-toh-**meg**-ah-loh-**VYE**-rus): A group of large, herpes-type viruses that cause a variety of diseases.

cytotoxic drug (**sigh**-toh-**TOK**-sick): Medication that kills or damages cells that is used as an immuno-suppressant and as an antineoplastic.

D

deafness: The complete or partial loss of the ability to hear.

debridement (day-breed-**MON**): The removal of dirt, foreign objects, damaged tissue, and cellular debris from a wound to prevent infection and to promote healing.

decubitus ulcer (dee-**KYOU**-bih-tus): An ulcerated area in which prolonged pressure causes tissue death; also known as a pressure ulcer or bedsore.

deep tendon reflexes: Testing of reflexes to diagnose disruptions of the nerve supply to the involved muscles.

deep vein thrombosis: The condition of having a thrombus attached to the wall of a deep vein.

defibrillation (dee-**fib**-rih-**LAY**-shun): The use of electrical shock to restore the heart's normal rhythm; also known as cardioversion.

dehydration: A condition in which fluid loss exceeds fluid intake and disrupts the body's normal electrolyte balance.

delirium (dee-**LIR**-ee-um): A condition of sudden onset in which the patient is confused, anxious, and unable to think clearly. This is often caused by a high fever, intoxication, or shock.

delirium tremens (dee-**LIR**-ee-um **TREE**-mens): An acute organic brain syndrome due to alcohol withdrawal that is characterized by sweating, tremor, restlessness, anxiety, mental confusion, and hallucinations.

delusion (dee-**LOO**-zhun): A false personal belief that is maintained despite obvious proof or evidence to the contrary.

dementia (dee-**MEN**-shee-ah): A slowly progressive decline in mental abilities including memory, thinking, and judgment that is often accompanied by personality changes.

dental calculus (**KAL**-kyou-luhs): Hardened dental plaque on the teeth that irritates the surrounding tissues; also known as tartar.

dental caries (**KAYR**-eez): An infectious disease that destroys the enamel and dentin of the tooth; also known as tooth decay or a cavity.

dental plaque (**PLACK**): A soft deposit consisting of bacteria and bacterial by-products that builds up on the teeth and is a major cause of dental caries and periodontal disease.

depression: A common mood disorder characterized by lethargy and sadness, as well as a loss of interest or pleasure in normal activities.

dermabrasion (**der**-mah-**BRAY**-zhun): A form of abrasion involving the use of a revolving wire brush or sandpaper to remove acne scars as well as for facial skin rejuvenation.

dermatitis (**der**-mah-**TYE**-tis): Inflammation of the skin.

dermatopathy (**der**-mah-**TOP**-ah-thee): Any disease of the skin.

dermatoplasty (**DER**-mah-toh-**plas**-tee): The replacement of damaged skin with healthy tissue taken from a donor site on the patient's body; also known as a skin graft.

dermatosis (**der**-mah-**TOH**-sis): A general term used to denote skin lesions or eruptions of any type that are *not* associated with inflammation.

detached retina: The condition in which the retina is pulled away from its normal position of being attached to the choroid in the back of the eye; also known as a retinal detachment.

diabetes insipidus (**dye**-ah-**BEE**-teez in-**SIP**-ih-dus): A condition caused by insufficient production of the antidiuretic hormone or by the inability of the kidneys to respond to this hormone.

diabetes mellitus (**dye**-ah-**BEE**-teez mel-**EYE**-tus *or* **MEL**-ih-tus): A group of metabolic diseases characterized by hyperglycemia resulting from defects in insulin secretion, insulin action, or both.

diabetic coma: A diabetic emergency caused by very high blood sugar (hyperglycemia).

diabetic nephropathy: A kidney disease that is the result of thickening and sclerosis of the glomeruli caused by long-term diabetes mellitus.

diabetic retinopathy (**ret**-ih-**NOP**-ah-thee) (**DR**): Injury to the eye that occurs when diabetes damages the tiny blood vessels in the retina of the eye.

diagnostic ultrasound: The imaging of deep body structures by recording the echoes of pulses of sound waves above the range of human hearing; also known as ultrasound and ultrasonography.

dialysis (dye-**AL**-ih-sis): A procedure to remove waste products from the blood of patients whose kidneys no longer function.

diaphragmatic breathing: A relaxation technique used to relieve anxiety; also called abdominal breathing.

diarrhea (dye-ah-**REE**-ah): The flow of frequent loose or watery stools.

digital rectal examination: A manual examination performed to screen for indications of prostate enlargement and of prostate cancer. As used here, *digital* means performed with a finger.

digital subtraction angiography: A diagnostic technique that makes it possible to view vascular structures without superimposed bone and soft tissue densities. As used here, *digital* means a number in a computer-enhanced image.

digitalis (dij-ih-**TAL**-is): Medication administered to treat atrial fibrillation and congestive heart failure by slowing and strengthening the heart muscle contractions; also known as digoxin.

digoxin (dih-**JOCK**-sin): Medication administered to treat atrial fibrillation and congestive heart failure by slowing and strengthening the heart muscle contractions; also known as digitalis.

dilation and curettage (dye-**LAY**-shun and **kyou**-reh-**TAHZH**): The expansion of the opening of the cervix and the removal of material from the surface of the uterus; also known as D & C.

diphtheria (dif-**THEE**-ree-ah): An acute bacterial infection of the throat and upper respiratory tract that can result in damage to the heart muscle and peripheral nerves.

diplopia (dih-**PLOH**-pee-ah): The perception of two images of a single object; also known as double vision.

dislocation: The total displacement of a bone from its joint; also known as luxation.

dissociative disorders: Conditions that occur when normal thought is separated from consciousness.

diuresis (dye-you-**REE**-sis): The increased excretion of urine.

diuretics (dye-you-**RET**-icks): Medications administered to increase urine secretion to rid the body of excess sodium and water.

diverticulectomy (**dye**-ver-**tick**-you-**LECK**-toh-mee): Surgical removal of a diverticulum.

diverticulitis (**dye**-ver-tick-you-**LYE**-tis): Inflammation of one or more diverticula in the wall of the colon.

diverticulosis (**dye**-ver-**tick**-you-**LOH**-sis): The presence of a number of diverticula in the wall of the colon.

diverticulum (**dye**-ver-**TICK**-you-lum): A pouch or sac occurring in the lining or wall of a tubular organ (plural, diverticula).

doppler echocardiogram: An ultrasonic diagnostic procedure that measures the speed and direction of the blood flow within the heart.

Down syndrome: A genetic syndrome characterized by varying degrees of mental retardation and multiple physical abnormalities; also known as trisomy 21.

drug interaction: Changes in the effect of one drug when it is administered at the same time as another drug.

dual x-ray absorptiometry (ab-**sorp**-shee-**OM**-eh-tree): A low-exposure radiographic measurement of the spine and hips that is able to detect early signs of osteoposoris.

Duchenne's muscular dystrophy (doo-**SHENZ**): A form of muscular dystrophy that appears in males from two to six years of age and progresses slowly.

ductal carcinoma in situ: Breast cancer at its earliest stage before the cancer has broken through the wall of the milk duct.

dyscrasia (dis-**KRAY**-zee-ah): Any pathologic condition of the cellular elements of the blood.

dyskinesia (**dis**-kih-**NEE**-zee-ah): Distortion or impairment of voluntary movement in which the movements appear purposeful but are not under voluntary control.

dyslexia (dis-**LECK**-see-ah): A learning disability characterized by substandard reading achievement due to the inability of the brain to process symbols; also known as a developmental reading disorder.

dysmenorrhea (**dis**-men-oh-**REE**-ah): Abdominal pain caused by uterine cramps during a menstrual period.

dyspepsia (dis-**PEP**-see-ah): Pain or discomfort in digestion; also known as indigestion.

dysphagia (dis-**FAY**-jee-ah): Difficulty in swallowing.

dysphonia (dis-**FOH**-nee-ah): Any change in vocal quality including hoarseness, weakness, or the cracking of a boy's voice in puberty.

dysplasia (dis-**PLAY**-see-ah). Abnormal tissue development.

dyspnea (**DISP**-nee-ah): Difficult or labored breathing; also known as shortness of breath.

dysrhythmia (dis-**RITH**-mee-ah): A change in the rhythm of the heartbeat; also known as cardiac arrhythmia.

dystaxia (dis-**TACK**-see-ah): Difficulty in controlling voluntary movement; also known as partial ataxia.

dysthymia (dis-**THIGH**-mee-ah): A chronic depression present at least 50 percent of the time for more than two years; also known as dysthymic disorder.

dystonia (dis-**TOH**-nee-ah): A condition of abnormal muscle tone.

dysuria (dis-**YOU**-ree-ah): Difficult or painful urination.

E

ecchymosis (**eck**-ih-**MOH**-sis): A large, irregular area of purplish discoloration larger than 10 mm in diameter (plural, ecchymoses).

echocardiography (**eck**-oh-**kar**-dee-**OG**-rah-fee): An ultrasonic diagnostic procedure used to evaluate the structures and motion of the heart; also known as ECHO.

echoencephalography (**eck**-oh-en-**sef**-ah-**LOG**-rah-fee): The use of ultrasound imaging to diagnose a shift in the midline structures of the brain.

eclampsia (eh-**KLAMP**-see-ah): During pregnancy, a more serious form of preeclampsia characterized by convulsions and sometimes coma.

E. coli: Severe watery diarrhea that may be bloody caused by the bacteria *Escherichia coli.*

ectopic pregnancy (eck-**TOP**-ick): The condition in which a fertilized egg is implanted and begins to develop outside of the uterus; also known as an extrauterine pregnancy.

ectropion (eck-**TROH**-pee-on): The turning outward of the edge of an eyelid.

eczema (**ECK**-zeh-mah): A form of dermatitis associated with severe itching, redness, blistering, and possibly oozing sores.

edema (eh-**DEE**-mah): Swelling caused by excess fluid in body tissues.

electrocardiogram (ee-**leck**-troh-**KAR**-dee-oh-**gram**): A record of the electrical activity of the myocardium that is produced by electrocardiography.

electrocardiography (ee-**leck**-troh-kar-dee-**OG**-rah-fee): The process of recording the electrical activity of the myocardium.

electroconvulsive therapy (ee-**leck**-troh-kon-**VUL**-siv): A controlled convulsion produced by the passage of an electric current through the brain used to treat certain mental disorders; also known as electroshock therapy.

electroencephalography (ee-**leck**-troh-en-**sef**-ah-**LOG**-rah-fee): The process of recording the electrical activity of the brain through the use of electrodes attached to the scalp.

electrolysis: The use of electric current to destroy hair follicles for the removal of undesired hair.

electromyography (ee-**leck**-troh-my-**OG**-rah-fee): A diagnostic procedure that measures the electrical activity within muscle fibers in response to nerve stimulation.

electroneuromyography (ee-**leck**-troh-**new**-roh-my-**OG**-rah-fee): A diagnostic procedure for testing and recording neuromuscular activity by the electric stimulation of the nerve trunk that carries fibers to and from the muscle; also known as nerve conduction studies.

ELISA: The acronym for enzyme-linked immunosorbent assay, a blood test that is used to screen for the presence of HIV antibodies.

emaciated (ee-**MAY**-shee-ayt-ed): Abnormally thin.

embolism (**EM**-boh-lizm): The sudden blockage of a blood vessel by an embolus.

embolus (**EM**-boh-lus): A foreign object, such as a blood clot, quantity of air or gas, or a bit of tissue or tumor, that is circulating in the blood (plural, emboli).

emesis (**EM**-eh-sis): To expel the contents of the stomach through the esophagus and out of the mouth; also known as vomiting.

emetic (eh-**MET**-ick): Medication that is administered to produce vomiting.

emphysema (**em**-fih-**SEE**-mah): The progressive loss of lung function that is commonly attributed to long-term smoking.

empyema (**em**-pye-**EE**-mah): An accumulation of pus or infected fluid in the pleural cavity; also known as pyothorax.

encephalitis (**en**-sef-ah-**LYE**-tis): Inflammation of the brain.

encephalocele (en-**SEF**-ah-loh-**seel**): A congenital herniation of brain substance through a gap in the skull; also known as a craniocele.

encephalomalacia (en-**sef**-ah-loh-mah-**LAY**-shee-ah): Abnormal softening of the brain.

encephalopathy (en-**sef**-ah-**LOP**-ah-thee): Any degenerative disease of the brain.

endarterectomy (**end**-ar-ter-**ECK**-toh-mee): The surgical removal of the lining of an artery that is clogged with plaque.

endocarditis (**en**-doh-kar-**DYE**-tis): Inflammation of the inner lining of the heart.

endocervicitis (**en**-doh-**ser**-vih-**SIGH**-tis): Inflammation of the mucous membrane lining of the cervix.

endocrinopathy (**en**-doh-krih-**NOP**-ah-thee): Any disease due to a disorder of the endocrine system.

endometrial biopsy: A diagnostic test in which a small amount of the tissue lining the uterus is removed for microscopic examination.

endometriosis (**en**-doh-**mee**-tree-**OH**-sis): A condition in which patches of endometrial tissue escape the uterus and become attached to other structures in the pelvic cavity

endometritis (**en**-doh-mee-**TRY**-tis): Inflammation of the endometrium.

endoscope (**EN**-doh-**skope**): A fiber optic instrument used for endoscopy and named for the body parts involved.

endoscopic surgery: A surgical procedure performed through very small incisions with the aid of an endoscope.

endoscopy (en-**DOS**-koh-pee): The visual examination of the interior of a body cavity or organ by means of an endoscope.

endotracheal intubation (**en**-doh-**TRAY**-kee-al **in**-too-**BAY**-shun): The passage of a tube through the nose or mouth into the trachea to establish or maintain an open airway.

endovaginal ultrasound (**en**-doh-**VAJ**-ih-nal): A diagnostic test utilizing ultrasound to image the uterus and fallopian tubes to determine the cause of abnormal vaginal bleeding.

end-stage coronary artery disease: The final stage of coronary artery disease characterized by unrelenting angina pain and a severely limited lifestyle.

end-stage renal disease: The late stages of chronic renal failure in which there is irreversible loss of the function of both kidneys.

enteritis (**en**-ter-**EYE**-tis): Inflammation of the small intestine caused by eating or drinking substances contaminated with viral or bacterial pathogens.

entropion (en-**TROH**-pee-on): The turning inward of the edge of an eyelid.

enuresis (**en**-you-**REE**-sis): The involuntary discharge of urine.

epicondylitis (**ep**-ih-**kon**-dih-**LYE**-tis): Inflammation of the tissues surrounding the elbow.

epididymitis (**ep**-ih-did-ih-**MY**-tis): Inflammation of the epididymis; also called epididymo-orchitis**.**

epidural anesthesia (**ep**-ih-**DOO**-ral **an**-es-**THEE**-zee-ah): Regional anesthesia produced by injecting a local anesthetic into the epidural space of the lumbar or sacral region of the spine.

epiglottitis (**ep**-ih-glot-**TYE**-tis): Inflammation of the epiglottis.

epilepsy (**EP**-ih-**lep**-see): A group of neurologic disorders characterized by recurrent episodes of seizures.

epinephrine: A hormone produced by the adrenal medulla that stimulates the sympathetic nervous system; a synthetic hormone used as a vasoconstrictor to treat conditions such as heart dysrhythmias and asthma attacks.

episiorrhaphy (eh-**piz**-ee-**OR**-ah-fee): Surgical suturing to repair an episiotomy.

episiotomy (eh-**piz**-ee-**OT**-oh-mee): A surgical incision of the perineum and vagina to facilitate delivery and prevent laceration of the tissues.

epispadias (**ep**-ih-**SPAY**-dee-as): A congenital abnormality affecting the opening of the urethral meatus. In the male this opening is located on the upper surface of the penis; in the female the urethral opening is in the region of the clitoris.

epistaxis (**ep**-ih-**STACK**-sis): Bleeding from the nose that is usually caused by an injury, excessive use of blood thinners, or bleeding disorders; also known as a nosebleed.

erectile dysfunction: The inability of the male to achieve or maintain a penile erection; also known as impotence.

erythema (**er**-ih-**THEE**-mah): Any redness of the skin due to dilated capillaries, including a nervous blush, inflammation, or sunburn.

erythrocyte sedimentation rate (eh-**RITH**-roh-site): A blood test based on the rate at which the red blood cells separate from the plasma and settle to the bottom of the container; also known as a sed rate.

erythroderma (eh-**rith**-roh-**DER**-mah): A condition in which there is widespread erythema accompanied by scaling of the skin; also known as exfoliative dermatitis.

esophagalgia (eh-**sof**-ah-**GAL**-jee-ah): Pain in the esophagus.

esophageal reflux (eh-**sof**-ah-**JEE**-al **REE**-flucks): The upward flow of stomach acid into the esophagus; also known as gastroesophageal reflux disease (GERD).

esophageal varices (eh-**sof**-ah-**JEE**-al **VAYR**-ih-seez): Enlarged and swollen veins at the lower end of the esophagus.

esophagogastrectomy (eh-**sof**-ah-goh-gas-**TRECK**-toh-mee): Surgical removal of all or part of the esophagus and stomach.

esophagogastroduodenoscopy (eh-**sof**-ah-goh-**gas**-troh-**dew**-oh-deh-**NOS**-koh-pee): The endoscopic examination of the esophagus, stomach, and upper duodenum.

esotropia (**es**-oh-**TROH**-pee-ah): Strabismus characterized by an inward deviation of one eye or both eyes; also known as cross-eyes.

essential hypertension: Consistently elevated blood pressure of unknown cause; also known as primary or idiopathic hypertension.

eustachitis (**you**-stay-**KYE**-tis): Inflammation of the eustachian tube.

Ewing's sarcoma (**YOU**-ingz sar-**KOH**-mah): A group of cancers that most frequently affects children or adolescents; also known as Ewing's family of tumors.

exfoliative cytology (ecks-**FOH**-lee-**ay**-tiv sigh-**TOL**-oh-jee): A biopsy technique in which cells are scraped from the tissue and examined under a microscope.

exophthalmos (**eck**-sof-**THAL**-mos): An abnormal protrusion of the eyes.

exotropia (**eck**-soh-**TROH**-pee-ah): Strabismus characterized by the outward deviation of one eye relative to the other; also known as walleye.

external fixation: A fracture treatment procedure in which pins are placed through the soft tissues and bone so that an external appliance can be used to hold the pieces of bone firmly in place during healing.

extraoral radiography: As used in dentistry, placement of the radiographic film outside of the mouth.

F

factitious disorder (fack-**TISH**-us): A condition in which a person acts as if he or she has a physical or mental illness when he or she is not really sick; previously known as Munchausen syndrome.

factitious disorder by proxy: A form of child abuse in which the abusive parent, although seeming very concerned about the child's well-being, falsifies an illness in a child by making up or creating symptoms and then seeking medical treatment, even surgery, for the child; previously known as Munchausen syndrome by proxy.

fasciectomy (fas-ee-**ECK**-toh-mee): Surgical removal of fascia.

fasciitis (**fas**-ee-**EYE**-tis): Inflammation of a fascia; fascitis is also an acceptable spelling.

fasciodesis (**fash**-ee-**ODD**-eh-sis): Binding fascia to a skeletal attachment.

fascioplasty (**FASH**-ee-oh-**plas**-tee): Surgical repair of a fascia.

fasciorrhaphy (**fash**-ee-**OR**-ah-fee): Surgical suturing of torn fascia.

fasciotomy (**fash**-ee-**OT**-oh-mee): A surgical incision through a fascia to relieve tension or pressure.

fasting blood sugar: A blood test to measure the glucose levels after the patient has not eaten for 8 to 12 hours.

fat embolus (**EM**-boh-lus): The release of fat cells from yellow bone marrow into the bloodstream when a long bone is fractured.

fecal occult blood test: A laboratory test for hidden blood in the stools; also known as the hemoccult test.

fenestration (**fen**-es-**TRAY**-shun): A surgical procedure in which a new opening is created in the labyrinth of the inner ear to restore hearing.

fetal monitoring: The use of an electronic device to record the fetal heart rate and the maternal uterine contractions during labor.

fibrillation (**fih**-brih-**LAY**-shun): Rapid, random, quivering, and ineffective contractions of the heart.

fibroadenomas: Small, benign lumps of fibrous and glandular tissue; also known as fibrous breast lumps.

fibrocystic breast disease (**figh**-broh-**SIS**-tick): The presence of single or multiple cysts in the breasts.

fibroid: A benign tumor composed of muscle and fibrous tissue that occurs in the wall of the uterus; also known as a leiomyoma.

fibromyalgia syndrome (**figh**-broh-my-**AL**-jee-ah): A chronic, often disabling, condition of unknown cause that is characterized by uncontrollable fatigue and widespread pain in the muscles, ligaments, and tendons.

fissure (**FISH**-ur): A groove or crack-like sore of the skin; also normal folds in the contours of the brain.

fistula (**FIS**-tyou-lah): An abnormal passage between two internal organs or leading from an organ to the surface of the body.

floaters: Particles of cellular debris that float in the vitreous fluid and cast shadows on the retina; also known as vitreous floaters.

fluorescein angiography (**flew**-oh-**RES**-ee-in **an**-jee-**OG**-rah-fee): A radiographic study of the blood vessels in the retina of the eye following the intravenous injection of a fluorescein dye that acts as a contrast medium.

fluorescein staining (**flew**-oh-**RES**-ee-in): A strain placed on the cornea that appears bright green when corneal abrasions are present.

fluoroscopy (**floo**-or-**OS**-koh-pee): An imaging technique used to visualize body parts in motion by projecting x-ray images on a luminous fluorescent screen.

folliculitis (foh-**lick**-you-**LYE**-tis): Inflammation of the hair follicles that is especially common on the limbs and in the beard area on men.

fracture: A broken bone.

fructosamine test (fruck-**TOHS**-ah-meen): A blood test that measures average glucose levels over the past three weeks.

functional disorder: A condition in which there are no detectable physical changes to explain the symptoms being experienced by the patient.

functional endoscopic sinus surgery: A surgical procedure performed using an endoscope in which chronic sinusitis is treated by enlarging the opening between the nose and sinus.

furuncles (**FYOU**-rung-kuls): Large, tender, swollen areas caused by a staphylococcal infection around hair follicles or sebaceous glands; also known as boils.

G

galactorrhea (gah-**lack**-toh-**REE**-ah): The production of breast milk in women who are not breast feeding that is caused by a malfunction of the thyroid or pituitary gland.

gallstone: A hard deposit that forms in the gallbladder and bile ducts; also known as biliary calculus.

gametic cell mutation: Changes within the genes found in the gametes (sex cells) that can be transmitted by parents to their children.

ganglion cyst: A harmless fluid-filled swelling that occurs most commonly on the outer surface of the wrist.

gangrene (**GANG**-green): Tissue death caused by a loss of circulation to the affected tissues.

gastralgia (gas-**TRAL**-jee-ah): Pain in the stomach.

gastrectomy (gas-**TRECK**-toh-mee): Surgical removal of all or a part of the stomach.

gastric bypass: A surgical procedure in which the size of the stomach is drastically reduced.

gastritis (gas-**TRY**-tis): Inflammation of the stomach.

gastroduodenostomy (**gas**-troh-**dew**-oh-deh-**NOS**-toh-mee): The removal of the pylorus of the stomach and the establishment of an anastomosis between the upper portion of the stomach and the duodenum.

gastrodynia (gas-troh-**DIN**-ee-ah): Pain in the stomach.

gastroenteritis (**gas**-troh-en-ter-**EYE**-tis): Inflammation of the mucous membrane lining the stomach and intestines.

gastroenterocolitis (gas-troh-**en**-ter-oh-koh-**LYE**-tis): Inflammation of the stomach, small intestine, and large intestine.

gastroesophageal reflux disease: The upward flow of stomach acid into the esophagus; also known as esophageal reflux.

gastropexy (**GAS**-troh-**peck**-see): Surgical fixation of the stomach to correct displacement.

gastrorrhaphy (gas-**TROR**-ah-fee): Suturing of the stomach.

gastrorrhea (**gas**-troh-**REE**-ah): The excessive secretion of gastric juice or mucus in the stomach.

gastrosis (gas-**TROH**-sis): Any abnormal condition of the stomach.

gastrostomy (gas-**TROS**-toh-mee): The surgical creation of an artificial opening into the stomach.

generalized anxiety disorder: A mental condition characterized by persistent, intrusive, excessive worry about multiple topics that is difficult to control.

generic drug: Medication named for its chemical structure that is not protected by a brand name or trademark.

genetic disorders: Diseases or conditions caused by a defective gene that are transmitted from the parents to their children; also known as hereditary disorders.

genital herpes (**HER**-peez): A sexually transmitted disease caused by the herpes simplex virus type 2 (HSV-2).

genital warts: A sexually transmitted disease caused by a chronic infection by the human papilloma virus.

gestational diabetes mellitus (jes-**TAY**-shun-al **dye**-ah-**BEE**-teez mel-**EYE**-tus *or* **MEL**-ih-tus): The form of diabetes that occurs during some pregnancies.

gigantism (jigh-**GAN**-tiz-em): Abnormal overgrowth of the body caused by excessive secretion of the growth hormone *before* puberty; also known as giantism.

gingivectomy (**jin**-jih-**VECK**-toh-mee): Surgical removal of diseased gingival tissue.

gingivitis (**jin**-jih-**VYE**-tis): Inflammation of the gums; the earliest stage of periodontal disease.

GI series: Radiographic studies of the digestive system.

Given Diagnostic Imaging System: A tiny video camera in a capsule swallowed by the patient that records images of the walls of the small intestine; also known as known as a capsule endoscopy.

glaucoma (glaw-**KOH**-mah): A group of eye diseases characterized by increased intraocular pressure (IOP) that causes damage to the optic nerve and retinal nerve fibers.

glomerulonephritis (gloh-**mer**-you-loh-neh-**FRY**-tis): A form of nephritis that involves primarily the glomeruli.

Glucophage: A medication administered to type 2 diabetics to aid the cells in combating insulin resistance.

glycosuria (**glye**-koh-**SOO**-ree-ah): The presence of glucose in the urine.

goiter (**GOI**-ter): An enlargement of the thyroid gland that produces a swelling in the front of the neck; also known as thyromegaly.

gonorrhea (**gon**-oh-**REE**-ah): A sexually transmitted disease caused by the bacterium *Neisseria gonorrhoeae*.

gouty arthritis (**GOW**-tee ar-**THRIGH**-tis): A type of arthritis caused by an excess of uric acid in the body; also known as gout.

grand mal epilepsy (**GRAN MAHL EP**-ih-**lep**-see): The more severe form of epilepsy that is characterized by generalized seizures.

granulation tissue: The tissue that forms during the healing of a wound that will become the scar tissue.

granuloma (**gran**-you-**LOH**-mah): A general term used to describe small knotlike swellings of granulation tissue in the epidermis.

Graves' disease (**GRAYVZ** dih-**ZEEZ**): An autoimmune disorder, which is a form of hyperthyroidism, that is characterized by goiter and/or exophthalmos.

greenstick fracture: A type of fracture that occurs primarily in children in which the bone is bent and only partially broken; also known as an incomplete fracture.

Guillain-Barré syndrome (gee-**YAHN**-bah-**RAY**): Inflammation of the myelin sheath of peripheral nerves, characterized by rapidly worsening muscle weakness that may lead to temporary paralysis; also known as infectious polyneuritis.

gynecomastia (**guy**-neh-koh-**MAS**-tee-ah): The condition of excessive mammary development in the male.

H

halitosis (hal-ih-**TOH**-sis): An unpleasant odor coming from the mouth that may be caused by dental diseases or respiratory or gastric disorders, also known as bad breath.

hallucination (hah-**loo**-sih-**NAY**-shun): A sense perception that has no basis in external stimulation.

hallux valgus (**HAL**-ucks **VAL**-guss): An abnormal enlargement of the joint at the base of the great toe; also known as a bunion.

hamstring injury: A strain or tear on any of the three hamstring muscles that straighten the hip and bend the knee.

Hashimoto's thyroiditis (hah-shee-**MOH**-tohz **thigh**-roi-**DYE**-tis): An autoimmune disorder in which the immune system mistakenly attacks thyroid tissue.

hearing aid: An external electronic device that amplifies sounds to reduce the effects of a sensorineural hearing loss.

heel spurs: Hardened deposits in the plantar fascia near its attachment to the heel.

hemangioma (hee-**man**-jee-**OH**-mah): A benign tumor made up of newly formed blood vessels.

hematemesis (**hee**-mah-**TEM**-eh-sis *or* **hem**-ah-**TEM**-eh-sis): Vomiting blood.

hematocrit (hee-**MAT**-oh-krit) (**Hct** or **HCT**): A blood test that measures the percentage by volume of packed red blood cells in a whole blood sample.

hematoma (**hee**-mah-**TOH**-mah): A swelling of clotted blood trapped in the tissues that is usually caused by an injury.

hematuria (**hee**-mah-**TOO**-ree-ah *or* **hem**-ah-**TOO**-ree-ah): The presence of blood in the urine.

hemianopia (**hem**-ee-ah-**NOH**-pee-ah): Blindness in one half of the visual field; sometimes spelled hemianopsia.

hemiparesis (**hem**-ee-pah-**REE**-sis): Slight paralysis of one side of the body.

hemiplegia (**hem**-ee-**PLEE**-jee-ah): Total paralysis of one side of the body.

hemoccult test (**HEE**-moh-kult): A laboratory test for hidden blood in the stools; also known as fecal occult blood test.

hemochromatosis (**hee**-moh-**kroh**-mah-**TOH**-sis): A genetic disorder in which the intestines absorb too much iron; also known as iron-overload disease.

hemodialysis (**hee**-moh-dye-**AL**-ih-sis): A procedure that filters waste products from the patient's blood to replace the function of damaged kidneys.

hemoglobin A1c testing (HbA1c): A blood test that measures the average blood glucose level over the previous three to four months.

hemolytic anemia (**hee**-moh-**LIT**-ick ah-**NEE**-mee-ah). The condition in which red blood cells are destroyed more rapidly than the bone marrow can replace them.

hemolytic reaction (**hee**-moh-**LIT**-ick): The destruction of red blood cells that occurs when a patient receives a transfusion of mismatched blood; also known as a transfusion reaction.

hemophilia (**hee**-moh-**FILL**-ee-ah): A group of hereditary bleeding disorders in which one of the factors needed to clot the blood is missing.

hemoptysis (hee-**MOP**-tih-sis): Coughing up of blood or bloodstained sputum.

hemorrhage (**HEM**-or-idj): The loss of a large amount of blood in a short time.

hemorrhagic stroke (**hem**-oh-**RAJ**-ick): Damage to the brain that occurs when a blood vessel in the brain leaks or ruptures; also known as a bleed.

hemorrhoidectomy (**hem**-oh-roid-**ECK**-toh-mee): The surgical removal of hemorrhoids.

hemorrhoids (**HEM**-oh-roids): A cluster of enlarged veins, near the anal opening; also known as piles.

hemostasis (**hee**-moh-**STAY**-sis): To stop or control bleeding.

hemothorax (**hee**-moh-**THOH**-racks): Blood in the pleural cavity.

hepatectomy (**hep**-ah-**TECK**-toh-mee): The surgical removal of all or part of the liver.

hepatitis (**hep**-ah-**TYE**-tis): Inflammation of the liver.

hepatomegaly (**hep**-ah-toh-**MEG**-ah-lee): Abnormal enlargement of the liver.

hepatorrhaphy (**hep**-ah-**TOR**-ah-fee): Surgical suturing of the liver.

hernia (**HER**-nee-ah): The protrusion of a part or structure through the tissues normally containing it.

herniated disk (**HER**-nee-**ayt**-ed): The breaking apart of a intervertebral disk that results in pressure on spinal nerve roots; also known as a ruptured disk.

herniorrhaphy (**her**-nee-**OR**-ah-fee): Surgical suturing of a defect in a muscular wall to repair a hernia.

herpes labialis (**HER**-peez **lay**-bee-**AL**-iss): Blister-like sores on the lips and adjacent tissue caused by the oral herpes simplex virus type 1; also known as cold sores or fever blisters.

herpes zoster (**HER**-peez **ZOS**-ter): An acute viral infection characterized by painful skin eruptions that follow the underlying route of the inflamed nerve.

hiatal hernia (high-**AY**-tal **HER**-nee-ah): The protrusion of part of the stomach through the esophageal sphincter in the diaphragm.

high-density lipoprotein cholesterol: The form of cholesterol that does not contribute to plaque buildup; is also known as good cholesterol.

hirsutism (**HER**-soot-izm): Excessive bodily and facial hair in women, usually occurring in a male pattern.

Hodgkin's lymphoma (**HODJ**-kinz lim-**FOH**-mah): A malignancy of the lymphatic system that is distinguished from non-Hodgkin's lymphoma by the presence of *Reed-Sternberg cells*; also known as Hodgkin's disease.

Holter monitor: A portable ECG worn by an ambulatory patient to continuously monitor the heart rates and rhythms over a 24-hour period.

hordeolum (hor-**DEE**-oh-lum): A pus-filled lesion on the eyelid resulting from an infection in a sebaceous gland; also known as a stye.

hormone replacement therapy: Synthetic hormones that are administered to replace the estrogen and progesterone that are no longer produced during perimenopause and after menopause.

human growth hormone therapy: A synthetic version of the growth hormone that is administered to stimulate growth when the natural supply of growth hormone is insufficient for normal development; also known as recombinant GH.

human immunodeficiency virus: A bloodborne pathogen that progressively damages or kills cells of the immune system, also known as HIV.

Huntington's disease: A hereditary disorder whose symptoms first appear in midlife and that causes the irreversible and progressive loss of muscle control and mental ability; also known as Huntington's chorea.

hydrocele (**HIGH**-droh-seel): A fluid-filled sac in the scrotum along the spermatic cord leading from the testicles.

hydrocephalus (high-droh-**SEF**-ah-lus): A condition in which there is an abnormally increased amount of cerebrospinal fluid within the ventricles of the brain.

hydrocortisone: The synthetic equivalent of corticosteroids produced by the body that are administered to suppress inflammation and to act as an immunosuppressant; also known as cortisone.

hydronephrosis (**high**-droh-neh-**FROH**-sis): The dilation of one or both kidneys that is the result of an obstruction of the flow of urine.

hydroureter (**high**-droh-you-**REE**-ter): The distention of the ureter with urine that cannot flow because the ureter is blocked.

hyperalbuminemia (**high**-per-al-**byou**-mih-**NEE**-mee-ah): Abnormally high level of albumin in the blood.

hypercalcemia (**high**-per-kal-**SEE**-mee-ah): Abnormally high concentrations of calcium circulating in the blood.

hypercapnia (**high**-per-**KAP**-nee-ah): The abnormal buildup of carbon dioxide in the blood.

hypercrinism (**high**-per-**KRY**-nism): A condition caused by excessive secretion of any gland, especially an endocrine gland.

hyperemesis (**high**-per-**EM**-eh-sis): Extreme, persistent vomiting that may lead to dehydration.

hyperesthesia (**high**-per-es-**THEE**-zee-ah): A condition of excessive sensitivity to stimuli.

hyperglycemia (**high**-per-glye-**SEE**-mee-ah): An abnormally high concentration of glucose in the blood.

hyperglycosuria (**high**-per-**glye**-koh-**SOO**-ree-ah): The presence of excess sugar in the urine.

hypergonadism (**high**-per-**GOH**-nad-izm): The excessive secretion of hormones by the sex glands.

hyperhidrosis (**high**-per-high-**DROH**-sis): A condition of excessive sweating in one area or over the whole body.

hyperinsulinism (**high**-per-**IN**-suh-lin-izm): A condition marked by excessive secretion of insulin.

hyperkinesia (**high**-per-kye-**NEE**-zee-ah): Abnormally increased motor function or activity; also known as hyperactivity.

hyperlipidemia (**high**-per-**lip**-ih-**DEE**-mee-ah): The condition of elevated plasma concentrations of cholesterol, triglycerides, and lipoproteins in the bloodstream; also known as hyperlipemia.

hyperopia (**high**-per-**OH**-pee-ah): A vision defect in which light rays focus beyond the retina; also known as farsightedness.

hyperparathyroidism (**high**-per-**par**-ah-**THIGH**-roid-izm): The overproduction of the parathyroid hormone that causes hypercalcemia and the formation of kidney stones.

hyperpituitarism (**high**-per-pih-**TOO**-ih-tah-rizm): Pathology that results in the excessive secretion by the anterior lobe of the pituitary gland.

hyperplasia (**high**-per-**PLAY**-zee-ah): The enlargement of an organ or tissue because of an abnormal increase in the number of cells.

hyperpnea (**high**-perp-**NEE**-ah): An increase in the depth and rate of the respiratory movements.

hyperproteinuria (**high**-per-**proh**-tee-in-**YOU**-ree-ah): The presence of abnormally *high* concentrations of protein in the urine.

hypertension: Abnormally elevated blood pressure.

hypertension, essential: Consistently elevated blood pressure of unknown cause; also known as primary or idiopathic hypertension.

hypertension, malignant: A condition characterized by the sudden onset of severely elevated blood pressure.

hypertension, secondary: Elevated blood pressure caused by a different medical problem such as a kidney disorder or a tumor on the adrenal glands.

hyperthermia (**high**-per-**THER**-mee-ah): An extremely high fever.

hyperthyroidism (**high**-per-**THIGH**-roid-izm): A condition of excessive thyroid hormones in the bloodstream.

hypertonia (**high**-per-**TOH**-nee-ah): A condition of excessive tone of the skeletal muscles.

hypertrophy (high-**PER**-troh-fee): A general increase in the bulk of a part or organ due to an increase in the size, but not in the number, of cells in the tissues.

hyperventilation (**high**-per-**ven**-tih-**LAY**-shun): An abnormally rapid rate of deep respiration that results in a change in blood gas levels due to a decrease in carbon dioxide at the cellular level.

hypnotherapy: The use of hypnosis to produce a relaxed state of focused attention in which the patient may be more willing to believe and act on suggestions.

hypnotic: Medication that depresses the central nervous system and usually produces sleep.

hypocalcemia (**high**-poh-kal-**SEE**-mee-ah): A condition characterized by abnormally low levels of calcium in the blood.

hypochondriasis (**high**-poh-kon-**DRY**-ah-sis): A condition characterized by misinterpretation of physical symptoms and fearing that one has a serious illness despite appropriate medical evaluation and reassurance.

hypocrinism (**high**-poh-**KRY**-nism): A condition caused by deficient secretion of any gland, especially an endocrine gland.

hypoglycemia (**high**-poh-glye-**SEE**-mee-ah). An abnormally low concentration of glucose in the blood.

hypogonadism (**high**-poh-**GOH**-nad-izm): The condition of deficient secretion of hormones by the sex glands.

hypohidrosis (**high**-poh-high-**DROH**-sis): Abnormal condition resulting in the diminished flow of perspiration.

hypokinesia (**high**-poh-kye-**NEE**-zee-ah): Abnormally decreased motor function or activity.

hypomenorrhea (**high**-poh-men-oh-**REE**-ah): A small amount of menstrual flow during a shortened regular menstrual period.

hypoparathyroidism (**high**-poh-**par**-ah-**THIGH**-roid-izm): A condition caused by an insufficient or absent secretion of the parathyroid glands that is usually accompanied by hypocalcemia and in severe cases leads to tetany.

hypoperfusion (**high**-poh-per-**FYOU**-zhun): A deficiency of blood passing through an organ or body part.

hypopituitarism (**high**-poh-pih-**TOO**-ih-tah-rizm): A condition of reduced secretion due to the partial, or complete, loss of the function of the anterior lobe of the pituitary gland.

hypoplasia (**high**-poh-**PLAY**-zee-ah): The incomplete development of an organ or tissue.

hypopnea (**high**-poh-**NEE**-ah): Shallow or slow respiration.

hypoproteinemia (**high**-poh-**proh**-tee-in-**EE**-mee-ah): The condition of the presence of abnormally *low* concentrations of protein in the blood.

hypospadias (**high**-poh-**SPAY**-dee-as): The congenital abnormality of the placement of the urethral opening. In the male the urethral opening is on the under surface of the penis; in the female the urethral opening is into the vagina.

hypotension (**high**-poh-**TEN**-shun): Lower than normal arterial blood pressure.

hypothermia (**high**-poh-**THER**-mee-ah): An abnormally low body temperature.

hypothyroidism (**high**-poh-**THIGH**-roid-izm): A deficiency of thyroid secretion; also known as an underactive thyroid.

hypotonia (**high**-poh-**TOH**-nee-ah): A condition in which there is diminished tone of the skeletal muscles.

hypoxemia (**high**-pock-**SEE**-mee-ah): A condition of having subnormal oxygen level in the blood.

hypoxia (high-**POCK**-see-ah): The condition of having subnormal oxygen levels in the body tissues and cells; less severe than anoxia.

hysterectomy (**hiss**-teh-**RECK**-toh-mee): The surgical removal of the uterus that may, or may not, include removal of the cervix.

hysterocele (**HISS**-ter-oh-seel): A hernia of the uterus, particularly during pregnancy.

hysterorrhaphy (**hiss**-ter-**OR**-ah-fee): Surgical suturing of the uterus.

hysterorrhexis (**hiss**-ter-oh-**RECK**-sis): Rupture of the uterus, particularly during pregnancy.

hysterosalpingography (**hiss**-ter-oh-**sal**-pin-**GOG**-rah-fee): A radiographic examination of the uterus and fallopian tubes following the instillation of radiopaque material.

hysteroscopy (**hiss**-ter-**OSS**-koh-pee): The direct visual examination of the interior of the uterus and fallopian tubes using the magnification of a hysteroscope.

I

iatrogenic illness (eye-**at**-roh-**JEN**-ick): A side effect or an unfavorable response arising from a prescribed treatment or medication.

ichthyosis (**ick**-thee-**OH**-sis): A group of genetic disorders characterized by dry, thickened, scaly skin.

idiopathic disorder (**id**-ee-oh-**PATH**-ick): An illness without known cause.

idiopathic pulmonary fibrosis (**id**-ee-oh-**PATH**-ick): A type of pulmonary fibrosis for which a cause cannot be identified.

idiosyncratic reaction (**id**-ee-oh-sin-**KRAT**-ick): An unexpected reaction to a drug.

ileectomy (**ill**-ee-**ECK**-toh-mee): The surgical removal of the ileum.

ileostomy (**ill**-ee-**OS**-toh-mee): The surgical creation of an artificial excretory opening between the ileum and the outside of the abdominal wall.

ileus (**ILL**-ee-us): The partial or complete blockage of the small and/or large intestine caused by the cessation of intestinal peristalsis.

immobilization: The act of holding, suturing, or fastening a bone in a fixed position with strapping or a cast; also known as stabilization.

immunodeficiency disorder (**im**-you-noh-deh-**FISH**-en-see): A condition that occurs when one or more parts of the immune system are deficient, missing, or not working properly.

immunofluorescence (**im**-you-noh-**floo**-oh-**RES**-ens): A method of tagging antibodies with a fluorescent dye to detect or localize antigen-antibody combinations.

immunosuppressant (**im**-you-noh-soo-**PRES**-ant): A substance that prevents or reduces the body's normal immune response.

immunosuppression (**im**-you-noh-sup-**PRESH**-un): Treatment used to interfere with the ability of the immune system to respond to stimulation by antigens.

immunotherapy (ih-**myou**-noh-**THER**-ah-pee): A treatment of disease by either stimulating or repressing the immune response.

impacted cerumen: An accumulation of earwax that forms a solid mass adhering to the walls of the external auditory canal.

impetigo (**im**-peh-**TYE**-goh): A highly contagious bacterial skin infection characterized by isolated pustules that become crusted and rupture.

impingement syndrome (im-**PINJ**-ment): Inflammation of tendons that get caught in the narrow space between the bones within the shoulder joint.

implantable cardioverter defibrillator (**KAR**-dee-oh-**ver**-ter dee-**fib**-rih-**LAY**-ter): A double-action pacemaker that regulates the heartbeat and acts as an automatic defibrillator.

impotence (**IM**-poh-tens): The inability of the male to achieve or maintain a penile erection; also known as erectile dysfunction.

incision and drainage: An incision into a lesion, such as an abscess, for the purpose of draining the contents; also known as I & D.

incontinence (in-**KON**-tih-nents): The inability to control excretory functions.

indwelling catheter: Placement of a catheter that is to remain inside the body for a prolonged time.

infection (in-**FECK**-shun): Invasion of the body by a pathogenic organism.

infectious disease (in-**FECK**-shus): An illness caused by a living pathogenic organism such as a bacterium, virus, or fungus.

infectious mononucleosis (**mon**-oh-**new**-klee-**OH**-sis): An infection caused by the Epstein-Barr virus that is characterized by fever, a sore throat, and enlarged lymph nodes.

infestation: The dwelling of microscopic parasites on external surface tissue.

infiltrating ductal carcinoma: Breast cancer that starts in the milk duct, breaks through the wall of that duct, and invades the surrounding fatty breast tissue; also known as invasive ductal carcinoma.

infiltrating lobular carcinoma: Breast cancer that starts in the milk glands, breaks through the wall of the gland, and invades the surrounding fatty tissue of the breast; also known as invasive lobular carcinoma.

inflammation (**in**-flah-**MAY**-shun): A localized response to an injury or destruction of tissues that is characterized by heat, redness, swelling, and pain.

inflammatory bowel disease: The general name for diseases that cause inflammation in the intestines.

influenza (**in**-flew-**EN**-zah): An acute, highly contagious viral respiratory infection that occurs most commonly in epidemics during the colder months; also known as flu.

inguinal hernia (**ING**-gwih-nal **HER**-nee-ah): The protrusion of a small loop of bowel through a weak place in the lower abdominal wall or groin.

inhalation administration: The administration of medication in the form of vapor and gases taken in through the nose or mouth and absorbed into the bloodstream through the lungs.

insomnia: The prolonged or abnormal inability to sleep.

insulinemia (**in**-suh-lih-**NEE**-mee-ah): Abnormally high levels of insulin in the blood.

insulinoma (**in**-suh-lin-**OH**-mah): A benign tumor of the pancreas that causes hypoglycemia.

insulin shock: A diabetic emergency caused by very low blood sugar.

intermittent claudication (**klaw**-dih-**KAY**-shun): Pain in the leg muscles that occurs during exercise and is relieved by rest.

internal fixation: Treatment of a fracture in which pins, or a plate, are placed directly into the bone to hold the broken pieces in place; also known as open reduction internal fixation.

interstitial cystitis (**in**-ter-**STISH**-al sis-**TYE**-tis): A chronic inflammation within the wall of the bladder.

interstitial lung diseases (**in**-ter-**STISH**-al): A group of diseases that cause inflammation and scarring of the alveoli and their supporting structures.

intestinal adhesions (ad-**HEE**-zhunz): Parts of the intestine that are abnormally held together where they normally should be separate.

intestinal obstruction: The partial or complete blockage of the small and/or large intestine caused by a physical obstruction.

intracranial pressure: The amount of pressure inside the skull; elevated levels may be due to a tumor, an injury, or improper drainage of cerebrospinal fluid.

intradermal injection: The administration of medication by injection into the middle layers of the skin.

intramuscular injection: The administration of medication by injection directly into muscle tissue.

intraocular lens: An artificial lens that is surgically implanted to replace the natural lens.

intraoral radiography: The placement of x-ray film within the mouth with the camera positioned next to the cheek.

intravenous injection: The administration of medication by injection directly into a vein.

intravenous pyelogram (**PYE**-eh-loh-**gram**): A series of timed radiographic studies of the kidneys and ureters used to diagnose changes in the urinary tract.

intravenous urography (you-**ROG**-rah-fee): Radiographic visualization of the urinary tract with the use of a contrast medium.

intussusception (**in**-tus-sus-**SEP**-shun): The telescoping of one part of the small intestine into the opening of an immediately adjacent part.

invasive ductal carcinoma: Breast cancer that starts in the milk duct, breaks through the wall of that duct, and invades the surrounding fatty breast tissue; also known as infiltrating ductal carcinoma.

invasive lobular carcinoma: Breast cancer that starts in the milk glands, breaks through the wall of the gland, and invades the surrounding fatty tissue of the breast; also known as infiltrating lobular carcinoma.

iridalgia (**ir**-ih-**DAL**-jee-ah): Pain in the iris of the eye.

iridectomy (**ir**-ih-**DECK**-toh-mee): The surgical removal of a portion of the iris tissue.

iridopathy (**ir**-ih-**DOP**-ah-thee): Any disease of the iris.

iridotomy (**ir**-ih-**DOT**-oh-mee): A surgical incision into the iris of the eye.

iritis (eye-**RYE**-tis): Inflammation of the iris.

iron-deficiency anemia: A decrease in the red cells of the blood that is caused by too little iron.

irritable bowel syndrome: A common condition of unknown cause with symptoms that may include intermittent cramping, abdominal pain, bloating, constipation, and/or diarrhea; also known as spastic colon.

ischemia (iss-**KEE**-mee-ah): A temporary deficiency in blood supply due to either the constriction or the obstruction of a blood vessel.

ischemic heart disease (iss-**KEE**-mick): A group of cardiac disabilities resulting from an insufficient supply of oxygenated blood to the heart.

ischemic stroke: Damage to the brain that occurs when the flow of blood to the brain is blocked by narrowing of the carotid artery or by a cerebral thrombosis.

J

jaundice (**JAWN**-dis): A yellow discoloration of the skin and eyes caused by greater-than-normal amounts of bilirubin in the blood; also known as icterus.

juvenile rheumatoid arthritis: The type of arthritis that affects children, causing pain and swelling in the joints, skin rash, fever, slowed growth, and fatigue.

K

Kaposi's sarcoma (**KAP**-oh-seez sar-**KOH**-mah): Malignant tumors that may affect the skin, mucous membranes, lymph nodes, and internal organs.

keloid (**KEE**-loid): An abnormally raised or thickened scar that expands beyond the boundaries of the incision.

keratitis (**ker**-ah-**TYE**-tis): Inflammation of the cornea.

keratoplasty (**KER**-ah-toh-**plas**-tee): The surgical replacement of a scarred or diseased cornea with clear corneal tissue from a donor; also known as corneal transplant.

keratosis (**kerr**-ah-**TOH**-sis): Any skin growth, such as a wart or a callus, in which there is overgrowth and thickening of the skin (plural, keratoses).

ketonuria (**kee**-toh-**NEW**-ree-ah): The presence of ketones in the urine.

kleptomania (**klep**-toh-**MAY**-nee-ah): A disorder characterized by repeatedly stealing objects neither for personal use nor for their monetary value.

koilonychia (**koy**-loh-**NICK**-ee-ah): A malformation of the nails in which the outer surface is concave or scooped out like the bowl of a spoon; also known as spoon nail.

KUB: A radiographic study of the kidneys, ureters, and bladder without the use of a contrast medium; also known as a flat-plate of the abdomen.

kyphosis (kye-**FOH**-sis): An abnormal increase in the outward curvature of the thoracic spine as viewed from the side; also known as humpback or dowager's hump.

L

labyrinthectomy (**lab**-ih-rin-**THECK**-toh-mee): The surgical removal of all or a portion of the labyrinth of the inner ear.

labyrinthitis (**lab**-ih-rin-**THIGH**-tis): Inflammation of the labyrinth that may result in vertigo and deafness.

labyrinthotomy (**lab**-ih-rin-**THOT**-oh-mee): A surgical incision between two of the fluid chambers of the labyrinth to allow the pressure to equalize.

laceration (**lass**-er-**AY**-shun): A torn, ragged wound or an accidental cut.

laminectomy (**lam**-ih-**NECK**-toh-mee): The surgical removal of a lamina from a vertebra.

laparoscopic adrenalectomy (ah-**dree**-nal-**ECK**-toh-mee): A minimally invasive procedure to surgically remove one or both adrenal glands.

laparoscopic cholecystectomy (**koh**-lee-sis-**TECK**-toh-mee): The surgical removal of the gallbladder using a laparoscope; also known as a lap choley.

laparoscopy (**lap**-ah-**ROS**-koh-pee): The visual examination of the interior of the abdomen with the use of a laparoscope.

laryngectomy (**lar**-in-**JECK**-toh-mee): The surgical removal of the larynx.

laryngitis (**lar**-in-**JIGH**-tis): Inflammation of the larynx.

laryngoplasty (lah-**RING**-goh-**plas**-tee): The surgical repair of the larynx.

laryngoplegia (**lar**-ing-goh-**PLEE**-jee-ah): Paralysis of the larynx.

laryngorrhagia (**lar**-ing-goh-**RAY**-jee-ah): Bleeding from the larynx.

laryngoscopy (**lar**-ing-**GOS**-koh-pee): The visual examination of the larynx using a laryngoscope

laryngospasm (lah-**RING**-goh-spazm): The sudden spasmodic closure of the larynx.

laser iridotomy (**ir**-ih-**DOT**-oh-mee): Treatment of closed-angle glaucoma in which a laser is used to create an opening in the iris to allow proper drainage.

laser trabeculoplasty (trah-**BECK**-you-loh-**plas**-tee): Treatment of open-angle glaucoma in which a laser is used to create an opening in the trabecular meshwork to allow fluid to drain properly.

LASIK: The acronym describing laser treatment of vision conditions that are caused by the shape of the cornea.

lateral projection: A radiographic projection that has the patient positioned at right angle to the film; also known as a side view.

legal blindness: The point at which, under law, an individual is considered to be blind.

leiomyoma (**lye**-oh-my-**OH**-mah): A benign tumor composed of muscle and fibrous tissue that occurs in the wall of the uterus; also known as a fibroid.

lensectomy (len-**SECK**-toh-mee): The surgical removal of a cataract-clouded lens.

lesion (**LEE**-zhun): A pathologic change of tissues due to disease or injury.

lethargy (**LETH**-ar-jee): A lowered level of consciousness marked by listlessness, drowsiness, and apathy.

leukemia (loo-**KEE**-mee-ah): A malignancy characterized by a progressive increase in the number of abnormal white blood cells found in hemopoietic tissues, other organs, and in the circulating blood.

leukorrhea (**loo**-koh-**REE**-ah): A profuse whitish mucus discharge from the uterus and vagina.

lipectomy (lih-**PECK**-toh-mee): The surgical removal of fat beneath the skin.

lipedema (lip-eh-**DEE**-mah): A chronic swelling caused by the collection of fat and fluid under the skin.

lipid tests: A blood test that measures the amounts of total cholesterol, high-density lipoprotein (HDL), low-density lipoprotein (LDL), and triglycerides; also known as a lipid panel.

lipoma (lih-**POH**-mah): A benign fatty deposit under the skin that causes a bump.

liposuction (**LIP**-oh-**suck**-shun *or* **LYE**-poh-**suck**-shun): The surgical removal of fat beneath the skin with the aid of suction; also known as suction-assisted lipectomy.

lithotomy (lih-**THOT**-oh-mee): A surgical incision for the removal of a stone, usually from the bladder.

lithotomy position (lih-**THOT**-oh-mee): An examination position in which the patient is supine with the feet and legs raised and supported in stirrups.

lithotripsy (**LITH**-oh-**trip**-see): The destruction of a kidney, urinary, or bladder stone with the use of high-energy ultrasonic waves traveling through water or gel; also known as extracorporeal shock-wave lithotripsy.

lobectomy (loh-**BECK**-toh-mee): The surgical removal of a lobe of the lung, liver, brain, or thyroid gland.

lordosis (lor-**DOH**-sis): An abnormal increase in the forward curvature of the lumbar spine; also known as swayback.

low-density lipoprotein cholesterol: The form of cholesterol that contributes to plaque buildup in the arteries; is also known as bad cholesterol.

lumbago (lum-**BAY**-goh): Pain of the lumbar region of the spine; also known as low back pain.

lumbar puncture: A procedure for obtaining a specimen of cerebrospinal fluid by inserting a needle into the subarachnoid space of the lumbar region; also known as a spinal tap.

lumbar radiculopathy: Nerve pain in the lower back.

lumpectomy: Surgical removal of only the cancerous tissue and a margin of surrounding normal breast tissue.

lupus erythematosus (**LOO**-pus er-ih-**thee**-mah-**TOH**-sus): An autoimmune disorder characterized by a red, scaly rash on the face and upper trunk that also attacks the connective tissue in other body systems; also known as systemic lupus erythematosus.

luxation (luck-**SAY**-shun): The total displacement of a bone from its joint; also known as dislocation.

Lyme disease: A bacterial infection caused by the spirochete *Borrelia burgdorferi* and transmitted to humans by the bite of an infected deer tick.

lymphadenectomy (lim-fad-eh-**NECK**-toh-mee): Surgical removal of a lymph node.

lymphadenitis (lim-**fad**-eh-**NIGH**-tis): Inflammation of the lymph nodes; also known as swollen glands.

lymphadenopathy (lim-**fad**-eh-**NOP**-ah-thee): Any disease process usually involving enlargement of the lymph nodes.

lymphangiogram (lim-**FAN**-jee-oh-**gram**): The record produced by lymphangiography.

lymphangiography (lim-**fan**-jee-**OG**-rah-fee): A radiographic examination of the lymphatic vessels after the injection of a contrast medium.

lymphangioma (lim-**fan**-jee-**OH**-mah): A benign tumor formed by an abnormal collection of lymphatic vessels.

lymphangiitis (lim-fan-**JIGH**-tis): Inflammation of the lymph vessels; also spelled *lymphangitis*.

lymphedema (**lim**-feh-**DEE**-mah): Swelling due to an abnormal accumulation of lymph within the tissues.

lymphedema, primary: A hereditary disorder in which swelling due to an abnormal accumulation of lymph within the tissues may appear at any time in life.

lymphedema, secondary: Swelling due to an abnormal accumulation of lymph within the tissues that is the result of the removal or destruction of lymph nodes or vessels, cancer treatments, burns, or trauma.

lymph node dissection: A diagnostic procedure in which all of the lymph nodes in a major group are removed to determine the spread of cancer.

lymphoma (lim-**FOH**-mah): A general term applied to malignancies that develop in the lymphatic system.

M

macular degeneration (**MACK**-you-lar): A progressive condition in which damages to the macula of the retina causes the loss of central vision; also known as age-related macular degeneration.

macule (**MACK**-youl): A discolored, flat spot, such as a freckle, that is less than 1 cm in diameter.

magnetic resonance angiography: A specialized MRI study using a contrast medium to locate problems with blood vessels throughout the body; also known as magnetic resonance angio or MRA.

magnetic resonance imaging: An imaging technique that uses a combination of radio waves and a strong magnetic field to create signals that are sent to a computer and converted into images of any plane through the body; also known as MRI.

malabsorption (**mal**-ab-**SORP**-shun): A condition in which the small intestine cannot absorb nutrients from the food passing through it.

malaria (mah-**LAY**-ree-ah): A disease caused by a parasite that lives within certain mosquitoes and is transferred to humans by the bite of an infected mosquito.

malignant: Harmful, tending to spread, becoming progressively worse, and life-threatening.

malignant hypertension: A condition characterized by the sudden onset of severely elevated blood pressure.

malingering (mah-**LING**-ger-ing): A condition characterized by the intentional creation of false or grossly exaggerated physical or psychological symptoms, motivated by external incentives, such as avoiding work.

malnutrition: A lack of proper food or nutrients in the body, due to either a shortage of food or the improper absorption or distribution of nutrients.

mammography (mam-**OG**-rah-fee): A radiographic screening examination of the breast to detect the presence of cancer.

mammoplasty (**MAM**-oh-**plas**-tee): Surgical repair or restructuring of the breast; also spelled mammaplasty.

manipulation: The attempted manual realignment of the bone involved in a fracture or joint dislocation; also known as closed reduction.

Mantoux PPD skin test: A diagnostic test for tuberculosis that is performed to confirm the results of a screening test.

mastalgia (mass-**TAL**-jee-ah): Pain in the breast; also known as mastodynia.

mastectomy (mas-**TECK**-toh-mee): Surgical removal of an entire breast.

mastitis (mas-**TYE**-tis): Inflammation of one or both breasts.

mastodynia (**mas**-toh-**DIN**-ee-ah): Pain in the breast.

mastoidectomy (**mas**-toy-**DECK**-toh-mee): The surgical removal of mastoid cells.

mastoiditis (**mas**-toy-**DYE**-tis): Inflammation of any part of the mastoid process.

mastopexy (**MAS**-toh-**peck**-see): Surgery to affix sagging breasts in a more elevated position.

maxillofacial surgery (mack-**sill**-oh-**FAY**-shul): Specialized surgery of the face and jaws to correct deformities, treat diseases, and repair injuries.

measles: An acute, highly contagious infection caused by the rubeola virus.

meatotomy (**mee**-ah-**TOT**-oh-mee): An incision of the urinary meatus to enlarge the opening.

megaloblastic anemia (**MEG**-ah-loh-**blas**-tick ah-**NEE**-mee-ah): A blood disorder in which red blood cells are larger than normal.

melanodermatitis (**mel**-ah-noh-**der**-mah-**TYE**-tis): Excess melanin present in an area of skin inflammation.

melanoma (mel-ah-**NOH**-mah): A type of skin cancer that occurs in the melanocytes; also known as malignant melanoma.

melanosis (**mel**-ah-**NOH**-sis): Any condition of unusual deposits of black pigment in different parts of the body.

melena (meh-**LEE**-nah *or* **MEL**-eh-nah): The passage of stools with a black and tarlike appearance that is caused by the presence of digested blood.

meningitis (**men**-in-**JIGH**-tis): Inflammation of the meninges of the brain or spinal cord.

meningocele (meh-**NING**-goh-**seel**): The congenital herniation of the meninges that surround the brain or spinal cord through a defect in the skull or spinal column.

meningoencephalitis (meh-**ning**-goh-en-**sef**-ah-**LYE**-tis): Inflammation of the meninges and brain.

meningoencephalomyelitis (meh-**ning**-goh-en-**sef**-ah-loh-**my**-eh-**LYE**-tis): Inflammation of the meninges, brain, and spinal cord.

meningomalacia (meh-**ning**-goh-mah-**LAY**-shee-ah): Abnormal softening of the meninges.

menometrorrhagia (**men**-oh-**met**-roh-**RAY**-jee-ah): Excessive uterine bleeding occurring both during the menses and at irregular intervals between periods.

menorrhagia (**men**-oh-**RAY**-jee-ah): An excessive amount of menstrual flow or flow over a period of more than seven days; also known as hypermenorrhea.

mental retardation: General intellectual functioning that is significantly below average and accompanied by a significant limitation in adaptive functioning.

metastasis (meh-**TAS**-tah-sis): The noun that describes a new cancer site that results from the spreading process (plural, metastases).

metastasize (meh-**TAS**-tah-sighz): The verb that describes the process by which cancer spreads from one place to another.

metered dose inhaler: A medical device that mixes a single dose of the medication with a puff of air and pushes it into the mouth via a chemical propellant.

metrorrhea (**mee**-troh-**REE**-ah): An abnormal discharge, such as mucus or pus, from the uterus.

migraine (**MY**-grayn): A headache syndrome characterized by sudden, throbbing, sharp pain that is usually more severe on one side of the head and is often accompanied by nausea and sensitivity to light or sound.

miliaria (**mill**-ee-**AYR**-ee-ah): An intensely itchy rash caused by blockage of the sweat glands by bacteria and dead cells; also known as heat rash and prickly heat.

minimally invasive direct coronary artery bypass: A bypass procedure performed with the aid of a fiberoptic camera through small openings between the ribs; also known as a keyhole or buttonhole bypass; also known as MIDCAB.

modified radical mastectomy: The surgical removal of the entire breast and axillary lymph nodes under the adjacent arm.

Mohs' surgery: A technique of excising skin tumors by removing tumor tissue, layer-by-layer, until the entire tumor has been removed.

moniliasis (mon-ih-**LYE**-ah-sis): Infections of the skin or mucous membranes caused by the pathogenic yeast *Candida albicans*.

monochromatism (**mon**-oh-**KROH**-mah-tizm): The inability to distinguish certain colors; also known as color blindness.

monoclonal antibodies: Medication to enhance a patient's immune response to some non-Hodgkin's lymphoma, melanoma, and breast and colon cancers.

morbid obesity: The condition of weighing two or three times, or more, the ideal weight; also known as clinically severe obesity.

multidrug-resistant tuberculosis: A dangerous form of tuberculosis in which the germs have become resistant to the effect of the primary TB drugs; also known as MDR-TB.

multiparous (mul-**TIP**-ah-rus): A woman who has given birth two or more times.

multiple dysplastic nevi (dis-**PLAS**-tick **NEE** vye): Atypical moles that may develop into skin cancer.

multiple sclerosis (skleh-**ROH**-sis): A progressive autoimmune disorder characterized by scattered patches of demyelination of nerve fibers of the brain and spinal cord.

mumps: An acute viral disease characterized by the swelling of the parotid glands.

muscle relaxant: Medication that acts on the central nervous system to relax the muscle tone and to relieve spasms of skeletal muscles.

muscular dystrophy (**DIS**-troh-fee): A group of more than 20 inherited muscle disorders that cause muscle weakness without affecting the nervous system.

myalgia (my-**AL**-jee-ah): Muscle tenderness or pain.

myasthenia gravis (**my**-as-**THEE**-nee-ah **GRAH**-vis): A chronic autoimmune disease that affects the neuromuscular junction and produces serious weakness of voluntary muscles.

mycoplasma pneumonia (**my**-koh-**PLAZ**-mah new-**MOH**-nee-ah): A milder but longer lasting form of pneumonia caused by the bacterium *Mycoplasma pneumoniae;* also known as atypical or walking pneumonia.

mycosis (my-**KOH**-sis): Any disease caused by a fungus.

mydriatic drops (**mid**-ree-**AT**-ick): Medication placed on the eyeball to produce temporary paralysis forcing the pupils to remain wide open even in the presence of bright light.

myectomy (my-**ECK**-toh-mee): Surgical removal of a portion of a muscle.

myelitis (**my**-eh-**LYE**-tis): Inflammation of the spinal cord; inflammation of bone marrow.

myelodysplastic syndrome (**my**-eh-loh-dis-**PLAS**-tick): A progressive condition of dysfunctional bone marrow that may eventually develop into leukemia; also known as preleukemia.

myelography (**my**-eh-**LOG**-rah-fee): A radiographic study of the spinal cord after the injection of a contrast medium through a lumbar puncture.

myeloma (my-eh-**LOH**-mah): A malignant tumor composed of blood-forming tissues of the bone marrow.

myelopathy (my-eh-**LOP**-ah-thee): Any pathologic condition of the spinal cord.

myelosis (my-eh-**LOH**-sis): A tumor of the spinal cord; an abnormal proliferation of bone marrow tissue.

myocardial infarction (**my**-oh-**KAR**-dee-al in-**FARK**-shun): The occlusion of one or more coronary arteries resulting in an infarct of the affected myocardium; also known as a heart attack or MI.

myocarditis (**my**-oh-kar-**DYE**-tis): Inflammation of the myocardium.

myocele (**MY**-oh-seel): The protrusion of a muscle through its ruptured sheath or fascia.

myoclonus (**my**-oh-**KLOH**-nus *or* my-**OCK**-loh-nus): A spasm or twitching of a muscle or group of muscles.

myofascial damage (**my**-oh-**FASH**-ee-ahl): Injury caused by overworking muscles that results in tenderness and swelling of the muscles and their surrounding fascia.

myolysis (my-**OL**-ih-sis): The deterioration or breaking down of muscle tissue.

myoma (my-**OH**-mah): A benign tumor made up of muscle tissue.

myomalacia (**my**-oh-mah-**LAY**-shee-ah): Abnormal softening of muscle tissue.

myonecrosis (**my**-oh-neh-**KROH**-sis): The death of individual muscle fibers.

myoparesis (**my**-oh-**PAR**-eh-sis): Weakness or slight paralysis of a muscle.

myopathy (my-**OP**-ah-thee): Any pathologic change or disease of muscle tissue.

myopia (my-**OH**-pee-ah): A defect in which light rays focus in front of the retina; also known as nearsightedness.

myoplasty (**MY**-oh-**plas**-tee): Surgical repair of a muscle.

myorrhaphy (my-**OR**-ah-fee): Surgical suturing a muscle wound.

myorrhexis (**my**-oh-**RECK**-sis): The rupture of a muscle.

myosarcoma (**my**-oh-sahr-**KOH**-mah): A malignant tumor derived from muscle tissue.

myosclerosis (**my**-oh-skleh-**ROH**-sis): Abnormal hardening of muscle tissue.

myositis (**my**-oh-**SIGH**-tis): Inflammation of a skeletal muscle.

myotomy (my-**OT**-oh-mee): A surgical incision into, or division of, a muscle.

myotonia (**my**-oh-**TOH**-nee-ah): The delayed relaxation of a muscle after a strong contraction.

myringitis (**mir**-in-**JIGH**-tis): Inflammation of the tympanic membrane.

myringotomy (**mir**-in-**GOT**-oh-mee): A surgical incision of the eardrum to create an opening for the placement of tympanostomy tubes.

myxedema (**mick**-seh-**DEE**-mah): A severe form of adult hypothyroidism.

N

narcolepsy (**NAR**-koh-**lep**-see): A sleep disorder consisting of recurring episodes of falling asleep during the day.

narcotic analgesics: Medication to relieve severe pain that may cause physical dependence or addiction.

nasogastric intubation (nay-zoh-**GAS**-trick **in**-too-**BAY**-shun): The placement of a tube through the nose and into the stomach.

nausea (**NAW**-see-ah): The sensation that leads to the urge to vomit.

nebulizer (**NEB**-you-lye-zer): A medical device that dispenses medication in the form of a mist that is inhaled via a face mask or mouthpiece.

necrotizing fasciitis (fas-ee-**EYE**-tis) (**NF**): An infection caused by group A strep that enters the body through a wound. If untreated, the infected body tissue can be destroyed and the illness may be fatal; also known as flesh-eating bacteria.

needle breast biopsy: A diagnostic technique in which an x-ray guided needle is used to remove small samples of tissue from the breast.

neoplasm (**NEE**-oh-plazm): A new and abnormal tissue formation in which the multiplication of cells is uncontrolled, abnormally rapid, and progressive; also known as a tumor.

nephrectasis (neh-**FRECK**-tah-sis): The distention of a kidney.

nephrectomy (neh-**FRECK**-toh-mee): Surgical removal of a kidney.

nephritis (neh-**FRY**-tis): Inflammation of the kidney.

nephrolith (**NEF**-roh-lith): A stone located in the kidney; also known as renal calculus or a kidney stone.

nephrolithiasis (**nef**-roh-lih-**THIGH**-ah-sis): A disorder characterized by the presence of a stone or stones in the kidney.

nephrolysis (neh-**FROL**-ih-sis): The freeing of a kidney from adhesions.

nephromalacia (nef-roh-mah-**LAY**-shee-ah): Abnormal softening of the kidney.

nephropathy (neh-**FROP**-ah-thee): Any disease of the kidney

nephropexy (**NEF**-roh-**peck**-see): The surgical fixation of a floating kidney.

nephroptosis (**nef**-rop-**TOH**-sis): The downward displacement of a kidney; also known as a floating kidney.

nephropyosis (**nef**-roh-pye-**OH**-sis): Suppuration of the kidney.

nephrosclerosis (**nef**-roh-skleh-**ROH**-sis): Abnormal hardening of the kidney.

nephrosis (neh-**FROH**-sis): Any degenerative kidney disease causing nephrotic syndrome *without* inflammation.

nephrostomy (neh-**FROS**-toh-mee): The establishment of an opening between the pelvis of the kidney and the exterior of the body.

nephrotic syndrome (neh-**FROT**-ick): A condition in which very high levels of protein are lost in the urine and low levels of protein are present in the blood.

nephrotomy (neh-**FROT**-oh-mee): A surgical incision into the kidney.

neuralgia (new-**RAL**-jee-ah): Pain in a nerve or nerves.

neuritis (new-**RYE**-tis): Inflammation of a nerve or nerves.

neuroma (new-**ROH**-mah): A benign tumor made up nerve tissue.

neuromalacia (**new**-roh-mah-**LAY**-shee-ah): Abnormal softening of a nerve or nerves.

neuromuscular blocker: A medication that causes temporary paralysis by blocking the transmission of nerve stimuli to the muscles; also known as a neuromuscular blocking agent.

neuropathy (new-**ROP**-ah-thee): Damage to the nerves.

neuroplasty (**NEW**-roh-**plas**-tee): The surgical repair of a nerve or nerves.

neurorrhaphy (new-**ROR**-ah-fee): Surgically suturing together the ends of a severed nerve.

neurotomy (new-**ROT**-oh-mee): A surgical incision into, or the dissection of, a nerve.

nevi (**NEE**-vye): Small dark skin growths that develop from melanocytes in the skin (singular, nevus); also known as moles.

nitroglycerin: A vasodilator that is prescribed to relieve the pain of angina pectoris.

nocturia (nock-**TOO**-ree-ah): Excessive urination during the night.

nocturnal enuresis: The involuntary discharge of urine during sleep; also known as bed-wetting.

nocturnal myoclonus (nock-**TER**-nal **my**-oh-**KLOH**-nus *or* my-**OCK**-loh-nus): Jerking of the limbs that may occur normally as a person is falling asleep.

nodule: A solid raised skin lesion that is larger than 0.5 cm in diameter and deeper than a papule.

noise-induced hearing loss: Nerve deafness caused by damage due to repeated exposure to very intense noise.

non-Hodgkin's lymphoma (non-**HODJ**-kinz lim-**FOH**-mah): The term used to describe all lymphomas *other than* Hodgkin's lymphoma.

nonnarcotic analgesics: Medications to control mild to moderate pain that do not cause physical dependence or addiction.

nonsteroidal anti-inflammatory drugs: Medications administered to control pain and to reduce inflammation and swelling; also known as NSAIDs.

nosocomial infection (**nos**-oh-**KOH**-mee-al): An infection acquired in a hospital or clinic.

nuclear scan: A diagnostic procedure that uses nuclear medicine technology to gather information about the structure and function of organs or systems.

nulligravida (**null**-ih-**GRAV**-ih-dah): A woman who has never been pregnant.

nullipara (nuh-**LIP**-ah-rah): A woman who has never borne a viable child.

nyctalopia (**nick**-tah-**LOH**-pee-ah): A condition in which an individual with normal daytime vision has difficulty seeing at night; also known as night blindness.

nystagmus (nis-**TAG**-mus): An involuntary, constant, rhythmic movement of the eyeball.

O

obesity (oh-**BEE**-sih-tee): An excessive accumulation of fat in the body.

oblique fracture: A fracture that occurs at an angle across the bone.

obsessive-compulsive disorder: A mental condition characterized by obsessions and/or compulsions that are recurrent, persistent, and excessive.

ocular prosthesis: A replacement for an eyeball that is either congenitally missing or has been surgically removed.

oligomenorrhea (ol-ih-goh-**men**-oh-**REE**-ah): Light or infrequent menstrual flow.

oligospermia (ol-ih-goh-**SPER**-mee-ah): An abnormally low number of sperm in the semen; also known as a low sperm count.

oliguria (ol-ih-**GOO**-ree-ah): Scanty urination.

onychectomy (on-ih-**KECK**-toh-mee): Surgical removal of a fingernail or toenail.

onychia (oh-**NICK**-ee-ah): Inflammation of the matrix of the nail; also known as onychitis.

onychitis (on-ih-**KYE**-tis): Inflammation of the matrix of the nail; also known as onychia.

onychocryptosis (on-ih-koh-krip-**TOH**-sis) Ingrown toenail.

onychoma (on-ih-**KOH**-mah): A tumor arising from the nail bed.

onychomalacia (on-ih-koh-mah-**LAY**-shee-ah): Abnormal softening of the nails.

onychomycosis (on-ih-koh-my-**KOH**-sis): A fungal infection of the nail.

onychophagia (on-ih-koh-**FAY**-jee-ah): Nail biting or nail eating.

oophorectomy (**oh**-ahf-oh-**RECK**-toh-mee): The surgical removal of an ovary; also known as an ovariectomy.

oophoritis (**oh**-ahf-oh-**RYE**-tis): Inflammation of an ovary.

oophoropexy (oh-**AHF**-oh-roh-**peck**-see): Surgical fixation of a displaced ovary.

oophoroplasty (oh-**AHF**-oh-roh-**plas**-tee): Surgical repair of an ovary.

open fracture: A fracture in which the bone is broken and there is an open wound in the skin; also known as a compound fracture.

open reduction internal fixation: The treatment of a fracture in which pins, or a plate, are placed directly into the bone to hold the broken pieces in place; also known as internal fixation.

ophthalmoscope (ahf-**THAL**-moh-skope): An instrument used to examine the interior of the eye.

ophthalmoscopy (ahf-thal-**MOS**-koh-pee): The visual examination of the fundus of the eye with ophthalmoscope; also known as funduscopy.

oral administration: Medication taken by mouth to be absorbed from the stomach or small intestine.

oral glucose tolerance test (**GLOO**-kohs): A series of blood tests that is performed to confirm a diagnosis of diabetes mellitus and to aid in diagnosing hypoglycemia.

oral hypoglycemics: Medications that lower blood sugar by causing the body to release more insulin.

oral rehydration therapy: Treatment to counteract the dehydration in which a solution of electrolytes is administered in a liquid preparation.

oral thrush: An infection in infants characterized by white spots inside the mouth that is cause by the fungus *Candida albicans*.

orbitotomy (or-bih-**TOT**-oh-mee): A surgical incision into the orbit for biopsy, abscess drainage, or the removal of a tumor or foreign object.

orchidectomy (or-kih-**DECK**-toh-mee): The surgical removal of one or both testicles; also known as an orchiectomy.

orchiectomy (**or**-kih-**ECK**-toh-mee): The surgical removal of one or both testicles; also known as an orchidectomy.

orchitis (or-**KYE**-tis): Inflammation of one or both testicles; also known as testitis.

organic disorder (or-**GAN**-ick): A pathological condition in which there are physical changes to explain the symptoms being experienced by the patient.

orthostatic hypotension (**or**-thoh-**STAT**-ick **high**-poh-**TEN**-shun): Low blood pressure that occurs in a standing posture; also known as postural hypotension.

ostealgia (**oss**-tee-**AL**-jee-ah): Pain in a bone; also spelled ostalgia or known as osteodynia.

ostectomy (oss-**TECK**-toh-mee): The surgical removal of bone.

osteitis (**oss**-tee-**EYE**-tis): Inflammation of bone; also spelled ostitis.

osteitis deformans (**oss**-tee-**EYE**-tis dee-**FOR**-manz): A disease of unknown cause that is characterized by extensive bone destruction followed by abnormal bone repair; also known as Paget's disease.

osteoarthritis (**oss**-tee-oh-ar-**THRIGH**-tis): The type of arthritis most commonly associated with aging; also known as wear-and-tear arthritis.

osteoarthropathy (**oss**-tee-oh-ar-**THROP**-ah-thee): Any disease involving the bones and joints.

osteochondroma (**oss**-tee-oh-kon-**DROH**-mah): A benign bone tumor characterized by a cartilage-capped bony growth that projects from the surface of the affected bone; also known as an exostosis.

osteoclasis (**oss**-tee-**OCK**-lah-sis): The surgical fracture of a bone to correct a deformity.

osteomalacia (**oss**-tee-oh-mah-**LAY**-shee-ah): Abnormal softening of bones in adults; also known as adult rickets.

osteomyelitis (**oss**-tee-oh-**my**-eh-**LYE**-tis): Inflammation of the bone marrow and adjacent bone.

osteonecrosis (**oss**-tee-oh-neh-**KROH**-sis): The death of bone tissue due to an insufficient blood supply, infection, malignancy, or trauma.

osteopenia (**oss**-tee-oh-**PEE**-nee-ah): Thinner-than-average bone density in a young person.

osteoplasty (**OSS**-tee-oh-**plas**-tee): The surgical repair of a bone or bones.

osteoporosis (**oss**-tee-oh-poh-**ROH**-sis): A marked loss of bone density and an increase in bone porosity that is frequently associated with aging.

osteoporotic hip fracture (**oss**-tee-oh-pah-**ROT**-ick): A fracture of a hip weaken by osteoporosis that can occur spontaneously or as the result of a fall.

osteorrhaphy (**oss**-tee-**OR**-ah-fee): Surgical suturing, or wiring together, of bones.

osteosarcoma (**oss**-tee-oh-sar-**KOH**-mah): A malignant tumor usually involving the upper shaft of long bones, the pelvis, or knee.

osteosclerosis (**oss**-tee-oh-skleh-**ROH**-sis): Abnormal hardening of bone.

osteotomy (**oss**-tee-**OT**-oh-mee): A surgical incision or sectioning of a bone.

ostomy (**OSS**-toh-mee): A surgical procedure to create an artificial opening between an organ and the body surface.

otalgia (oh-**TAL**-gee-ah): Pain in the ear; also known as an earache.

otitis (oh-**TYE**-tis): Inflammation of the ear.

otitis media (oh-**TYE**-tis **MEE**-dee-ah): Inflammation of the middle ear.

otomycosis (**oh**-toh-my-**KOH**-sis): A fungal infection of the external auditory canal, also known as swimmer's ear.

otoplasty (**OH**-toh-**plas**-tee): Surgical repair of the pinna of the ear.

otopyorrhea (**oh**-toh-**pye**-oh-**REE**-ah): The flow of pus from the ear.

otorrhagia (**oh**-toh-**RAY**-jee-ah): Bleeding from the ear.

otosclerosis (**oh**-toh-skleh-**ROH**-sis): Ankylosis of the bones of the middle ear resulting in a conductive hearing loss.

otoscope (**OH**-toh-skope): An instrument used to visually examine the external ear canal and tympanic membrane.

ovarian cancer: Cancer that begins within the cells of the ovaries.

ovariectomy (**oh**-vay-ree-**ECK**-toh-mee): The surgical removal of an ovary; also known as an oophorectomy.

ovariorrhexis (**oh**-**vay**-ree-oh-**RECK**-sis): The rupture of an ovary.

overactive bladder: A condition that occurs when the detrusor muscle in the wall of the bladder is too active.

over-the-counter drug: Medication that may be dispensed without a written prescription.

overuse injuries: Injuries that occur when minor tissue injuries resulting from overuse have not been given time to heal.

P

pacemaker: An electronic device attached externally or implanted under the skin to regulate the heartbeat.

Paget's disease (**PAJ**-its): A disease of unknown cause that is characterized by extensive bone destruction followed by abnormal bone repair: also known as osteitis deformans.

palatoplasty (**PAL**-ah-toh-**plas**-tee): Surgical repair of a cleft palate.

palliative (**PAL**-ee-**ay**-tiv *or* **PAL**-ee-ah-tiv): A substance that eases the pain or severity of a disease but does not cure it.

palpation (pal-**PAY**-shun): An examination technique in which the examiner's hands are used to feel the texture, size, consistency, and location of certain body parts.

palpitation (**pal**-pih-**TAY**-shun): A pounding or racing heart with or without irregularity in rhythm.

pancreatalgia (**pan**-kree-ah-**TAL**-jee-ah): Pain in the pancreas.

pancreatectomy (**pan**-kree-ah-**TECK**-toh-mee): Surgical removal of the pancreas.

pancreatitis (**pan**-kree-ah-**TYE**-tis): Inflammation of the pancreas.

pancreatotomy (**pan**-kree-ah-**TOT**-oh-mee): A surgical incision into the pancreas.

panic disorder: A condition characterized by having more than one panic attack, resulting in persistent fear of the attacks.

Papanicolaou test (**pap**-ah-**nick**-oh-**LAY**-ooh): An exfoliative biopsy to screen for early indications of cervical cancer; also known as a Pap smear.

papilledema (**pap**-ill-eh-**DEE**-mah): Swelling and inflammation of the optic nerve at the point of entrance into the eye through the optic disk; also known as choked disk.

papilloma (**pap**-ih-**LOH**-mah): A benign, superficial wartlike growth on the epithelial tissue or elsewhere in the body, such as in the bladder.

papule (**PAP**-youl): A small, raised red lesion, such as an insect bite, that is less than 0.5 cm in diameter.

paradoxical drug reaction: The effect caused by a medication that is the exact opposite of that which was therapeutically intended.

paralysis (pah-**RAL**-ih-sis): The loss of sensation and voluntary muscle movements in a muscle through disease or injury to its nerve supply (plural, paralyses).

paraplegia (**par**-ah-**PLEE**-jee-ah): Paralysis of both legs and the lower part of the body.

paraspadias (**par**-ah-**SPAY**-dee-as): A congenital abnormality in males in which the urethral opening is on one side of the penis.

parathyroidectomy (**par**-ah-**thigh**-roi-**DECK**-toh-mee): Surgical removal of one or more of the parathyroid glands.

parenteral administration (pah-**REN**-ter-al): The administration of medication by injection through a hypodermic syringe.

paresthesia (**par**-es-**THEE**-zee-ah): An abnormal sensation, such as burning or prickling, in the extremities that may be caused by a wide range of neurological diseases or nerve damage.

Parkinson's disease: A chronic, degenerative central nervous system disorder in which there is a progressive loss of control over movement resulting in tremors and a shuffling gait.

paronychia (**par**-oh-**NICK**-ee-ah): An infection of the skin fold around a nail.

paroxysmal atrial tachycardia (**par**-ock-**SIZ**-mal **tack**-ee-**KAR**-dee-ah): An episode that begins and ends abruptly during which there are very rapid and regular heartbeats that originate in the atrium.

pathogen (**PATH**-oh-jen): A microorganism that causes a disease.

patulous eustachian tube (**PAT**-you-lus): Distention of the eustachian tube.

peak flow meter: A handheld device often used to measure how quickly a person with asthma can expel air.

pediculosis (pee-**dick**-you-**LOH**-sis): An infestation with lice.

pelvic inflammatory disease: Any inflammation of the female reproductive organs not associated with surgery or pregnancy.

pelvimetry (pel-**VIM**-eh-tree): A radiographic study to measure the dimensions of the pelvis to determine its capacity to allow passage of the fetus through the birth canal.

peptic ulcers (**UL**-serz): Erosions of the mucous membranes of the digestive system.

percussion (per-**KUSH**-un): A diagnostic procedure to determine the density of a body area that uses the sound produced by tapping the surface with the finger or an instrument.

percutaneous diskectomy (**per**-kyou-**TAY**-nee-us dis-**KECK**-toh-mee): Treatment of a herniated disk that

polyarteritis (**pol**-ee-**ar**-teh-**RYE**-tis): Inflammation of several arteries.

polyarthritis (**pol**-ee-ar-**THRIGH**-tis): Inflammation of more than one joint.

polycystic kidney disease (**pol**-ee-**SIS**-tick): An inherited kidney disorder in which the kidneys become enlarged because of multiple cysts.

polycystic ovary syndrome (**pol**-ee-**SIS**-tick): Enlargement of the ovaries caused by the presence of many cysts formed by incompletely developed follicles; also known as Stein-Leventhal syndrome.

polydipsia (**pol**-ee-**DIP**-see-ah): Excessive thirst.

polymenorrhea (**pol**-ee-**men**-oh-**REE**-ah): Abnormally frequent menstruation.

polymyalgia (pol-ee-my-AL-jee-ah): Pain in several muscle groups.

polymyositis (**pol**-ee-**my**-oh-**SIGH**-tis): Inflammation of several skeletal muscles at the same time.

polyneuritis (**pol**-ee-new-**RYE**-tis): Inflammation affecting many nerves.

polyp (**POL**-ip): A mushroom-like growth from the surface of a mucous membrane.

polyphagia (**pol**-ee-**FAY**-jee-ah): Excessive hunger.

polysomnography (**pol**-ee-som-**NOG**-rah-fee): The diagnostic measurement of physiological activity during sleep; also known as a sleep apnea study.

polyuria (**pol**-ee-**YOU**-ree-ah): Excessive urination.

port-wine stain: A large, reddish purple discoloration of the face or neck; also known as a birthmark.

positive pressure ventilation: Treatment of sleep apnea by pumping a steady supply of air into the nose all night through a tube and mask.

positron emission tomography: An imaging technique that combines tomography with radionuclide tracers to produce enhanced images of selected body organs or areas.

posttraumatic stress disorder: The development of characteristic symptoms after a major traumatic event.

postural drainage: A procedure in which the patient is tilted head or chest downward to allow gravity to help drain secretions from the lungs.

potentiation (poh-**ten**-shee-**AY**-shun): A drug interaction that occurs when the effect of one drug is increased by another drug; also known as synergism.

preeclampsia (**pree**-ee-**KLAMP**-see-ah): A complication of pregnancy characterized by hypertension, edema, and proteinuria; also known as toxemia or pregnancy-induced hypertension (PIH).

pregnancy test: A diagnostic test to is determine if a woman is pregnant.

premature ejaculation: A condition in which the male reaches climax too soon, usually before, or shortly after, penetration.

premature infant: A neonate born before the thirty-seventh week of gestation; also known as a preemie.

premature menopause: A condition in which the ovaries cease functioning before age 40.

premenstrual dysphoric disorder: A condition associated with severe emotional and physical problems linked to the menstrual cycle.

premenstrual syndrome: A group of symptoms experienced by some women within the two-week period before menstruation.

presbycusis (**pres**-beh-**KOO**-sis): A gradual sensorineural hearing loss that occurs as the body ages.

presbyopia (**pres**-bee-**OH**-pee-ah): Changes in the eyes that are commonly associated with aging.

prescription: An order for medication, therapy, or a therapeutic device that is given by one authorized person to another authorized person to properly dispense or perform the order.

priapism (**PRYE**-ah-**piz**-em): A painful erection lasting four hours or more, not accompanied by sexual excitement.

primary aldosteronism: An abnormality of electrolyte balance caused by disorders of the adrenal glands; also known as Conn's syndrome.

primary lymphedema: A hereditary disorder in which swelling due to an abnormal accumulation of lymph within the tissues may appear at any time in life.

primigravida (**prye**-mih-**GRAV**-ih-dah): A woman during her first pregnancy.

primipara (prye-**MIP**-ah-rah): A woman who has borne one viable child.

proctalgia (prock-**TAL**-jee-ah): Pain in and around the anus and rectum.

proctectomy (prock-**TECK**-toh-mee): Surgical removal of the rectum.

proctopexy (**PROCK**-toh-**peck**-see): Surgical fixation of a prolapsed rectum to an adjacent tissue or organ.

proctoplasty (**PROCK**-toh-**plas**-tee): Surgical repair of the rectum.

prolactinoma (proh-**lack**-tih-**NOH**-mah): A benign tumor of the pituitary gland that causes it to produce too much prolactin; also known as a prolactin-producing adenoma.

prophylaxis (**proh**-fih-**LACK**-sis): Professional cleaning of the teeth to remove plaque and tartar; also treatment, such as vaccination, intended to prevent a disease or stop it from spreading.

prostatectomy (**pros**-tah-**TECK**-toh-mee): Surgical removal of all or part of the prostate gland.

prostate-specific antigen: A diagnostic blood test that is used to screen for prostate cancer.

prostatitis (**pros**-tah-**TYE**-tis): Inflammation of the prostate gland.

prostatomegaly (**pros**-tah-toh-**MEG**-ah-lee): An abnormal enlargement of the prostate gland; also known as benign prostatic hypertrophy or an enlarged prostate.

prosthesis (pros-**THEE**-sis): A substitute for a diseased or missing part of the body.

proteinuria (**proh**-tee-in-**YOU**-ree-ah): The presence of an abnormal amount of protein in the urine.

prothrombin time (proh-**THROM**-bin): A blood test used to diagnose conditions associated with abnormal bleeding and to monitor anticoagulant therapy; also known as pro time.

pruritus (proo-**RYE**-tus): Itching.

pruritus vulvae (proo-**RYE**-tus **VUL**-vee): Severe itching of the external female genitalia.

pseudophakia (**soo**-doh-**FAY**-kee-ah): An eye in which the natural lens has been replaced with an intraocular lens.

psoriasis (soh-**RYE**-uh-sis): A skin disorder characterized by flare-ups in which red papules covered with silvery scales occur on the elbows, knees, scalp, back, or buttocks.

psychoanalysis (**sigh**-koh-ah-**NAL**-ih-sis): Treatment based on the concept that mental disorders have underlying causes stemming from childhood and can only be overcome by gaining insight into one's feelings and patterns of behavior.

psychotic disorder (sigh-**KOT**-ick): A condition characterized by the loss of contact with reality and deterioration of normal social functioning.

psychotropic drugs (**sigh**-koh-**TROP**-pick): Drugs that are capable of affecting the mind, emotions, and behavior and are used in the treatment of mental illness.

pterygium (teh-**RIJ**-ee-um): A noncancerous growth that develops on the cornea and may grow large enough to distort vision.

pulmonary edema (eh-**DEE**-mah): An accumulation of fluid in the lung tissues.

pulmonary fibrosis (figh-**BROH**-sis): The formation of scar tissue in the lung, resulting in decreased lung capacity and increased difficulty in breathing.

pulmonary function tests: A group of tests used to measure the capacity of the lungs to hold air as well as their ability to move air in and out and to exchange oxygen and carbon dioxide.

pulse oximeter (ock-**SIM**-eh-ter): An external monitor that measures the oxygen saturation level in the blood.

puncture wound: A deep hole made by a sharp object such as a nail.

purpura (**PUR**-pew-rah): A condition that causes spontaneous bruises that are 2 mm to 10 mm in diameter, as well as hemorrhages in the internal organs and other tissues.

purulent (**PYOU**-roo-lent): Producing or containing pus.

pustule (**PUS**-tyoul): A small, circumscribed lesion containing pus; also known as a pimple.

putrefaction (**pyou**-treh-**FACK**-shun): Decay that produces foul-smelling odors.

pyelitis (**pye**-eh-**LYE**-tis): Inflammation of the renal pelvis.

pyelonephritis (**pye**-eh-loh-neh-**FRY**-tis): Inflammation of the renal pelvis and of the kidney.

pyeloplasty (**PYE**-eh-loh-**plas**-tee): The surgical repair of the renal pelvis.

pyelotomy (**pye**-eh-**LOT**-oh-mee): A surgical incision into the renal pelvis.

pyemia (pye-**EE**-mee-ah): The presence of pus-forming organisms in the blood.

pyoderma (**pye**-oh-**DER**-mah): Any acute, inflammatory, pus-forming bacterial skin infection such as impetigo.

pyosalpinx (**pye**-oh-**SAL**-pinks): An accumulation of pus in the fallopian tube.

pyothorax (**pye**-oh-**THOH**-racks): An accumulation of pus in the pleural cavity; also known as empyema.

pyromania (**pye**-roh-**MAY**-nee-ah): A disorder characterized by repeated, deliberate fire setting.

pyrosis (pye-**ROH**-sis): The burning sensation caused by the return of acidic stomach contents into the esophagus; also known as heartburn.

pyuria (pye-**YOU**-ree-ah): The presence of pus in the urine.

Q

quadriplegia (**kwad**-rih-**PLEE**-jee-ah): Paralysis of all four extremities.

R

rabies (**RAY**-beez): A viral infection transmitted to humans by the blood, tissue, or saliva of an infected animal.

radial keratotomy (**ker**-ah-**TOT**-oh-mee): A surgical procedure to correct myopia.

radiation therapy: The treatment of cancers through the use of x-rays.

radiculitis (rah-**dick**-you-**LYE**-tis): Inflammation of the root of a spinal nerve; also known as a pinched nerve.

radiograph: The image produced by the use of radiant energy to visualize conditions such as bone fractures; also known as x-rays.

radiography: The use of x-radiation to visualize hard-tissue internal structures.

radioimmunoassay (**ray**-dee-oh-**im**-you-noh-**ASS**-ay): A laboratory technique in which a radioactively labeled substance is mixed with a blood specimen; also known as radioassay.

radiology (**ray**-dee-**OL**-oh-jee): The use of radiant energy and radioactive substances in medicine for diagnosis and treatment.

radiolucent (**ray**-dee-oh-**LOO**-sent): A substance that allows x-rays to pass through and appears black or dark gray on the resulting film.

radionuclide tracer: A radioactive substance that is specific to the body system being examined; also known as a radioactive tracer.

radiopaque (**ray**-dee-oh-**PAYK**): A substance that does not allow x-rays to pass through and appears white or light gray on the resulting film.

rale (**RAHL**): An abnormal rattle or crackle-like respiratory sound heard while breathing in.

range of motion testing: A diagnostic procedure to evaluate joint mobility and muscle strength.

Raynaud's phenomenon (ray-**NOHZ**): Intermittent attacks of pallor, cyanosis, and redness of the fingers and toes.

rectal administration: The insertion of medication into the rectum as either suppositories or liquid solutions.

red blood cell count: A blood test that is performed to determine the number of erythrocytes in the blood.

refraction: An examination procedure to determine an eye's refractive error and the best corrective lenses to be prescribed.

refractive disorder: A focusing problem caused when the lens and cornea do not bend light so that it focuses properly on the retina.

regurgitation (ree-**gur**-jih-**TAY**-shun): The return of swallowed food into the mouth.

renal colic (**REE**-nal **KOLL**-ick): Acute pain in the kidney area that is caused by blockage during the passage of a kidney stone.

renal failure: The inability of one or both of the kidneys to perform their functions; also known as kidney failure.

renal transplantation: The grafting of a donor kidney into the body to replace the recipient's failed kidneys; also known as a kidney transplant.

repetitive motion disorders: A variety of muscular conditions that result from repeated motions performed in the course of normal activities; also known as repetitive stress disorders.

respirator: A machine used for prolonged artificial respiration when the patient is unable to breathe without assistance.

retinal detachment: Pulling away of the retina from its normal position of being attached to the choroid in the back of the eye; also known as a detached retina.

retinitis (**ret**-ih-**NIGH**-tis): Inflammation of the retina.

retinopathy (**ret**-ih-**NOP**-ah-thee): Any disease of the retina.

retinopexy (**RET**-ih-noh-**peck**-see): Treatment to reattach the detached area in a retinal detachment.

retrograde urography: A radiographic study of the urinary system taken after dye has been placed in the urethra and caused to flow upward through the urinary tract.

Reye's syndrome: A condition that has been linked to giving aspirin to children suffering from viral infections; affects all organs of the body but is most harmful to the brain and the liver and is potentially fatal.

rheumatoid arthritis (**ROO**-mah-toyd ar-**THRIGH**-tis): An autoimmune disorder in which the synovial membranes, and other body tissues, are inflamed and thickened.

rhinitis (rye-**NIGH**-tis): Inflammation of the nose.

rhinophyma (**rye**-noh-**FIGH**-muh): Hyperplasia of the tissues of the nose; also known as bulbous nose.

rhinoplasty (**RYE**-noh-**plas**-tee): Plastic surgery to change the shape or size of the nose.

rhinorrhea (**rye**-noh-**REE**-ah): An excessive flow of mucus from the nose; also known as a runny nose.

rhonchus (**RONG**-kus): An added musical sound occurring during breathing that is caused by a partially obstructed airway (plural, rhonchi); also known as wheezing.

rhytidectomy (**rit**-ih-**DECK**-toh-mee): The surgical removal of excess skin and fat for the elimination of wrinkles; also known as a facelift.

rickets (**RICK**-ets): A disorder occurring in children involving softening and weakening of the bones primarily caused by lack of Vitamin D, calcium, or phosphate.

Rocky Mountain spotted fever: A bacterial infection caused by *Rickettsia rickettsii* and transmitted to humans by the bite of an infected tick.

rosacea (roh-**ZAY**-shee-ah): A chronic condition of unknown cause that produces redness, tiny pimples, and broken blood vessels.

rotator cuff tendinitis (**ten**-dih-**NIGH**-tis): Inflammation of the tendons of the rotator cuff of the shoulder.

rubella (roo-**BELL**-ah): A viral infection characterized by fever and a diffuse, fine, red rash; also known as German measles or 3-day measles.

S

salmonella (**sal**-moh-**NEL**-ah): Severe diarrhea, nausea, and vomiting accompanied by a high fever that are caused by the bacteria *Salmonella.*

salpingectomy (**sal**-pin-**JECK**-toh-mee): Surgical removal of a fallopian tube.

salpingitis (**sal**-pin-**JIGH**-tis): Inflammation of a fallopian tube.

salpingo-oophorectomy (sal-**ping**-goh oh-**ahf**-oh-**RECK**-toh-mee): The surgical removal of a fallopian tube and ovary.

sarcoma (sar-**KOH**-mah): A malignant tumor that arises from connective tissue (plural, sarcomas or sarcomata).

sarcopenia (**sar**-koh-**PEE**-nee-ah): The age-related reduction in skeletal muscle mass in the elderly.

SARS: A sometimes fatal viral respiratory disorder that begins with a fever and progresses to a dry nonproductive cough, dyspnea, or hypoxemia; full name severe acute respiratory syndrome.

scabies (**SKAY**-beez): A skin infection caused by an infestation with the itch mite that produces distinctive brown lines and an itchy rash.

scales: Flakes or dry patches made up of excess dead epidermal cells.

schizophrenia (**skit**-soh-**FREE**-nee-ah): A psychotic disorder characterized by two or more of the following: delusions, hallucinations, disorganized speech, disorganized or catatonic behavior, and/or negative symptoms.

sciatica (sigh-**AT**-ih-kah): Inflammation of the sciatic nerve.

scintigram (**SIN**-tih-gram): A nuclear medicine diagnostic procedure to gather information about the structure and function of organs or systems that cannot be seen on conventional x-rays; also known as a nuclear scan.

scleritis (skleh-**RYE**-tis): Inflammation of the sclera of the eye.

scleroderma (**sklehr**-oh-**DER**-mah): An autoimmune disorder in which the connective tissues become thickened and hardened, causing the skin to become hard and swollen.

sclerotherapy (**sklehr**-oh-**THER**-ah-pee): Treatment involving injections of a sclerosing solution to cause spider veins to collapse and disappear.

scoliosis (**skoh**-lee-**OH**-sis): An abnormal lateral curvature of the spine.

scotoma (skoh-**TOH**-mah): An abnormal area of absent or depressed vision surrounded by an area of normal vision; also known as blind spot.

scratch test: A diagnostic test to identify commonly troublesome allergens such as tree pollen and ragweed.

sebaceous cyst (seh-**BAY**-shus): A sebaceous gland containing yellow, fatty material.

seborrhea (**seb**-oh-**REE**-ah): Any of several common skin conditions in which there is an overproduction of sebum:

seborrheic dermatitis (**seb**-oh-**REE**-ick **der**-mah-**TYE**-tis): Inflammation that causes scaling and itching of the upper layers of the skin or scalp.

seborrheic keratosis (**seb**-oh-**REE**-ick **kerr**-ah-**TOH**-sis): A benign skin growth that has a waxy or "pasted-on" look. These growths, which can vary in color from light tan to black, occur most commonly in the elderly.

secondary aldosteronism: An abnormality of electrolyte balance that is not caused by a disorder of the adrenal gland.

secondary hypertension: Elevated blood pressure caused by a different medical problem, such as a kidney disorder or a tumor on the adrenal glands.

secondary lymphedema: Swelling due to an abnormal accumulation of lymph within the tissues that is the result of the removal or destruction of lymph nodes or vessels, cancer treatments, burns, or trauma.

sedative: Medication that depresses the central nervous system to produce calm and diminished responsiveness without producing sleep.

seizure (**SEE**-zhur): A disturbance in the brain that can be caused by extreme high fever or by brain injury or lesions; also known as a convulsion.

sensorineural hearing loss: Hearing loss due to damage to the hair cells or nerves in the inner ear; also known as nerve deafness.

sentinel-node biopsy: A technique used during cancer surgery that limits the number of lymph nodes required to be removed for biopsy.

septicemia (**sep**-tih-**SEE**-mee-ah): A systemic disease caused by the spread of microorganisms and their toxins via the circulating blood; also known as blood poisoning.

septoplasty (**SEP**-toh-**plas**-tee): The surgical repair or alteration of parts of the nasal septum.

serum enzyme tests: Blood tests that measure the blood enzymes and provide useful evidence of a myocardial infarction.

serum bilirubin test: A blood test that measures how well red blood cells are being broken down.

sexually transmitted diseases: Diseases transmitted through sexual intercourse or other genital contact that affect both males and females; also known as venereal diseases and STDs.

shin splint: Pain caused by the muscle tearing away from the tibia.

sickle cell anemia: A genetic disorder that causes abnormal hemoglobin, resulting in red blood cells that assume an abnormal sickle shape.

sigmoidectomy (**sig**-moi-**DECK**-toh-mee): Surgical removal of all or part of the sigmoid colon.

sigmoiditis (**sig**-moi-**DYE**-tis): Inflammation of the sigmoid colon.

sigmoidoscopy (**sig**-moi-**DOS**-koh-pee): The endoscopic examination of the interior of the rectum, sigmoid colon, and possibly a portion of the descending colon.

sign: Objective evidence of disease, such as a fever.

silicosis (**sill**-ih-**KOH**-sis): The form of pneumoconiosis caused by inhaling silica dust in the lungs.

Sims' position: An examination position in which the patient is lying on the left side with the right knee and thigh drawn up with the left arm placed along the back.

singultus (sing-**GUL**-tus): Myoclonus of the diaphragm that causes the characteristic hiccup sound with each spasm; also known as hiccups.

sinusitis (**sigh**-nuh-**SIGH**-tis): An inflammation of the sinuses.

skin tags: Benign small flesh-colored or light-brown polyps that hang from the body by fine stalks.

sleep apnea syndromes: A group of potentially fatal disorders in which breathing repeatedly stops during sleep for long enough periods to cause a measurable decrease in blood oxygen levels.

slit-lamp ophthalmoscopy (**ahf**-thal-**MOS**-koh-pee): A diagnostic procedure in which a narrow beam of light is focused to permit the ophthalmologist to examine the structures at the front of the eye including the cornea, iris and lens.

SNRI: Medication that is thought to work by inhibiting the reuptake of serotonin and norepinephrine; full name is serotonin and norepinephrine reuptake inhibitor.

somatic cell mutation: Change within the cells of the body that affect the individual but cannot be transmitted to the next generation.

somatization disorder (**soh**-muh-ti-**ZAY**-shun): A condition characterized by years of physical complaints of many types that can not be explained by a medical condition.

somatoform disorders (soh-**MAT**-oh-**form**): Conditions that are characterized by physical complaints or concerns about one's body which are out of proportion to any physical findings or disease.

somnambulism (som-**NAM**-byou-lizm): The condition of walking or performing some other activity without awakening; also known as noctambulism or sleepwalking.

somnolence (**SOM**-noh-lens): A condition of unnatural sleepiness or semiconsciousness approaching coma from which the individual usually can be aroused by verbal stimuli.

spasm: A sudden, violent, involuntary contraction of one or more muscles.

spasmodic torticollis (spaz-**MOD**-ick **tor**-tih-**KOL**-is): A stiff neck due to spasmodic contraction of the neck muscles that pull the head toward the affected side; also known as wryneck.

SPECT: A nuclear imaging technique in which pictures are taken by one to three gamma cameras after a radionuclide tracer has been injected into the blood; full name single photon emission computerized tomography.

speculum (**SPECK**-you-lum): An instrument used to enlarge the opening of any canal or cavity to facilitate inspection of its interior.

speech audiometry: The threshold of hearing and understanding speech sounds.

sperm analysis: A test performed on freshly ejaculated semen to determine the volume plus the number, shape, size, and motility of the sperm; also known as a sperm count.

sphincterotomy (**sfink**-ter-**OT**-oh-mee): An incision into or division of a sphincter muscle.

sphygmomanometer (**sfig**-moh-mah-**NOM**-eh-ter): An instrument used to measure blood pressure.

spina bifida (**SPY**-nah **BIF**-ih-dah) (**SB**): The congenital defect that occurs during early pregnancy in which the spinal canal fails to close around the spinal cord.

spinal cord injury: Paralysis resulting from damage to the spinal cord that prevents nerve impulses from being transmitted below the level of the injury.

spinal fusion: A technique to immobilize part of the spine by joining together two or more vertebrae.

spiral fracture: A fracture in which the bone has been twisted apart.

spirometry (spy-**ROM**-eh-tree): A noninvasive test in which a patient breathes into a device that measures airflow, the length of time of each breath, and air volume.

splenectomy (splee-**NECK**-toh-mee): Surgical removal of the spleen.

splenitis (splee-**NIGH**-tis): Inflammation of the spleen.

splenomegaly (**splee**-noh-**MEG**-ah-lee): An abnormal enlargement of the spleen.

splenorrhagia (**splee**-noh-**RAY**-jee-ah): Bleeding from the spleen.

splenorrhaphy (splee-**NOR**-ah-fee): Surgical suturing of the spleen.

spondylolisthesis (**spon**-dih-loh-liss-**THEE**-sis): The slipping forward of the body of one of the lower lumbar vertebrae on the vertebra below it.

spondylosis (**spon**-dih-**LOH**-sis): Any degenerative disorder that may cause loss of normal spinal structure and function.

sprain: An injury to a joint, such as ankle, knee, or wrist, that usually involves a stretched or torn ligament.

sputum (**SPYOU**-tum): Phlegm ejected through the mouth that may be examined for diagnostic purposes.

squamous cell carcinoma (**SKWAY**-mus): A malignant tumor of the thin, scaly squamous cells of the epithelium that can quickly spread to other body systems.

SSRI: Medication that is thought to work by reducing the re-entry of serotonin into nerve cells, thus allowing serotonin to build up in the nerve synapse; full name is selective serotonin reuptake inhibitor.

staging: The process of classifying tumors with respect to how far the disease has progressed, the potential for its responding to therapy, and the patient's prognosis.

stapedectomy (**stay**-peh-**DECK**-toh-mee): The surgical removal of the top portion of the stapes bone and the insertion of a prosthetic device that conducts sound vibrations to the inner ear.

stent: A wire-mesh tube that is implanted in a coronary artery to provide support to the arterial wall to prevent restenosis.

stethoscope (**STETH**-oh-skope): An instrument used to listen to sounds within the body and during the measurement of blood pressure.

stillbirth: The birth of a fetus that died before, or during, delivery.

stimulants: Substances that work by increasing activity in certain areas of the brain, thus increasing concentration and wakefulness.

stoma (**STOH**-mah): An opening on a body surface that can occur naturally (for example, a pore in the skin) or may be created surgically.

strabismus (strah-**BIZ**-mus): A disorder in which the eyes point in different directions or are not aligned correctly because the eye muscles are unable to focus; also known as squint.

strain: An injury to the body of a muscle or the attachment of a tendon.

strangulated hernia: A condition that occurs when a portion of the intestine is constricted inside the hernia and its blood supply is cut off.

strangulating obstruction: Blockage that occurs when the blood flow to a segment of the intestine is cut off.

strawberry hemangioma (hee-**man**-jee-**OH**-mah *or* heh-**man**-jee-**OH**-mah): A dark, reddish benign tumor made up of newly formed blood vessels; also known as a birthmark.

stress fracture: A small crack in a bone that often develops from chronic, excessive impact.

stress incontinence: The inability to control the voiding of urine under physical stress such as running, sneezing, laughing, or coughing.

stress test: The use of electrocardiography to assess cardiovascular health and function during and after stress such as exercise on a treadmill.

stridor (**STRYE**-dor): An abnormal, high-pitched, harsh or crowing sound heard during inspiration that results from a partial blockage of the pharynx, larynx, and trachea.

stupor (**STOO**-per): A state of impaired awareness in which the mind and senses are dulled to environmental stimuli.

subcutaneous injection: The administration of medication by injection into the fatty layer just below the skin.

sublingual administration: The administration of medication by placing it under the tongue where it dissolves and is absorbed through the sublingual tissue directly into the bloodstream.

subluxation (**sub**-luck-**SAY**-shun): The partial displacement of a bone from its joint.

substance abuse: The addictive use of tobacco, alcohol, medications, or illegal drugs.

sudden infant death syndrome: The sudden and unexplainable death of an apparently healthy infant between the ages of two weeks and one year that typically occurs while the infant is sleeping; also known as SIDS or crib death.

supine (**SUE**-pine): Lying on the back with the *face up*.

suppuration (**sup**-you-**RAY**-shun): The formation or discharge of pus.

suprapubic catheterization (**soo**-prah-**PYOU**-bick): The placement of a catheter into the bladder through a small incision made through the abdominal wall above the pubic bone.

symptom (**SIMP**-tum): Subjective evidence, such as pain or a headache.

syncope (**SIN**-koh-pee): The brief loss of consciousness caused by the decreased flow of blood to the brain; also known as fainting.

syndrome (**SIN**-drohm): A set of the signs and symptoms that occur together as part of a specific disease process.

synechia (sigh-**NECK**-ee-ah): An adhesion that binds the iris to an adjacent structure such as the lens or cornea (plural, synechiae).

synergism (**SIN**-er-jizm): A drug interaction that occurs when the effect of one drug is increased by another drug; also known as potentiation.

synovectomy (sin-oh-**VECK**-toh-mee): The surgical removal of a synovial membrane from a joint.

synovitis (sin-oh-**VYE**-tiss): Inflammation of the synovial membrane that results in swelling and pain of the affected joint.

synthetic immunoglobulins: A postexposure preventive measure against certain viruses including rabies and some types of hepatitis; also known as immune serum.

synthetic interferon: Medication administered to treat multiple sclerosis, hepatitis C, and some cancers.

syphilis (**SIF**-ih-lis): A sexually transmitted disease that is caused by the bacterium *Treponema pallidum*.

systemic lupus erythematosus: An autoimmune disorder characterized by a red, scaly rash on the face and upper trunk that also attacks the connective tissue in other body systems; also known as lupus erythematosus.

T

tachycardia (**tack**-ee-**KAR**-dee-ah): An abnormally fast heartbeat usually at a rate of more than 100 beats per minute.

tachypnea (**tack**-ihp-**NEE**-ah): An abnormally rapid rate of respiration usually of more than 20 breaths per minute.

talipes (**TAL**-ih-peez): A congenital deformity in which the foot is turned outward or inward; also known as clubfoot.

tarsorrhaphy (tahr-**SOR**-ah-fee): The partial or complete suturing together of the upper and lower eyelids.

Tay-Sachs disease: A hereditary disease in which a missing enzyme in the brain causes progressive physical degeneration, mental retardation, and early death.

teletherapy (**tel**-eh-**THER**-ah-pee): Radiation therapy administered at a distance from the body that is precisely targeted with the use of three-dimensional computer imaging.

temporomandibular disorders (**tem**-poh-roh-man-**DIB**-you-lar): A group of complex symptoms including pain, headache, or difficulty in chewing that are related to the functioning of the temporomandibular joint.

tendonitis (**ten**-doh-**NIGH**-itis): Inflammation of the tendons caused by excessive or unusual use of the joint; also known as tendinitis, tenonitis, and tenontitis.

tenectomy (teh-**NECK**-toh-mee): Surgical removal of a portion of a tendon or tendon sheath; also known as a tenonectomy.

tenodesis (ten-**ODD**-eh-sis): Surgical suturing of the end of a tendon to bone.

tenodynia (**ten**-oh-**DIN**-ee-ah): Pain in a tendon.

tenolysis (ten-**OL**-ih-sis): Freeing a tendon from adhesions.

tenoplasty (**TEN**-oh-**plas**-tee): The surgical repair of a tendon; also known as tendinoplasty.

tenorrhaphy (ten-**OR**-ah-fee): Surgical suturing of a divided tendon.

tenotomy (teh-**NOT**-oh-mee): The surgical division of a tendon for relief of a deformity caused by the abnormal shortening of a muscle, such as in strabismus; also known as a tendotomy.

testicular self-examination: A self-care manual examination that is performed to detect testicular cancer.

testitis (test-**TYE**-tis): Inflammation of one or both testicles; also known as orchitis.

tetanus (**TET**-ah-nus): An acute and potentially fatal infection of the central nervous system caused by a toxin produced by the tetanus bacteria; also known as lockjaw.

tetany (**TET**-ah-nee): An abnormal condition characterized by periodic painful muscle spasms and tremors.

thalamotomy (**thal**-ah-**MOT**-oh-mee): A surgical incision into the thalamus performed to quiet the tremors of Parkinson's disease and to treat some psychotic disorders or uncontrollable pain.

thalassemia (thal-ah-**SEE**-mee-ah): A diverse group of genetic blood diseases characterized by absent or decreased production of normal hemoglobin; also known as Cooley's anemia.

thallium stress test (**THAL**-ee-um): The assessment of the flow of blood through the heart during activity with the use of the radiopharmaceutical thallium during a stress test.

therapeutic ultrasound: The use of high frequency sound waves to treat muscle injuries by generating heat deep within muscle tissue.

thermal capsulorrhaphy (**kap**-soo-**LOR**-ah-fee): An arthroscopic technique in which heat is used to shrink and tighten the tissues involved in shoulder instability disorders.

thoracentesis (**thoh**-rah-sen-**TEE**-sis): The surgical puncture of the chest wall with a needle to obtain fluid from the pleural cavity.

thoracostomy (**thoh**-rah-**KOS**-toh-mee): The surgical creation of an opening into the chest cavity to establish drainage of empyema.

thoracotomy (**thoh**-rah-**KOT**-toh-mee): A surgical incision through the chest wall into the pleural space for the visual examination of internal organs and the procurement of tissue specimens.

thrombolytic (**throm**-boh-**LIT**-ick): Medication that slows coagulation and prevents new clots from forming; also known as an anticoagulant or clot-busting drug.

thrombosis (throm-**BOH**-sis): The abnormal condition of having a thrombus (plural, thromboses).

thrombotic occlusion (throm-**BOT**-ick ah-**KLOO**-zhun): The blocking of an artery by a thrombus.

thrombus (**THROM**-bus): A blood clot attached to the interior wall of an artery or vein.

thymectomy (thigh-**MECK**-toh-mee): The surgical removal of the thymus gland.

thymitis (thigh-**MY**-tis): Inflammation of the thymus gland.

thymoma (thigh-**MOH**-mah): A usually benign tumor derived from the tissue of the thymus.

thymopathy (thigh-**MOP**-ah-thee): Any disease of the thymus gland.

thyroiditis (thigh-roi-**DYE**-tis): Inflammation of the thyroid gland.

thyroidotomy (thigh-roi-**DOT**-oh-mee): A surgical incision into the thyroid gland.

thyroid scan: A specialized nuclear scan to evaluate thyroid function.

thyroid-stimulating hormone assay: A diagnostic test that measures circulating blood levels of thyroid-stimulating hormone that may indicate abnormal thyroid activity.

thyromegaly (**thigh**-roh-**MEG**-ah-lee): An abnormal enlargement of the thyroid gland; also known as goiter.

thyrotoxicosis (**thy**-roh-**tock**-sih-**KOH**-sis): A life-threatening condition resulting from the release of excessive quantities of the thyroid hormones into the bloodstream; also known as thyroid storm.

tic douloureux (**TICK** doo-loo-**ROO**): Inflammation of the fifth cranial nerve that is characterized by sudden, intense, brief attacks of sharp pain on one side of side of the face; also known as trigeminal neuralgia.

tinea (**TIN**-ee-ah): A fungal infection of the skin, hair, or nails; also known as ringworm.

tinnitus (tih-**NIGH**-tus): A ringing, buzzing, or roaring sound in one or both ears.

tissue plasminogen activator (**TISH**-you plaz-**MIN**-oh-jen **ACK**-tih-**vay**-tor): A thrombolytic administered to some patients having a heart attack or stroke to dissolve damaging blood clots.

tonometry (toh-**NOM**-eh-tree): The part of a routine eye examination in which intraocular pressure is measured.

tonsillectomy (**ton**-sih-**LECK**-toh-mee): The surgical removal of the tonsils.

tonsillitis (**ton**-sih-**LYE**-tis): Inflammation of the tonsils.

torsion of the testis: A sharp pain in the scrotum brought on by a twisting of the vas deferens and blood vessels leading into the testis.

total hemoglobin test: A blood test that measures the amount of hemoglobin found in whole blood.

tracheobronchoscopy (**tray**-kee-oh-brong-**KOS**-koh-pee): The endoscopic inspection of both the trachea and bronchi with the use of a bronchoscope.

tracheoplasty (**TRAY**-kee-oh-**plas**-tee): Surgical repair of the trachea.

tracheorrhagia (**tray**-kee-oh-**RAY**-jee-ah): Bleeding from the mucous membranes of the trachea.

tracheostenosis (**tray**-kee-oh-steh-**NOH**-sis): Abnormal narrowing of the lumen of the trachea.

tracheostomy (**tray**-kee-**OS**-toh-mee): The creation of an opening into the trachea and inserting a tube to facilitate the passage of air or the removal of secretions.

tracheotomy (**tray**-kee-**OT**-oh-mee): An emergency procedure in which an incision is made into the trachea to gain access to the airway below a blockage.

traction: A pulling force exerted on a limb in a distal direction in an effort to return the bone or joint to normal alignment.

transcutaneous electronic nerve stimulation: A method of pain control by the application of electronic impulses to the nerve endings through the skin; also known as TENS.

transdermal medications: The administration of medication through the unbroken skin so that it is absorbed continuously to produce a systemic effect.

transesophageal echocardiography (**trans**-eh-**sof**-ah-**JEE**-al **eck**-oh-**kar**-dee-**OG**-rah-fee): An ultrasonic imaging technique that is performed from inside the esophagus to evaluate heart structures.

transient ischemic attack (iss-**KEE**-mick): The temporary interruption in the blood supply to the brain.

transverse fracture: A fracture that occurs straight across the bone.

trauma (**TRAW**-mah): Wound or injury.

triage (tree-**AHZH**): Screening of patients to determine their relative priority of need and the proper place of treatment.

trichomonas (**trick**-oh-**MOH**-nas): A sexually transmitted disease caused by the protozoan parasite *Trichomonas vaginalis*.

trichotillomania (**trick**-oh-**till**-oh-**MAY**-nee-ah): A disorder characterized by the repeated pulling out of one's hair resulting in noticeable hair loss.

tricyclic antidepressants: Medications named for their chemical structure that are also administered to treat depression.

trigeminal neuralgia: Inflammation of the fifth cranial nerve that is characterized by sudden, intense, brief attacks of sharp pain on one side of side of the face and affecting the lips, gum or cheek; also known as tic douloureux.

tubal ligation: A surgical procedure performed for the purpose of female sterilization.

tuberculin skin testing: A screening test for tuberculosis in which the skin of the arm is injected with a harmless antigen extracted from the TB bacterium.

tuberculosis (too-**ber**-kew-**LOH**-sis): An infectious disease caused by *Mycobacterium tuberculosis* that usually attacks the lungs; also known as TB.

tumor: A new and abnormal tissue formation in which the multiplication of cells is uncontrolled, abnormally rapid, and progressive; also known as a neoplasm.

tympanocentesis (**tim**-pah-noh-sen-**TEE**-sis): The surgical puncture of the tympanic membrane with a needle to remove fluid from the middle ear.

tympanometry (**tim**-pah-**NOM**-eh-tree): The measurement of acoustical energy absorbed or reflected by the middle ear through the use of a probe placed in the ear canal.

tympanoplasty (**tim**-pah-noh-**PLAS**-tee): The surgical correction of a damaged middle ear that is performed either to cure chronic inflammation or to restore function.

tympanostomy tubes (**tim**-pan-**OSS**-toh-mee): Tiny ventilating tubes placed through the eardrum to provide ongoing drainage for fluids and to relieve pressure that can build up after childhood ear infections; also known as pediatric ear tubes.

type 1 diabetes: An autoimmune insulin deficiency disorder that involves the destruction of pancreatic islet beta cells, which results in the inability of the cells to produce insulin.

type 2 diabetes: An insulin resistance disorder in which, although insulin is being produced, the body does not use it effectively.

typhoid fever: Headache, delirium, cough, watery diarrhea, rash, and a high fever that are caused by the bacterium *Salmonella typhi;* also known as enteric fever.

U

ulcer (**UL**-ser): An open lesion of the skin or mucous membrane resulting in tissue loss around the edges.

ulcerative colitis (koh-**LYE**-tis): A chronic condition of unknown cause in which repeated episodes of inflammation in the rectum and large intestine cause ulcers and irritation.

ultrasonic bone density testing: A screening test for osteoposoris or other conditions that cause a loss of bone mass.

ultrasonography (**ul**-trah-son-**OG**-rah-fee): The imaging of deep body structures by recording the echoes of pulses of sound waves above the range of human hearing; also known as ultrasound and diagnostic ultrasound.

unconscious: A state of being unaware, with the inability to respond to normal stimuli.

upper respiratory infection: A term used to describe the common cold; also known as acute nasopharyngitis.

uremia (you-**REE**-mee-ah): A toxic condition caused by excessive amounts of urea and other waste products in the bloodstream; also known as uremic poisoning.

ureterectasis (you-**ree**-ter-**ECK**-tah-sis): The distention of a ureter.

ureterectomy (**you**-ree-ter-**ECK**-toh-mee): The surgical removal of a ureter.

ureterolith (you-**REE**-ter-oh-**lith**): A stone located in the ureter.

ureterolysis (you-**ree**-ter-**OL**-ih-sis): A procedure performed to separate adhesions around a ureter.

ureteroplasty (you-**REE**-ter-oh-**plas**-tee): The surgical repair of a ureter.

ureterorrhagia (you-**ree**-ter-oh-**RAY**-jee-ah): The discharge of blood from the ureter.

ureterorrhaphy (**you**-ree-ter-**OR**-ah-fee): Surgical suturing of a ureter.

ureterostenosis (you-**ree**-ter-oh-steh-**NOH**-sis): Narrowing of the ureter due to a stricture caused by scar tissue.

urethral catheterization: The insertion of a tube along the urethra and into the bladder.

urethritis (**you**-reh-**THRIGH**-tis): Inflammation of the urethra.

urethrocele (you-**REE**-throh-seel): A hernia in the urethral wall.

urethropexy (you-**REE**-throh-**peck**-see): Surgical fixation of the urethra usually for the correction of urinary stress incontinence.

urethrorrhagia (you-**ree**-throh-**RAY**-jee-ah): Bleeding from the urethra.

urethrorrhea (you-**ree**-throh-**REE**-ah): An abnormal discharge from the urethra.

urethrostenosis (you-**ree**-throh-steh-**NOH**-sis): Abnormal narrowing of the urethra.

urethrostomy (you-**reh**-**THROS**-toh-mee): The surgical creation of a permanent opening between the urethra and the skin.

urethrotomy (you-**reh**-**THROT**-oh-mee): A surgical incision into the urethra.

urinalysis (**you**-rih-**NAL**-ih-sis): The examination of urine to determine the presence of abnormal elements.

urinary catheterization (**kath**-eh-ter-eye-**ZAY**-shun): The use of a catheter to obtain a sterile specimen for diagnostic purposes; also used to instill medication.

urinary hesitancy: Difficulty in starting a urinary stream.

urinary incontinence: The inability to control the voiding of urine.

urinary retention: The inability to empty the bladder.

urinary tract infection: An infection involving the structures of the urinary system that usually begins in the bladder.

urticaria (**ur**-tih-**KAR**-ree-ah): Wheals caused by an allergic reaction; also known as hives.

uterine cancer: Cancer of the uterus that occurs most commonly after menopause.

uterine prolapse (proh-**LAPS**): The condition in which the uterus sags from its normal position and moves part way, or all of the way, into the vagina; also known as a pelvic floor hernia.

uveitis (you-vee-**EYE**-tis): Inflammation anywhere in the uveal tract of the eyes.

V

vaginal candidiasis (**kan**-dih-**DYE**-ah-sis): A fungal infection of the vagina caused by *Candida albicans;* also known as vaginal thrush or as a yeast infection.

vaginitis (**vaj**-ih-**NIGH**-tis): Inflammation of the lining of the vagina; also known as colpitis.

vaginocele (**VAJ**-ih-noh-**seel**): A hernia protruding into the vagina.

vaginodynia (vaj-ih-noh-**DIN**-ee-ah): Pain in the vagina.

valvoplasty (**VAL**-voh-**plas**-tee): The surgical repair or replacement of a heart valve; also known as valvulozplasty.

valvular prolapse: The abnormal protrusion of a heart value that results in the inability of the valve to close completely.

valvulitis (**val**-view-**LYE**-tis): An inflammation of a heart valve.

valvuloplasty (**VAL**-view-loh-**plas**-tee): The surgical repair or replacement of a heart valve; also known as valvoplasty.

varicella (**va**r-ih-**SEL**-ah): An infection caused by the herpes virus *Varicella zoster*; also known as chickenpox.

varicocele (**VAR**-ih-koh-**seel**): A knot of varicose veins in one side of the scrotum.

varicocelectomy (**var**-ih-koh-sih-**LECK**-toh-mee): The removal of a portion of an enlarged vein to relieve a varicocele.

varicose veins (**VAR**-ih-kohs **VAYNS**): Abnormally swollen veins usually occurring in the legs.

vasculitis (**vas**-kyou-**LYE**-tis): Inflammation of a blood or lymph vessel; also known as angiitis.

vasectomy (vah-**SECK**-toh-mee): The male sterilization procedure in which a small portion of the vas deferens is surgically removed.

vasoconstrictor (**vas**-oh-kon-**STRICK**-tor): Medication that constricts the blood vessels.

vasodilator (**vas**-oh-dye-**LAYT**-or): Medication that dilates the blood vessels.

vasovasostomy (**vas**-oh-vah-**ZOS**-toh-mee *or* **vay**-zoh-vay-**ZOS**-toh-mee): A procedure performed as an attempt to restore fertility to a vasectomized male; also known as a vasectomy reversal.

venereal diseases (veh-**NEER**-ee-ahl): Diseases transmitted through sexual intercourse or other genital contact that affect both males and females; also known as sexually transmitted diseases.

venipuncture (**VEN**-ih-**punk**-tyour): The puncture of a vein for the purpose of drawing blood; also known as phlebotomy.

venography: An x-ray image of veins after the injection of a contrast medium; also known as phlebography.

ventilator: A mechanical device for artificial ventilation of the lungs that is used to replace or supplement the patient's natural breathing function.

ventricular fibrillation (ven-**TRICK**-you-ler **fih**-brih-**LAY**-shun): The rapid, irregular, and useless contractions of the ventricles that is usually fatal unless reversed by electric defibrillation; also known as V fib.

verrucae (veh-**ROO**-see): Small, hard skin lesions caused by the human papilloma virus; also known as warts (singular, verruca).

vertebral crush fractures: The spontaneous collapse of weakened vertebrae; also known as compression fractures of the spine.

vertigo (**VER**-tih-goh): A sense of whirling, dizziness, and the loss of balance, often combined with nausea and vomiting.

vesicle (**VES**-ih-kul): A small blister, less than 0.5 cm in diameter, containing watery fluid.

vesicovaginal fistula (**ves**-ih-koh-**VAG**-ih-nahl **FIS**-tyou-lah): An abnormal opening between the bladder and vagina.

viral (**VYE**-ral): Pertaining to a virus.

visual acuity measurement (ah-**KYOU**-ih-tee): Evaluation of the eye's ability to distinguish object details and shape.

visual field testing: A diagnostic test to determine losses in peripheral vision; also known as perimetry.

vitiligo (**vit**-ih-**LYE**-goh): An autoimmune disorder characterized by a loss of melanin resulting in whitish areas of skin, usually on the face and hands.

vitrectomy (vih-**TRECK**-toh-mee): The removal the vitreous fluid and its replacement with a clear solution.

voiding cystourethrography (**sis**-toh-you-ree-**THROG**-rah-fee) (**VCUG**): A diagnostic procedure in which a fluoroscope is used to examine the flow of urine from the bladder and through the urethra.

volvulus (**VOL**-view-lus): Twisting of the intestine on itself that causes an obstruction.

vulvitis (vul-**VYE**-tis): Inflammation of the vulva.

vulvodynia (vul-voh-**DIN**-ee-ah): A nonspecific syndrome of unknown cause characterized by chronic burning, pain during sexual intercourse, itching, or stinging irritation of the vulva.

vulvovaginitis (**vul**-voh-**vaj**-ih-**NIGH**-tis): Inflammation of the vulva and the vagina.

W

Western blot test: A blood test to confirm the diagnosis of HIV.

West Nile virus: A viral infection that causes flulike symptoms, which is carried by birds and transmitted to humans by mosquito or tick bites.

wheal (**WHEEL**): A small bump, which itches, that appears as a symptom of an allergic reaction; a welt.

white blood cell count: A blood test to determine the number of leukocytes in the blood.

white blood cell differential: A blood test to determine what percentage of the total white blood cell count is composed of each of the five types of leukocyte.

X

xeroderma (zee-roh-**DER**-mah): Excessively dry skin; also known as xerosis.

xerophthalmia (**zeer**-ahf-**THAL**-mee-ah): Drying of the eye surfaces, including the conjunctiva; also known as dry eye.

xerostomia (**zeer**-oh-**STOH**-mee-ah): The lack of adequate saliva due to the absence of or diminished secretions by the salivary glands; also known as dry mouth.

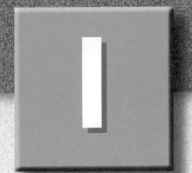

Index

Note: Page numbers in **boldface** indicate tables/figures.

C

G

M

O

S

License Agreement for Thomson Delmar Learning

IMPORTANT! READ CAREFULLY: This End User License Agreement ("Agreement") sets forth the conditions by which Thomson Delmar Learning, a division of Thomson Learning Inc. ("Thomson") will make electronic access to the Thomson Delmar Learning-owned licensed content and associated media, software, documentation, printed materials, and electronic documentation contained in this package and/or made available to you via this product (the "Licensed Content"), available to you (the "End User"). BY CLICKING THE "I ACCEPT" BUTTON AND/OR OPENING THIS PACKAGE, YOU ACKNOWLEDGE THAT YOU HAVE READ ALL OF THE TERMS AND CONDITIONS, AND THAT YOU AGREE TO BE BOUND BY ITS TERMS, CONDITIONS, AND ALL APPLICABLE LAWS AND REGULATIONS GOVERNING THE USE OF THE LICENSED CONTENT.

1.0 SCOPE OF LICENSE

1.1   Licensed Content. The Licensed Content may contain portions of modifiable content ("Modifiable Content") and content which may not be modified or otherwise altered by the End User ("Non-Modifiable Content"). For purposes of this Agreement, Modifiable Content and Non-Modifiable Content may be collectively referred to herein as the "Licensed Content." All Licensed Content shall be considered Non-Modifiable Content, unless such Licensed Content is presented to the End User in a modifiable format and it is clearly indicated that modification of the Licensed Content is permitted.

1.2   Subject to the End User's compliance with the terms and conditions of this Agreement, Thomson Delmar Learning hereby grants the End User, a nontransferable, non-exclusive, limited right to access and view a single copy of the Licensed Content on a single personal computer system for noncommercial, internal, personal use only. The End User shall not (i) reproduce, copy, modify (except in the case of Modifiable Content), distribute, display, transfer, sublicense, prepare derivative work(s) based on, sell, exchange, barter or transfer, rent, lease, loan, resell, or in any other manner exploit the Licensed Content; (ii) remove, obscure, or alter any notice of Thomson Delmar Learning's intellectual property rights present on or in the Licensed Content, including, but not limited to, copyright, trademark, and/or patent notices; or (iii) disassemble, decompile, translate, reverse engineer, or otherwise reduce the Licensed Content.

2.0 TERMINATION

2.1   Thomson Delmar Learning may at any time (without prejudice to its other rights or remedies) immediately terminate this Agreement and/or suspend access to some or all of the Licensed Content, in the event that the End User does not comply with any of the terms and conditions of this Agreement. In the event of such termination by Thomson Delmar Learning, the End User shall immediately return any and all copies of the Licensed Content to Thomson Delmar Learning.

3.0 PROPRIETARY RIGHTS

3.1   The End User acknowledges that Thomson Delmar Learning owns all rights, title and interest, including, but not limited to all copyright rights therein, in and to the Licensed Content, and that the End User shall not take any action inconsistent with such ownership. The Licensed Content is protected by U.S., Canadian and other applicable copyright laws and by international treaties, including the Berne Convention and the Universal Copyright Convention. Nothing contained in this Agreement shall be construed as granting the End User any ownership rights in or to the Licensed Content.

3.2   Thomson Delmar Learning reserves the right at any time to withdraw from the Licensed Content any item or part of an item for which it no longer retains the right to publish, or which it has reasonable grounds to believe infringes copyright or is defamatory, unlawful, or otherwise objectionable.

4.0 PROTECTION AND SECURITY

4.1   The End User shall use its best efforts and take all reasonable steps to safeguard its copy of the Licensed Content to ensure that no unauthorized reproduction, publication, disclosure, modification, or distribution of the Licensed Content, in whole or in part, is made. To the extent that the End User becomes aware of any such unauthorized use of the Licensed Content, the End User shall immediately notify Thomson Delmar Learning. Notification of such violation may be made by sending an e-Email to delmarhelp@thomson.com.

5.0 MISUSE OF THE LICENSED PRODUCT

5.1   In the event that the End User uses the Licensed Content in violation of this Agreement, Thomson Delmar Learning shall have the option of electing liquidated damages, which shall include all profits generated by the End User's use of the Licensed Content plus interest computed at the maximum rate permitted by law and all legal fees and other expenses incurred by Thomson Delmar Learning in enforcing its rights, plus penalties.

6.0 FEDERAL GOVERNMENT CLIENTS

6.1 Except as expressly authorized by Thomson Delmar Learning, Federal Government clients obtain only the rights specified in this Agreement and no other rights. The Government acknowledges that (i) all software and related documentation incorporated in the Licensed Content is existing commercial computer software within the meaning of FAR 27.405(b)(2); and (2) all other data delivered in whatever form, is limited rights data within the meaning of FAR 27.401. The restrictions in this section are acceptable as consistent with the Government's need for software and other data under this Agreement.

7.0 DISCLAIMER OF WARRANTIES AND LIABILITIES

7.1 Although Thomson Delmar Learning believes the Licensed Content to be reliable, Thomson Delmar Learning does not guarantee or warrant (i) any information or materials contained in or produced by the Licensed Content, (ii) the accuracy, completeness or reliability of the Licensed Content, or (iii) that the Licensed Content is free from errors or other material defects. THE LICENSED PRODUCT IS PROVIDED "AS IS," WITHOUT ANY WARRANTY OF ANY KIND AND THOMSON DELMAR LEARNING DISCLAIMS ANY AND ALL WARRANTIES, EXPRESSED OR IMPLIED, INCLUDING, WITHOUT LIMITATION, WARRANTIES OF MERCHANTABILITY OR FITNESS OR A PARTICULAR PURPOSE. IN NO EVENT SHALL THOMSON DELMAR LEARNING BE LIABLE FOR: INDIRECT, SPECIAL, PUNITIVE OR CONSEQUENTIAL DAMAGES INCLUDING FOR LOST PROFITS, LOST DATA, OR OTHERWISE. IN NO EVENT SHALL THOMSON DELMAR LEARNING'S AGGREGATE LIABILITY HEREUNDER, WHETHER ARISING IN CONTRACT, TORT, STRICT LIABILITY OR OTHERWISE, EXCEED THE AMOUNT OF FEES PAID BY THE END USER HEREUNDER FOR THE LICENSE OF THE LICENSED CONTENT.

8.0 GENERAL

8.1 <u>Entire Agreement.</u> This Agreement shall constitute the entire Agreement between the Parties and supercedes all prior Agreements and understandings oral or written relating to the subject matter hereof.

8.2 <u>Enhancements/Modifications of Licensed Content.</u> From time to time, and in Thomson Delmar Learning's sole discretion, Thomson Delmar Learning may advise the End User of updates, upgrades, enhancements and/or improvements to the Licensed Content, and may permit the End User to access and use, subject to the terms and conditions of this Agreement, such modifications, upon payment of prices as may be established by Thomson Delmar Learning.

8.3 <u>No Export.</u> The End User shall use the Licensed Content solely in the United States and shall not transfer or export, directly or indirectly, the Licensed Content outside the United States.

8.4 <u>Severability.</u> If any provision of this Agreement is invalid, illegal, or unenforceable under any applicable statute or rule of law, the provision shall be deemed omitted to the extent that it is invalid, illegal, or unenforceable. In such a case, the remainder of the Agreement shall be construed in a manner as to give greatest effect to the original intention of the parties hereto.

8.5 <u>Waiver.</u> The waiver of any right or failure of either party to exercise in any respect any right provided in this Agreement in any instance shall not be deemed to be a waiver of such right in the future or a waiver of any other right under this Agreement.

8.6 <u>Choice of Law/Venue.</u> This Agreement shall be interpreted, construed, and governed by and in accordance with the laws of the State of New York, applicable to contracts executed and to be wholly preformed therein, without regard to its principles governing conflicts of law. Each party agrees that any proceeding arising out of or relating to this Agreement or the breach or threatened breach of this Agreement may be commenced and prosecuted in a court in the State and County of New York. Each party consents and submits to the non-exclusive personal jurisdiction of any court in the State and County of New York in respect of any such proceeding.

8.7 <u>Acknowledgment.</u> By opening this package and/or by accessing the Licensed Content on this Web site, THE END USER ACKNOWLEDGES THAT IT HAS READ THIS AGREEMENT, UNDERSTANDS IT, AND AGREES TO BE BOUND BY ITS TERMS AND CONDITIONS. IF YOU DO NOT ACCEPT THESE TERMS AND CONDITIONS, YOU MUST NOT ACCESS THE LICENSED CONTENT AND RETURN THE LICENSED PRODUCT TO DELMAR LEARNING (WITHIN 30 CALENDAR DAYS OF THE END USER'S PURCHASE) WITH PROOF OF PAYMENT ACCEPTABLE TO THOMSON DELMAR LEARNING, FOR A CREDIT OR A REFUND. Should the End User have any questions/comments regarding this Agreement, please contact Thomson Delmar Learning at delmarhelp@thomson.com.

Flash Cards

INSTRUCTIONS

- Carefully remove the flash card pages from the book and cut them apart to create 160 flash cards.

- There are three types of cards: **prefixes** (such as **a-** and **hyper-**), **suffixes** (such as **-graphy** and **-rrhagia**), and **combining forms** (such as **gastr/o** and **arthr/o**). For the prefixes and suffixes, the type of word part is listed on the front on each card. The definition is on the back.

- The combining form cards are arranged by body system. This allows you to sort out the cards you want to study based on where you are in the book. Use the "general" cards as they apply throughout your course.

- Use the flash cards to memorize word parts, to test yourself, and to periodically review the material.

- By putting cards together, you can create terms, just as you did in the challenge word-building exercises.

WORD PART GAMES

Here are games you can play with one or more partners to help you learn word parts using your flash cards.

The Review Game

Word Parts Up: Shuffle the deck of flash cards. Put the pile, *word parts up*, in the center of the desk. Take turns choosing a card from anywhere in the deck and giving the definition of the word part shown. If you get it right, you get to keep it. If you miss, it goes into the discard pile. When the draw pile is gone, whoever has the largest pile wins.

Definitions Up: Shuffle the deck of flash cards and place them with the *definition side up*. Play the review game, this time giving the word for the definition.

The Create-a-Word Game

Shuffle the deck and deal each person 14 cards, *word parts up*. Place the remaining draw pile in the center of the desk, *word parts down*.

Each player should try to create as many legitimate medical words as possible using the cards he or she has been dealt. Then take turns discarding one card (word part up, in the discard pile) and taking one. When it is your turn to discard a card, you may choose either the card the previous player discarded, or a "mystery card" from the draw pile. Continue working on words until all the cards in the draw pile have been taken.

To score, each player must define every word created correctly. If the definition is correct, the player receives one point for each card used. If it is incorrect, two points are deducted for each card in that word. Cards left unused each count as one point off. Whoever has the highest score wins. *Note:* Use your medical dictionary if there is any doubt that a word is legitimate!

prefix

A-, AN-

prefix

END-, ENDO-

prefix

ANTE-

prefix

HEMI-

prefix

ANTI-

prefix

HYPER-

prefix

BRADY-

prefix

HYPO-

prefix

DYS-

prefix

INTER-

within, in, inside	without, away from, negative, not
half	before, toward
excessive, increased	against, counter
deficient, decreased	slow
between, among	bad, difficult, painful

prefix

INTRA-

prefix

POST-

prefix

NEO-

prefix

PRE-

prefix

PER-

prefix

SUB-

prefix

PERI-

prefix

SUPER-, SUPRA-

prefix

POLY-

prefix

TACHY-

after	within, inside
before	new, strange
below	excessive, through
above, excessive	surrounding, around
fast, rapid	many

-AC, -AL

-CYTE

-ALGIA

-DESIS

-ARY

-ECTOMY

-CELE

-ECTASIS

-CENTESIS

-EMIA

cell

pertaining to, relating to

surgical fixation of bone or
joint, to bind, tie together

pain, suffering

surgical removal

pertaining to

stretching, enlargement

hernia, tumor, swelling

blood, blood condition

surgical puncture to
remove fluid

-ESTHESIA

-ITIS

-GRAM, -GRAPH

-LYSIS

-GRAPHY

-MALACIA

-IA

-MEGALY

-IC

-NECROSIS

inflammation	sensation, feeling
breakdown, separation, setting free, destruction, loosening	a picture or record
abnormal softening	the process of recording a picture or record
enlargement	state or condition
tissue death	pertaining to

-OLOGIST

-OTOMY

-OLOGY

-PATHY

-OMA

-PAUSE

-OSIS

-PEXY

-OSTOMY

-PLASTY

surgical incision

specialist

disease, suffering, feeling, emotion

the science or study of

stopping

tumor

surgical fixation, to put in place

abnormal condition

surgical repair

surgical creation of an opening

-PLEGIA

-RRHEA

-PNEA

-RRHEXIS

-PTOSIS

-SCLEROSIS

-RRHAGIA, -RRHAGE

-SCOPE

-RRHAPHY

-SCOPY

flow or discharge

paralysis

rupture

breathing

abnormal hardening

prolapse, drooping forward

instrument for visual
examination

bleeding, abnormal
excessive fluid
discharge

to see, visual examination

surgical suturing

-STENOSIS

ARTER/O, ARTERI/O

-TRIPSY

ATHER/O

-URIA

CARD/O, CARDI/O

ANGI/O

HEM/O, HEMAT/O

AORT/O

PHLEB/O

artery

abnormal narrowing

plaque, fatty substance

to crush

heart

urination, urine

blood, pertaining to
the blood

pertaining to blood
or lymph vessels

vein

aorta

Cardiovascular System	**Digestive System**
THROMB/O	**COL/O,** **COLON/O**
Cardiovascular System	**Digestive System**
VEN/O	**DUODEN/I,** **DUODEN/O**
Diagnostic Procedures	**Digestive System**
ECH/O	**ENTER/O**
Diagnostic Procedures	**Digestive System**
RADI/O	**ESOPHAG/O**
Digestive System	**Digestive System**
CHOLECYST/O	**GASTR/O**

colon, large intestine	clot
duodenum	vein
small intestine	sound
esophagus	radiation, x-rays
stomach	gallbladder

Digestive System	**Endocrine System**
# HEPAT/O	# THYR/O, THYROID/O
Digestive System	**General**
# SIGMOID/O	# ADIP/O
Endocrine System	**General**
# ADREN/O, ADRENAL/O	# ALBIN/O
Endocrine & Reproductive Systems	**General**
# GONAD/O	# CEPHAL/O
Endocrine & Digestive Systems	**General**
# PANCREAT/O	# CERVIC/O

thyroid gland	liver
fat	sigmoid colon
white	adrenal glands
head	sex gland
neck, cervix (neck of uterus)	pancreas

CORON/O

LAPAR/O

CYAN/O

LEUK/O

CYT/O

LIP/O

ERYTHR/O

MELAN/O

HIST/O

MYC/O

abdomen, abdominal wall

coronary, crown

white

blue

fat, lipid

cell

black, dark

red

fungus

tissue

General	**Immune System**
PATH/O	ONC/O
General	**Integumentary System**
PY/O	CUTANE/O
General	**Integumentary System**
PYR/O	DERM/O, DERMAT/O
General	**Integumentary System**
SARC/O	HIDR/O
Immune System	**Integumentary System**
CARCIN/O	SEB/O

tumor	disease, suffering, feeling, emotion
skin	pus
skin	fever, fire
sweat	flesh (connective tissue)
sebum	cancerous

Integumentary System	Muscular System
UNGU/O	**MY/O**

Integumentary System	Muscular System
XER/O	**TEN/O, TEND/O, TENDIN/O**

Lymphatic System	Nervous System
ADEN/O	**ENCEPHAL/O**

Lymphatic System	Nervous System
SPLEN/O	**MENING/O**

Muscular System	Nervous System
FASCI/O	**NEUR/I, NEUR/O**

muscle	nail
tendon, stretch out, extend, strain	dry
brain	gland
meninges, membranes	spleen
nerve, nerve tissue	fascia, fibrous band

Reproductive Systems

COLP/O

Reproductive Systems

OOPHOR/O, OVARI/O

Reproductive Systems

HYSTER/O

Reproductive Systems

ORCH/O, ORCHI/O, ORCHID/O

Reproductive Systems

MEN/O

Reproductive Systems & Special Senses

SALPING/O

Reproductive Systems

METR/O, METRI/O

Reproductive Systems

UTER/O

Reproductive Systems

OO/O, OV/I, OV/O

Reproductive Systems

VAGIN/O

ovary

vagina

testicles, testis, testes

uterus

uterine (fallopian) tube,
auditory (eustachian) tube

menstruation, menses

uterus

uterus

vagina

egg

Respiratory System	Respiratory System
BRONCH/O, BRONCHI/O	**PULM/O, PULMON/O**

Respiratory System	Respiratory System
LARYNG/O	**TRACHE/O**

Respiratory System	Skeletal System
PHARYNG/O	**ANKYL/O**

Respiratory System	Skeletal System
PLEUR/O	**ARTHR/O**

Respiratory System	Skeletal System
PNEUM/O, PNEUMON/O	**CHONDR/O**

lung	bronchial tube, bronchus
trachea, windpipe	larynx, voice box
crooked, bent, stiff	throat, pharynx
joint	pleura, side of the body
cartilage	lung, air

Skeletal System

COST/O

Skeletal & Respiratory Systems

THORAC/O

Skeletal System

CRANI/O

Special Senses & Integumentary System

KERAT/O

Skeletal System & Nervous System

MYEL/O

Special Senses

MYRING/O

Skeletal System

OSS/E, OSS/I, OST/O, OSTE/O

Special Senses

OPTIC/O, OPT/O

Skeletal System

SPONDYL/O

Special Senses

OT/O

chest	rib
horny, hard, cornea	skull
tympanic membrane, eardrum	spinal cord, bone marrow
eye, vision	bone
ear, hearing	vertebrae, vertebral column, back bone

Special Senses	Urinary System
RETIN/O	**NEPHR/O**
Special Senses & Integumentary System	Urinary System
SCLER/O	**PYEL/O**
Special Senses	Urinary System
TYMPAN/O	**REN/O**
Urinary System	Urinary System
CYST/O	**URETER/O**
Urinary System & Digestive System	Urinary System
LITH/O	**URETHR/O**

kidney	retina
renal pelvis, bowl of kidney	sclera, white of eye, hard
kidney	tympanic membrane, eardrum
ureter	urinary bladder, cyst, sac of fluid
urethra	stone, calculus